Adult CCRN®
Certification Review

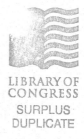

Kendra Menzies Kent, MS, RN, CENP, CCRN, CNRN, SCRN, TCRN, graduated from the University of Texas in Arlington in 1985 with her BSN. She successfully completed and graduated from Parkland Memorial Hospital's Critical Care and Trauma Internship. She has worked in the Surgery/Trauma, Thoracic and Neurosurgical ICU at Parkland Memorial Hospital as a staff nurse and nurse educator. Ms. Kent has been a manager on a trauma floor and the director of critical care at Zale Lipshy University Hospital in Dallas. She has her master's of nursing from Texas Women's University as a clinical nurse specialist (CNS) and has worked as a CNS in the surgical trauma ICU at Parkland Memorial Hospital. Ms. Kent moved to Florida and is currently the director of the Marcus Neuroscience Institute associated with Boca Raton Regional Hospital. Ms. Kent has presented seminars throughout the United States, Canada, and Oman. She has also published multiple chapters and books, including the books *Adult CCRN® Certification Review, Trauma Certified Registered Nurse (TCRN®) Examination Review,* and *Neuroscience Certification Review for Nurses,* published by Springer Publishing Company. Ms. Kent has been known to be engaging and supportive of nurses desiring certification. She receives emails from nurses who are excited that they have successfully passed their examinations.

Adult CCRN®
Certification Review

Think in Questions, Learn by Rationales

SECOND EDITION

Kendra Menzies Kent, MS, RN, CENP, CCRN, CNRN, SCRN, TCRN

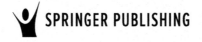

SPRINGER PUBLISHING

Springer Publishing Company, LLC
11 West 42nd Street, New York, NY 10036
www.springerpub.com
connect.springerpub.com/

Acquisitions Editor: Jaclyn Koshofer
Compositor: diacriTech

ISBN: 9780826151469
ebook ISBN: 9780826151476
DOI: 10.1891/9780826151476

21 22 23 24 / 5 4 3 2 1

The author and the publisher of this Work have made every effort to use sources believed to be reliable to provide information that is accurate and compatible with the standards generally accepted at the time of publication. Because medical science is continually advancing, our knowledge base continues to expand. Therefore, as new information becomes available, changes in procedures become necessary. We recommend that the reader always consult current research and specific institutional policies before performing any clinical procedure or delivering any medication. The author and publisher shall not be liable for any special, consequential, or exemplary damages resulting, in whole or in part, from the readers' use of, or reliance on, the information contained in this book. The publisher has no responsibility for the persistence or accuracy of URLs for external or third-party Internet websites referred to in this publication and does not guarantee that any content on such websites is, or will remain, accurate or appropriate.

CCRN® is a registered trademark of the American Association of Critical-Care Nurses (AACN) Certification Corporation. The AACN is the sole owner of its certification programs. AACN does not endorse this exam preparation resource, nor do they have a proprietary relationship with Springer Publishing Company.

Library of Congress Control Number: 2021912667

Contact sales@springerpub.com to receive discount rates on bulk purchases.

Publisher's Note: **New and used products purchased from third-party sellers are not guaranteed for quality, authenticity, or access to any included digital components.**

Printed in the United States of America.

To my wonderful husband, Robby, and to my parents, Sid and Judy,
for all the love and support they have given me.

Contents

Preface

Welcome to the second edition of *Adult CCRN® Certification Review*. This book was created specifically for critical care nurses as a comprehensive review book to prepare for successful completion of the national certification examination. It presents question styles and content material used by the American Association of Critical Care Nurses (AACN).

This book can be used to enhance study habits, hone test-taking skills, prepare for the Adult Acute/ Critical Care Nursing Certification exam, reinforce knowledge, and avoid test-taking errors. This book can also be used for continuing education for all critical care nurses, even if they are not planning on taking the examination.

The book provides an overview of the certification exam. Distinctive to this book is a format of asking a question and thinking through a response with rationales. This review book is unique in its "think in questions" format, which helps readers to anticipate the kinds of questions that might be asked and to promote critical thinking throughout the exam. The content review comprises bite-sized sections for easier learning and memorization that include thousands of unfolding questions, answers, and hints.

The book contains practice questions in content areas that are tested on the exams. To reinforce your knowledge, each question is associated with a rationale explaining why it is correct. A practice exam that is representative in length, variety, and complexity of the board exam questions is provided and can be taken in a timed format to assess your abilities under pressure.

I am eager to receive feedback on this book regarding the questions and rationales and offering suggestions for additions so that we can make the next edition even more superior. Please send any comments, suggestions, feedback, or criticisms to Kendra Kent at kendrakentcr@aol.com.

Kendra Menzies Kent

Introduction:
Think in Questions

Welcome to the journey toward certification. This book was written to help guide the reader on the pathway of the journey. It is written in a question/answer format to encourage you to think in questions when studying for the examination. When you study, I encourage you to ask yourself, "What can be asked about this particular topic?" "What would be a good question?" "What is important in this disease?" "What makes it different from other disorders?" This prepares you to anticipate the kinds of questions that might be asked and not just attempt to memorize content for the certification examination.

The book also provides multiple-choice questions similar to the questions that are found on the Adult Acute/Critical Care Nursing Certification (CCRN®) examination. These questions allow the nurse to practice taking an examination and also assist the nurse in determining areas that require further study prior to taking the CCRN examination. The answers and rationale, including some test-taking skills, are provided for each question, further preparing the nurse for the real examination.

▶ WHY CERTIFICATION?

The most important reason for certification is to do it for yourself (Box I.1). Certification is viewed as a mark of excellence in an area of specialty. It is an achievement and qualification that can be seen by peers, physicians, leaders of health care institutes, and patients/families. Becoming certified takes a certain dedication to critical care nursing and demonstrates a level of competency. The CCRN examination is developed to verify knowledge in critical care nursing.

Box I.1 Reasons to Become Certified

- Validates your knowledge of critical care to your hospital and peers
- Validates your knowledge of critical care to the patients
- Validates your knowledge of critical care to the physician
- Promotes continuing excellence in the nursing profession
- Demonstrates competency
- Assists with hospital credentialing
- Provides monetary benefit (from some hospitals)

▶ ADULT CCRN EXAMINATION INFORMATION

The CCRN examination follows the blueprint developed by the American Association of Critical Care Nurses (AACN). The test is developed and reviewed by experts in critical care. The CCRN Application Handbook can be accessed from the website www.certcorp.org. The examination application may be completed online or can be printed and mailed or faxed to the AACN Certification Corporation. The Adult CCRN provides a 3-year certification for critical care nurses.

▶ EXAMINATION

The Adult CCRN examination consists of 150 multiple-choice questions, of which 25 questions will not count for or against you. These 25 questions are being tested for use in future examinations. You will not know which questions count, so complete all 150 questions as if they count. The test is not arranged per system, and it is randomized. You may have one question on the renal system and the next one on the cardiovascular system. The time allowed to complete the examination is 3 hours (50 questions per hour).

Eligibility requirements to take the Adult CCRN examination are RN licensure and 1,750 hours of direct bedside care of critically ill patients during the previous 2 years with 875 of those hours obtained in the year preceding application to take the examination. Or, one must have been practicing as an RN for 5 years with a minimum of 2,000 hours of direct care of critically ill patients, with 144 of those hours logged during the preceding year. Nurse educators and managers in the adult critical care areas may apply hours spent at the bedside supervising nurses and nursing students.

The Adult CCRN examination is offered year-round as a computer-based test (CBT) and is also given as paper–pencil in certain circumstances. Once AACN receives your application and approves it, they send a confirmation email and postcard. Once confirmed, there is a 90-day window to take the examination. You will need to schedule your examination at an approved testing center. These centers can be found at www.goAMP.com. Immediate test results with score breakdown are available with the CBT.

HINT Do not schedule your exam at the end of the 90-day window. If, for some reason, you are unable to take the examination on the scheduled date, you will have to pay an extra $100 to reschedule.

Renewal of your CCRN license can be made through continuing education recognition points (CERPs) or retaking the examination. The CERP requirement is 100 hours in various categories (A, B, and C). For more details on renewal, use the AACN's website for renewal by the CERPs brochure.

▶ TEST PLAN

The Adult CCRN test plan is a blueprint for the exam content. Each major system is divided into subheadings and topics, and clinical judgment, professional caring, and ethical practice.

The amount of coverage in each of the systems is:

- Cardiovascular, 17%
- Respiratory, 15%
- Endocrine/Hematology/Gastrointestinal/Renal/Integumentary, 20%
- Musculoskeletal/Neurological/Psychosocial, 14%
- Multisystem, 14%
- Professional Caring and Ethical Practice, 20%

The CCRN blueprint also has a list of "testable nursing actions," which are nursing actions under each body system that may be tested. Nursing assessment, monitoring, and pharmacology are included in each body system and should be reviewed in preparation for the examination.

For additional, detailed information, please consult the Adult CCRN Exam Handbook (www.aacn.org).

▶ PREPARATION

Be positive!! Avoid any negative thoughts about passing the examination. These thoughts can cause a self-fulfilling prophecy. Set the test date, then establish a realistic schedule for preparing for the examination. Set your priorities; study those areas you are less familiar with first. Look at the percentage of each body system and establish timelines based on the largest to smallest percentage. Know how you study best, by yourself or in study groups. Study in a manner that works best for you. There are flash cards, practice questions, review courses, and study books in outline format and narrative format available for studying. Practice your test questions within a set time limit to familiarize yourself with the time limitations. Allow 2 minutes or less per question (remember the 50-questions-per-hour rule).

When using the practice test questions to study, determine several things when the answers and rationale are being reviewed. Analyze why you missed the question: Did you simply not know the content? Go back and restudy this section. Did you misread the question? Did you misread the answers? Did you miss an important element in the question or scenario? Was there a clue based on age, timeline, or symptoms?

Study those areas that you are least comfortable with, or those that are not in your specialty area. As adult learners, we tend to want to read and study what we like, or what we can use on a daily basis. For this examination, do not spend as much time in your area of specialty (you already know it) but focus on other areas you are not familiar with in your clinical practice.

▶ DAY OF THE TEST

Before the examination eat a healthy meal and limit the amount of liquids (to avoid the need for breaks during the exam). Remember, restroom breaks are allowed, but the testing time does not stop!

Do not try to cram immediately before the test; this will increase your anxiety. After the exam, make plans to do something special for yourself.

Know where you have to go for the test before the actual day of the test, and also know how long it will take you to get there at the appointed time. Running late and feeling hurried will increase your anxiety and can poorly affect your test-taking skills. Remember, if you are more than 15 minutes late, you will not be allowed to take the examination.

Bring your letter of approval and two forms of identification (one picture ID). You cannot bring any personal effects into the testing room, so leave everything in the car or at home (usually a locker is provided for you to put your personal items in).

You are allowed to do a tutorial on the computer before you start your exam if you need some assistance with CBT. The test time begins as soon as you start the first question of the actual exam. Leaving the testing site without authorization results in an automatic voiding of the test. You will be allowed only 3 hours from the time the test is started.

Results of the examination will be presented onsite at the completion of your exam following a test evaluation.

▶ TEST-TAKING SKILLS

Frequently, the difference between pass or fail depends on one's test-taking skills. An important reminder: Do not read into the questions; take the question and information provided at face value. Answer all questions; do not leave any questions blank. A blank answer will be counted against you. Answering the question, even if it is an "educated" guess, will give you a one out of four chance of being correct.

Key words are important phrases or words used to focus attention on what the question is specifically asking. Examples include always, earliest, first, on admission, best, least, immediately, and initial.

HINT If the question asks for the "best" response, this is an indication that all answers are probably correct and you will have to determine the best answer for that particular scenario.

Eliminate incorrect options first. Sometimes, you will immediately see an answer that is incorrect. Mark through it to narrow down your choices and improve your odds. Frequently you can get the choices down to two that are more correct than others.

HINT Eliminating options gives a 50/50 chance for an educated guess of the correct answer.

Avoid those answers with words such as "always" or "never." There is rarely a time in the medical field in which you will always or never take a particular action. If three of the four answers are similar, choose the answer that does not sound similar.

Do not change answers unless absolutely sure. You can "bookmark" a question that you are not sure about and return to it at the end of the test. Sometimes, you will feel more comfortable with the answer after you come back to it.

HINT First impressions are usually good! Do not spend too much time on any one question.

XVI   ADULT CCRN CERTIFICATION REVIEW

Do not let it worry you if you do not know all the answers. Take a deep breath and keep going. Rejoice in those answers you know and find easy!

HINT   You are not really supposed to know all the answers.

Do not try to establish patterns, such as using "two as in a row" for answers.

If there is a long scenario with a large amount of data, read the question first, then read the scenario, then reread the question. Sometimes there will be erroneous data that is not required to answer the question. Too much time may be spent trying to comprehend the whole scenario.

HINT   Do not forget to reread the question to make sure you read it correctly the first time.

Read all answers before you make a choice; there may be more than one correct answer, but one will be the better answer for the question.

HINT   Do not choose the first one that appears to be correct. Use the most correct answer.

Read the question carefully and answer only the question asked. Do not read into the question or think you need more information/data to answer the question.

HINT   The question will provide you with all the information needed to correctly answer the question.

Time frame questions are frequently used in the test. Use the time frame to assist with making the correct choice. Example: Which complication of subarachnoid hemorrhage is seen 7 to 10 days after the bleed?

HINT   All answers may be correct, but only one will occur more commonly during the time frame provided in the question.

Questions may be worded using the lead-in, "What is the gold standard . . .?" This is not asking what is the most common routine, but what is the most reliable and accurate.

Scenarios: Read the patient's description, word for word. Read the question, then formulate an answer. Read answers and choose the one closest to your formulated answer. Reread the question after answering to ensure you understood the question correctly.

HINT   When the question is answered, you are done. Move on to the next question. Do not second-guess yourself.

Look for answers that facilitate the care of the patient. Facilitative words include nurture, aid, support, reinforce, encourage, and assist.

▶ SUMMARY

Certification is a great path toward personal growth and professionalism. You have taken the first step and are on your way to a great journey. Learning is an amazing thing, and you will learn new information, remember things you may have previously learned, and apply this to your practice while studying for this examination. Good luck on your journey, and stay positive and excited about the learning process.

Pretest Questions and Answers

▶ QUESTIONS

1. The nurse notes that the ICU patient's pulse oximetry saturation is 100% and the arterial blood gas (ABG) oxygen saturation is 88%. Which of the following disorders best accounts for this discrepancy?

   A. Hypotension
   B. Chronic obstructive pulmonary disease (COPD)
   C. Anemia
   D. Carbon monoxide poisoning

2. A learned skill in which a person has an awareness of, and appreciation for, another's cultural uniqueness is called what?

   A. Cultural diversity
   B. Cultural paradigms
   C. Cultural sensitivity
   D. Ethnocentrism

3. A patient experiences a near-death experience and wants to talk to the nurse about the experience. What is the best response by the nurse?

   A. Encourage the patient to talk about her experiences and listen actively.
   B. Explain to the patient that she had hallucinations due to the pain medications.
   C. Reorient the patient to the actual events of the resuscitation.
   D. Tell the patient it is important to talk to her family about the issue.

4. Which of the following diagnostic tests is the most definitive for the diagnosis of a pulmonary embolism (PE)?

   A. Ventilation quotient (VQ) scan
   B. CT angiogram
   C. Pulmonary angiogram
   D. Duplex scanning

5. A patient in the ICU is complaining of muscle cramps. The ICU nurse assesses for Chvostek and Trousseau's signs, which were both positive. Which electrolyte abnormality is the most likely cause for the findings?

    A. Hypernatremia
    B. Hypercalcemia
    C. Hypomagnesemia
    D. Hypoglycemia

6. A patient was brought to the ICU unresponsive. He is noted to be "cherry" red and has a significant oxygen discrepancy between pulse oximetry and arterial blood gas. Which of the following is the most appropriate care?

    A. Administer 100% oxygen
    B. Administer N-Acetylcysteine (NAC)
    C. Alkalinize the urine with bicarbonate infusion
    D. Prepare the patient for hemodialysis

7. A significant Q wave without ST elevation in two contiguous leads indicates which of the following?

    A. Myocardial injury
    B. Myocardial ischemia
    C. Acute myocardial infarction (MI)
    D. MI, age undetermined

8. Which of the following disorders is classified as a constrictive cardiomyopathy?

    A. Amyloidosis
    B. Aortic regurgitation
    C. Postirradiation fibrosis
    D. Pericardial tamponade

9. Delay in which of the following treatments of sepsis is associated with the greatest increase in mortality?

    A. Fluid administration
    B. Blood cultures
    C. Antibiotic therapy
    D. Initiation of steroids

10. Which of the following is the most effective method of establishing the learning needs of a family member?

    A. Literacy assessment to determine level of education
    B. Informal assessment with open-ended questions
    C. Formal assessment tools with questions about health beliefs and learning styles
    D. An in-depth interview to determine learning styles

11. Which of the following nursing interventions has been found to be the most effective preventative method for ventilator-associated pneumonia (VAP)?

    A. Administration of prophylactic antibiotics
    B. Oral decontamination
    C. Use of a silver-coated endotracheal (ET) tube
    D. A saline lavage ET tube

12. A patient presents with a glucose level of 845 mg/dL in diabetic ketoacidosis (DKA). An insulin infusion and hourly monitoring of glucose were ordered. What complication of overly rapid glucose correction should the ICU nurse be aware of when managing DKA?

    A. Subdural hematoma
    B. Cerebral edema
    C. Epidural hematoma
    D. Osmotic diuresis

13. A patient in sepsis develops multisystem organ dysfunction (MODS). Which of the following indicators is used to define respiratory failure?

    A. PaO_2 < 80 mm Hg
    B. FEV1/FVC ratio < 49% predicted
    C. PaO_2/FiO_2 ratio < 200
    D. SaO_2/PaO_2 ratio < 100

14. Which of the following signs is considered the hallmark of compartment syndrome?

    A. Paralysis of extremity
    B. Pain beyond pain meds
    C. Loss of pulse
    D. Pallor of distal extremity

15. A patient has been in the ICU for 5 days following a drug overdose. The patient is not responding and exhibits no reflexes, but does overbreathe the ventilator. The physician is continuing to order hemodialysis daily to treat the metabolic acidosis. The nurse caring for the patient is frustrated and believes that the physician should talk to the family regarding a DNR status. Which of the following is the most accurate statement?

    A. The nurse is correct and needs to initiate the conversation with the family.
    B. The nurse is experiencing moral distress.
    C. The physician is the final decision maker regarding medical interventions.
    D. This situation should be brought to the ethics committee immediately for review.

16. Following an inferior wall myocardial infarction (IWMI) with right ventricular (RV) involvement, which of the following medications should be avoided?

    A. Aspirin
    B. Nitrostat (nitroglycerin)
    C. Tenormin (atenolol)
    D. Plavix (clopidogrel)

17. Which of the following lab values is MOST specific to disseminated intravascular coagulation (DIC)?

    A. Thrombocytopenia
    B. Elevated activated partial thromboplastin time (aPTT)
    C. Elevated prothrombin time (PT) with international normalized ratio (INR)
    D. Elevated D-dimer

18. A patient with a history of pancreatic cancer is newly diagnosed with metastasis to the lungs. The patient complains of severe chronic pain and is expressing feelings of helplessness. Which of the following is the most appropriate response by the nurse?

    A. Reassure the patient that the pain will get better.
    B. Ask the family to come in and stay for longer periods of time with the patient.
    C. Ask the patient direct questions regarding death and suicide thoughts.
    D. Refer the patient to a cancer support group.

19. A patient presents with a wound rapidly progressing from an initial redness to ecchymosis with enlarging bullae. Which of the following is the most likely cause of these symptoms?

    A. Cellulitis
    B. Abscess
    C. Necrotizing fasciitis
    D. Tunneling

20. Which of the following electrolyte abnormalities will most likely result in ventilatory muscle weakness and hypoventilation?

    A. Hyperkalemia
    B. Hypophosphatemia
    C. Hypocalcemia
    D. Hyperchloremia

21. The thoracic surgeon states that the patient's current hemodynamic problems following a coronary artery bypass grafting (CABG) were probably due to a stunned myocardium. Which phrase best describes a stunned myocardium?

    A. Infiltrative changes of the myocytes
    B. A constrictive disorder of the heart
    C. Transient depression of left ventricular (LV) function
    D. Chronically impaired yet viable myocardial tissue

22. A patient presents with headache and fever. The physician evaluating her passively flexed her neck and her knees flexed automatically. This is called what?

    A. Cullen's sign
    B. Brudzinski's sign
    C. Kernig's sign
    D. Kehr's sign

23. A patient develops a fever, tachycardia, and elevated white blood cell (WBC) count. The sepsis bundles are initiated and cultures are obtained. Within what time period should the resuscitation bundle of interventions be completed for improved success in managing sepsis?

    A. 3 hours
    B. 6 hours
    C. 9 hours
    D. 12 hours

24. A preceptor observes that a new orientee is performing a task using a different method than the preceptor has used. What is the appropriate response by the preceptor?

   A. Tell the orientee he is doing it incorrectly and should perform the task as taught by the preceptor.
   B. Survey other nurses in the unit on their method of performing the task.
   C. Perform a literature review to determine if the orientee's method is appropriate.
   D. Ignore the difference and assume that the orientee is aware of the correct method.

25. Which of the following statements regarding the abdominal infection *Clostridium difficile* is TRUE?

   A. Proton pump inhibitors (PPIs) have been found to lower the incidence of *C. difficile*.
   B. Colonization of *C. difficile* is common in healthy subjects in the community.
   C. A severe, but uncommon, complication is circulatory shock.
   D. A colonoscopy is commonly used to diagnose *C. difficile*.

▶ ANSWERS

1. **D) Carbon monoxide poisoning**
   Standard pulse oximeters do not detect carboxyhemoglobin (COHb). With high levels of COHb, arterial oxygen saturations decrease due to competition with carbon monoxide. Pulse oximeters overestimate arterial oxygenation in carbon monoxide poisoning. Anemia and COPD affect the hemoglobin (Hgb) level but do not cause discrepancies. Hypotension can affect reliability and may have to be monitored more centrally due to vasoconstriction, but it does not cause the discrepancies that are seen with carbon monoxide poisoning.

2. **C) Cultural sensitivity**
   Cultural sensitivity is the learned skill in which one person develops an awareness of and appreciation for another's culture and views. Cultural diversity refers to the difference between cultures in beliefs, values, and practices. Cultural paradigms are abstract explanations used by a cultural group to account for major life events. Ethnocentrism means judging another culture solely by the values and standards of one's own culture.

3. **A) Encourage the patient to talk about her experiences and listen actively**
   Allowing the patient time to talk about an experience helps the patient to work through thoughts and emotions regarding the event. The nurse should listen actively to the patient. Downplaying a patient's experience as a hallucination or attempting to reorient her to the actual events is not beneficial to the patient and may actually be counterproductive. Telling the patient to talk to the family instead of the nurse may cause the patient to lose trust in the healthcare provider.

4. **C) Pulmonary angiogram**
   A pulmonary angiogram is the most definitive diagnostic test for a PE and is considered the "gold standard" for diagnosing PE. It is not commonly used, due to a higher complication rate. The VQ scan and CT angiogram are frequently used, but have higher false positive and negative findings than a pulmonary angiogram. Duplex scanning is used to assess for DVT but not a PE.

5. **C) Hypomagnesemia**
   Hypomagnesemia symptoms cause muscle twitching and muscle spasms. A positive Chvostek and/or Trousseau's sign can occur with a low magnesium level. The other electrolyte abnormality that can cause the same symptoms is hypocalcemia (not hypercalcemia). Neither hypernatremia nor hypoglycemia causes these symptoms.

6. **A) Administer 100% oxygen**
   The patient likely has carbon monoxide toxicity. Administration of 100% oxygen increases the elimination of carboxyhemoglobin (COHb) and can lower the COHb levels within several hours. NAC is used as an antidote to acetaminophen overdose, and bicarbonate administration is used to treat salicylate toxicity. Hemodialysis is used in some drug overdoses to remove the drug from the system but will not be effective in lowering COHb levels.

7. **D) MI, age undetermined**
   A significant Q wave without ST elevation indicates an old MI. This is frequently called MI of undetermined age. A significant Q wave with ST elevation in the same leads indicates an acute MI. Myocardial injury does not have a Q wave, and myocardial ischemia is specific to ST elevation.

8. **D) Pericardial tamponade**
   Pericardial tamponade causes a constriction around the heart (like a boa constrictor) and so is classified as a constrictive cardiomyopathy. Amyloidosis and postirradiation fibrosis are both classified as restrictive cardiomyopathies. Aortic regurgitation frequently results in dilated/hypertrophic cardiomyopathy.

9. **C) Antibiotic therapy**
   Delays in administering antibiotics in sepsis have been associated with an increase in mortality. The goal is to start antibiotic therapy within 1 hour of the diagnosis of severe sepsis and septic shock. Blood cultures should be obtained prior to the initiation of antibiotics, but antibiotic administration

should not be delayed while attempting to obtain blood cultures. Fluid administration follows if lactate levels are elevated or the patient is hypotensive. Steroids are not indicated until the patient is unresponsive to vasoconstrictive therapy.

10. **B) Informal assessment with open-ended questions**
An informal assessment of learning needs using open-ended questions is the best method to determine learning needs. It may also be used to validate understanding of the concepts being taught. Example: "What is your understanding of your loved one's condition?" Formal assessment tools use generic questions regarding health beliefs and learning styles, and are not individualized for the learner. Talking with the family member and asking open-ended questions provides an informal assessment of the individual's education and literacy level. This assessment requires sensitivity because adults will usually try to hide illiteracy. In-depth interviews to determine learning styles do not provide the information needed to provide education to family members. Informal, short sessions at the bedside may be the most effective teaching method.

11. **B) Oral decontamination**
Oral decontamination, with frequent and good mouth care, has been found to lower the incidence of VAP. Aspiration of pathogens in the oropharynx is considered to be the inciting event for most VAPs. The pathogens that colonize the oral airway are gram-negative aerobic bacilli, which are the predominant cause of VAP. Prophylactic antibiotics are not recommended and can lead to greater bacterial antibiotic resistance. Use of silver-coated ET tubes may lower the incidence of infection, but this is not a nursing intervention. Saline lavage down the ET tube may actually increase the incidence of VAP.

12. **B) Cerebral edema**
Correcting the serum glucose too rapidly causes a sudden drop in osmolality and fluid shift interstitially. This results in cerebral edema. Correcting hyponatremia too rapidly causes central pontine demyelinolysis. Osmotic diuresis has already occurred with the hyperglycemia and subdural or epidural hematoma are not complications of DKA.

13. **C) PaO_2/FiO_2 ratio < 200**
PaO_2/FiO_2 ratio is used to define acute respiratory distress syndrome (ARDS). A ratio of <200 indicates lung injury and is used to determine organ failure. PaO_2 < 80 mm Hg indicates hypoxia but is not used to define ARDS or organ failure. FEV1/FVC ratio is used to assess asthma. SaO_2/PaO_2 ratio is not used to evaluate lung involvement.

14. **B) Pain beyond pain meds**
Pain beyond pain medications a hallmark sign of compartment syndrome while pain on passive movement is an early sign of compartment syndrome. Paralysis of the extremity can occur but is not considered the hallmark. Pallor and loss of pulses are very late signs in compartment synrdome.

15. **B) The nurse is experiencing moral distress**
Moral distress occurs when the nurse believes that she or he knows the ethically correct action to take in a situation, but a conflicting action is being pursued by other members of the healthcare team or family. There is more than one option in an ethical dilemma, with each option having an equally compelling alternative. A moral argument can be made for and against each alternative. A discussion or conference with the physician and the family would be indicated before sending the situation to the ethics committee. The physician does not have final decision-making power if the course of action is against the patient's or family's wishes.

16. **B) Nitrostat (nitroglycerin)**
Nitroglycerin is a venodilator that causes venous pooling, a decrease in venous return, and a lowering of preload. Treatment of an acute MI with RV involvement may involve all but the nitroglycerin. RV dysfunction is managed by increasing preload to improve stroke volume.

17. **D) Elevated D-dimer**
DIC does involve thrombocytopenia, elevated aPTT, and PT, but so do several other coagulopathies. None of those lab findings would specifically indicate DIC. Elevated D-dimer occurs due

to breakdown of fibrin (clot) and release of fibrin degradation products. DIC is the only coagulopathy that would increase D-dimer.

18. **C) Ask the patient direct questions regarding death and suicide thoughts.**
Patients at high risk for suicide include those experiencing chronic pain. This patient's risk increased with the new diagnosis of metastasis and talk about feeling hopeless. Asking specific questions about death, self-harm, and suicide is recommended to identify patients with plans of suicide. Falsely reassuring the patient may create greater feelings of hopelessness. Involving the family and referring the patient to a support group are good interventions, but the most important intervention is suicide risk assessment.

19. **C) Necrotizing fasciitis**
Necrotizing fasciitis symptoms progress rapidly. Ecchymosis with bullae that can enlarge and rupture and a dusky color is common wound appearance in necrotizing fasciitis. Cellulitis appears as redness and does not progress. An abscess is a contained infection and will not present with enlarging bullae. Tunneling occurs in the subcutaneous tissue of a wound and would not be described as progressive ecchymosis with developing bullae.

20. **B) Hypophosphatemia**
Hypophosphatemia causes muscle weakness and hypoventilation in the ICU. Hypocalcemia causes an increase in muscle tone. Hyperkalemia may cause apathy and generalized weakness but does not typically result in hypoventilation.

21. **C) Transient depression of LV function**
A stunned myocardium describes a transient depression of LV function due to temporary reduction of myocardial blood flow after a myocardial infarction (MI) or CABG. Hibernating myocardium describes a chronically impaired yet viable myocardial tissue. Pericardial tamponade is a constrictive disorder. Amyloidosis involves infiltrative changes of the myocytes.

22. **B) Brudzinski's sign**
Brudzinski's sign and Kernig's sign are indicative of meningitis. The Brudzinski's sign is obtained by passively flexing the neck and observing for spontaneous flexing of the knees. Kernig's sign is performed by flexing the hip at a 90-degree angle and then extending the knee. Pain and spasm of the hamstring indicate a positive test. Kehr's sign and Cullen's sign are not used to evaluate a patient for meningitis or meningeal irritation.

23. **B) 6 hours**
The current recommendation is to complete the resuscitation interventions, including cultures, antibiotics, fluid boluses, lactate levels, and vasopressin (if required) within 6 hours of sepsis onset.

24. **C) Perform a literature review to determine if the orientee's method is appropriate**
Professionalism includes mentoring others, as well as being mentored. The preceptor is mentoring and teaching the orientee but can learn from the orientee as well. If there is a difference in methods for performing a procedure, perform a literature review to determine best practice. There is more than one way to do some procedures, and one way is not always the best way. Stating that the orientee is wrong, without appropriate research, does not acknowledge the nurse as having a base of knowledge and skills. Surveying other nurses can be done in certain circumstances but is not the best answer in this scenario. Ignoring the identified problem does not allow for growth in either the preceptor or the orientee.

25. **C) A severe, but uncommon, complication is circulatory shock**
An uncommon but severe complication can be circulatory failure and multiorgan failure. This is called megacolon and presents with abdominal distention and circulatory shock. PPIs have been found to be associated with a higher incidence of *C. difficile* infections. Healthy subjects in the community do not typically colonize *C. difficile*. A colonoscopy may be used but is not the most common diagnostic for *C. difficile*.

Cardiovascular System Review

2

In this chapter, you will review:

- Acute coronary syndrome
  - ○ Non-ST-segment elevation myocardial infarction (NSTEMI)
  - ○ ST-segment elevation myocardial infarction (STEMI)
  - ○ Unstable angina
- Cardiogenic shock
- Dysrhythmias
- Heart failure
- Aortic aneurysm/Aortic dissection/Aortic rupture
- Cardiac tamponade
- Cardiomyopathies
  - ○ Dilated
  - ○ Hypertrophic
  - ○ Idiopathic
  - ○ Restrictive
- Hypertensive crisis
- Structural heart defects (acquired and congenital, including valvular disease)
- Acute peripheral vascular insufficiency
  - ○ Carotid artery stenosis
  - ○ Endarterectomy
  - ○ Fem-pop bypass
  - ○ Arterial venous occlusion
- Cardiac surgery
  - ○ Coronary artery bypass graft (CABG)
  - ○ Valve replacement or repair
- Acute pulmonary edema
- Cardiac/vascular catheterization
- Myocardial conduction system defects
- Papillary muscle rupture
- Transcatheter aortic valve replacement (TAVR)

●) ACUTE CORONARY SYNDROME

Q What are acute coronary syndromes (ACSs)?

A Unstable angina (UA), ST-segment elevation myocardial infarction (STEMI), and non-ST-segment elevation myocardial infarction (NSTEMI)

UA, STEMI, and NSTEMI are typically considered to be complications of ACS (Table 2.1).

HINT The findings on the 12-lead EKG make the initial differentiation between STEMI and NSTEMI/UA. It is important to obtain an EKG immediately when there is chest pain.

Table 2.1 Acute Coronary Syndromes

ACS	Echocardiogram Findings	Cardiac Enzyme Results
Unstable angina	Normal or nonspecific T-wave changes	Normal
Non-ST-segment elevation MI	Normal or new onset ST-segment depression	Elevated
ST-segment elevation MI	Elevated ST-segment in two or more contiguous leads	Elevated

ACS, acute coronary syndromes; MI, myocardial infarction.

▶ PATHOPHYSIOLOGY

Q What are the characteristics of a "vulnerable" plaque in the coronary artery?

A Large lipid-rich core, thin fibrous cap over the lipid core, and activated smooth muscle cells and macrophages

Vulnerable plaque, also called "unstable plaque," is more likely to cause ACS. It is more likely to rupture than a "stable plaque." The development of a thrombus at the site causes a sudden occlusion of the coronary artery and distal ischemia. The stable plaque has a thinner lipid-rich core and a thicker fibrous cap. When plaque is more stable and narrows the vessel diameter over time, the heart develops collateral circulation. This collateral circulation allows for perfusion distal to the narrowing, even when it nears almost complete occlusion.

HINT A patient presents with UA but is ruled out for an acute myocardial infarction (AMI). The patient is then typically referred for a cardiac catheterization. The most common finding will be a near-complete obstruction of the involved coronary artery. This is a stable plaque. The patient did not have an AMI.

Q What is plaque erosion?

A The endothelium erodes, exposing the intimal layer to the components of the circulating blood

Plaque rupture is the most common cause of ACS, but erosion of the plaque can also initiate AMI. Both the rupture and erosion lead to the release of tissue factor, proinflammatory factors, and procoagulants, causing intracoronary thrombosis.

Q A patient presents with a myocardial infarction (MI), which is called a type 2 MI. Does this patient have coronary artery disease (CAD)?

A No

MI type 2 typically results from an imbalance between oxygen supply and delivery to the myocardial muscle with anatomically stable coronary arteries. MI is a result of other factors that cause the oxygen imbalance (Box 2.1).

HINT The cause of Prinzmetal's angina is coronary artery spasms. Persistent spasm can result in MI.

Box 2.1 Other Causes of AMI (Type 2)

Coronary artery spasm	Pulmonary hypertension
Coronary artery embolism	Coronary vasculitis
Hypertrophic cardiomyopathy	Congenital coronary abnormalities
Dilated cardiomyopathy	Trauma injury coronary artery
Restricted cardiomyopathy	Hypotension
Acute blood loss	Aortic stenosis

AMI, acute myocardial infarction.

▶ PREVENTION OF ACS

Q What is a commonly prescribed cholesterol-lowering drug?

A Statin

Statins are hydroxy-3-methylglutaryl-coenzyme A (HMG-CoA) reductase inhibitors and are commonly prescribed to lower cholesterol. Other cholesterol-lowering therapies include omega-3 fatty acids, fibrates, and lifestyle changes (Box 2.2).

Box 2.2 Prevention of ACS

Lifestyle changes	Smoking cessation
	Dietary Approaches to Stop Hypertension (DASH)-like diet
	Regular physical activity
	Weight management
Class I recommendation	Blood pressure control
	LDL-C lowering therapy
	Beta blocker
	ACE inhibitor/ARB
Class II recommendation	Glycemic control in diabetes mellitus
	ASA/antiplatelet agent
	Omega-3 fatty acids
Other	Influenza vaccination

ACE, angiotensin-converting enzyme; ARB, angiotensin-converting enzyme; ASA, aspirin; LDL-C, low-density lipoprotein cholesterol.

HINT   Stains also stabilize the atherosclerotic plaque and can reduce the risk of secondary ischemic events.

▶ SYMPTOMS/ASSESSMENT

Q What is a positive Levine sign?

A Clenched fist held over the chest wall in association with angina chest pain

The chest pain is described as a pressure, heaviness, squeezing, burning, or choking sensation. Typical locations for radiation of pain are the arms, shoulders, and neck. The intensity of angina does not change with respiration, cough, or change in position.

HINT   Sharp pain that worsens with movement and deep breathing may be caused by pericarditis.

Q What is the most common atypical sign of ACS?

A Shortness of breath (SOB)

SOB is the most common atypical sign of ACS. Other atypical signs include epigastric discomfort, nausea and vomiting, diaphoresis, dyspnea, and generalized weakness.

HINT A question on atypical symptoms would most likely involve a woman in the scenario because women often experience the atypical symptoms of AMI.

Q Which abnormal heart sound accompanies chest pain caused by AMI?

A S_4 gallop

An S_4 gallop is caused by a ventricle resistant to filling during the late diastolic phase. The S_4 is typically present with chest pain and disappears when chest pain is alleviated. An S_3 gallop is associated with congestive heart failure (CHF) or volume overload. It occurs during the early diastolic phase (Box 2.3).

Box 2.3 Associated Symptoms of Angina

Cool, clammy skin	Heart rate changes (tachy or brady)
S_3 gallop	Arrhythmias
S_4 gallop	Diaphoresis
Blood pressure changes (hyper- or hypo-)	Dyspnea
Leukocytosis	Low-grade fever

HINT An S_3 or S_4 may be used in the scenario as a hint for the answer. Remember, S_3 is CHF and S_4 is angina.

Q Which patient population may have a "silent" MI?

A Diabetics

Patients with diabetes mellitus may experience an MI without significant chest pain. This may be attributed to their autonomic neuropathy leading to sensory denervation.

HINT A patient with diabetes may not have been aware of having a previous MI, but pathological Q waves are found on 12-lead indicating a history of an MI.

Q Which two locations for an AMI may result in bradycardia?

A Inferior wall AMI and posterior wall AMI

The sinoatrial (SA) node is perfused by the proximal right coronary artery (RCA) in 55% of the population and by the left circumflex artery (LCX) in 45% of the population. A loss of blood flow through the RCA or the LCX, depending on the dominance, will result in bradycardia.

HINT The presence of a first-degree heart block (prolongation of the PR interval) indicates ischemia at the level of the atrioventricular (AV) node, which is mostly supplied by RCA.

▶ DIAGNOSIS

Q What is the initial diagnostic test obtained with the onset of chest pain?

A 12-lead EKG

A 12-lead EKG is performed and interpreted within 10 minutes of arrival in the ED with chest pain. If the initial 12-lead shows ST-segment elevation in two contiguous leads, then reperfusion strategies are initiated. If the initial 12-lead does not show significant finding, but if the patient continues to have chest pain, then an EKG may be obtained as often as every 10 minutes.

HINT   Remember that a person can be having an AMI without elevating ST segments. The differentiation between UA and NSTEMI is cardiac enzymes.

| **Q** The finding of ST-segment elevation in leads II, III, and aVF indicates the need for what follow-up EKG?

| **A** Right precordial lead placement (right-sided EKG)

An inferior wall AMI (leads II, III, and aVF) may also involve the wall of the right ventricle (RV). The best diagnostic for RV involvement is to obtain a right precordial EKG and look for ST-segment changes in V_{3R} and V_{4R}. Another change in lead placement may be to extend the left precordial leads laterally toward the left posterior chest to better view the posterior-lateral infarction.

HINT   The best EKG lead placement for the diagnosis of a posterior wall AMI is on the back even though this is not commonly performed. Typically, look for reciprocal changes in the anterior leads. The changes include tall R waves and ST depression in V_1 and V_2 (sometimes V_3). This is a reciprocal change of ST-segment elevation and Q waves (or loss of R wave height). Posterior infarcts are mirror images of anterior infarcts.

| **Q** Which leads are used to recognize lateral wall ischemia and infarction?

| **A** Leads I, aVL, V_5, V_6

Leads I, aVL, V_5 and V_6 all view the lateral aspect of the left ventricle (LV) (Table 2.2).

HINT   ST elevation in leads I and aVL only indicate a high lateral STEMI

Table 2.2 Localizing the Infarct

Wall Involvement	Leads of Monitor	Involved Coronary Artery
AWMI	V3–V4 or loss of R-wave progression	LAD
Septal wall	V1–V2	LAD
LWMI	I, aVL, V5, V6	LCX
IWMI or RV infarct	II, III, aVF	RCA

AWMI, anterior wall myocardial infarction; IWMI, inferior wall myocardial infarction; LAD, left anterior descending; LWMI, lateral wall myocardial infarction; LCX, left circumflex; RCA, right coronary artery; RV, right ventricle.

| **Q** Which EKG change indicates an acute myocardial injury?

| **A** An elevated ST segment

An elevated ST segment indicates a potentially reversible injury. An ST-segment elevation of ≥1 mm in two contiguous leads is considered significant. ST segments return to normal after reperfusion. STEMI is commonly associated with a transmural wall ischemia/injury.

HINT   Q wave without ST-segment changes indicate a previous MI and are usually noted to be of an "undetermined" age. It is important to compare a patient's EKG with an old one, if available, to evaluate for old or new changes.

| **Q** What is considered to be a "significant" Q wave?

| **A** A Q wave of 2 mm or more in depth or longer than 0.04-second duration or greater than a third of the height of the QRS complex

Significant Q waves indicate irreversible myocardial damage (infarction). Q waves may develop within several hours of injury or may take up to several days to weeks to occur. Q waves can persist for the lifetime of a patient.

HINT   Inferior leads on 12-lead EKG typically have small Q waves but are not significant.

> **Q** Which of the cardiac enzymes is the preferred biomarker for diagnosing an AMI?
>
> **A** Troponin levels

Troponin levels are more sensitive and specific to AMI than creatine phosphokinase-myocardial band (CPK-MB).

HINT There are other causes of elevated troponin levels, so an elevated troponin is not diagnostic of MI alone (Box 2.4).

Box 2.4 Causes of Elevated Troponins

Acute myocardial infarction	Cardiac contusions
Congestive heart failure	Myocarditis
Acute cardiomyopathy	Chronic kidney disease
Rhabdomyolysis	Sepsis

> **Q** How long after the onset of myocardial injury will an increase in cardiac enzymes occur?
>
> **A** 4 to 6 hours

CPK-MB and troponin increase within 4 to 6 hours after ischemia. To rule out MI, cardiac enzymes are commonly drawn every 8 hours for 24 hours. CPK-MB levels return to baseline within 36 to 40 hours. Troponin levels remain elevated for up to 10 days.

HINT Prolonged days of chest pain prior to presentation in ED can use these markers to identify if acute or subacute MI based upon which markers are elevated.

> **Q** Which cardiac protein elevates first?
>
> **A** Myoglobin

Myoglobin levels elevate within 1 hour of ischemia and return to normal within 24 hours. It is a sensitive marker for muscle damage but is not specific to myocardial muscle.

HINT Elevated myoglobin increases suspicion of AMI in patients presenting with anginal-type chest pain.

▶ MANAGEMENT OF AMI

> **Q** Name two emergency treatments for STEMI.
>
> **A** Emergency coronary balloon angioplasty with stenting and intravenous (IV) thrombolytic agent

Primary percutaneous coronary intervention (PCI) is the recommended therapy for STEMI, but thrombolytic therapy remains an important option for treatment in hospitals without PCI capabilities.

HINT IV thrombolytics is indicated in a STEMI and is not a treatment for NSTEMI or UA.

> **Q** What is the standard for "door-to-balloon" time?
>
> **A** Less than 90 minutes

Current standards mandate that the time to primary PCI should be less than 90 minutes. PCI includes angioplasty, aspiration thrombectomy, and/or stent placement. Stents are either bare-metal stents (BMS) or drug-eluting stents (DES).

HINT Stent determination may be based upon the length of required antiplatelet therapy.

> **Q** For which types of ACS is PCI indicated?
>
> **A** STEMI, NSTEMI, and UA

PCI is indicated if ischemic symptoms started less than 12 hours ago, clinical evidence of ongoing ischemia is between 12 and 24 hours after onset of symptoms, or if there is cardiogenic shock/severe heart failure (HF) regardless of time delay from onset.

HINT PCI should not be performed in a noninfarct artery at the time of primary PCI in patients with STEMI who are hemodynamically stable.

High-risk MI has better outcomes with primary PCI therapy (Box 2.5).

Box 2.5 High-Risk Myocardial Infarctions

Elderly patients	Systolic BP <100
Anterior wall STEMI Serious ventricular arrhythmias	Signs of acute heart failure or low CO
	Cardiogenic shock

BP, blood pressure; CO, cardiac output; STEMI, ST-segment elevation myocardial infarction.

Q Which drug therapy is recommended to support primary PCI?

A Anticoagulant and/or antiplatelet agent

Aspirin (ASA) and thienopyridine (clopidogrel, prasugrel, or ticagrelor) should be given as early as possible or at the time of the PCI. A glycoprotein (GP) IIb/IIIa receptor antagonist may also be used at the time of the primary PCI if receiving unfractionated heparin (UFH). These include abciximab, tirofiban, and eptifibatide. Bivalirudin monotherapy may be used instead of the combination of UFH and a GP IIb/IIIa receptor antagonist.

HINT Prasugrel should not be administered to patients with a history of prior stroke or transient ischemic attack (TIA).

Q What is the minimal time required for dual antiplatelet drug therapy in DES?

A 1 year

A dual antiplatelet therapy is recommended for a minimum of 1 year after a DES and 1 month (4–6 weeks) after placement of a BMS. A BMS is recommended for high risk of bleeding, predicted compliance issues, and known need for a surgical procedure.

HINT The dual antiplatelet is an ASA and a thienopyridine (P2Y$_{12}$ receptor inhibitor). Thienopyridines include clopidogrel (Plavix), prasugrel (Effient), or ticagrelor.

Q What are the clinical indications for fibrinolytic therapy?

A STEMI, hyperacute T wave, posterior infarction (reciprocal ST-segment depression V$_1$–V$_3$), and new-onset left bundle branch block (LBBB)

Fibrinolytic therapy is a treatment option and should be given, if not contraindicated, within 12 hours of onset of ischemic symptoms if PCI cannot be performed within 120 minutes.

HINT Peaked T waves are tall and narrow and develop at the onset of the infarction. These are called "peaking" or "hyperacute" T waves. Rule out peaked T waves due to hyperkalemia.

Q What is the recommendation for "door-to-needle" time when administering a fibrinolytic agent?

A 30 minutes or less

If fibrinolytic therapy is used, the goal for "door-to-needle" time is less than 30 minutes from presentation to medical facility.

Q When would a fibrinolytic agent be administered to a patient with STEMI beyond the 12-hour window?

A Ongoing signs of ischemia

A fibrinolytic agent may be administered when PCI is not available, and the patient has clinical evidence of ongoing ischemia (symptoms and/or EKG changes), hemodynamic instability, or when a large area of myocardium is at risk. This should still occur within 12 to 24 hours of the onset of symptoms.

HINT   If the scenario is a STEMI patient in cardiogenic shock or acute severe HF, immediate transfer is recommended to a hospital with PCI capabilities, irrespective of the time of onset of symptoms.

Q Which ACS patients would not be a candidate for fibrinolytic therapy?

A NSTEMI and UA

Fibrinolytic therapy is not indicated in NSTEMI or UA, and transfer to a hospital with PCI capabilities is mandated (Box 2.6 and Table 2.3).

Box 2.6 Absolute Contraindications of Fibrinolytic Therapy

Prior intracranial hemorrhage	Suspected aortic dissection
Known intracranial vascular lesion (e.g., aneurysm, AVM)	Active bleeding
Known malignant intracranial tumor	Ischemic stroke within 3 months
Significant traumatic brain injury within 3 months	

AVM, arteriovenous malformation.

Table 2.3 Fibrinolytic Agents

	Streptokinase	tPA	rPA	TNK
Dose	1.5 million units over 30–60 minutes	15 mg bolus followed by 0.75 mg/kg given over 30 minutes, then 0.5 mg/kg over 1 hour	Two 10 U boluses given 30 minutes apart	Based on kilograms of body weight
Half-life	20 minutes	4–6 minutes	18 minutes	20 minutes
90-minute patency	50%	75%	60%–70%	75%
Fibrin specificity	– –	++	+	+++

rPA, reteplase; TNK, tenecteplase; tPA, alteplase.

HINT   A patient with an NSTEMI or ST depression (unless confirmed posterior MI) is not a candidate for thrombolytic therapy.

Q Following the administration of a fibrinolytic agent, what medications should be given to prevent early reinfarction?

A Antiplatelet and anticoagulation therapy

Early reinfarction following thrombolytic therapy may be prevented with the administration of antiplatelet and anticoagulation medications. An ASA (81–325 mg) should continue indefinitely. Clopidogrel (Plavix) should be continued for at least 14 days and up to 1 year. Anticoagulation therapy is recommended for a minimum of 48 hours and may continue throughout hospitalization (up to 8 days). Anticoagulation therapy can include one of the following: UFH, enoxaparin (Lovenox), or fondaparinux.

HINT   Clopidogrel (Plavix) is administered initially as a loading dose except in patients older than 75 years of age.

Q What are the four signs of reperfusion following the administration of a fibrinolytic agent or PCI?

A Relief of chest pain, ST-segment return to baseline, abrupt onset of ventricular arrhythmias, and increased levels of cardiac enzymes (washout effect)

When the myocardium is reperfused, there is a relief of chest pain and return of ST-segment toward baseline due to the reversal of the ischemic injury. Recannulation of the previously obstructed coronary artery allows the washout of cardiac enzymes accumulated distal to the obstruction with accompanying ventricular arrhythmias and short runs of ventricular tachycardia (VT).

HINT   The most important sign is the relief of chest pain and ST-segment improvement of more than 50%.

Q What is the most sensitive continuous monitor used to recognize MI or efficacy of treatment for STEMI?

A ST-segment monitoring

ST-segment monitoring is recommended for patients with ACS. If the patient suffered an STEMI, use the best lead with the ST elevation as the "fingerprint" to monitor for changes in the elevation of the ST segment. If the patient does not have ST-segment elevation, monitor leads III and V_5. ST-segment monitoring can also recognize a "silent MI" and may be more sensitive than a patient reporting chest pain in some situations.

HINT   High-risk surgical patients may also benefit from continuous ST-segment monitoring. Lead V_5 is the most valuable for identifying demand-related ischemia.

Q What is the indication of a CABG in a patient with an STEMI?

A Coronary artery anatomy not amendable by PCI

An urgent CABG is indicated in patients with an STEMI experiencing ongoing or recurrent ischemia, cardiogenic shock, and severe HF, and when coronary artery anatomy is not amendable by PCI. Another indication is a patient who presents within 6 hours of onset of symptoms and is not considered to be a candidate for PCI or fibrinolytic therapy.

Q What is the primary intervention for an RV infarction?

A Fluid bolus

The RV pumps differently from the LV. The LV has both spiral and circular muscles. The spiral muscles wrap around in such a manner that contributes to the contraction or "wringing" out of the blood of the heart. Volume overload worsens LV HF. In patients with LV involvement, fluid intake is limited, and venodilators such as nitrates and morphine are administered to lower the preload. The RV pumps by using a bellows-type mechanism with the free wall moving toward the septum. Volume in the RV is required to produce an adequate stroke volume (SV). With RV involvement, fluid boluses are indicated.

HINT   Nitrates should not be used in RV infarction. Inotropic agents and intra-aortic balloon counterpulsations may also be indicated.

Q Which class of anticoagulation therapy is not recommended in UA or NSTEMI?

A Vitamin K antagonist

An ASA is recommended immediately and must be continued indefinitely. Clopidogrel (Plavix) may also be used as a substitute or as dual antiplatelet therapy. GP IIb/IIIa inhibitors may also be administered to patients at higher risk and may be used as a third antiplatelet drug. UFH has been found to be beneficial for patients with UA. Factor Xa inhibitors have been shown to produce favorable outcomes in UA/NSTEMI and direct thrombin inhibitors may be an alternative. Warfarin (Coumadin), a vitamin K antagonist, has shown no benefit and may increase bleeding risk.

Q Which two drugs administered after ACS have been found to reduce LV remodeling?

A Beta blockers and ACE inhibitors

Beta blockers blunt the effects of the sympathetic nervous system, thereby reducing heart rate (HR), blood pressure (BP), and contractility. They may also reduce the risk of serious arrhythmia by preventing maladaptive remodeling of the LV. ACE inhibitors can also prevent the adverse remodeling of the LV following an MI. They should be initiated during hospitalization and continued long term (unless contraindicated).

HINT   Beta blockers are contraindicated if signs of cardiogenic shock or severe HF are present.

> **Q** Which medication is indicated within the first 24 hours of anterior wall myocardial infarction (AWMI) with a ventricular ejection fraction (EF) of less than 40%?
>
> **A** ACE inhibitor

This is an American College of Cardiology (ACC) and American Heart Association (AHA) Class I recommendation for AWMI. An ACE inhibitor may also be indicated for other types of AMI within the first 24 hours in the absence of hypotension. ACE inhibitors function as arterial vasodilators, decreasing LV afterload, lowering BP, and preventing adverse LV remodeling. Following an AMI, ventricular remodeling can result in sudden cardiac death (SCD) from ventricular arrhythmias.

HINT High-intensity statin therapy should be administered in all patients with STEMI (unless contraindicated).

> **Q** Which clinical situations would be contraindicated to administer an aldosterone blocker?
>
> **A** Elevated serum creatinine levels and hyperkalemia

Inspra (Eplerenone) is an aldosterone blocker used in acute MI and HF with a left ventricular ejection fraction (LVEF) of less than 40%. Contraindications include serum creatinine levels greater than 2.5 mg/dL in men and greater than 2.0 mg/dL in women. It is also contraindicated to administer if potassium levels are greater than 5.0 mEq/L.

▶ COMPLICATIONS

> **Q** Acute pulmonary edema following an inferior MI with new-onset holosystolic murmur indicates which complication?
>
> **A** Acute severe mitral regurgitation

Acute severe mitral regurgitation usually occurs within 24 hours of the infarction but may occur up to 3 to 5 days later. Early recognition and management with inotropic therapy, intra-aortic balloon counterpulsation, and surgery can improve outcomes. Urgent surgical repair of the mitral valve is a Class I recommendation by the ACC/AHA.

HINT Mitral regurgitation causes a holosystolic murmur. Look at the type of murmur given as a hint in the scenario.

> **Q** What is the recommended treatment for pericarditis after STEMI?
>
> **A** ASA

ASA is the recommended drug therapy following a STEMI. If ASA—even at higher doses—is ineffective, then administration of acetaminophen, colchicine, or opioid analgesics may be ordered.

HINT If pericarditis is due to STEMI, do not administer glucocorticoids and nonsteroidal anti-inflammatory drugs. These are potentially harmful in this situation.

> **Q** Which type of AMI is most likely to result in development of an LV mural thrombus?
>
> **A** AWMI

A large AWMI develops LV regional wall akinesia or dyskinesia with blood stasis. The contributing factors of a thrombus include inflammation of the endocardium and a hypercoagulable state. The presentation is an embolic stroke, and symptoms depend on the location of the embolus. An echocardiogram can be used to identify the thrombus in the LV. Anticoagulation therapy is used to manage the thrombus (heparin followed by warfarin for 3–6 months).

HINT This complication of an LV mural thrombus typically occurs within the first 10 days of AMI.

> **Q Following ventricular septal rupture (VSR), what type of murmur does the patient suddenly develop?**
>
> **A Loud, harsh holosystolic murmur**

The other symptoms of VSR include SOB, biventricular failure, chest pain, and hypotension. This complication may occur within 24 hours of the AMI and then peaks again 3 to 5 days after the AMI. Very rarely would it present after 2 weeks. Treatment would be to manage the patient with vasodilators (reduce afterload), inotropic agents, diuretics, or mechanical support with an intra-aortic balloon pump (IABP) until the defect can be repaired surgically.

HINT   The complication of cardiogenic shock does not produce a murmur, and mitral regurgitation has a soft systolic murmur.

> **Q What is the most common arrhythmia or cause of death in an LV free wall rupture?**
>
> **A Pulseless electrical activity (PEA)**

LV free wall rupture may occur with large, transmural infarctions. Clinical presentation may include sudden, severe chest pain with abrupt hemodynamic collapse, and PEA. This is due to the rapid development of pericardial tamponade (Box 2.7).

Box 2.7 Complications of AMI

Cardiogenic shock	Arrhythmias
Pericarditis	Ventricular free wall rupture
Post–myocardial infarction syndrome (Dressler's syndrome)	Cardiac tamponade
Left ventricular aneurysm	Ventricular septal rupture
Papillary muscle rupture/mitral regurgitation	Left ventricular mural thrombus

AMI, acute myocardial infarction.

HINT   Rupture of the ventricular free wall will result in signs of pericardial tamponade and PEA.

⬤ CARDIOGENIC SHOCK

> **Q What is the most severe form of HF?**
>
> **A Cardiogenic shock**

Cardiogenic shock is the most severe form of HF and requires emergency management.

HINT   Cardiogenic shock and pericardial tamponade are life-threatening conditions.

▶ PATHOPHYSIOLOGY

> **Q What is the primary cause of cardiogenic shock?**
>
> **A Myocardial ischemia**

Cardiogenic shock remains the leading cause of mortality in AMI. Ischemic cardiomyopathy is the primary cause of cardiogenic shock. Cardiogenic shock is defined as hypoperfusion due to cardiac failure (Box 2.8).

Box 2.8 Other Causes of Cardiogenic Shock

Hypertrophied cardiomyopathy	Stress-induced cardiomyopathy (takotsubo cardiomyopathy)
Aortic dissection with aortic insufficiency	Acute valvular regurgitation (endocarditis or chordal rupture)
Aortic or mitral stenosis (increases myocardial stress)	Cardiac tamponade
Acute myopericarditis	Massive pulmonary embolism

HINT STEMI patients are more likely to experience cardiogenic shock compared to NSTEMI.

Q Which location of AMI is most likely associated with cardiogenic shock?

A AWMI

Risk factors for the development of cardiogenic shock following an AMI include AWMI, multiple-vessel disease, older age, hypertension, prior MI, STEMI, and the presence of LBBB.

HINT May use these risk factors as hints in a scenario to assist with recognizing cardiogenic shock.

Q What is the initial physiological change which results in the clinical signs of cardiogenic shock?

A Decreased myocardial contractility

The decreased myocardial contractility leads to decreased cardiac output, hypotension, and systemic vasoconstriction. The vasoconstriction may initially improve perfusion but results in increased afterload and workload of the heart causing significant myocardial ischemia.

HINT Insufficient circulatory leads to multisystem organ failure.

▶ SYMPTOMS/ASSESSMENT

Q What are the characteristic hemodynamic parameters of cardiogenic shock?

A Low cardiac output (CO)/cardiac index (CI), high systemic vascular resistance (SVR), and high filling pressures

Cardiogenic shock demonstrates persistent hypotension with severe reduction in CO/CI and adequate or elevated filling pressures. Compensatory mechanisms for low CO/CI include vasoconstriction (elevates SVR) and tachycardia, which actually worsens the CO/CI due to high resistance and increased workload of the heart, causing a vicious cycle to develop (Box 2.9).

HINT Severe reduction of CI is defined as less than 1.8 L/min/m^2 without support and less than 2.0 to 2.2 L/min/m^2 with support.

Box 2.9 Other Symptoms of Cardiogenic Shock

Tachycardia	Altered mental status
Cool, clammy skin	Tachypnea
Pale nail beds with delayed capillary refill	Presence arrhythmias
Decreased urine output	Pulmonary congestion
Hypotension	

HINT Presentation with cool extremities and pulmonary congestion is identified as "cold and wet" presentation.

▶ DIAGNOSIS

> **Q** Which monitoring device may be used to assist with the diagnosis of cardiogenic shock?
>
> **A** Pulmonary artery catheter (PAC)

A PAC provides information on the CO/CI, filling pressures and enables the calculation of SVR. These readings are used to define and recognize cardiogenic shock. Newer hemodynamic monitors that are minimally invasive and that use the arterial waveform may also be used to assist with the diagnosis.

HINT An echocardiogram may be used to confirm the diagnosis of high filling pressures and to rule out other causes of hypotension following an AMI.

▶ MEDICAL MANAGEMENT

> **Q** What is the greatest concern when administering an inotropic agent to a patient in cardiogenic shock?
>
> **A** Increase in myocardial workload and oxygen consumption

Inotropic agents are frequently needed to increase CO and reduce filling pressures in the RV and LV, but they can increase the oxygen demand in a heart with limited oxygen supply. This may increase the ischemic injuries to the myocardium. Inotropes are recommended in hypoperfusion states with or without pulmonary congestion but may be initiated at a lower dose in cardiogenic shock to limit complications.

HINT Inotropes can also induce arrhythmias in ischemic hearts and should be closely monitored.

> **Q** What is a first-line intervention in managing hypotension in cardiogenic shock?
>
> **A** Inotropes

Vasoconstrictors (e.g., norepinephrine) should not be used initially to treat hypotension in cardiogenic shock due to the presence of increased SVR. Other interventions for managing hypotension in cardiogenic shock include a combination of inotropic agents with vasodilators, fluid challenges with inotropic agents, and mechanical circulatory assist devices (IABP, left ventricular assist device [LVAD]). These devices may offer significant advantages over vasopressor therapy. (Box 2.10)

Box 2.10 Mechanical Circulatory Assist Devices

IABP
Axial flow pumps (Impella)
Left atrial-to-femoral arterial ventricular assist devices (Tandem Heart)
Venous-arterial ECMO

ECMO, extracorporeal membrane oxygenation; IABP, intra-aortic balloon pump.

HINT If vasoconstrictors are needed, it is recommended that norepinephrine be used with caution instead of dopamine.

▶ SURGICAL MANAGEMENT

> **Q** What is the surgical procedure for managing cardiogenic shock?
>
> **A** Revascularization

Emergency revascularization with a CABG procedure is indicated to improve survival. It may not improve the 30-day survival, but it has been shown to improve long-term survival (6-month and 6-year outcome studies).

HINT   Mechanical circulatory assist devices (e.g., IABP) may be used as a bridge to stabilize the patient prior to surgery.

 DYSRHYTHMIAS ASSOCIATED WITH AMI

▶ PATHOPHYSIOLOGY

Q What is the most common reason for atrial arrhythmias following an AMI?

A Left atrial (LA) distension

LA distention is frequently caused by high pressure in the LV. Atrial arrhythmias (PACs, atrial flutter, atrial fibrillation [AF]) are frequently a result of LA distention following an AMI.

HINT   Atrial arrhythmias are also common after CABG or valve surgeries.

▶ DIAGNOSIS

Q What is the EKG finding of a first-degree heart block?

A PR interval prolonged greater than 0.20

A prolonged PR interval without loss of ventricular conduction indicates that the block is above the bundle of His. Calcium channel blockers and beta blockers may exacerbate the prolonging of the PR interval but should only be stopped if hemodynamically unstable or a higher degree of block occurs.

Q What EKG change determines whether the block is above or below the nodal area?

A Width of the QRS

Supranodal or intranodal blocks produce a narrow QRS pattern. Blocks that occur below the nodal area produce a wide QRS complex.

▶ MEDICAL MANAGEMENT

Q Are rate-control drugs more effective in atrial flutter or AF?

A AF

Atrial flutter is managed similarly to AF, except ventricular rate control in the atrial flutter is not as responsive to rate-control drugs. A patient who develops an atrial flutter and is hemodynamically compromised requires synchronized electrical cardioversion.

Q What complication of AMI would limit the use of IV diltiazem in the treatment of AF?

A Moderate to severe HF

The use of IV diltiazem in managing ventricular rate should be done cautiously following an AMI due to the complication of HF.

HINT   Remember that some calcium channel blockers have negative inotropic effects.

▶ COMPLICATIONS

Q Following an inferior AMI, the patient presents with HR less than 40 bpm and hypotension. If BP is unresponsive to atropine, what complication may be the cause?

A RV infarction and/or volume depletion

An RV infarction can be present with an inferior wall MI. The presence of RV involvement and/or volume depletion will frequently result in continued hypotension, despite treatment with atropine. Obtain right-sided 12-lead EKG and administer fluids for RV involvement to correct the hypotension.

HINT Remember: Bradycardia does not require treatment if the patient is hemodynamically stable (Table 2.4). Review Advanced Cardiovascular Life Support (ACLS) certification.

Table 2.4 Arrhythmias

Arrhythmia	Causes	Treatment/Management
PSVT	LA distention from elevated LV pressures Inflammation (pericarditis)	Adenosine when hypotension not present If hypotensive, may use IV diltiazem or beta blocker If severe hypotension, perform synchronized electrical cardioversion
Atrial flutter	Sympathetic overstimulation of LA (usually transient)	Similar to AF except not responsive to rate-control drugs If symptomatic, perform synchronized electrical cardioversion If refractory medical management, may overdrive atrial pace
AF	LV failure Ischemia to atria RV infarction Pericarditis	If unstable, immediate synchronized electrical cardioversion If stable, control the ventricular rate IV amiodarone or digoxin Beta blocker may be used if not hypotensive Anticoagulation therapy
Bradycardia	Inferior or posterior wall myocardial infarction Vagal stimulation	If unstable, administer atropine 0.5 to 1 mg External or transvenous pacing
First-degree atrioventricular block	Inferior wall myocardial infarction	No treatment required
Second-degree Mobitz Type I AV block	Inferior wall myocardial infarction	No treatment required if hemodynamically stable
Second-degree Mobitz Type II AV block	Anterior wall MI	Transcutaneous or transvenous pacing Atropine Possibly permanent demand pacemaker
Third-degree AV block	Anterior wall MI Inferior wall MI	Atropine if inferior wall MI Temporary transcutaneous or transvenous pacing Permanent demand pacemaker
VT	Monomorphic VT most likely caused by myocardial scar Polymorphic VT most likely caused by ischemia Electrolyte abnormalities Hypoxia Acid–base disturbances	If unstable, unsynchronized cardioversion If stable, administer amiodarone Maintain K^+ > 4 mEq/L and Mg^+ > 2.0 mEq/L
Ventricular fibrillation (VF)	MI Cardiogenic shock	Unsynchronized electrical countershock

AF, atrial fibrillation; AV, atrioventricular; IV, intravenous; LA, left atrial; LV, left ventricular; MI, myocardial infarction; PSVT, paroxysmal supraventricular tachycardia; RV, right ventricular; VT, ventricular tachycardia.

HEART FAILURE

> **Q** During admission history, a patient with HF tells you that he is comfortable at rest but becomes short of breath during activities of daily living. In which New York Heart Association (NYHA) class is this patient?
>
> **A** NYHA Class II

NYHA Class II is described as a person that is asymptomatic at rest but becomes dyspneic during normal activities of daily living.

The NYHA classification system was devised to classify the extent of HF based on functional capacity. It lists four categories of cardiac disease (Classes I–IV) ranging from mild to severe with progressively increasing symptoms of physical limitation associated with each class. For more information, please see www.my.americanheart.org.

> **Q** At which stage is a patient with normal EF, but a history of mitral regurgitation, according to the ACC/AHA stages?
>
> **A** Stage B

The ACC/AHA stages of HF were developed for early identification of at-risk patients for HF (Table 2.5). The stages are not meant to replace the NYHA classification system. Patients in stages A and B are at risk for HF but are currently not symptomatic. The staging system includes therapy recommendations for each stage (Table 2.6).

Table 2.5 ACC/AHA Stages in Development of HF

Stage	Definition	Patients at risk
Stage A	At high risk for HF but without structural heart disease or symptoms of HF	Hypertension Atherosclerotic disease Diabetes Obesity Metabolic syndrome Using cardiotoxins Family history of cardiomyopathy
Stage B	Structural heart disease but without signs or symptoms of HF	Previous MI LV remodeling, including LVH and low EF Asymptomatic valvular disease
Stage C	Structural heart disease with prior or current symptoms of HF	Known structural heart disease Shortness of breath Fatigue, reduced exercise tolerance
Stage D	Refractory HF requiring specialized interventions	Marked symptoms at rest despite maximal medical therapy

ACC, American College of Cardiology; AHA, American Heart Association; EF, ejection fraction; HF, heart failure; LV, left ventricle; LVH, Left ventricular hypertrophy; MI, myocardial infarction.

Source: Data from the ACC/AHA practice guidelines.

Table 2.6 ACC/AHA-Recommended Therapy by Stage

Stage	Goals	Drugs	Devices/Options
Stage A	Treat hypertension Encourage smoking cessation Treat lipid disorders Encourage regular exercise Discourage alcohol intake, illicit drug use Control metabolic syndrome	ACE inhibitor or ARB in appropriate patients for vascular disease or diabetes	

(continued)

Table 2.6 ACC/AHA-Recommended Therapy by Stage (*continued*)

Stage	Goals	Drugs	Devices/Options
Stage B	Same as Stage A	ACEI or ARB in appropriate patients Beta blockers in appropriate patients	
Stage C	All measures under Stages A and B Dietary salt restriction	Diuretics for fluid retention ACEI Beta blockers Selected patients Aldosterone antagonist ARBs Digitalis Hydralazine/nitrates	Biventricular pacing Implantable defibrillators
Stage D	Appropriate measures under Stages A, B, and C. Decision regarding appropriate level of care		Compassionate end-of-life care/hospice Extraordinary measures Heart transplant Chronic inotropes Permanent mechanical support Experimental surgery or drugs

ACC, American College of Cardiology; ACEI, angiotensin-converting enzyme inhibitor; AHA, American Heart Association; ARB, angiotensin receptor blocker.

Source: Data from the ACC/AHA practice guidelines.

▶ PATHOPHYSIOLOGY

Q Which type of HF is caused by a difficulty in filling the ventricles?

A Diastolic dysfunction

HF caused by diastolic dysfunction is a result of a difficulty with the filling of the ventricles. The difficulty with the ventricular filling may be caused by an incomplete ventricular relaxation, increased stiffness, pericardial restraint, or high intrathoracic pressure.

HINT The new term is HF with preserved EF.

Q What is the most common underlying etiology of a heart failure with preserved ejection fraction (HFpEF)?

A Hypertrophic cardiomyopathy

Hypertrophic cardiomyopathy is the most common cause of HFpEF. It may be congenital or caused by chronic hypertension or aortic stenosis (Box 2.11).

Box 2.11 HF Classification

HFrEF	LV EF of 40% or lower
HFpEF	LV EF of 50% or higher
HFpEF Borderline	LV EF between 41% and 49%

HFpEF heart failure preserved ejection fraction; HFrEF, heart failure reduced ejection fraction; LV, left ventricular.

> **Q** Which commonly used drug classification in HF is contraindicated if the underlying abnormality is a diastolic dysfunction?
>
> **A** Inotropic agents

The problem is not with the contractility of the pump (most patients with diastolic dysfunction actually have normal EF) but with a small ventricular chamber. An inotropic agent will constrict the chamber, limiting the filling capability even more. Calcium channel blockers or beta blockers are typically used to manage diastolic dysfunction. The goal is afterload reduction and relaxation of the ventricles.

HINT Diastolic dysfunction HF frequently exhibits symptoms of failure but has a high EF.

> **Q** Which type of HF is associated with decreased EF?
>
> **A** Systolic dysfunction

Systolic dysfunction is caused by poor contractility or reduction in CO. It is commonly defined as an EF less than 40%. It is the most common cause of HF (Box 2.12).

HINT This is called HFrEF

Box 2.12 Etiology of HFrEF

Myocardial ischemia	Obstructive cardiomyopathy
Myocardial infarction	Infection
Valvular heart disease	Toxin exposure
Chronic volume overload	Congenital heart defects
Dilated cardiomyopathy	

HFrEF, heart failure reduced ejection fraction.

The goal is to decrease preload and afterload.

HINT Remember:
Preload = Volume
Afterload = Resistance

> **Q** Drugs used to manage HF typically inhibit which neurohormonal compensatory mechanism?
>
> **A** Renin-angiotensin system (RAS)

Aldosterone blockers, ACE inhibitors, and angiotensin receptor blockers (ARBs) all work on the RAS (Figure 2.1).

> **Q** What compensatory mechanism increases blood flow to the kidneys, thus decreasing the release of renin?
>
> **A** Brain natriuretic peptide (BNP)

Pro-BNP is an inactive peptide secreted by stretched myocytes during HF then is converted to an active BNP. The BNP will increase glomerular filtration rates, increase renal blood flow, decrease the release of renin, and decrease Na^+ reabsorption by the kidneys.

HINT Pro-BNP and BNP levels are used for the diagnosis of acute and chronic HF.

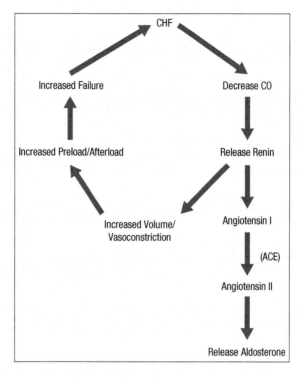

Figure 2.1 Renin–angiotensin system.

▶ SYMPTOMS/ASSESSMENT

Q Which abnormal heart sound is commonly associated with HF?

A S_3

S_3 is a gallop that occurs during early diastole and is frequently caused by ventricular overload (Box 2.13). An S3 occurs in early diastole, immediately after the mitral valve closes. ~çf

HINT   A patient scenario with an S_3 is typically HF, whereas an S_4 is angina.

Box 2.13 Symptoms of HF

Left-Sided Failure	Right-Sided Failure	Other Symptoms
Crackles	Jugular venous distention	Fatigue
Tachypnea	Hepatomegaly	Weakness
Dyspnea	Splenomegaly	Decreased exercise tolerance
Hypoxemia	Elevated CVP	Unexplained confusion
Cough	Peripheral edema	
Pink, frothy sputum	Decreased CO	
Decreased CO	Tachycardia	
Orthopnea		
Tachycardia		

CO, cardiac output; CVP, central venous pressure; HF, heart failure.

▶ DIAGNOSIS

> **Q** What is the single most useful diagnostic test in the evaluation of a patient with HF?
>
> **A** Comprehensive two-dimensional (2-D) echocardiogram coupled with Doppler flow

The 2-D echocardiogram can determine whether the abnormality is with the myocardium, heart valves, or pericardium. SV can be determined with the use of echocardiogram by measuring the LV outflow tract and the amount of blood that goes through it. In cases of valvular etiology, valve area, valvular gradient, and regurgitant severity can be determined (Table 2.7).

HINT An echocardiogram is the recommended diagnostic test for new-onset HF.

Table 2.7 Other Diagnostic Tests

Test	Advantage	Disadvantage
Radionuclide ventriculography	Accurate measurements of LV function and RVEF	Unable to assess valve abnormalities or cardiac hypertrophy
MRI	Evaluate chamber size, ventricular mass, RV dysplasia, and pericardial disease	
CXR	Estimate degree of cardiac enlargement and pulmonary edema	Unable to determine LV function or valvular abnormalities
12-lead EKG	Demonstrate evidence of prior myocardial infarction, LV hypertrophy, cardiac conduction abnormality, or cardiac arrhythmia	Unable to determine the mechanical function of the ventricles

CXR, chest x-ray; LV, left ventricular; RV, right ventricular; RVEF, right ventricular ejection fraction.

> **Q** Which laboratory test may be used to determine the severity of HF?
>
> **A** BNP levels

BNP levels may also be used to differentiate between HF and pulmonary disease in dyspneic patients. Elevated BNP levels accurately detect CHF in 95% to 97% of patients (100 pg/mL). The diagnostic "gray area" is between 100 and 500 pg/mL, and anything greater than 500 pg/mL is positive.

HINT BNP levels may be falsely low in obese patients.

> **Q** Are there false positives with elevated BNP levels?
>
> **A** Yes

There are disease processes, both cardiac and noncardiac, that can falsely elevate BNP levels (Box 2.14).

Box 2.14 Causes of False Elevation of BNP Levels

Cardiac	Noncardiac
Acute coronary syndrome	Elderly
Myocarditis	Renal failure
Pericardial disease	Severe brain injury
Cardioversion	Bacterial sepsis
Atrial fibrillation	
Hypertension	

BNP, brain natriuretic peptide.

> **Q** What is the primary difference between BNP and N-terminal (NT)-ProBNP levels?
>
> **A** Half-life of NT-ProBNP is longer than BNP

The half-life of NT-ProBNP is 1 to 2 hours versus 20 minutes with BNP. The NT-ProBNP levels correlate to the NYHA classifications:

NYHA I = mean 1,015
NYHA II = mean 1,666
NYHA III = mean 3,029
NYHA IV = mean 3,465

▶ MANAGEMENT

> **Q** A patient on an ACE inhibitor is noncompliant. Which side effect of the ACE inhibitor is the most likely cause?
>
> **A** Dry, nonproductive cough

Some patients who cough while taking ACE inhibitors have this symptom because of CHF rather than ACE inhibitor intolerance and might improve with further diuresis. Others develop a dry, hacking cough that can interfere with activities of daily living (i.e., eating, talking, sleeping) and may require changing to an ARB.

HINT Recognize the drug is an ACE inhibitor when it ends in "-pril."

> **Q** What electrolyte abnormality is common with an ACE inhibitor?
>
> **A** Hyperkalemia

ACE inhibitors promote the excretion of Na^+ and water, thus increasing the reabsorption of K^+. Hyperkalemia may occur when patients are on ACE inhibitors, ARBs, and aldosterone antagonists. Serum potassium levels should be monitored closely in HF patients. Diuretics are commonly used in HF and can lead to hypokalemia. Hypokalemia may adversely affect cardiac conduction and lead to arrhythmias and sudden death.

HINT Remember hypokalemia may increase the risk of digitalis toxicity.

> **Q** Which class of drugs is used if a patient is ACE-inhibitor intolerant?
>
> **A** ARB

ARBs allow the conversion of angiotensin I to angiotensin II but block the receptor sites of angiotensin II. These drugs have side effects similar to an ACE inhibitor but less cough or cases of angioedema. Following an episode of angioedema, the patient should have the ACE inhibitor changed to an ARB. ARBs may be used as a first-line treatment with mild to moderate HF and reduced LVEF.

> **Q** A person with symptomatic HF on an ACE inhibitor and beta blocker has persistent symptoms. Which combinations of medications are recommended at this time?
>
> **A** Hydralazine and nitrate

The addition of a combination of hydralazine and nitrate is reasonable for patients with reduced LVEF, who are already taking an ACE inhibitor and beta blocker but have persistent symptoms. These can improve symptoms of HF by afterload reduction.

HINT The combination of hydralazine and nitrate is also recommended to improve outcomes for African Americans with moderate to severe symptoms.

> **Q** Which EKG finding indicates the need for cardiac resynchronization therapy?
>
> **A** QRS duration 0.12 seconds or longer

Other indications include patients with LVEF 35% or less, sinus rhythm, and NYHA functional Class III or ambulatory IV. Pacemakers depolarize the RV then the left. This results in dyssynchronization and can decrease EF. Cardiac resynchronization therapy paces both the left and the RV, allowing for synchronization and improved EF.

HINT   Resynchronization therapy is biventricular pacing.

AORTIC ANEURYSM/AORTIC DISSECTION/ AORTIC RUPTURE

> **Q What is an aortic dissection?**
>
> **A Lengthwise separation of the medial layer of the aorta**

An aortic dissection involves the medial layer of the aorta. There is a lengthwise separation of the medial layer due to a tear in the intima with extravasation. Blood flows between the intimal and medial layers creating a double lumen, called a false lumen and a true lumen (aorta). Dissection can be acute, present within the first 14 days of initial injury, or chronic, with presentation longer than 14 days.

HINT   A traumatic aortic aneurysm is a disruption of the intimal, medial, and adventitial layers. This is called an aortic transection.

> **Q What happens if blood flows into the false lumen, forming a large hematoma?**
>
> **A Partial to complete obstruction of the true lumen**

Following the intimal tear, blood enters the medial layer and can form a large hematoma, obstructing the true lumen and affecting distal perfusion. Shearing forces can also cause further tears, producing exit sites and flow back into the true lumen (Box 2.15).

HINT   Thoracic aortic aneurysm occurs above the diaphragm, and abdominal aortic aneurysm occurs below.

Box 2.15 Sites of Aortic Dissections

Ascending aorta	Descending aorta
Aortic arch	Thoracoabdominal aorta

> **Q What genetic disorder of connective tissue resulting in above-average height causes risk for an aortic dissection?**
>
> **A Marfan's syndrome**

Marfan's syndrome is inherited as a dominant trait, and symptoms vary from mild to severe. People with Marfan's syndrome tend to be very tall, with long limbs and fingers. They are at risk for aortic aneurysms and dissections (Box 2.16).

HINT   Other connective tissue diseases that may be used in the scenario include Ehlers–Danlos or Loeys–Dietz

Box 2.16 Causes/Risk Factors of Aortic Dissection

Hypertension, especially uncontrolled	Chronic corticosteroid or immunosuppressive use
Pheochromocytoma	Congenital factors (bicuspid valve)
Cocaine or other stimulant use	Inflammatory vasculitis
Weight lifting or other Valsalva maneuvers	Atherosclerosis (e.g., PVD, coronary artery disease)
Pregnancy	Infections of the vascular wall
Genetic	Iatrogenic (e.g., aortic valve manipulation)
Polycystic kidney disease	

PVD, peripheral vascular disease.

▶ PATHOPHYSIOLOGY

> **Q** **What leads to the complication of organ ischemia with an aortic dissection?**
>
> **A** **Obstruction of arterial branches off the aorta**

The dissection can propagate through the arteries that branch off of the aorta, leading to stenosis or obstruction. The obstruction of arterial flow leads to organ ischemia and end-organ failure. Dissections can extend retrograde and antegrade (Box 2.17).

Box 2.17 Branch Arteries of the Aorta

Coronary	Renal
Brachiocephalic (e.g., subclavian, carotid)	Visceral (e.g., superior and inferior mesenteric arteries)
Intercostal	

HINT   May present with symptoms of end-organ ischemia from loss of blood flow through these arteries.

> **Q** **What part of the aorta is involved in a DeBakey Type II dissection?**
>
> **A** **Ascending aorta**

There are two major classification systems used in aortic dissections: DeBakey and Stanford systems. The DeBakey system uses Type I to Type III, whereas the Stanford system uses Type A and B (Table 2.8).

Table 2.8 Classifications of Aortic Dissections

	Type I	Type II	Type III
DeBakey System	Ascending and also involvement of descending aorta	Ascending aorta only	Only the descending is involved: IIIA: distal to the left subclavian artery to the diaphragm IIIB: descending aorta below the diaphragm
Stanford System	Ascending involved	Descending involved	NA

HINT   Most common location for abdominal aortic aneurysm (AAA) is infrarenal.

▶ SYMPTOMS/ASSESSMENT

> **Q** **How is the pain of an aortic dissection frequently described?**
>
> **A** **Ripping or tearing sensation**

The quality and severity of pain are frequently used to assist with the diagnosis of a dissection. The pain is initially described as a "ripping or tearing" sensation. It is of abrupt onset and severe intensity. There is sometimes a "latency" period during which the pain will get better after the initial onset, but then it returns as a "knife-like" severe pain.

HINT   These patients typically report 10/10 pain despite pain management and will typically be agitated.

> **Q** **What specific physical examination should be performed in a suspected thoracic aortic dissection?**
>
> **A** **Obtain BP in both arms**

Compare BPs obtained in each arm. A high-risk feature would be a discrepancy of systolic BP greater than 20 mmHg between upper extremities. Another assessment includes assessing pulses in the upper limbs compared to the lower limbs. A significant pulse deficit in the lower extremity should also increase level of suspicion (Box 2.18).

HINT   An associated new-onset diastolic murmur (aortic regurgitation) may indicate dissection of the ascending aorta.

Box 2.18 Signs of Aortic Dissection

Chest or abdominal pain (refers to the back)	Bruit (carotid, brachial, femoral)
Tracheal compression	Focal neurological deficits
Laryngeal hoarseness (pressure on recurrent laryngeal nerve)	Hemothorax
Dysphagia	Anxiety and premonition of death
Abdominal mass (pulsating)	Fever
Diastolic murmur (high-pitched blowing)	Hypertension
Pulse deficit	Manifestations of pericardial tamponade
Syncope	

Q What are the three signs of Horner's syndrome?

A Ptosis, miosis, and anhidrosis

Horner's syndrome is caused by an interruption in the cervical sympathetic ganglia and manifests as ptosis, miosis, and anhidrosis. This can occur with a dissection of the aortic arch.

HINT Horner's syndrome is the loss of sympathetic nervous system innervation.

▶ DIAGNOSIS

Q What diagnostic test is best used in an unstable patient with suspected aortic dissection?

A Echocardiogram

A chest x-ray (CXR) is frequently the initial evaluation but may not reveal any significant findings. A CT scan is used in hemodynamically stable patients, whereas an echocardiogram is preferred if unstable. It is performed at the bedside, is rapid and noninvasive (unless a transesophageal echocardiogram [TEE] is used, which is minimally invasive). An emergency CT angiography with three-dimensional (3-D) reconstruction is being used to obtain a view of the aorta without the potential complications of the more invasive aortogram. The aortogram can pinpoint the site of intimal tear, the true and false lumen entry site, appearance of dye outside of the aorta, and bulging of aorta.

HINT The gold standard is still considered to be the aortogram for diagnosis of aortic dissection.

Q What is the disadvantage of a TEE in diagnosing thoracic aortic dissection?

A Limited ability to visualize the distal ascending aorta

TEE has limited ability to visualize the distal ascending aorta and proximal arch because of the air-filled trachea and main stem bronchus.

HINT TEE can be used to identify an endoleak and is a valuable tool in evaluating aortic dissections.

▶ MEDICAL MANAGEMENT

Q What class of drugs is recommended for the initial management of a thoracic aortic dissection?

A Beta blocker

The initial treatment goal is to decrease the aorta wall stress by slowing the HR and lowering the BP. Esmolol (Brevibloc) is frequently used in acute management. If contraindicated to use a beta blocker, the second choice of drugs is nondihydropyridine calcium channel-blocking agents, which should be utilized as an alternative for rate control. Beta blockers should be used cautiously in acute aortic regurgitation due to the block on compensatory tachycardia.

HINT   Vasodilator therapy, such as Nipride, should not be used until after HR control has been achieved to avoid reflex tachycardia.

Q What is the target BP and HR in an acute aortic dissection?

A Systolic rate between 110 and 120 mmHg and HR between 60 and 80 bpm

During an acute aortic dissection, aggressive management of BP and HR should be initiated to lower the intraluminal pressure to limit extension of dissection. The end-organ perfusion also needs to be evaluated when managing BP to prevent hypoperfusion.

HINT   Most patients will be hypertensive; a hypotensive presentation may indicate pericardial tamponade or hemorrhage into the pleural or retroperitoneal space.

▶ SURGICAL MANAGEMENT

Q When is surgical repair recommended in an asymptomatic patient with a descending aortic aneurysm?

A Aneurysm greater than 5.5 cm

A patient with a stable chronic dissection may be observed for signs of progressive enlargement of the aorta. Surgical intervention is recommended with an aneurysm in the descending aorta greater than 5.5 cm. It is reasonable to follow up with CT scans or ultrasonography every 12 months to evaluate the size of the aneurysm, if less than 5.5 cm. Other indications for surgery include a saccular aneurysm or postsurgical pseudoaneurysm.

HINT   If the patient is symptomatic with acute dissection of any size, surgical intervention may be recommended.

Q What technique is used in the operating room to protect organs from ischemia during repair of the aorta?

A Cardiopulmonary bypass (CPB)

Other correct answers include partial left heart bypass, deep hypothermic circulatory arrest, and retrograde perfusion. Goals of surgery include repair of aorta as well as prevention of ischemic insult to distal organs. Surgical procedures can include intimal flap repair, removal of thrombosis and false lumen, replacement of dilated aorta with a graft, repair of aortic root, and replacement of aortic valve. Endovascular repair may also be used in descending aortic dissections through femoral access.

HINT   CPB requires heparinization. Postoperative management includes assessing for signs of coagulopathy and continued reversing of heparin.

Q What technique may be used to protect the spinal cord during surgical or endovascular repair of descending aorta?

A Cerebrospinal fluid (CSF) drainage

CSF drainage is recommended in patients with high risk for spinal cord ischemia during surgical repair of the descending aorta. They may also use other spinal cord perfusion techniques such as proximal aortic pressure maintenance and distal aortic perfusion to optimize spinal cord perfusion (Box 2.19).

Box 2.19 Other Treatments Used in the Prevention of Spinal Cord Ischemia

Intraoperative systemic hypothermia	Intrathecal papaverine
Epidural irrigation with hypothermic solution	Metabolic suppression with anesthetic agents
High-dose glucocorticosteroids	Reimplantation of intercostal arteries
Osmotic diuretic (i.e., Mannitol)	Distal perfusion

HINT   A postoperative patient should be assessed for any motor or sensory abnormalities.

> **Q** What is the priority in the postoperative care of an aortic repair with graft placement?
>
> **A** BP management

BP management is important in postoperative (as well as preoperative) care to prevent disruption of the graft, dissection, and hemorrhage. Antihypertensive agents used preoperatively may be continued in the postoperative period. Hemodynamic monitoring, prevention of fluid overload, correct coagulopathy, and administration of antibiotics to prevent graft infections are components of postoperative management.

> **Q** Which of the following is considered the surgical treatment of choice for repair of an uncomplicated infrarenal AAA?
>
> **A** Endovascular aneurysm repair (EVAR)

EVAR has some advantages over open technique for repair of AAA including lower early risk of complications. EVAR is recommended for an uncomplicated infrarenal AAA.

HINT   Patients with pararenal or juxta-renal AAA may require open technique with graft placement due to the location.

> **Q** Where does an embolism from catheter manipulation during interventional graft placement typically travel?
>
> **A** Legs and viscera

The internal surface of the aorta can be covered by atheromas. Manipulation of the catheter during interventional stent placement can break loose debris and become a distal embolism. This may involve the lower extremities or the abdominal viscera. Another complication can be migration of the graft.

HINT   May involve the renal, mesenteric, or iliac arteries. Assess for signs of organ hypoperfusion postprocedure.

▶ COMPLICATIONS

> **Q** What part of the aorta is at the highest risk for aortic rupture?
>
> **A** Ascending aorta

A high-risk aortic injury for rupture involves the ascending portion of the aorta and should be referred for emergent surgery to prevent life-threatening complications.

HINT   Ascending aortic dissections can dissect through the aortic valve resulting in acute aortic regurgitation and acute onset HF.

> **Q** Three days after the repair of a descending aortic dissection (Type B) with a graft placement, a patient develops severe abdominal pain and shows occult blood in stool. What is the most likely cause of the abdominal pain?
>
> **A** Bowel ischemia/infarction

Dissection of the aorta can involve the branch arteries. The superior and inferior mesenteric arteries may be involved in a descending aortic dissection. Signs of malperfusion of the bowel with ischemia and infarction include new-onset severe abdominal pain, elevated lactate and CPK levels, and sometimes the presence of occult blood in stool. The diagnostic procedure is typically abdominal CT.

HINT   Most postoperative complications will involve the malperfusion of organs from branch artery occlusion (Box 2.20).

Box 2.20 Complications

Perioperative MI	Graft occlusion
Stroke	Arterial embolism to extremities
Hypertension	Aortic thrombosis/stenosis
Low cardiac output syndrome	Wound infection
Renal failure	Bowel ischemia
Dysrhythmias	Paraplegia
Coagulopathies/DIC	Hemorrhage (retroperitoneal, intraperitoneal)
Graft infections	

DIC, disseminated intravascular coagulopathy; MI, myocardial infarction.

 CARDIAC TAMPONADE

> Q **What is the most common mechanism for a traumatic pericardial tamponade?**
>
> A **Penetrating injury**

Pericardial tamponade is caused by bleeding into the pericardial sac due to a ruptured coronary artery, lacerated pericardium, or an injury to the myocardium (Box 2.21).

HINT   Rapid accumulation of blood in the pericardium exceeds the pericardium's ability to stretch causing an increase in intrapericardial pressure.

Box 2.21 Causes of Pericardial Tamponade

Iatrogenic from cardiac catheterization
Post-cardiac surgery
Aortic dissection
Cardiac neoplasm
Severe pericardial effusions
Trauma

▶ PATHOPHYSIOLOGY

> Q **Is pericardial tamponade considered a diastolic or systolic dysfunction?**
>
> A **Diastolic dysfunction**

The pericardial sac usually contains 25 to 50 mL of fluid. Following an injury, blood accumulates within the pericardial sac, causing a constriction on the heart. The pericardial pressure becomes higher than the ventricular filling pressures, interfering with the ability of the ventricles to fill with blood (diastolic phase). The amount of blood required to impair filling depends upon the rate of the accumulation of blood and the compliance of the pericardial sac.

HINT   Pericardial tamponade is considered a constrictive cardiomyopathy.

▶ SYMPTOMS/ASSESSMENT

> Q **What is the first sign of a traumatic pericardial tamponade?**
>
> A **Tachycardia**

A significant decrease in ventricular filling results in a decrease in SV. Tachycardia is a compensatory mechanism, an attempt to maintain a normal CO.

HINT Suspect a pericardial tamponade in chest trauma if shock symptoms are unresponsive to fluid administration.

Q What is the Beck's triad?

A Increased jugular venous distention, hypotension, and muffled heart sounds

The pressure caused by the blood in the pericardial sac limits the filling of the heart, backing the blood up into the venous circulation. This produces jugular venous distention. The decreased filling results in a decrease in SV, leading to hypotension. The accumulation of blood in the pericardial sac muffles the heart sounds. The presentation of a classical Beck's triad occurs with an acute cardiac tamponade.

HINT Look for distended jugular veins as a clue of the elevated central venous pressure (CVP). Trauma patients typically have flat neck veins due to hypovolemia (Box 2.22).

Box 2.22 Other Symptoms of Pericardial Tamponade

Dyspnea	Pericardial friction rub
Cyanosis	Agitation
Diaphoresis	Feelings of impending doom
Cold, clammy skin	Electrical alternans
Pulsus paradoxus	

HINT Scenario of a penetrating chest wound in which the patient insists on sitting bolt upright, is agitated and confused, or has air hunger is more likely to be a condition of pericardial tamponade.

Q What is the most common type of cardiac arrest following a pericardial tamponade?

A PEA

PEA occurs in cardiac tamponade due to the constriction interfering with the mechanical activity of the heart, but the electrical activity continues.

HINT Cardiac tamponade is one of the differential diagnoses of PEA in a trauma patient.

▶ DIAGNOSIS

Q What CXR changes would you expect to find in a pericardial tamponade?

A Enlarged cardiac silhouette

Not all patients with a traumatic pericardial tamponade will demonstrate CXR findings and therefore it should not be used alone to rule out the injury. A CT scan may also be used to identify pericardial fluid but only on a stable patient.

HINT The heart may also have the appearance of a water-bottle shape on CXR.

Q Which diagnostic test is frequently used in the ED to screen for a pericardial tamponade?

A Ultrasonography

Ultrasonography is one of the most important tools for recognizing a tamponade. The classical pattern is a "swinging" heart. The heart oscillates within the pericardium side to side (this produces the pulsus alternans seen on the EKG). It may also detect pericardial fluid, thrombus, and collapsing of the ventricular wall during diastole.

HINT Focused assessment sonography for trauma (FAST) is used to assess the abdomen and may frequently be used to assess the chest for pericardial tamponade in a trauma patient.

▶ MEDICAL MANAGEMENT

> **Q** A patient is found to have a pericardial tamponade following a stab wound to the anterior chest. He is hypotensive. What would be the immediate medical management of this patient?
>
> **A** Oxygen, fluid bolus, inotropic agent

Remember the ABCs of trauma. Oxygen should be administered, and pulse oximetry should be monitored. The effects of hypovolemia are profound in a cardiac tamponade, and fluid bolus may be used to increase SV and perfusion. Volume overload may worsen the ventricular contractility and should be avoided. Passive elevation of the legs may also be used to increase venous return and improve ventricular filling. Positive inotropic drugs (i.e., dobutamine) may improve contractility without increasing SVR.

HINT Avoid positive pressure ventilation, if possible. If intubated and ventilated, minimize positive end-expiratory pressure (PEEP) levels due to the decrease in venous return.

▶ SURGICAL MANAGEMENT

> **Q** What is the definitive care for a pericardial tamponade?
>
> **A** Remove the blood/fluid from the pericardial space

This can be done with an emergency subxiphoid percutaneous aspiration in an unstable patient in the ED. Pericardiocentesis can also be performed using landmarks or guided by echocardiogram and by placing a drain tube. Pericardotomy may be performed using a balloon to create the pericardial window. Open thoracotomy is required in some cases.

HINT A minimally invasive technique commonly used is the video-assisted thorascopic (VAT) procedure.

> **Q** What is a life-threatening complication of a pericardiocentesis?
>
> **A** Rupture of the myocardium or coronary arteries

During the procedure, the myocardium can be accidentally punctured, resulting in a myocardial rupture. Other complications include arrhythmias, puncture of the lungs, liver, or stomach.

HINT Continuous EKG monitoring to detect ventricular arrhythmias is recommended.

 CARDIAC TRAUMA

▶ PATHOPHYSIOLOGY

> **Q** What is the new term for cardiac contusion?
>
> **A** Blunt cardiac injury

Cardiac contusion is hemorrhage within the myocardium, marked by cellular injury and extravasation of red blood cells (RBCs) into the muscle fibers. Contusion severity ranges from subepicardial to intramural hemorrhage into the intraventricular septum. The hemorrhage can extend up to varying depths into the myocardium. But due to the severity ranges of blunt cardiac trauma from silent, to arrhythmias to cardiac rupture, the new term is blunt cardiac injury (BCI).

HINT Commotio cordis is sudden death following BCI due to cardiac arrest with no known risk for cardiac disease.

> **Q Which mechanism of injury is the most common cause for BCI?**
>
> **A Motor vehicle crash (MVC)**

MVC is the most common cause of BCI (Box 2.23). The sternum, ribs, and spine are protective of the heart, but a significant force with direct impact to the chest can cause BCI.

HINT   Fracture of sternum and ribs 1 to 2 indicate significant enough force to cause BCI.

Box 2.23 Causes of Blunt Cardiac Injury

Motor vehicle crash
Falls
Blast injuries
Assaults
Sports injuries

> **Q Which ventricle is the most susceptible to injury following a blunt chest trauma?**
>
> **A RV**

The RV is the most vulnerable because of its location under the sternum being more anterior. The mitral and aortic valves are more likely to be injured than the tricuspid and pulmonic because of higher pressures in the LV, especially during diastole.

HINT   Deceleration mechanism can cause the heart to move in the thoracic cavity lacerating valves, and coronary arteries.

▶ SYMPTOMS/ASSESSMENT

> **Q What is the most common patient complaint of a BCI?**
>
> **A Chest pain or SOB**

The chest pain is precordial and is frequently unrelieved by analgesics. The symptoms and presentation vary following a myocardial contusion. Some patients may present without symptoms.

HINT   A bruise across the chest from a seatbelt should increase the suspicion level of the critical care nurse for a BCI.

> **Q What is the most common arrhythmia following a BCI?**
>
> **A Sinus tachycardia**

Following a trauma, most patients will present with sinus tachycardia, which is a sympathetic nervous system response. The most lethal arrhythmias of a myocardial contusion are VT and VF. Other arrhythmias include AF, heart blocks, right bundle branch block, and right bundle branch block with hemiblock. The severity of the arrhythmia does not correlate with the severity of the contusion (Box 2.24).

HINT   Tachycardia beyond expectation for hypovolemia based upon calculated blood loss is a high suspicion for BCI.

Box 2.24 Other Symptoms of BCI

Bruising on chest wall	Pericardial friction rub/murmurs
Crackles	Presence of associated injuries
S_3 gallop	Hypotension

BCI, blunt cardiac injury.

Q When does a patient require cardiac monitoring?

A Abnormal findings

Monitoring is not required if the echocardiogram, EKG, and troponin levels are normal in a hemodynamically stable patient. It has been reported for patients to develop arrhythmias after 24 hours, even with an initial normal EKG and troponin. This is a delayed presentation of BCI.

HINT   If EKG or troponin levels are abnormal, an echocardiogram is recommended.

▶ DIAGNOSIS

Q Which of the cardiac markers is most specific to injury caused by BCI?

A Troponin levels

CPK-MB levels will elevate following skeletal muscle trauma and myocardial injury and are nonspecific for myocardium. Troponin levels are more specific to myocardial injury.

HINT   Also important to determine the patients risk factors for experiencing an MI before BCI is diagnosed.

Q An echocardiogram is used to identify which specific change found in a BCI?

A Abnormal wall motion

Transthoracic and esophageal echocardiograms can be used to identify abnormalities in cardiac function that can be used in diagnosing myocardial contusions. It is also used to identify patients requiring cardiac monitoring and the presence of complications, such as pericardial effusion. The abnormal wall motion results in a decrease in SV, CO, and BP.

HINT   Chest CT or MRI is not as useful in evaluating the patient for BCI as an echocardiogram.

▶ MANAGEMENT

Q Within what time period following a BCI would arrhythmias most commonly occur?

A Within 24 to 48 hours

A patient sustaining a blunt chest trauma with a high suspicion or abnormal cardiac findings should have cardiac monitoring for 24 to 48 hours. Other management issues include hemodynamic stabilization and treatment of associated injuries.

HINT   BCI can cause ventricular arrhythmias or transient bundle branch blocks (BBBs).

▶ COMPLICATIONS

Q Following a blunt chest trauma, a patient develops a new-onset systolic murmur. Which valve abnormality is most likely the cause?

A Mitral regurgitation

The two most common valves to be damaged following a blunt chest injury are the mitral and aortic valves. A rupture (regurgitation) of the mitral valve results in a systolic murmur, whereas a rupture of the aortic valve would cause a diastolic murmur (Box 2.25).

HINT   Valve regurgitation causes a murmur to be heard during the cardiac cycle when the valve should be closed. The mitral valve should be closed during systole (systolic murmur) and the aortic valve must close during diastole (diastolic murmur).

Box 2.25 Complications of BCIs

Arrhythmias	Cardiac rupture
LV dysfunction with CHF	Ventricular thrombosis
Acute valvular regurgitation (valve rupture) Ventricular aneurysm	Chronic constrictive pericarditis
Pericardial effusion (with or without tamponade)	Coronary vasospasm, thrombosis, or rupture
Intracardiac structural damage	Atrial fistula

BCI, blunt cardiac injury; CHF, congestive heart failure; LV, left ventricle.

TRAUMATIC AORTIC ANEURYSM

Q What is a common cause of death at the scene of a high-speed MVC?

A Traumatic aortic transection

Traumatic aortic transection is a common cause of death at the scene due to a high-speed sudden deceleration mechanism. The aorta is completely transected (intimal, medial, and adventitia layers).

HINT If the patient survives to the ED, he or she will usually have a small tear or a partial-thickness tear of the aorta forming an aneurysm.

▶ PATHOPHYSIOLOGY

Q A traumatic aortic aneurysm is most likely to be caused by what mechanism of injury?

A Sudden deceleration

A sudden deceleration may be either horizontal (i.e., high-speed motor vehicle crash [MVC]) or vertical (i.e., fall). The aorta is relatively mobile in the chest and will continue to travel after the sudden deceleration except where it is secured by a ligament.

HINT The scenario given will usually be a high-speed MVC with a sudden deceleration on impact.

Q What is the most common site of the aorta for a traumatic aortic aneurysm?

A Level of the isthmus

The level of the isthmus is distal to the great vessels, where the aorta begins to descend. The ligamentum arteriosum secures the proximal descending thoracic aorta, just distal to the arch (called the "level of the isthmus"). During the sudden deceleration, this ligament holds the aorta back while the arch of the aorta continues to travel. This causes the aorta to transect at the level of the isthmus.

HINT Other sites of fixation include the ascending aorta, the aortic root, and the diaphragmatic hiatus are less likely to cause a transection.

▶ SYMPTOMS/ASSESSMENT

Q What is the classic diagnostic sign of a traumatic aortic aneurysm?

A Widened mediastinum on CXR

Patients may be relatively asymptomatic for a traumatic aortic aneurysm. The CXR is used as a screening device. The patient may also present as hemodynamically unstable if there is bleeding into the thoracic cavity or in the presence of associated injuries. The patient may present with a cyclic pattern of responding to a fluid bolus, then becoming hypotensive again (Box 2.26).

Box 2.26 Other Symptoms of Aortic Aneurysm

Retrosternal or intracapsular chest pain	Swelling at base of neck
Hoarseness (tracheal compression)	Paraplegia
Dysphagia (esophageal compression)	Pseudocoarctation syndrome
Systolic murmur over base of neck	

HINT   Hemodynamic stability needs to be determined to guide management of these patients.

> **Q** What are the signs of pseudocoarctation syndrome?
>
> **A** Hypertension in upper extremities and hypotension in lower extremities

The patient may present with bounding pulses in the upper extremities and hypertension. The pulses are diminished in the lower extremities and hypotensive. This is due to the formation of a hematoma, narrowing the lumen of the aorta. The narrowing creates a high pressure above and low pressure below the site. This can occur following a traumatic transection but is not common.

HINT   The question may also have the nurse check BP in both arms, assessing for a significant difference in BP between the two to identify signs of aortic dissection.

> **Q** A chest tube is placed for left-sided hemothorax in a trauma patient. What finding following chest tube placement is a sign of an aortic injury?
>
> **A** Large volume of bright-red blood from the chest tube

A rupture of the aorta frequently results in bleeding into the left pleural space and a resulting hemothorax. The sign is a large-volume hemorrhage from the chest tube, typically bright-red blood.

▶ DIAGNOSIS

> **Q** What are three findings on a CXR that would lead to suspicion of a thoracic aortic aneurysm?
>
> **A** Widened mediastinum, loss of aortic knob, or left apical cap

A widened mediastinum is the most classic sign found on a CXR. The loss of the aortic knob (also called superior widened mediastinum) and an apical cap may also be commonly seen in a thoracic aortic aneurysm.

HINT   Other CXR signs include a deviated nasogastric (NG) tube to the right, an obvious double lumen contour of the aorta, or depression of the left-stem bronchus.

> **Q** Which radiographic procedure has the most definitive diagnosis for a thoracic aortic aneurysm?
>
> **A** Arteriogram

The CXR is used as a screening device and is used in combination with the mechanism of injury to warrant further workup for a traumatic aneurysm. A multidetector helical CT scan is the best diagnostic tool. The angiogram has been the gold standard for diagnosing an aortic injury but is being replaced with a CT scan. If the CT scan findings are equivocal or do not visualize branch vessels or surrounding structures, an angiogram is used as a follow-up prior to surgery.

HINT   If the test question asks what the gold standard is for diagnosing thoracic aneurysm, "angiogram" is the answer.

▶ MEDICAL MANAGEMENT

> **Q** Where should the systolic blood pressure (SBP) be maintained in a patient with thoracic aortic aneurysm?
>
> **A** Between 90 and 120 mmHg

Allowing an increase in SBP above 120 mmHg will increase the risk of free rupture of the aneurysm. Lowering the SBP below 90 mmHg will cause hypoperfusion and may contribute to organ dysfunction. Short-acting antihypertensives may be used in the acute period to maintain BP within the acceptable range.

HINT Avoid aggressive fluid resuscitation even in hemodynamically unstable patients due to risk of rupture.

▶ SURGICAL MANAGEMENT

Q What is the definitive management of an aortic aneurysm?

A Graft replacement of the aorta

Open thoracotomy is the most commonly used route to repair an aortic injury from a trauma. The endovascular route has also been used. Surgery may involve placing the patient on CPB or partial left heart bypass to maintain perfusion distal to the area of injury (Box 2.27).

Box 2.27 Indications for Surgical Management

Hemodynamically unstable
Large-volume hemorrhage from chest tubes
Contrast extravasation on CT scan or rapidly expanding mediastinal hematoma
Penetrating aortic injury

● CARDIOMYOPATHIES

Q Which of the cardiomyopathies have a high incidence of SCD due to lethal arrhythmias?

A Hypertrophic cardiomyopathy

The hypertrophied LV wall places the patient at risk for increased myocardial oxygen consumption and fatal arrhythmias. The thickening of the ventricular wall is called remodeling. Remodeling causes an increase in ventricular arrhythmias and SCD.

HINT A hypertrophic cardiomyopathy may be an indication for the placement of automatic internal cardiac defibrillator (AICD).

Q What are the two classifications of hypertrophic cardiomyopathy?

A Obstructive and nonobstructive

The obstructive hypertrophic cardiomyopathy has an obstruction to outflow from the LV in combination with ventricular hypertrophy. The obstruction to outflow is due to the enlarged septal wall causing the mitral valve to interfere with outflow during mid-systole through the aortic valve.

HINT A midsystolic ejection murmur may be auscultated.

Q Your patient has a history of chronic alcoholism. Which type of cardiomyopathy would you suspect due to his history?

A Dilated cardiomyopathy

Dilated cardiomyopathy is the most common nonischemic cardiomyopathy. An etiology of dilated cardiomyopathy is chronic alcoholism (Box 2.28).

HINT Dilated cardiomyopathy is classified as a systolic dysfunction

Box 2.28 Causes of Dilated Cardiomyopathy

Peripartum	Volume overload
Viral infection	Chemotherapeutic agents
Alcohol-induced	Idiopathic/genetic
Cocaine-induced	
Ischemia/infarction (previous myocardial infarction)	

Q Which cardiomyopathy demonstrates a reduced diastolic volume but near-normal wall thickness?

A Restrictive cardiomyopathy

A restrictive cardiomyopathy is characterized by restrictive filling and reduced diastolic volume of either or both ventricles with normal to near-normal systolic function and wall thickness. A restrictive cardiomyopathy needs to be differentiated from a constrictive cardiomyopathy, which may be curable with surgical intervention. A restrictive cardiomyopathy is the least common form of cardiomyopathy.

HINT   A constrictive cardiomyopathy is caused by constriction around the heart (e.g., pericardial tamponade), whereas a restrictive cardiomyopathy is caused by stiffness of the ventricles.

Q What causes the ventricles to become noncompliant or stiff in a restrictive cardiomyopathy?

A Interstitial fibrosis or amyloid deposits

A restrictive cardiomyopathy is characterized by intracellular accumulation of amyloid material sufficient to impair myocardial function. Deposits of protein fibrils throughout the myocardium create a rubbery consistency of the ventricular wall. Amyloid deposits are the most common cause (Box 2.29).

HINT   On autopsy, in a restricted cardiomyopathy, the heart does not collapse when removed from the chest cavity.

Box 2.29 Causes of Restrictive Cardiomyopathy

Idiopathic	
■ Heart muscle disease ■ Amyloidosis ■ Hemochromatosis ■ Malignancy	Eosinophilic fibrosis Postirradiation fibrosis

▶ PATHOPHYSIOLOGY

Q In an obstructive hypertrophic cardiomyopathy, what causes the obstruction to outflow tract from the LV?

A Leaflet of the mitral valve

During systole, there is an anterior motion of the mitral valve toward the hypertrophied septal wall. This abnormal motion of the mitral valve results in further narrowing of the outflow tract of the aortic valve. The outflow tract may already be narrowed from the hypertrophied septal wall.

HINT   A common cause of hypertrophied cardiomyopathy is congenital.

Q Which cardiomyopathy is associated with a high EF?

A Hypertrophic cardiomyopathy

Hypertrophic cardiomyopathy is characterized by increased contractility due to increased ventricular muscle mass. This increase in contractility results in near emptying of the LV at the end of systole. On echocardiogram, it is sometimes called a "kissing ventricle."

HINT Hypertrophic cardiomyopathy is the only cardiomyopathy with a high EF, whereas the others have a low EF.

> **Q** Is hypertrophied cardiomyopathy a diastolic or systolic dysfunction?
>
> **A** Diastolic dysfunction

The LV chamber is small, decreasing the preload capability, and limiting the filling of the ventricle during diastole. The hypertrophic LV has increased contractility without significant systolic dysfunction.

HINT This is called HFrEF.

> **Q** What effect does a dilated cardiomyopathy have on the CO?
>
> **A** Decreases the CO

Dilated cardiomyopathy has a decrease in CO and an increase in pulmonary pressures caused by abnormal contractility, volume overload, and HF. It is characterized by an increase in end-diastolic and end-systolic volumes with a low EF.

HINT Dilated cardiomyopathies are classified as a systolic dysfunction in HF or HFrEF.

> **Q** Progressive dilation of the LV can lead to which valve abnormalities?
>
> **A** Mitral or aortic regurgitation

The dilation of the LV stretches the leaflets of the valve, resulting in loss of integrity of the aortic and mitral valves. The regurgitation across these valves contributes to volume overload and further dilation of the ventricle (Table 2.9).

HINT Aortic regurgitation produces diastolic murmur and mitral regurgitation a systolic murmur.

Table 2.9 Comparison of LV Dysfunction Cardiomyopathies

Type of Dysfunction	Hypertrophy Cardiomyopathy	Dilated Cardiomyopathy	Restricted Cardiomyopathy
Systolic dysfunction		X	
Diastolic dysfunction	X		X

LV, left ventricle.

▶ SYMPTOMS/ASSESSMENT

> **Q** What is the most common presenting symptom of a hypertrophied cardiomyopathy?
>
> **A** Dyspnea

Dyspnea is caused by elevated diastolic pressures (impaired diastolic compliance) and may occur in about 90% of people with hypertrophied cardiomyopathy.

HINT SCD may be the first presentation of a person with hypertrophied cardiomyopathy.

> **Q** What is the most common cause of SCD in hypertrophied cardiomyopathies?
>
> **A** VF

VF accounts for about 80% of SCDs of hypertrophied cardiomyopathies. Atrial arrhythmias (i.e., AF, paroxysmal supraventricular tachycardia, Wolff–Parkinson–White [WPW] syndrome) may degenerate to VF as well.

> **Q** Which cardiomyopathy frequently produces an S4 gallop?
>
> **A** Hypertrophy cardiomyopathy

An S_4 is produced during atrial contraction against a noncompliant hypertrophied ventricle. A dilated cardiomyopathy is more likely to produce an S_3 due to volume overload. Atrial contraction against a noncompliant ventricle can also produce a double apical impulse and a double carotid arterial pulse.

HINT   Remember, an S_3 occurs during passive filling of the ventricle and an S_4 occurs during the atrial kick. An S_3 is commonly caused by volume overload and an S_4 occurs with ventricle noncompliance.

> **Q** What is a common 12-lead EKG finding in hypertrophied cardiomyopathy?
>
> **A** Left-axis deviation

The left-axis deviation is caused by the thicker LV wall mass. Other EKG changes include ST–T-wave changes, prolonged PR interval, sinus bradycardia, and atrial enlargement.

HINT   An LBBB with a right-axis deviation is suggestive of a dilated cardiomyopathy.

> **Q** What is the most common arrhythmia associated with a restrictive cardiomyopathy?
>
> **A** Complete heart block and AF

The amyloid and fibrous deposits within the SA and AV node can result in a complete heart block. Amyloid deposits within the bundle branches are rare. Ventricular arrhythmias are not as common as atrial arrhythmias (Table 2.10).

Table 2.10 Comparative Chart: Symptoms of Cardiomyopathies

	Hypertrophic Cardiomyopathy	Dilated Cardiomyopathy	Restrictive Cardiomyopathy
Clinical Findings	Sudden cardiac death	Atrial fibrillation	Fatigue
	Dyspnea	Dyspnea	Shortness of breath
	Presyncope/syncope	Chest pain	Peripheral edema (pitting)
	Fatigue	Syncope (due to arrhythmia)	Abdominal ascites
	Angina Palpitations Orthopnea and paroxysmal nocturnal dyspnea Congestive heart failure Dizziness	JVD Tachycardia (loss of parasympathetic control)	Chest pain Syncope (due to low CO syndrome) Pleural effusions Hepatomegaly (splenomegaly rare)
Heart Sounds	Split S_2	S_3 gallop	Loud S_3
	S_3 and S_4 gallop		Rare S_4
	Systolic murmur (mitral regurgitation)		Systolic murmur (mitral and tricuspid regurgitation)
	Diastolic decrescendo murmur (aortic regurgitation)		

CO, cardiac output; JVD, jugular venous distension.

HINT   SCD with restrictive cardiomyopathy is usually caused by PEA.

> **Q** What abnormal lab value is a predictor of poor outcomes in dilated cardiomyopathy?
>
> **A** Hyponatremia

Hyponatremia parallels severity of HF. It is due to release of antidiuretic hormone (ADH) and volume overload (dilutional hyponatremia).

HINT The degree of hyponatremia is related to the severity of HF caused by cardiomyopathy.

▶ DIAGNOSIS

Q Which lab value is found elevated in a dilated cardiomyopathy?

A BNP

BNP levels are increased in dilated cardiomyopathy due to the overstretched ventricle. Restrictive cardiomyopathy will also significantly elevate BNP levels.

HINT BNP levels will be normal in constrictive cardiomyopathy but grossly elevated in a restrictive cardiomyopathy.

Q In a restrictive cardiomyopathy, how would the atria appear on an echocardiogram?

A Dilated bilateral atrium

The ventricles are noncompliant and restrictive to filling, so blood backs up in the atrium, causing dilation of both the right and left atria. The echocardiogram would also show bilateral ventricular thickening with restrictive filling patterns, normal systolic function and EF (until later in the disease), and abnormal myocardial texture (amyloid deposits).

Q What is the confirmation diagnosis of a restrictive cardiomyopathy due to amyloid deposits?

A Cardiac biopsy

A cardiac biopsy is used to confirm the diagnosis. A fine-needle aspiration of abdominal fat may also be used and is easier and safer for the diagnosis of amyloidosis.

HINT A liver biopsy may be performed to diagnosis hemochromatosis (another cause of restrictive cardiomyopathy).

▶ MEDICAL MANAGEMENT

Q Which antiarrhythmic agent has been found to lower the incidence of arrhythmogenic SCD in hypertrophied cardiomyopathy?

A Amiodarone (Cordarone)

Amiodarone is the only agent proven to reduce the incidence and risk of SCD, with or without obstruction to LV outflow. It is very effective at converting AF and flutter to sinus rhythm and at suppressing the recurrence of these arrhythmias. Disopyramide (Norpace) may be used to raise the atrial and ventricular arrhythmia threshold but is not recommended without concomitant beta-blockade.

HINT Monitoring of QTc interval is recommended with the administration of Norpace.

Q Is the goal in managing hypertrophic cardiomyopathy to increase or decrease the inotropic state of the LV?

A Decrease the inotropic state

Hypertrophied cardiomyopathy is a diastolic dysfunction with a small LV chamber. An increase in the inotropic state of the LV will further limit the size of the LV chamber and filling capabilities. Agents that decrease the inotropic state of the LV and result in relaxation of the LV chamber are indicated to improve ventricular filling. First-line agents include beta blockers and calcium channel blockers.

HINT Beta blockers have also been shown to reduce the gradient across the LV outflow tract.

> **Q Which type of calcium channel blocker would be contraindicated in managing hypertrophied cardiomyopathy?**
>
> **A Dihydropyridine calcium channel blockers**

An example of a dihydropyridine calcium channel blocker is nifedipine (Procardia). Cardiac glycosides (Digoxin) and other positive inotropic agents should also be avoided in patients with hypertrophic cardiomyopathy. The positive inotropic effect will increase the contractility and make the LV chamber size even smaller. This will worsen the filling capability of the ventricles, thus worsening CO and HF.

HINT   Verapamil (Calan) is an L-type calcium channel blocker and is indicated if beta-blockade is not effective.

> **Q What is the indication for anticoagulation therapy in dilated cardiomyopathy?**
>
> **A Severe LV dysfunction or at risk of AF**

Dilated cardiomyopathy presents as LV systolic dysfunction. As the LV dysfunction becomes severe with a low EF, a thrombus can form in the LV. Anticoagulation therapy is recommended to prevent a cardioembolic stroke or pulmonary embolism (from the RV). Dilated cardiomyopathy patients are at risk for the development of AF and should also be anticoagulated (Box 2.30).

Box 2.30 Pharmacological Management of Cardiomyopathies

Hypertrophic Cardiomyopathy	Dilated Cardiomyopathy	Restricted Cardiomyopathy
Amiodarone (Cordarone)	ACE inhibitor	Diuretics
Beta blocker	Beat blocker	Nitrates
Ca+ channel blocker (L-type only)	Angiotensin receptor blocker	Anticoagulation therapy (AF)
Anticoagulation therapy (AF)	Cardiac glycosides	Antiplasma cell therapy
	Diuretics	Corticosteroids
	Antiarrhythmic	Interferon
	Vasodilator	
	Aldosterone antagonist	
	Inotropic agents	
	Anticoagulation therapy (AF)	
	Nesiritide (Natrecor)	

ACE, angiotensin-converting enzyme; AF, atrial fibrillation.

▶ SURGICAL MANAGEMENT

> **Q What is the surgical option for a restrictive cardiomyopathy?**
>
> **A Cardiac transplant**

A cardiac transplant may be considered if symptoms are refractory to treatment in idiopathic, familial, and amyloidosis cases of restrictive cardiomyopathy.

> **Q What is the surgical option for an obstructive hypertrophic cardiomyopathy?**
>
> **A LV myomectomy**

An LV myomectomy is a procedure to remove the septal muscle, thus managing the obstruction to outflow in a hypertrophic cardiomyopathy. LV myomectomy is indicated for patients with severe symptoms refractory to therapy and outflow gradient greater than 50 mmHg. It is usually successful in abolishing the outflow gradient and can provide symptomatic relief for at least 5 years. The gradient outflow may increase gradually over time and return to the same level as before, requiring a repeat procedure. Other options to manage the outflow obstruction include mitral valve replacement, transcatheter septal alcohol ablation, and a dual-chamber pacemaker.

HINT A patient with hypertrophic cardiomyopathy will have an implanted cardioverter-defibrillator (ICD) to prevent SCD.

▶ COMPLICATIONS

Q What is the primary complication of all of cardiomyopathies?

A HF

Whether the cardiomyopathy is hypertrophied, dilated, restrictive, or constrictive, HF is the common complication. AF can also complicate all types of cardiomyopathies (Box 2.31).

Box 2.31 Other Complications of Cardiomyopathies

Hypertrophic Cardiomyopathy	Dilated Cardiomyopathy	Restrictive Cardiomyopathy
SCD (due to arrhythmias)	Hypertrophy (remodeling)	MI
	Mitral and tricuspid regurgitation	Low output syndrome
	Pulmonary embolism	

MI, myocardial infarction; SCD, sudden cardiac death.

● HYPERTENSIVE CRISIS

Q What BP is considered to be a hypertensive crisis?

A Systolic greater than 180 mmHg and diastolic greater than 110 mmHg

Hypertensive crisis is acute, severe hypertension typically defined as an SBP greater than 180/110 mmHg but this can vary based upon the individual. About 1% to 3% of people with hypertension will experience a hypertensive crisis.

Q What makes the hypertensive crisis a "hypertensive emergency" instead of "hypertensive urgency"?

A Evidence of acute damage of organs

Acute hypertension can cause acute end-organ damage. When there is evidence of acute or ongoing injury to target organs, rapid reduction of BP is recommended. Hypertensive urgency, without evidence of organ involvement, can be treated less aggressively. It is not defined by the absolute BP but by the presentation (Box 2.32).

HINT The risk of a hypertensive emergency may not be the absolute BP but how rapidly the BP increases.

Box 2.32 Clinical Presentation of Organ Damage for Hypertensive Emergencies

Hypertensive intracranial hemorrhage	Aortic dissection
Hypertensive encephalopathy	Acute kidney injury
Angina/myocardial ischemia	Eclampsia/pre-eclampsia
Left ventricular failure with pulmonary edema	Retinal hemorrhage

▶ PATHOPHYSIOLOGY

Q **What is the most common cause of a hypertensive emergency?**

A **Preexisting hypertension**

The most common history following a hypertensive emergency is noncompliance with antihypertensive medications or uncontrolled hypertension (Box 2.33).

HINT   The test question may focus on a complete medication history assessment by the nurse on admission.

Box 2.33 Common Causes Hypertensive Crisis

Chronic hypertension
Sympathomimetic drugs
Stimulant diet supplements
Pheochromocytoma
Pregnancy-induced

Q **Which hemodynamic change initiates hypertensive crisis?**

A **Increase in SVR**

An abrupt increase in SVR initiates a hypertensive crisis. There is a loss of autoregulation causing greater sympathetic nervous system involvement. The vasoconstriction may be a result of release of vasoactive substances from the endothelium.

HINT   Remember that the diastolic pressure is the resistance the heart is pumping against (afterload).

▶ SYMPTOMS/ASSESSMENT

Q **What is a common presentation of hypertensive emergency?**

A **Chest pain, dyspnea, and neurological deficits**

The three most common presentations of hypertensive emergencies include chest pain, dyspnea, and neurological deficits. Other symptoms may include fatigue, nasal congestion, or a new-onset cough. The cardiac evaluation includes signs of ACS. If the presentation is consistent with aortic dissection, immediate evaluation is required.

Q **What is the usual presentation of hypertensive encephalopathy or posterior reversible encephalopathy syndrome (PRES)?**

A **Headache and altered level of consciousness**

A syndrome presents with headache, altered mental status, visual changes, and seizures due to hypertensive crisis. A focused neurological examination is required to assess for any focal neurological changes including visual changes. Ocular/fundal examination finding of advanced retinopathy, hemorrhages, or papilledema assists with the recognition of hypertensive encephalopathy.

HINT   If present, it indicates potential hemorrhagic stroke. A sudden onset, "worst headache of my life" presentation may indicate an aneurysm rupture and subarachnoid hemorrhage.

▶ DIAGNOSIS

Q **What type of hemodynamic monitoring is recommended during the management of hypertension?**

A **Arterial BP monitoring**

Arterial BP monitoring allows for continuous monitoring of BP during the management of hypertensive emergencies. It is recommended when titrating infusions for targeted BP.

▶ MANAGEMENT

Q **What is the percentage of decrease of mean arterial pressure (MAP) typically used as a goal in managing hypertensive emergencies?**

A **25% decrease in MAP**

Multiple organizations have developed guidelines for the management of hypertension. The typical recommendation is to decrease MAP by 25% within 2 to 6 hours or to decrease diastolic pressure by 10% to 15% or below 110 mmHg within 30 to 60 minutes.

HINT After the first hour, a more gradual decrease is recommended.

Q **What is a commonly used goal for systolic pressure in a hypertensive emergency?**

A **Less than 160 mmHg**

The goal in a hypertensive patient should be to control the lowering of BP but should not be to "normalize" the BP. Chronic hypertension resets the autoregulation range for organ perfusion. A normal BP can cause hypoperfusion to vital organs (i.e., brain, heart, kidneys) in a chronic hypertensive patient.

HINT Continue to monitor for signs of organ hypoperfusion while managing the BP.

Q **What is the mechanism of action of Labetalol?**

A **Nonselective beta blocker and alpha$_1$ blocker**

Labetalol is frequently used in hypertensive emergencies and can be administered as a bolus or continuous IV infusion. It is a nonselective beta blocker (blocks both beta$_1$ and beta$_2$ receptors) as well as a selective alpha$_1$ blocker. It is not a pure beta-adrenergic blocker, so does not decrease CO like other beta blockers. Potential adverse effects are AV nodal dysfunction (heart block) and bronchospasm.

HINT If the hypertensive scenario presents a patient with a significant history of asthma, avoid labetalol (or any beta blockers) as the answer for the appropriate antihypertensive therapy due to bronchodilation.

Q **Which antihypertensive, administered as a continuous infusion, has a rapid onset of 1 minute and a potential side effect of bradycardia?**

A **Esmolol**

Esmolol is a cardioselective beta blocker. It has a very rapid onset of 1 minute with duration of 10 to 20 minutes (ultra-short acting). It is administered as a continuous infusion, titrated to a goal BP. It is a beta blocker, thus it decreases rate and contractility of the heart. It is frequently used in acute aortic dissection patients as an antihypertensive agent. It is contraindicated in patients with decompensated HF and bradycardia.

HINT Esmolol would be a good answer for a hypertensive patient with acute pulmonary edema and underlying diastolic dysfunction.

Q **How is esmolol metabolized?**

A **Hydrolysis**

Esmolol is metabolized by hydrolysis of ester linkages by RBC esterases. This agent may be administered to patients with hepatic dysfunction and kidney failure. This accounts for esmolol's rapid metabolism and ultra-short half-life.

HINT Esmolol is a good answer for antihypertensive agent in hepatic or renal failure patients.

Q Which antihypertensive has a vasodilatory effect in both coronary and cerebral vasculature?

A Nicardipine

Nicardipine is a dihydropyridine-derivative calcium channel blocker. It produces antihypertensive effects by blocking the influx of calcium, thus resulting in relaxation of smooth muscle in the vasculature. It also a coronary and cerebral vasodilator and has been shown to increase coronary and cerebral blood flow. Nicardipine is used as a continuous infusion with onset of 5 to 15 minutes, half-life of 1 hour, and duration of action of 4 to 6 hours.

HINT   Nicardipine is frequently used as an antihypertensive agent in a hemorrhagic stroke or in patients with CAD.

Q What is the advantage of using fenoldopam in hypertensive emergencies?

A Produces natriuresis

Fenoldopam (Corlopam) is an IV antihypertensive used to manage hypertensive emergencies. It is a dopamine-1-receptor agonist producing vasodilation by acting on dopamine type 1 receptors in the peripheral. It also activates dopaminergic receptors in the renal tubules, resulting in sodium excretion (natriuresis). This agent improves creatinine clearance, urine output, and sodium excretion in patients with and without normal renal function. The onset is within 5 minutes and has duration of 30 to 60 minutes.

HINT   Fenoldopam is a good answer as an antihypertensive agent in patients with acute renal failure.

Q What is the greatest risk of using fenoldopam in hypertensive emergencies?

A Hypersensitivity reactions

Fenoldopam solution contains sodium metabisufate. Patients with sulfite allergies may have an allergic reaction to fenoldopam. It is metabolized rapidly and extensively in the liver.

HINT   Look at the scenario. If the patient has an allergy to sulfite, avoid fenoldopam as an appropriate antihypertensive agent.

Q Which drug may be used as an adjunctive agent in a hypertensive patient with MI?

A Nitroglycerin

Nitroglycerin, at high doses, is an arterial dilator. It is both a venodilator and an arterial dilator. It is not considered a first-line drug for a hypertensive emergency, but it can be used as an adjunctive agent in a myocardial ischemic patient experiencing a hypertensive emergency.

HINT   Remember that the mechanism of nitroglycerin is dose-dependent. Lower doses affect preload and higher doses affect afterload.

Q What is the toxin that can accumulate with Nipride at higher doses?

A Cyanide

Sodium nitroprusside (Nipride) can lead to cyanide poisoning. The potential amount of cyanide accumulation depends on the dose and duration of the Nipride infusion. Typically, infusions more than 4 mcg/kg/min for 2 to 3 hours have led to toxic levels of cyanide. If higher infusions of Nipride are required, thiosulfate may be administered to prevent accumulation of cyanide.

HINT   Nipride can also cause a "steal" phenomenon in the lungs and heart.

Q Does Nipride affect preload, afterload, or both?

A Both preload and afterload

Sodium nitroprusside (Nipride) dilates both the arterial and venous circulation, thus producing an effect on both preload and afterload. It has a rapid onset of 1 to 2 minutes and a half-life of 3 to 4 minutes. Due to the quick onset and short duration, Nipride is easily titrated. It should be avoided in patients with renal and hepatic failure due to dependence on these organs for metabolism. Nipride can cause a reduction in coronary blood flow to areas of ischemia (steal phenomenon), an increase in intracranial pressure (ICP), and may worsen hypoxia in acute respiratory failure.

HINT Avoid Nipride as an answer in patients with ACS, acute respiratory failure, and in neurological patients with increased ICP.

> **Q** Which of the IV dihydropyridine calcium channel blockers has the shortest half-life?
>
> **A** Clevidipine (Cleviprex)

Clevidipine's half-life is 1 to 2 minutes with rapid onset within 2 to 4 minutes and a duration of 5 to 15 minutes. Nicardipine, in comparison, has a half-life of 1 hour and a duration of 4 to 6 hours. They are both administered as a continuous infusion and are titrated to target BP. Clevidipine is more titratable due to its shorter half-life. It is metabolized by esterases in the blood and accounts for the ultra-short half-life of the drug. Clearance of the drug should not be affected by renal or hepatic impairment but requires more research.

HINT When titrating a drug for a targeted BP, clevidipine may be used as the answer over nicardipine, due to the shorter half-life.

> **Q** Clevidipine is contraindicated in patients with what allergies?
>
> **A** Allergies to soy products and egg or egg products

Clevidipine is a milky, white emulsion that is high in lipids. It is contraindicated in patients who are allergic to soy products, eggs, or egg products. The lipid solutions provide 2 kcal/mL of clevidipine, so it needs to be counted in caloric intake.

> **Q** What antihypertensives should be avoided in hypertensive emergencies?
>
> **A** Nifedipine and hydralazine

Nifedipine used by oral or sublingual route can cause a sudden, uncontrolled, and severe drop in BP and should not be administered for hypertensive emergencies. Hydralazine is a direct-acting vasodilator. It has a half-life of 3 hours and a half-life of approximately 10 hours. Hydralazine should be avoided because of its prolonged, unpredictable effects and difficulty in titration to target BP.

▶ COMPLICATIONS

> **Q** What is a potential complication of antihypertensive therapy?
>
> **A** Hypotension and hypoperfusion of organs

The targeted BP is 160/110 to prevent hypoperfusion to vital organs due to the resetting of autoregulation in chronic hypertensive patients. A shorter-acting antihypertensive is recommended to prevent long periods of hypotension and is more titratable to targeted BPs.

⬤ STRUCTURAL HEART DEFECTS

> **Q** Would a rapid onset of symptoms with valvular structural defect be a stenosis or regurgitation?
>
> **A** Regurgitation

The stenosis of a valve occurs over time and is a more gradual process. Regurgitation can present with a sudden onset of symptoms of HF. In acute regurgitation, the heart has not compensated for the added volume in the ventricles or atria, so atrial and ventricular pressures can rise drastically in a short period of time. This results in HF.

HINT   If the scenario provides a "sudden onset" of HF, look for valvular abnormality of regurgitation. The most common is acute mitral regurgitation.

▶ PATHOPHYSIOLOGY

> **Q What is the most common cause of aortic stenosis?**
>
> **A Calcification of the aortic valve**

The most common cause of an aortic valve stenosis in adults is calcification of the valve, eventually causing reduction in leaflet motion.

HINT   Mitral valve abnormalities (both stenosis and regurgitation) are most commonly associated with rheumatic disease.

> **Q Which cardiomyopathy can be caused by an aortic stenosis?**
>
> **A Hypertrophied cardiomyopathy**

Over time, the LV has been contracting against greater resistance as the aortic valve area decreases and there is a reduction in leaflet motion. The heart compensates by increasing the wall thickness.

HINT   This is like a body builder. The more weight you lift, the more muscle development.

> **Q What are the complications that a patient with acute aortic regurgitation can typically develop?**
>
> **A Pulmonary edema and cardiogenic shock**

There is a sudden large increase in blood volume in the LV due to the incompetence of the aortic valve. This results in a rapid increase in LV pressure with blood backing up into the LA. The elevated LA pressures cause congestion in pulmonary arteries. The LV is unable to compensate with the rapid volume overload and will decrease the CO. So, a patient with acute aortic regurgitation typically presents with either pulmonary edema or cardiogenic shock.

HINT   A dissection of the ascending thoracic aorta can damage the aortic valve, causing sudden onset of pulmonary edema.

> **Q What is the compensatory mechanism of the LV during chronic aortic regurgitation?**
>
> **A Dilated followed by hypertrophy of LV**

The initial response of the ventricles is to dilate to hold the increase in end-diastolic volume following the onset of aortic regurgitation. The LV then begins to hypertrophy to maintain the high EF (due to the large volume or preload). There is an increase in systolic wall stress causing an increase in afterload, thus causing further hypertrophy. Initially, the EF is maintained. Eventually, the hypertrophic response may become inadequate and the preload reserve fails, resulting in a low EF and signs of dyspnea.

HINT   Chronic aortic regurgitation occurs over time so the heart compensates and patients may remain asymptomatic for a time period.

> **Q What is the most common cause of mitral stenosis?**
>
> **A Rheumatic carditis**

Rheumatic heart disease and a history of rheumatic fever may be found in 40% to 60% of the patients diagnosed with mitral stenosis. Rheumatic disease causes thickening and calcification of the mitral valve leaflets, resulting in a funnel-shaped mitral apparatus that narrows the orifice.

HINT   This results in mitral stenosis but can have a combination of stenosis and regurgitation.

> **Q Does mitral valve prolapse (MVP) always result in mitral regurgitation?**
>
> **A No**

MVP is the billowing of one or both the mitral valve leaflets back up in the LA. It may or may not be associated with mitral regurgitation. An echocardiogram is used to identify the MVP and determine the presence of mitral regurgitation (Box 2.34).

HINT The tricuspid valve may also have prolapse in 40% of patients with MVP.

Box 2.34 Causes of Mitral Valve Abnormalities

Rheumatic heart disease
Coronary artery disease
Infective endocarditis
Ruptured chordae tendineae or papillary muscle

Q What is the most common arrhythmia induced by mitral regurgitation?

A AF

During mitral regurgitation, blood is pushed back up into the LA during systole. This causes LA overload and LA dilation. The dilating of the LA triggers the onset of AF.

HINT Pulmonary hypertension may also occur with CHF in later signs of mitral regurgitation.

▶ DIAGNOSIS

Q What is the most widely used screening for valvular heart disease (VHD)?

A Auscultation for murmurs

Murmurs are produced by three mechanisms:
1. High flow through normal or abnormal valve
2. Forward flow through a narrowed orifice (stenosis)
3. Backward flow through incompetent valve (regurgitation)

HINT Know the physiology of which valves are opened and closed during systole and diastole. This will help you determine whether a valve abnormality causes a systolic or diastolic murmur (Table 2.11).

Table 2.11 Valvular Murmurs

Questions to Ask Yourself	Answer	Potential Valve Abnormalities
Which two valves open during *diastole*?	Mitral and tricuspid	Mitral or tricuspid stenosis
Which two valves close during *diastole*?	Aortic and pulmonic	Aortic or pulmonic regurgitation
Which two valves are open during *systole*?	Aortic and pulmonic	Aortic or pulmonic stenosis
Which two valves close during *systole*?	Mitral and tricuspid	Mitral or tricuspid regurgitation

Q What are the characteristics that describe a cardiac murmur?

A Timing, quality, loudness, location, and radiation

The timing is in relation to the cardiac cycle and may use exact descriptions (i.e., holosystolic or throughout systole). It is also described on the configuration of the murmur (i.e., crescendo, decrescendo, and crescendo–decrescendo). The loudness is written with the bottom number being the scale used and the top number being the loudness of the murmur itself (i.e., 3/6 murmur—murmur is rated a 3 out of 6 for loudness). Typically, the loudness of the murmur indicates the severity of the structural defect (Table 2.12). The location of the chest sounds heard best assists with determining the valve producing the murmur (Table 2.13).

Table 2.12 Abnormal Valve Characteristics

Valve Abnormalities	Murmur Characteristics	Other Associated Abnormal Heart Sounds	Hemodynamic Changes
Aortic stenosis	Crescendo–decrescendo systolic murmur	Paradoxical splitting of the S_2	Decreased CO
Aortic regurgitation	Short and/or soft diastolic murmur	S_3 due to increased volume	Tachycardia Decreased CO Widened pulse pressure Exaggerated "A" wave in PAOP tracing
Mitral stenosis	Mid-diastolic murmur		Large "V" wave in PAOP tracing
Mitral regurgitation	Late systolic or holosystolic murmur	S_3 systolic clicks	Exaggerated "A" waves

CO, cardiac output; PAOP, pulmonary artery occlusive pressure.

Table 2.13 Location of Auscultation

Chest Wall Landmarks	Referred Valve Sounds
Second ICS right sternal border	Aortic valve
Second ICS left sternal border	Pulmonic valve
Fifth ICS midclavicular left side	Mitral valve
Fourth ICS left of sternal border	Tricuspid valve

ICS, intercostal space.

HINT   Use the location and timing of the murmur to determine the cause of the murmur. For example, a systolic murmur heard best at the second ICS right of the sternal border is most likely caused by aortic stenosis.

Q Which diagnostic test is recommended for patients with cardiac murmurs and signs of HF?

A Echocardiogram

The presence of murmurs in symptomatic patients requires further evaluation of the cardiac structures. This includes patients with signs of HF, ACS, syncope, infectious endocarditis, and other evidence of structural heart disease. Other diagnostics include CT angiogram (CTA) of chest, cardiac catheterization, and exercise testing.

HINT   A suspected aortic root dissection with aortic valve involvement may require a thoracic CT scan for more rapid diagnosis.

Q Which arrhythmia can trigger the onset of symptoms in a patient with mitral stenosis?

A AF

In mitral stenosis, the narrowed orifice decreases the speed of filling the LV during diastole. The LV diastolic volume is dependent on the gradient pressure caused by the atrial contraction. AF causes a significant decrease in LV end-diastolic volume due to loss of the atrial kick and onset of dyspnea. Exercise-induced dyspnea may also be found in patients with mitral stenosis due to the tachycardia and decreased ventricular filling time that occurs with exercise.

Aortic stenosis can also become symptomatic with new-onset AF. The hypertrophied ventricle has a greater resistance to filling and requires a strong atrial contraction to fill the chamber. A person may be asymptomatic until the onset of AF. The atrial contraction is lost in AF, resulting in less filling of the LV during diastole and a decrease in CO and clinical deterioration in symptoms.

> **HINT**   Symptoms of HF with exercise or new-onset AF should be red flags for the diagnosis of mitral stenosis, but aortic stenosis may also be a differential diagnosis.

> **Q**   While obtaining BP, you notice that Korotkoff sounds continue down to zero. Which valve abnormality would be the cause of loss of diastolic pressure?
>
> **A**   Aortic regurgitation

The aortic valve does not close completely during diastole, allowing for the equilibration of pressures in the aorta and LV during diastole. This frequently presents with a loss of diastolic pressure being obtained when auscultating BP.

> **HINT**   Arterial BP may demonstrate a widened pulse pressure (very low diastolic pressure).

> **Q**   Which EKG change may contribute to SCD in patients with MVP?
>
> **A**   Prolongation of QT interval

SCD is not common in mitral regurgitation but is more likely in familial versus nonfamilial forms of MVP. They have been frequently found to have prolongation of the QT interval, which may result in VT and SCD.

> **HINT**   Prolonged QT interval results in Torsades

▶ MEDICAL MANAGEMENT

> **Q**   What is the drug therapy of choice in severe acute aortic regurgitation?
>
> **A**   Vasodilator and positive inotropic support

Definitive treatment of severe acute aortic regurgitation is surgery. The goal for medical management temporarily before surgery is to augment the forward flow by increasing contractility and decreasing LV end-diastolic pressures (or afterload). Nipride with dobutamine may be used in combination. Vasodilator therapy may also be used in severe chronic aortic regurgitation to lower LV resistance (afterload).

> **HINT**   Remember, an IABP is contraindicated in a patient with aortic valve incompetence, so it is not a choice to reduce afterload in this scenario.

> **Q**   Which drug therapy should be avoided in severe acute regurgitation?
>
> **A**   Beta blockers

Beta blockers will block the compensatory tachycardia, which may benefit the patient by increasing CO. Beta blockers are typical drugs for managing an aortic dissection but should be avoided if the dissection involves the aortic root and aortic valve.

> **HINT**   The scenario may use an ascending thoracic dissection with aortic valve involvement, giving esmolol as a potential answer. In this scenario, Nipride may be the better answer.

> **Q**   What is the HR goal in managing mitral stenosis?
>
> **A**   Slow the HR

Medical management involves the use of drugs, which may slow the HR, allowing for greater time for the LV to fill during diastole. Agents with negative chronotropic effects, including beta blockers and HR regulating calcium channel blockers, are recommended.

> **HINT**   Avoid any medication that will increase the HR and worsen diastolic filling.

> **Q**   What are the treatment recommendations in patients with mitral stenosis and acute-onset AF or atrial flutter?
>
> **A**   Anticoagulation and control of HR response

Anticoagulation is to prevent systemic or pulmonary embolism during AF. Control of rapid ventricular response to AF includes the use of IV digoxin, HR-regulating calcium channel blockers, and beta blockers. If unable to use these previous agents, the second-line drug is an IV or oral amiodarone. If hemodynamically unstable, urgent electrical cardioversion is recommended.

HINT If the scenario indicates a need for electrical cardioversion, IV heparin is recommended before, during, and after the procedure.

Q What is the drug of choice to stabilize acute mitral regurgitation in preparation for surgery?

A Nitroprusside (Nipride)

Medical management of acute mitral regurgitation is limited and is typically used to stabilize and prepare the patient for surgery. Nitroprusside increases forward flow and reduces pulmonary congestion.

HINT Nipride should not be used alone if the patient is hypotensive. May combine with a positive inotropic agent.

▶ SURGICAL MANAGEMENT

Q What would be the indication for aortic valve replacement in aortic stenosis?

A Presence of symptoms

The decision to replace the aortic valve in aortic stenosis depends upon the severity of symptoms more than on the actual aortic valve area (size of the orifice). Some people have very severe stenosis but are asymptomatic. Others have mild stenosis but are symptomatic.

HINT The greater severity of aortic stenosis presents with HF and decreased CO and perfusion.

Q What symptoms would indicate the need to evaluate a patient with chronic aortic regurgitation for surgery?

A Dyspnea, angina, or syncope

It is recommended that symptomatic patients with severe aortic regurgitation undergo aortic valve replacement instead of long-term medical management.

HINT Signs of HF and decreased perfusion.

Q What echocardiogram finding would be a contraindication for percutaneous mitral balloon valvotomy?

A LA thrombus

An echocardiogram is recommended before percutaneous mitral balloon valvotomy to assess for the presence of an LA thrombus. If an LA thrombus is found, the patient should be anticoagulated with warfarin for 3 months for the resolution of the thrombi.

Q What can be used as a "bridge" for a hypotensive patient with acute mitral regurgitation caused by papillary muscle rupture?

A IABP counterpulsation

An acute mitral regurgitation may be treated with Nipride, but if hypotensive, an IABP may be beneficial. The IABP will increase forward flow and MAP while decreasing regurgitant volume and LV filling pressures.

▶ COMPLICATIONS

Q What is the primary complication of acute valvular dysfunction in left-sided valves?

A HF

Acute aortic and mitral valve dysfunction result in higher pressures within the LV and/or LA. The high pressures result in congestion and pulmonary edema. Other complications include cardiomyopathy, low CO syndrome, and thrombus formation.

HINT Both increased resistance outflow (aortic stenosis) and increased volume in LV (aortic regurgitation) can result in HF.

ACUTE PERIPHERAL VASCULAR INSUFFICIENCY

▶ PATHOPHYSIOLOGY

Q What is the primary cause of peripheral arterial disease (PAD)?

A Atherosclerosis

PAD is atherosclerosis of the extremities causing ischemia. The risk factors are the same as for CAD (Box 2.35).

Box 2.35 Risk Factors of PAD

Hypertension	Male
Diabetes	Obesity
Dyslipidemia	High homocysteine levels
Cigarette smoking	

PAD, peripheral arterial disease.

Q What is the most common location of a thrombus in the peripheral vascular system of the lower extremities?

A Popliteal bifurcation

Obstruction of the thrombus occurs at arterial bifurcations just distal to the common femoral bifurcation and at the popliteal bifurcation.

▶ SYMPTOMS/ASSESSMENT

Q What is the most classic symptom of PAD in the lower extremities?

A Intermittent claudication

Intermittent claudication is painful cramping or ache in the legs with exercise that is alleviated by rest. The most common site of claudication is the calves, but it can also occur in thighs, hips, buttocks, or feet. Claudication is exercise-induced reversible ischemia, similar to a stable angina. Some have atypical pain, including exercise intolerance, hip pain, and other joint pain.

HINT Pain at rest may indicate irreversible muscle ischemic injury and requires immediate intervention.

Q What aggravates the pain at rest?

A Elevating the leg

Pain worsens when the leg is elevated and improves when lowered (below the level of the heart). The pain may be described as cramping, burning, aching, or tightening (Box 2.36).

HINT This is due to decreased blood flow when the leg is raised.

Box 2.36 Other Signs of PAD in the Lower Extremities

Diminished or absence of peripheral pulses	Cyanotic
Dependent rubor	Increased sweating in extremities
Prolonged capillary refill (dependent)	Extremity cool to touch
Edema (if immobile)	Leg ulcers
Thin, pale (atrophic) skin	Erectile dysfunction (Leriche's syndrome)

PAD, peripheral arterial disease.

▶ DIAGNOSIS

Q What is the noninvasive test used to recognize PAD?

A Ankle–brachial index (ABI)

A low ABI indicates the presence of PAD. A normal index is between 1.00 and 1.40. ABI values of 0.91 to 0.99 are considered "borderline" and values greater than 1.40 indicate noncompressible arteries (Boxes 2.37 and 2.38). Ultrasonography is also used to evaluate noninvasively by determining pressure gradients and pulse–volume waveforms.

HINT   The lower the index, the more severe the PAD.

Box 2.37 How to Measure ABI

Obtain SBP in bilateral arms
Obtain SBP in bilateral ankles (may use a Doppler probe)
Calculate ankle-to-arm ratio (divide SBP of ankle by SBP of brachial)

SBP, systolic blood pressure.

Box 2.38 ABI Severity

Mild	Moderate	Severe
0.71–0.90	0.41–0.70	<0.40

ABI, ankle–brachial index.

Q What is the diagnostic test obtained prior to surgery for PAD?

A Arteriogram

An arteriogram provides details of the location and extent of arterial occlusion. It is typically performed before surgery or percutaneous transluminal angioplasty (PTA). It does not provide information about the functional significance of the abnormal findings.

Q When measuring transcutaneous oximetry (TcO$_2$), what level is predictive of poor wound healing?

A Less than 40 mmHg

TcO$_2$ may also be used to evaluate peripheral arterial insufficiency. A value less than 40 mmHg is predictive of poor wound healing and less than 20 mmHg indicates critical limb ischemia.

▶ MEDICAL MANAGEMENT

Q What is the primary pharmacological management of PAD?

A Antiplatelet therapy

Antiplatelet therapy is used to modify atherogenesis and reduce the risk of CAD, stroke, and vascular death. In lower extremity PAD, it may also lessen the symptoms and improve the walking distance. Antiplatelet therapy is also used after lower extremity revascularization (endovascular or surgical bypass). ASA is the recommended antiplatelet therapy and clopidogrel (Plavix) is an effective alternative. The combination of ASA and clopidogrel may be considered in a high-risk patient for CAD or loss of a limb who is not at increased risk of bleeding.

HINT ACE inhibitor may also be used to relieve symptoms of claudication by improving blood flow.

▶ SURGICAL/INTERVENTIONAL MANAGEMENT

Q What is the nonsurgical intervention for the treatment of PAD?

A PTA

Angioplasty, with and without stent placement, is recommended in patients with severe PAD that is amendable by the nonsurgical route. Stents may keep the arteries open with a lower restenosis rate over angioplasty alone. Stents work best in larger arteries with a higher flow, such as iliac and renal arteries (Table 2.14).

HINT PTA is not as useful in diffuse disease or long occlusions (typically >3–5 cm).

Table 2.14 Indications for PTA

Indications	Suitable Lesions
Claudication inhibiting daily activities	Short iliac stenosis (<3 cm)
Rest pain	Short, single, or multiple lesions that are superficial on the femoropopliteal segment
Gangrene	Complete occlusions superficial on the femoral artery
	Iliac stenosis proximal to bypass femoropopliteal artery

PTA, percutaneous transluminal angioplasty.

Q What is a complication of PTA?

A Loss of blood flow distal to the extremity

Complication following a PTA is loss of blood flow distal to the site of angioplasty and stent placement. Postprocedural assessment includes frequent neurovascular checks on the involved extremity. The loss of blood flow may be due to a thrombosis at the site of dilation, distal embolization, or the dissection of intimal lining causing an obstruction to flow.

HINT Sudden arterial occlusion may require immediate revascularization surgery or thrombolytic therapy.

Q What is the recommended conduit in surgical bypass procedures of the lower extremities?

A Autogenous vein

Surgical bypass procedures with an autogenous vein conduit are recommended in severe PAD with critical limb ischemia in patients with life expectancies longer than 2 years. Outcomes using a prosthetic bypass are poor, and balloon angioplasty with stent placement may be recommended over the use of a prosthetic conduit.

▶ COMPLICATIONS

Q What is a common complication of PAD?

A Foot or heal ulcers

Lower extremity ulcers that are not healing can indicate PAD. Skin ulcerations and presence of gangrene in the extremities meet the criteria for critical limb ischemia.

HINT Amputation of the extremity is also a resulting complication of severe PAD and critical limb ischemia.

⬤ CAROTID STENOSIS/CAROTID ENDARTERECTOMY

Carotid stenosis is the significant narrowing of carotid arteries and is frequently classified as symptomatic or asymptomatic, and treatment is determined by severity of occlusion. The higher degree of stenosis is a higher risk of stroke. Carotid stenosis can be unilateral, bilateral, or tandem lesions (lesion in common carotid and internal carotid on one side).

▶ PATHOPHYSIOLOGY

> **Q What is the descriptor for plaque that has an irregular or ulcerated surface?**
>
> **A Unstable plaque**

Unstable plaque has a greater risk of rupturing and forming a thrombosis. Unstable plaque is described as rapidly progressing lesion, intraplaque hemorrhage, irregular or ulcerated surface, or signs of inflammation or revascularization. Ischemic strokes are caused either by distal embolism from the unstable plaque or hypoperfusion due to the significant narrowing and limited collaterals.

HINT Carotid bifurcation is the most common site for plaque in the carotid artery.

▶ SYMPTOMS/ASSESSMENT

> **Q Would a TIA be considered symptomatic in a patient found to have significant carotid artery stenosis?**
>
> **A Yes**

Even though the symptoms resolved, if the patient exhibited focal neurological deficits that correlate to the site of stenosis, it is considered symptomatic carotid stenosis. TIAs are considered warnings for impending stroke.

What is considered common signs of ischemic stroke caused by carotid artery stenosis?

Motor weakness or paralysis of face, arm, and leg

The carotid artery supplies blood to the anterior circulation. Common presentations include motor weakness of face (facial droop), arm, and leg contralateral to involved carotid artery. Speech abnormalities are also commonly involved.

HINT Transient blindness in one eye can also be a sign of carotid stenosis with distal embolization to the retinal artery.

▶ DIAGNOSIS

> **Q Which diagnostic examination is most commonly used to screen for carotid stenosis?**
>
> **A Doppler ultrasound**

Carotid ultrasound is the most common screening diagnostic study used to determine carotid stenosis and severity. Alternatives or additional studies include CTA and MR angiogram (MRA) and can visualize more specifically the morphology of the plaque.

▶ MEDICAL MANAGEMENT

> **Q What is the pharmacological medical management for patients with known carotid stenosis?**
>
> **A Antiplatelet therapy and statins**

Medical management may be used in asymptomatic and chronic carotid stenosis. This includes antiplatelet therapy and statins. Lifestyle changes and risk management are also recommended to lower the risk factors of stroke.

HINT BP recommendation for nondiabetic asymptomatic carotid stenosis is below 140/90.

▶ SURGICAL MANAGEMENT

> **Q What is the recommended surgical management of symptomatic carotid stenosis?**
>
> **A Carotid endarterectomy (CEA) or Carotid artery stents (CAS)**

A patient that is symptomatic and has significant high-grade stenosis is recommended to have either CEA or CAS procedure to lower the long-term risk of having a stroke. Symptomatic carotid stenosis is diagnosed in patients who have experienced TIA or ischemic stroke that are found to have stenosis >50% on ipsilateral side. Patients are typically placed on dual antiplatelet therapy after CEA or CAS for minimum of 1 month followed by lifelong single antiplatelet therapy.

HINT Signs of unstable plaque has a higher risk for ischemic stroke and may be candidate for revascularization.

▶ COMPLICATIONS

> **Q What high-risk complication is associated with the CAS procedure?**
>
> **A Periprocedural stroke**

During the placement of the stent, distal embolization can occur resulting in stroke. This can be mitigated with the use of embolic protection devices.

HINT CEA is associated with higher risks of periprocedural acute MI.

> **Q Following CEA what should be performed before initiating the diet post-op?**
>
> **A Dysphagia screen**

A more common complication following CEA is cranial nerve (CN) injury due to the location of the CNs alongside the carotid artery. CN IX, X, XII can be affected and are involved in the patient's ability to swallow (Box 2.39).

HINT CN VII may also be injured and would result in unilateral facial droop.

Box 2.39 Complication of CEA

CN injury
Neck hematoma or bleeding
Hypotension and hypoperfusion
Hypertension
Cerebral hyperperfusion syndrome
Stroke
Infection

CEA, carotid endarterectomy; CN, cranial nerve.

HINT   Carotid baroreceptors are commonly involved in area of plaque and can cause hypotension, hypertension, and bradycardia.

⬤ HYPOVOLEMIC SHOCK

Q **What is the major component in defining shock?**

A **Hypoperfusion**

Shock is the pathophysiological state in which there is defective vascular perfusion of tissues and organs. It is a state of inadequacies between delivery of oxygen and the removal of end products of metabolism from peripheral tissues. This results in widespread reduction in tissue perfusion, hypoxia, and conversion of cellular respiration to an anaerobic form of metabolism, which produces lactate as a by-product. Rapid restoration of oxygen delivery can be a major factor in preventing the development of multiple organ dysfunction syndrome.

HINT   Remember, shock is defined by hypoperfusion, not hypotension. A patient can be in shock with a normal BP.

▶ PATHOPHYSIOLOGY

Q **During hypovolemic shock, which compensatory mechanism decreases urine output in an attempt to restore circulating blood volume?**

A **RAS**

During periods of hypovolemia and hypoperfusion, the kidneys release renin, which converts angiotensin I to angiotensin II. Angiotensin II is a potent vasoconstrictor, shunting blood away from nonvital organs. Angiotensin II stimulates the release of aldosterone, which results in reabsorption of sodium and water. This decreases the urine output while increasing vascular volume. The sympathetic nervous system (SNS) is another compensatory system activated during hypovolemic shock. It results in tachycardia, increased myocardial contractility, and vasoconstriction.

HINT   Vasoconstriction may maintain a BP during hypovolemic shock. Vital signs may not reflect the presence or severity of shock.

Q **What are the hemodynamic findings of hypovolemic shock that differentiate it from other types of shock?**

A **Low filling pressures and high SVR**

Hypovolemic shock is due to a decrease in circulating blood volume causing a low SV/CO ratio. Hypovolemia can be caused by blood loss, poor intake, increased fluid losses, or redistribution of fluid (third spacing).

HINT   Both the CVP and pulmonary artery occlusive pressure (PAOP) are low.

Q **What compartmental fluid shift occurs with hemorrhagic shock?**

A **Extravascular to intravascular**

In hemorrhagic shock, fluid shifts from the extravascular space into the intravascular space in an attempt to replace volume due to acute blood loss. In disease states in which plasma volume is lost, the fluid shifts from intravascular to the interstitial space. This is frequently called third spacing and can result in hypovolemic shock. Examples include peritonitis, burns, and crush injuries.

HINT   Replacement fluids should initially replace intravascular losses with isotonic fluids then changed to hypotonic to replace interstitial losses.

▶ SYMPTOMS/ASSESSMENT

> **Q** Following a trauma, a patient presents with the following vital signs on admission: HR 124, RR 32, BP 94/60, and UO 15 cc/hour. Based on these vital signs, what is the class of hemorrhagic shock?
>
> **A** Class III hemorrhagic shock

The American College of Surgeons has developed a classification of hemorrhagic shock based on vital signs to indicate the severity of blood loss. This is not exact and patient presentation can vary.

HINT A pregnant woman has a significantly greater normal circulating blood volume so can lose more blood before becoming symptomatic.

> **Q** A Class III hemorrhagic shock would indicate what percentage of blood loss?
>
> **A** 30% to 40%

A 30% to 40% total blood volume (TBV) loss (Class III) would be approximately 1,500 to 2,000 mL (Table 2.15).

HINT The classification is based on the percentage of TBV. The estimated amount of blood volume loss is based on a 70-kg male (TBV approximately 5 L).

Table 2.15 American College of Surgeons Classification of Hemorrhage

	Class I	Class II	Class III	Class IV
Blood loss (mL)	<750	750–1,500	1,500–2,000	>2,000
Blood loss (%)	<15	15–30	30–40	>40
Systolic blood pressure	Normal	Normal	Decreased	Decreased
Heart rate (bpm)	<100	>100	>120	>140
Respiratory rate (breaths/min)	14–20	20–30	30–40	>35
Mental status	Anxious	Agitated	Confused	Lethargic

Source: Data from the American College of Surgeons on Trauma. (1993). *Advanced trauma life support for physicians*. Students and Instructor Manual. Chicago, American College of Surgeons.

HINT Young patients may have normal BP/HR in the presence of significant blood loss due to the effectiveness of their compensatory mechanisms. Elderly patients may be hypotensive with minimal blood loss.

> **Q** What classification of drugs limits tachycardic response that occurs during hemorrhagic shock?
>
> **A** Beta blockers

Blocking beta-receptors of the heart results in a limited ability to respond to the sympathetic nervous system with tachycardia. The lack of tachycardia does not rule out hemorrhagic shock in patients taking beta blockers (Box 2.40).

HINT Hypovolemic/hemorrhagic shock patient may narrow the pulse pressure before decreasing systolic BP.

Box 2.40 Signs of Hypovolemic Shock

Tachycardia	Decreased urine output
Narrowed pulse pressure	Anxiety to altered mentation
Decreased blood pressure	Diminished distal pulses
Cool, clammy to touch	

▶ DIAGNOSIS

> **Q** Which laboratory studies may be used to identify the presence of shock in a normotensive patient?
>
> **A** Lactate and base deficit

Vital signs are not reliable in identifying all patients in shock. Cellular metabolism is limited by inadequate tissue hypoperfusion and results in mandatory changes from an aerobic to an anaerobic metabolism. In anaerobic metabolism, the production of lactic acid is an end product that creates lactic acidosis.

HINT   Elevated lactate levels and the presence of a base deficit are used to identify anaerobic metabolism.

> **Q** What is a base deficit?
>
> **A** Amount of base needed to titrate 1 L of whole blood to pH 7.40

The base deficit reflects the extent of anaerobic metabolism and the severity of the metabolic acidosis. This value is obtained from an arterial blood gas. The normal base is +2 to −2 mEq/L with positive numbers indicating a base excess and negative numbers indicating a base deficit.

HINT   Base deficit is used as an end point of resuscitation.

> **Q** Why does the hgb/hct not accurately reflect the RBC mass during an acute hemorrhage?
>
> **A** Equal loss of all blood components

Hematocrit (hct) and hemoglobin (Hgb) concentration are indices of balance between loss of blood and movement of extravascular fluid to intravascular space. During an acute hemorrhage, there is loss of whole blood with a decrease in all blood components in a similar ratio. If the initial hgb is low, it is caused by fluid administration and hemodilution. The rate of change in hgb over time is more predictive of the severity of bleeding.

HINT   A normal Hgb/hct does not rule out active bleeding in acute situations.

▶ MANAGEMENT

> **Q** What is the primary treatment for hypovolemic/hemorrhagic shock?
>
> **A** IV fluids

IV fluids are the mainstay treatment for hypovolemia. In the case of trauma or acute bleeding, finding the source of blood loss and stopping the bleeding surgically may be required. If the patient is hypothermic, the resuscitation fluids should be warmed prior to or during infusion.

HINT   Remember airway and breathing are still priority of care in all hemorrhagic shock patients.

> **Q** What is the greatest disadvantage of resuscitating with crystalloids?
>
> **A** Fluid shifts from intravascular to interstitial space

Crystalloids are electrolyte solutions with small molecules, which can shift across the spaces. A large amount of infused crystalloids will shift from the intravascular to the interstitial space within minutes of administration. This requires larger volumes of fluids to be administered to replace vascular losses. Frequently used crystalloids for resuscitation include lactated Ringer's (LR) and normal saline (NS). These fluids are both isotonic solutions.

HINT   A 3:1 replacement rule has been used to determine the amount required for crystalloid resuscitation (3 L of crystalloids for every 1 L of blood loss).

> **Q** Which acid–base imbalance is caused by large-volume infusions of NS?
>
> **A** Metabolic acidosis

A 1-L bag of NS contains 154 mEq/L of sodium and chloride. Large amounts of NS administered during resuscitation can cause hyperchloremic metabolic acidosis. An LR solution is a more balanced salt solution and may be used in large-volume resuscitations to prevent metabolic acidosis (Table 2.16).

HINT The patient's respiratory rate may be rapid to compensate for metabolic acidosis.

Table 2.16 Crystalloids Versus Colloids

	Crystalloids	Colloids
Advantages	Replaces interstitial fluid losses that may have occurred Cheaper Easier to store	Uses less fluid to resuscitate May draw fluid into the vascular space from interstitial space Albumin may have anti-inflammatory effects
Disadvantages	Uses larger amounts of fluid to resuscitate	During periods of increased capillary permeability, albumin will third-space into the extravascular space. Synthetic colloids (i.e., Dextran) activate immune response May cause hypersensitivity reaction Synthetic colloids increase bleeding tendencies More expensive Difficult to store

Q Which crystalloid is used to increase serum osmolality and rapidly expands the intravascular space?

A Hypertonic saline

Small amounts of hypertonic saline (4–5 mL/kg) can decrease the total amount of crystalloids used during resuscitation. Hypertonic saline increases serum osmolality and draws fluid from the extravascular space into the intravascular space. It may improve blood flow to organs and has been found to lower ICP.

HINT Metabolic acidosis and hypernatremia are complications of a hypertonic saline because of large amounts of chloride, even greater than an NS.
  Na^+ in 3% NS is 513 with Cl^- of 513
  Na^+ in 7.5% NS is 1,283 with Cl^- of 1,283

Q What is a benefit of "hypotensive resuscitation" in a bleeding patient?

A Limited blood loss

Avoiding aggressive fluid resuscitation to increase BP may limit the amount of blood volume loss in a bleeding patient prior to surgery. Hypotensive resuscitation aims to maintain the systolic BP between 80 and 90 mmHg with smaller boluses of fluid (200-mL bolus). Higher systolic BPs will increase intravascular hydrostatic pressure thus worsening blood loss in a bleeding patient. The risk of this strategy is hypoperfusion.

HINT The exception is traumatic brain injured patients. They require an SBP greater than 90 mmHg. Maintain the systolic BP more than 90 for those with traumatic brain injury.

Q When giving multiple units of packed red blood cells (PRBCs), what other blood products need to be administered?

A Fresh frozen plasma (FFP) and platelets

Administering PRBCs and fluid causes a dilutional coagulopathy. PRBCs are void of clotting factors and platelets. Transfusion practice is changing by adding more FFP and platelet transfusions into the resuscitation. Some practitioners are using the 1:1 replacement rule. For every one unit of blood, one unit of FFP is administered.

HINT Whole blood contains clotting factors and may be used by some in resuscitation to prevent coagulopathies.

> **Q** A patient without a history of cardiac problems was given PRBCs for acute blood loss. Within 4 hours of the transfusion, the patient became hypoxic, febrile, showing pulmonary edema on a CXR, requiring intubation. What is the most likely cause of this change in clinical status?
>
> **A** Transfusion-related acute lung injury (TRALI)

TRALI is the most common cause of transfusion-related deaths. The theory behind TRALI is a "two-hit" insult. The first hit is a stressful situation (such as trauma, sepsis, massive transfusion, CPB surgery), which causes the neutrophils to be "primed" and adhere to the pulmonary endothelial bed. The second hit is the actual transfusion of the blood. The transfused blood contains donor antibodies against neutrophil antigens and human leukocyte antigens. These antibodies activate the "primed" neutrophils and monocytes, resulting in increased capillary permeability and noncardiogenic pulmonary edema.

HINT Think of TRALI if there is a sudden onset of hypoxia, fever, and cough within 1 to 6 hours after a blood transfusion.

> **Q** What is the laboratory value that can be used as an end point of resuscitation?
>
> **A** Base deficit

The base deficit has been found to be a better prediction of metabolic dysfunction during hypovolemic shock and correlates with lactate levels and SvO_2 (guide to determine magnitude of volume deficit). Lactate levels are used to determine the presence of anaerobic metabolism but do demonstrate rapid adjustments to identify the return to aerobic metabolism.

HINT A base deficit of –3 to –5 may be seen on a postoperative patient and may indicate the need for further fluids (Box 2.41). A base deficit of more than –15 may indicate an ongoing blood loss.

Box 2.41 Base Deficit Determines Severity Hypovolemia

Mild	–3 to –5
Moderate	–6 to –14
Severe	>–15

▶ COMPLICATIONS

> **Q** What is the "lethal triad" that can occur with hemorrhagic shock and resuscitation?
>
> **A** Coagulopathy, hypothermia, acidosis

A worsening of one of these can lead to a cycle that results in rapid deterioration and ultimately death in a bleeding patient. All IV fluids should be warmed during the resuscitation, adequate replacement of clotting factors and platelets must be done to limit the coagulopathy, and maintaining perfusion of tissues and organs to help prevent these complications.

HINT Remember hypothermia worsens coagulopathy, and tissue hypoxia (shifts oxyhemoglobin dissociation curve), and decreases CO (decreasing myocardial contractility).

> **Q** What are the electrolyte abnormalities commonly found after a massive resuscitation?
>
> **A** Hypocalcemia, hypomagnesemia, hypo- or hyperkalemia

Blood transfusions contain citrate to increase the shelf-life of stored blood. Citrate binds calcium and magnesium, lowering the ionized levels of both. Multiple transfusions of blood can also increase potassium levels due to cell lysis, but frequently potassium levels are low after resuscitation. The low potassium may be caused by the release of aldosterone. The kidneys hold on to sodium and excrete potassium.

HINT Signs of low magnesium are similar to that of low calcium. Look for either answer if the scenario provides symptoms of muscle spasms, Chvostek's sign, or Trousseau's sign following blood transfusions.

Q What is the abdominal complication associated with aggressive fluid resuscitation?

A Abdominal compartment syndrome (ACS)

Excessive fluid administration increases the third spacing, resulting in compartment syndromes (cranium, thoracic, abdominal). The elevated pressure in the abdominal cavity results in pulmonary and renal complications, elevated ICP, and decreased venous return. Abdominal compartment syndrome affects almost all organ functions.

HINT Bladder pressure measurements are used to monitor abdominal compartment syndrome.

 # CARDIAC SURGERIES

Q What is an indication for a CABG surgery?

A Left main coronary artery occlusion

Other indications include severe triple vessel disease, recurrent HF due to ischemia, multiple coronary artery occlusions, and any contraindication to angioplasty/stent procedures (Box 2.42).

Box 2.42 Cardiac Surgeries

CABG	Repair or replacement of aorta root
Valve repair or replacement	Intracardiac tumors
Repair congenital or acquired defects (ASD and VSD)	LV aneurysmectomy

ASD, atrial septal defect; CABG, coronary artery bypass graft; VSD, ventricular septal defect.

Q What is the purpose of the use of cardioplegic hyperkalemic solution in open heart procedures?

A Induce asystole

The induction of asystole with cardioplegic hyperkalemic solutions on the heart during the surgery decreases myocardial metabolism and oxygen consumption. This potentially protects the heart during the period of ischemia.

HINT Produces cardiac standstill.

▶ PATHOPHYSIOLOGY

Q What aspects of CPB stimulate the release of the inflammatory system?

A Nonpulsatile flow and exposure to bypass circuit

CPB can cause a systemic reaction with the release of inflammatory mediators similar to sepsis. This inflammatory response is responsible for many of the adverse effects that can occur with CPB, including multisystem organ failure.

Q What are the potential advantages of "off-pump" CABG?

A Lowers risk of bleeding and multisystem organ failure

The development of off-pump or "beating heart" CABG procedures lower the incidence of complications attributed to CPB. This technique does not require CPB to be used.

HINT The greatest risk of off-pump CABG is the requirement of early revascularization procedures.

▶ SYMPTOMS/ASSESSMENT

Q What is the major focus of hemodynamic monitoring on a postoperative cardiac patient?

A Ventricular function

Ventricular function must be continuously assessed postoperatively in a cardiac surgery patient. Hemodynamic monitoring is used to determine ventricular function. Even after the heart abnormality is repaired, the ventricular function may continue to be affected for a period of time. Cardiac function has been found to be depressed postoperatively, peaking at 4 to 6 hours after surgery and typically improving within 24 hours.

HINT Interventions will be aimed at improving ventricular function pharmacologically or mechanically.

▶ DIAGNOSIS/POSTOPERATIVE MONITORING

Q Following a CABG procedure in which the left internal mammary artery (LIMA) was grafted to the left anterior descending (LAD) artery, what would ST elevation in all anterior leads indicate?

A LIMA spasm

ST elevation in all anterior leads following the procedure of grafting the LIMA to the LAD indicates spasm of the LIMA. This 12-lead EKG finding should be reported to the physician immediately. It is important for a post-CABG patient to perform ST-segment monitoring. The lead frequently used for continuous monitoring is a lead in the territory of the graft.

HINT ST elevation in two or more contiguous leads in a territory that was grafted indicates acute graft failure.

Q Which electrolytes are commonly monitored closely in a post–cardiac surgery patient?

A Potassium and magnesium

Hypokalemia and hypomagnesemia are frequent electrolyte abnormalities encountered in a post–cardiac surgical patient and require careful monitoring to treat. Hypokalemia and hypomagnesemia can significantly increase the likelihood of postoperative arrhythmias.

HINT Remember, to effectively treat the low potassium, the magnesium needs to be corrected first.

▶ MANAGEMENT

Q What is the hemodynamic complication that occurs during the rewarming of a post–cardiac surgery patient?

A Hypotension

Hypothermia causes vasoconstriction and an increase in SVR. Most postcardiac patients have been cooled in the operating room (usually <34°C). Vasodilation occurs during the rewarming process resulting in hypotension. Patients are rewarmed with the use of air convection that blows warm air over the patient.

HINT Rewarming is important in the management of patients to prevent complications of hypothermia (Box 2.43).

Box 2.43 Complications of Hypothermia

Myocardial contractility depression	Causes shivering and increased oxygen consumption
Predisposes to ventricular arrhythmias	Decreases CO_2 production
Increases afterload and myocardial workload	Causes coagulopathy

> **Q** Which of the inotropic agents is a phosphodiesterase inhibitor?
>
> **A** Milrinone (Primacor)

Inotropic agents are used in post-cardiac surgery patients to increase the contractility of the ventricles. Milrinone, being a phosphodiesterase inhibitor, does not rely on either alpha or beta stimulation for inotropic effects. Milrinone increases the levels of cyclic adenosine monophosphate (CMP) and intracardiac calcium, which promote increased contractility. The influx of calcium in the vascular beds leads to vasodilation and lowering of SVR.

HINT If the patient develops tolerance due to catecholamine depletion, milrinone is the drug of choice (Box 2.44).

Box 2.44 Other Inotropic Agents

Dopamine	Epinephrine
Dobutamine	Norepinephrine

> **Q** What hemodynamic profile needs to be assessed before administering a vasopressor?
>
> **A** Fluid status

Vascular fluid status needs to be assessed before administering a vasopressor. The vascular volume should be replaced before administering a vasoconstricting drug. The vasoconstriction and increased afterload can result in organ hypoperfusion in a hypovolemic patient. Adequate volume status during the administration of a vasoconstrictor will limit the hypoperfusion.

HINT Do not attempt to squeeze an empty vessel. Replace fluid volume first, then vasoconstrict with pharmacological agents to increase MAP.

> **Q** Which vasoconstrictor is a pure alpha-agonist drug?
>
> **A** Phenylephrine

Phenylephrine is a pure alpha-agonist that has no beta-receptor effects. Norepinephrine is both an alpha- and beta-receptor agonist. Vasopressin may also be used as a vasoconstrictor. It is an exogenous production of ADH.

▶ COMPLICATIONS

> **Q** Why is bleeding a common postoperative complication of open-heart surgery with the use of CPB?
>
> **A** Heparinization

During the period of CPB, the patient is heparinized, and the activated clotting times (ACT) must be maintained at more than 400 seconds to prevent clotting in the bypass circuit. Longer CPB times result in greater incidence of bleeding complications, even with the reversal of heparin at the end of the surgery with protamine. If the ACT is elevated, administer protamine to further reverse the heparin. The patient may not have been completely reversed (inadequate dose) or received additional heparin at the time of discontinuation from the pump (Box 2.45).

HINT An ACT test should be performed on admission to the ICU to assure adequate reversal of heparin (normal values between 100 and 120 seconds). Always consider a surgical source of bleeding with sudden onset of fresh, rapid bleeding from mediastinal chest tubes.

Box 2.45 Other Causes of Postoperative Bleeding

Thrombocytopenia and abnormal function of platelets	Bleeding from small arteries or veins
Hypothermia	Leaks at vascular anastomosis
Preoperative anticoagulation or antiplatelet drugs	

Q What are the signs of a protamine reaction?

A Hypoxia and hypotension

A protamine reaction can occur with any administration of protamine, even if the patient had tolerated the drug previously. Pulmonary hypertension with resulting hypoxia and systemic hypotension are the signs of a protamine reaction. Monitor for this adverse reaction when administering protamine.

HINT Excessive use of protamine can also cause coagulopathy.

Q Administration of five units of platelets should increase the platelet count by how much?

A 25,000 to 50,000

Correction of the bleeding complication includes administration of platelets, FFP, cryoprecipitate, and PRBCs. Monitoring PT/PTT will guide the replacement of FFP. Cryoprecipitate contains fibrinogen and factor VIII. Other methods to control small venous bleeding in the thoracic cavity include raising the head of the bed and adding PEEP on the ventilator to increase pleural and mediastinal pressures. There are no definitive studies on these methods.

HINT The main purpose of giving PRBC in a postcardiac bleeding patient is to improve oxygen delivery. Otherwise, a stable patient may tolerate Hgb of 7.0 g/dL.

Q When would aminocaproic (Amicar) be indicated in a postoperative cardiac patient?

A Actively bleeding

Rescue Amicar may be used in a postoperative cardiac patient who is actively bleeding when all other causes of bleeding have been addressed. Amicar and tranexamic acid (TXA) are frequently administered to cardiac surgical patients in the operating room to reduce the amount of blood loss and limit the number of required blood transfusions. They are antifibrinolytic agents that inhibit conversion of plasminogen to plasmin thus preventing activation of fibrinolysis. The major risk of both drugs is thrombosis, including complete occlusion of the new graft.

HINT Amicar may cause renal failure, and TXA may increase the risk of seizures.

Q How does desmopressin acetate potentially work to prevent bleeding complications?

A Improves platelet function

Desmopressin acetate elevates the levels of factor VII and von Willebrand's factor. This may improve the platelet function following cardiac surgery.

Q Following an aortic valve replacement, a patient suddenly becomes hypotensive and decreases output from the mediastinal chest tubes. What complication would you suspect?

A Cardiac tamponade

Cardiac tamponade can be a complication of cardiac surgeries. It is more common in open-heart procedures such as valvular surgeries. The classic signs of pericardial tamponade may not be present, but the presence of hypotension needs to be evaluated for potential cardiac tamponade. Decreasing or abrupt cessation of output from the mediastinal chest tubes should increase the suspicion of a cardiac tamponade. TEE may be used to diagnose the cardiac tamponade. Volume resuscitation, inotropes, and vasopressors may be temporary measures until surgery.

HINT Cardiac tamponade can have a regional effect such as compression of RV with the onset of symptoms of RV failure.

Q Which arrhythmia commonly presents in elderly patients 2 to 3 days post cardiac surgery?

A AF

AF is common following cardiac surgeries, in particular, valve surgeries. It may be seen in patients of all ages but occurs most frequently in the older population. Other common arrhythmias that occur after cardiac surgery are heart blocks and ventricular arrhythmias.

HINT   New-onset AF should be immediately converted to prevent the formation of intracardiac thrombi.

Q What type of stroke is more common following CPB surgeries?

A Watershed stroke

Watershed strokes are ischemic strokes, which occur between major cerebral vascular territories. Periods of hypotension or hypoperfusion during the nonpulsatile flow state of CPB leads to the ischemia. Other causes of stroke following CPB include showing atherosclerotic emboli mobilized by surgical manipulation of the aorta and embolic strokes with the development of AF.

HINT   Neurological assessment is important for post-cardiac patients especially following CPB.

Q What is the primary symptom of an air embolus following CPB surgeries?

A Seizures

An air embolus is a risk when the surgery requires aortotomy or when an open heart procedure is performed. The symptoms include seizures, delayed emergence from anesthesia, and focal neurological deficits. In contrast to strokes, an air embolus rarely shows changes on CT or MRI (Box 2.46).

HINT   A scenario with valve replacement in a post-op patient who is not waking up, but shows nothing on CT/MRI, would most likely be caused by an air embolus.

Box 2.46 Neurological Complications of CPB

Stroke	Seizures
Coma	Memory deficits
Paralysis	

CPB, cardiopulmonary bypass.

Q Following a mitral valve replacement, what signs would indicate an acute dehiscence of the valve repair?

A New systolic murmur and new "V" wave

Acute dehiscence of a valve repair is rare. The signs would be a new regurgitant murmur. A mitral regurgitation produces a systolic murmur, whereas aortic valve regurgitation produces a diastolic murmur. A new "V" wave develops in the PAOP waveform due to high pressures in the LA during ventricular systole due to the backflow of blood into the LA.

● HEMODYNAMIC MONITORING

See Table 2.17.

Q A patient develops hypotension. The CVP is 14 and PAOP is 7. What is the most likely cause of these hemodynamic findings?

A RV failure

RV failure will result in an elevation of CVP due to backward flow and a lower PAOP due to less blood flow to the left side of the heart. This may be caused by RV infarct, pulmonary hypertension, or pulmonary embolism.

HINT   A high CVP with low to normal PAOP indicates right ventricular involvement.

Table 2.17 Hemodynamic Profiles

Parameter	Method Calculation	Normal
MAP	(Systolic BP—diastolic BP/3) + Diastolic	70–105 mmHg
CO	Liters per minute	4–8 L
Cardiac index	CO/body surface area	2.5–4.0 L/min/m²
SV	CO/HR	50–100 mL/beat
SI	SV ÷ BSA	25–45 mL/m²/beat
SVR	(MAP – CVP) × 80 ÷ CO	800–1,200
PVR	(Mean PA – PAOP) × 80 ÷ CO	50–250
LVSWI	SI × (MAP – PAOP) × 0.0136	40–65 g·m/m²
RVSWI	SI × (Pam – CVP) × 0.0136	5–12 g·m/m²
PA pressure	(MPAP = 9–18)	25/10
PAOP		4–12
CVP		2–6

BP, blood pressure; BSA, Body surface area; CO, cardiac output; CVP, central venous pressure; HR, heart rate; LVSWI, left ventricular stroke work index; MAP, mean arterial pressure; MPAP, mean pulmonary artery pressure; PA, pulmonary artery; PAOP, pulmonary artery occlusion pressure; PVR, pulmonary vascular resistance; RVSWI, right ventricular stroke work index; SI, stroke index; SV, stroke volume; SVR, systemic vascular resistance.

HINT If both the CVP and PAOP are elevated, it could be because of LV failure or volume overload (see Figure 2.2).

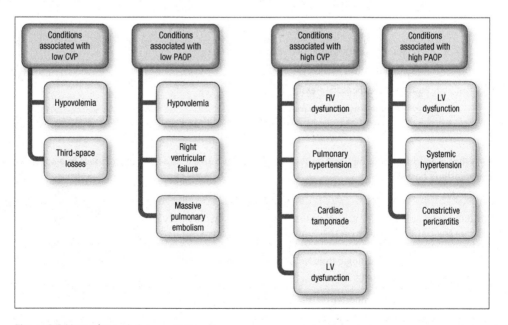

Figure 2.2 Hemodynamic interpretation.

Q Which valve abnormality interferes with the ability to obtain an accurate PAOP?

A Mitral stenosis

For the LA pressure to be equal to the LV end-diastolic pressure (LVEDP), the mitral valve must be open for the pressures to equalize. In mitral stenosis, the valve does not open completely, thus limiting the ability of the LA pressure to accurately reflect LV pressure. This is the same on the right side of the heart, obtaining a CVP reading, the tricuspid valve must be open completely for the RA to accurately reflect RV at end diastole.

HINT An accurate pressure reading can be obtained in mitral regurgitation if wave is read during the A wave only (when the mitral valve is open).

Q PAOP and CVP readings in patients with hypertrophied cardiomyopathy are falsely high or low?

A High

PAOP and CVP are readings of pressures in the heart chambers. Pressure is not always equal to volume and can cause an erroneous reading. Hypertrophied cardiomyopathies will read the pressures higher than the actual volume. This is due to the high pressure of the thickened myocardial muscle placed on the heart chambers. Dilated cardiomyopathies exert little pressure but are dilated chambers that hold large volumes of blood. In dilated cardiomyopathy, CVP and PAOP readings are lower than the actual volume.

HINT Pressure is not always equal to volume. Read the scenario and interpret findings based on the patient case study presented in the question.

Q What is strove volume variance (SVV) an indicator of?

A Preload responsiveness

SVV is frequently used to determine the need for fluid. SVV is not an indicator of actual volume (preload) but of relative preload responsiveness. The goal is to maintain SVV less than 13%.

HINT The patient must be ventilated for accuracy of measurement (Box 2.47).

Box 2.47 Limitations of SVV

Requires mechanical ventilation (improves accuracy)
Arrhythmias (affect accuracy)
Positive end-expiratory pressure (increase SVV)
Vascular tone (vasodilation may increase SVV)

SVV, strove volume variance.

Q What maneuver could be used instead of SVV to determine fluid responsiveness in a spontaneous breathing patient?

A Passive leg raising

Without the availability of SVV, raising the legs has proven clinically to act like a "self volume challenge" to indicate the patient's status on the Frank–Starling curve.

HINT This provides a physiologic fluid bolus and may be performed if the patient has arrhythmias or spontaneous breathing.

Q What are the three components of oxygen delivery (DO_2)?

A Oxygen saturation, Hgb, and CO

DO_2 is the amount of oxygen leaving the heart per minute and delivered to the tissue level. The components of DO_2 include oxygen saturation, Hgb, and CO. If DO_2 decreases, the body compensates by offloading more oxygen from the hgb to the tissues. CO is the most important component of this equation.

HINT If the tissues take more oxygen from the Hgb, then less oxygen is returned to the right side of the heart.

Q What is oxygen consumption (VO$_2$) equal to in a normal situation?

A Oxygen demand

In a normal situation with adequate oxygen delivery, an increase in oxygen demand will increase oxygen consumption. VO$_2$ will vary based on the metabolic needs of the tissues.

HINT Intervention may be to increase the delivery of oxygen or decrease the demand for oxygen (Box 2.48).

Box 2.48 Causes of Increased VO$_2$

Fever	Anxiety
Shivering	Hyperthermia
Increase in work of breathing	Response to major illness or surgeries
Pain	Seizures

VO$_2$, oxygen consumption.

Q Are critically ill patients usually supply independent or supply dependent?

A Supply dependent

VO$_2$ is a good measurement of the overall aerobic metabolism but by itself is an unreliable indicator of adequacy of tissue perfusion. Adding DO$_2$ in relation to VO$_2$ tells more about oxygen use. Supply independency occurs when the VO$_2$ remains constant during a period of increased demand or decreased supply. This indicates that DO$_2$ is sufficient for the demand, indicating adequate tissue perfusion. In critically ill patients, it is difficult to achieve this supply independency. Supply dependency occurs as the tissue demand increases and requires an increase in blood flow. This indicates that the DO$_2$ was not sufficient for the tissue demands.

HINT An increase in VO$_2$ after increasing DO$_2$ indicates an oxygen debt (see Figure 2.3).

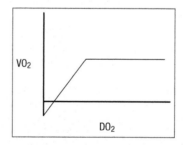

Figure 2.3 Supply dependence curve

Q What is a normal SvO$_2$ obtained from a PAC?

A 60% to 80%

SvO$_2$ monitoring is used to allow for continuous monitoring of O$_2$ supply and demand. SvO$_2$ measures oxygen saturation of the venous blood from the right side of the heart (it is the amount of oxygen returning to the right side after tissue extraction). A change in SvO$_2$ may indicate a change in either DO$_2$ or VO$_2$ or both.

HINT If the question gives a change in the SvO$_2$, look at both the demand and delivery to determine the cause.

Q What is the difference between SvO$_2$ and ScvO$_2$ monitoring?

A SvO$_2$ is a true mixed venous gas

ScvO$_2$ is obtained from a central line (central venous circulation), whereas SvO$_2$ is obtained from the PAC (pulmonary artery). ScvO$_2$ is not a true "mixed" venous gas but can be used to determine oxygen consumption.

HINT The goal is to maintain ScvO$_2$ at greater than 70%.

INTRA-AORTIC BALLOON PUMP COUNTERPULSATION

Q Where is the balloon positioned in the aorta?

A Descending thoracic aorta

The tip of the catheter should be positioned just distal to the left subclavian artery and above the renal and mesenteric arteries.

HINT Sudden cessation of urine may indicate migration of the balloon distally, obstructing the renal arteries.

Q When does inflation of the balloon occur?

A Beginning of diastole

The inflation of the balloon just after the closure of the aortic valve, the beginning of diastole, increases the aortic pressure and augments perfusion. It elevates the diastolic pressure in the aorta, thus improving coronary perfusion.

HINT Remember coronary perfusion pressure (CPP) is the difference between aortic diastolic pressure (ADP) and right atrial pressure (RAP):

CPP = ADP − RAP

Q What is the purpose of balloon deflation immediately prior to systole?

A Decreased afterload

The balloon should deflate just before the opening of the aortic valve, immediately prior to systole. This results in a sudden decrease in aortic pressure and decreases the afterload or resistance of the LV.

HINT If the balloon deflates after the onset of systole, it will increase the workload of the heart. It is important that deflation occurs immediately prior to systole.

Q Which of the following provides the most support to the heart: the 1:1, 1:2, or 1:3 cycle?

A 1:1

A 1:1 cycle indicates that the balloon inflates and deflates with every heartbeat. It provides support with every contraction. A 1:2 cycle provides support with every second cardiac cycle, and the 1:3 cycle every third.

HINT Weaning the IABP is typically performed by decreasing the cycle frequency from 1:1 to 1:2, then to 1:3 before removing the balloon.

Q Which valve abnormality would be a contraindication for the use of IABP?

A Aortic insufficiency

Inflates after closure of the aortic valve. An aortic insufficiency would cause the blood to flow back into the LV during balloon inflation, increasing the LV volume. This would increase the workload of the heart and worsen LV failure. Other contraindications include aortic dissection and severe peripheral vascular disease (due to placement of the catheter in femoral location).

HINT IABP is indicated for mitral valve insufficiency to lower the resistance of the LV (Box 2.49).

Box 2.49 Indications for an IABP

Cardiogenic shock: medically refractory	Acute ventricular septal rupture
AMI: medically refractory	Bridge to cardiac transplantation
Acute mitral regurgitation	

IABP, intra-aortic balloon pump.

Q A common complication of IABP is lower extremity ischemia. What should be performed routinely to assess for this potential complication?

A Check distal pulses hourly

The catheter is placed in the femoral artery and can diminish or occlude blood flow distally. It is recommended to assess distal pulses hourly for as long as the balloon is in place. Hematomas can occur at the insertion site contributing to a decrease in distal flow. Assessment of the insertion site hourly for the presence of hematoma is recommended (Box 2.50).

Box 2.50 Other Complications of Using an IABP

Occlusion of the renal, superior mesenteric, or subclavian artery	Thrombocytopenia
Acute aortic dissection or perforation with retroperitoneal hemorrhage	Thromboembolism
Wound infection	

IABP, intra-aortic balloon pump.

 PACEMAKERS

Q According to the pacemaker code, where does a DVI pacemaker sense and pace?

A Senses in ventricles, paces in both atrium and ventricles

A DVI pacemaker paces in both the atrium and ventricles and senses in the ventricles only. The first letter in the code is chamber paced, and the second letter is chamber sensed (Box 2.51).

Box 2.51 ICHD Pacemaker Codes

I	II	III
Chamber Paced	**Chamber Sensed**	**Mode of Response(s)**
V = Ventricle	V = Ventricle	T = Triggered
A = Atrium	A = Atrium	I = Inhibited
D = Double	D = Double	D = Double
O = None	O = None	O = None

ICHD, Inter-Society Commission for Heart Disease.

HINT   A fourth letter would indicate whether the pacemaker is rate responsive.
          For example, VVIR.

Q Following placement of a permanent pacemaker, the patient's BP decreased from 142/76 to 99/40 on admission to the ICU. What is the most likely cause of the hypotension?

A Cardiac tamponade

During placement of lead, manipulation or fixation of the screw into the wire causes bleeding into the pericardial space. The most common symptom is hypotension.

HINT   Emergency pericardiocentesis is required to manage pericardial tamponade (Box 2.52).

Box 2.52 Potential Complications of an Implanted Pacemaker

Rejection phenomena	Surgical complications (hematoma, infection, thrombosis)
Skin erosion	Lead problems (fractured, compressed, dislodgement)
Muscle or nerve simulation	Cardiac perforation, cardiac tamponade

Q Which pacemaker would be contraindicated in a patient with a complete AV heart block?

A Atrial pacemaker (AAI)

An atrial pacemaker senses and paces in the atrium only. The impulse travels to the AV junction and requires an intact pathway to travel down to the ventricles. A patient with an AV block requires either a ventricular (VVI) or dual chamber pacemaker (DDD) to pace below the level of the block.

HINT   Ventricular pacemakers (VVI) sense and pace only in the ventricles. Without any coordination with the atrium, the atrial kick is lost and can decrease the SV.

Q If the patient does not know what type of pacemaker he or she has, what test should be ordered?

A CXR

A CXR can identify the types of leads, the number of leads, and their positions. This indicates what system the patient has implanted. The shape of the pacemaker and manufacturer can assist with further identifying the type of pacemaker.

HINT   Two wires would indicate a dual-chamber pacemaker.

Q If CXR reveals three leads, what type of pacemaker does the patient have?

A Biventricular pacemaker (three-chamber pacemaker)

A biventricular pacemaker is also called cardiac resynchronization therapy (CRT). Single- and dual-chamber pacemakers pace in the right side of the heart. Depolarization of the LV occurs after the RV, resulting in dyssynchronization of the ventricles and can decrease CO. Pacing both LV and RV will resynchronize the ventricular contraction and improve CO. It is indicated for the reduction of the symptoms of moderate to severe HF (NYHA Functional Class III or IV) in those patients who remain symptomatic despite stable, optimal medical therapy and have an LVEF of 35% or less and a prolonged QRS duration.

HINT   The paced QRS complex on a triple-chamber pacemaker has a normal width compared to the wide QRS complex on a paced beat with ventricular or dual-chamber pacemaker.

Q What pacemaker problem can lead to competition between the pacemaker and the heart?

A Undersensing

Failure of the heart to sense the underlying electrical activity (P wave or QRS complex) is called "undersensing." The pacemaker sends electrical impulses when the heart does not need it. This results in competition.

HINT   Competition can cause an R-on-T phenomenon resulting in deadly arrhythmias, such as VT (torsades de pointes).

Q What is it called when the pacemaker detects other activities besides the intended P wave or QRS complex?

A Oversensing

Oversensing results in the chamber not being paced when indicated because the pacemaker sensed other activity. Unwanted signals commonly sensed can be T wave (sensed as a QRS), skeletal muscle myopotential, and signals from the pacemaker (cross-talking) in which the pacemaker senses the pacemaker spike as intrinsic activity.

HINT   On an EKG strip, this can look like a failure to pace.

> **Q What does a "failure to capture" look like on an EKG strip?**
>
> **A Pacer spike without electrical activity**

Capture is the depolarization of the paced chamber. This is influenced by the amplitude and duration of the stimulus.

HINT   To correct failure to capture, the milliamps (mA) are increased.

1. Which of the following drug classes is indicated to limit remodeling of the left ventricle following an acute myocardial infarction (AMI)?

   A. Beta blockers
   B. Statins
   C. Angiotensin-converting enzyme (ACE) inhibitors
   D. Calcium channel blockers

2. A patient is 2 days post ST-elevation myocardial infarction (STEMI) and has sudden-onset pulmonary congestion and a decrease in cardiac output. Upon further assessment, she is noted to have a new-onset holosystolic murmur. Which of the following is the most likely cause?

   A. Rupture of the ventricular wall
   B. Cardiac tamponade
   C. Cardiogenic shock
   D. Acute mitral regurgitation

3. A patient with atrial fibrillation (AF) requires rate reduction pharmacologic management. Which of the following medications used to slow the ventricular rate of AF is an ultra-short beta blocker?

   A. Brevibloc (esmolol)
   B. Lopressor (metoprolol)
   C. Cardizem (diltiazem)
   D. Cordarone (amiodarone)

4. During the initial assessment of a patient admitted to the ICU, the patient states that he experienced a ripping sensation in the chest and now has 10/10 chest pain. The nurse notes a diastolic murmur and pulmonary congestion on auscultation. Which of the following is the most likely cause of the symptoms?

   A. Ascending thoracic dissection
   B. Descending thoracic dissection
   C. Transection of the aorta at the level of the isthmus
   D. Dissection of the aorta at the level of the great vessels

5. Your patient is on captopril and metoprolol. Which of the following electrolyte abnormalities would you suspect may occur?

   A. Hyperkalemia
   B. Hyponatremia
   C. Hypercalcemia
   D. Hyperphosphatemia

6. Which of the following is the most useful finding to differentiate diastolic from systolic heart failure (HF)?

   A. Stroke volume (SV)
   B. Ejection fraction (EF)
   C. Blood pressure
   D. Heart rate

1. C) ACE inhibitors
ACE inhibitors prevent left ventricular (LV) hypertrophy, called remodeling. They are indicated following an AMI and have been found to lower the incidence of sudden cardiac death due to remodeling. Statins and beta blockers are also indicated following an AMI, but have not been found to limit remodeling. Calcium channel blockers are typically not indicated following AMI, due to their negative inotropic effects.

2. D) Acute mitral regurgitation
Acute mitral regurgitation can be caused by rupture of the papillary muscle following a STEMI and present with sudden onset of pulmonary edema and holosystolic murmur. A ventricular wall rupture characteristically demonstrates a step-up oxygen saturation from right atrium (RA) to pulmonary artery. Cardiogenic shock and cardiac tamponade demonstrate decreased cardiac output (CO) but without significant pulmonary edema.

3. A) Brevibloc (esmolol)
All four medications can be used to slow the ventricular rate in AF, but esmolol is an ultra-short-acting beta blocker commonly administered as a continuous infusion. Metoprolol is a beta blocker but not ultra-short acting, and is administered as intermittent boluses. Diltiazem is a calcium channel blocker and amiodarone is an antiarrhythmic drug able to both slow the rate and potentially convert to sinus rhythm.

4. A) Ascending thoracic dissection
An aortic dissection along the ascending aorta can tear retrograde into the aortic valve, causing an aortic insufficiency. This would account for pulmonary congestion and diastolic murmur, along with the chest pain commonly associated with an aortic dissection.

5. A) Hyperkalemia
Both angiotensin-converting enzyme (ACE) inhibitors and beta blockers can cause hyperkalemia. ACE inhibitors block release of aldosterone, so the kidneys excrete sodium and retain potassium. Beta blockers shift potassium from intracellular to intravascular, thus increasing potassium levels.

6. B) EF
Both diastolic and systolic HF result in a low SV, but diastolic HF is most commonly due to a hypertrophied cardiomyopathy, which has a high EF. This is called heart failure with preserved ejection fraction (HFpEF). With systolic HF, the primary problem is decrease in contractility and a low EF. This is called heart failure with reduced ejection fraction (HFrEF).

7. A 28-year-old man develops tachycardia and chest pain following a blunt injury to the chest. Which of the following should the nurse suspect is the most likely cause of his clinical signs?

   A. Myocardial infarction (MI)
   B. Cardiac tamponade
   C. Aortic dissection
   D. Cardiac contusion

8. A patient is readmitted to the ICU. He had experienced an acute myocardial infarction (AMI) 2 weeks prior. He currently has chest pain, fever, malaise, and an elevated white blood cell (WBC) count. Which of the following would account for the current presentation?

   A. Idiopathic thrombocytopenia purpura (ITP)
   B. Dressler's syndrome
   C. Endocarditis
   D. Vasculitis

9. A patient is admitted from the operating room (OR) following a gunshot to the abdomen. The patient received multiple units of packed red blood cells (PRBCs) and 8 L of normal saline (NS). Which of the following would be an expected finding due to the large volume of NS?

   A. Elevated potassium
   B. Metabolic acidosis
   C. Decreased calcium
   D. Decreased sodium

10. A 12-lead EKG demonstrates ST depression and large R waves in leads V1–V4. Which of the following is the most likely cause of the finding?

    A. Inferior wall myocardial infarction (MI)
    B. Anterior wall MI
    C. Lateral wall MI
    D. Posterior wall MI

11. The physician has ordered a 12-lead EKG on a patient suspected of having pericarditis. What EKG changes would the nurse expect to find in pericarditis?

    A. Left bundle branch block (LBBB)
    B. ST segment elevation in all leads
    C. Significant Q waves in the anterior leads
    D. Right axis deviation

12. A patient in the ICU requires hemodynamic monitoring. An arterial line with the capability of pulse pressure waveform analysis is placed and a stroke volume variance (SVV) is obtained. What does an SVV measure?

    A. Preload
    B. Afterload
    C. Fluid responsiveness
    D. Vascular resistance

7. D) Cardiac contusion
Cardiac contusion would be more likely than MI due to the patient's age and trauma. The most common sign of a blunt cardiac injury is tachycardia. Aortic dissection can occur following chest trauma but usually presents with hypotension and widened mediastinum on a chest x-ray (CXR). Cardiac tamponade presents with hypotension and jugular venous distention.

8. B) Dressler's syndrome
Dressler's syndrome is a complication of an AMI in the form of pericarditis. It is also called postmyocardial infarction syndrome. Symptoms can occur weeks to months after AMI; patients present with fever, malaise, elevated WBC count, and pericarditis. It is believed to result from an autoimmune reaction. ITP causes a decrease in platelets. Endocarditis is more likely to cause an AMI than be caused by one. Presentation is not one of vasculitis.

9. B) Metabolic acidosis
NS has a higher amount of sodium and chloride than the body's normal sodium/chloride levels. This increase in chloride levels can cause metabolic acidosis from large volumes of NS infusion. It would result in hypernatremia not hyponatremia.

10. D) Posterior wall MI
ST depression and large R waves in the anterior leads indicate the presence of a posterior wall MI. These are reciprocal changes found in the anterior leads. An anterior MI will elevate the ST segment and produce Q waves in the anterior leads (V1–V4). Inferior wall MI is identified in leads II, III, and aVF, whereas lateral wall MI involves leads I, V5–V6, and aVL.

11. B) ST segment elevation in all leads
ST segment elevation with an upward concavity in all leads indicates pericarditis. Acute myocardial infarction demonstrates ST segment elevation with an upward convexity in contiguous leads only. Pericarditis would not present with significant Q waves or new-onset LBBB.

12. C) Fluid responsiveness
SVV is a measurement used to determine the patient's responsiveness to fluid. If the reading is greater than 10%, the patient would be more likely to benefit from a fluid bolus. SVV does not measure preload (volume) directly or afterload.

13. What is the most common site for a thoracic aortic aneurysm following a blunt decelerating chest trauma?

   A. The level of the isthmus
   B. The ascending aorta
   C. The level of the great vessels
   D. Above the renal arteries

14. A patient has been in the ICU for 3 days following a motorcycle collision. The nurse notes unresolved pneumothorax and progressive mediastinal emphysema. Which of the following would be the best explanation for these findings?

   A. Tension pneumothorax
   B. Tracheal injury
   C. Diaphragmatic injury
   D. Flail chest

15. Which of the following best describes the physiology of patients presenting with near-complete occlusion of coronary artery with plaque but without sustaining a myocardial infarction?

   A. Remodeling of the myocardial muscle
   B. Bradycardia allowing improved coronary perfusion
   C. Decrease in wall stress
   D. Development of collateral circulation

16. A patient presents to the ED with chest pain. Upon further assessment, the nurse notes the patient is dyspneic, has a low-grade fever, slight elevation in white blood cells (WBCs), and states the chest pain worsens on inspiration. Which of the assessment findings is less likely to be associated with acute myocardial infarction (AMI)?

   A. Chest pain worsens with inspiration
   B. Dyspnea
   C. Low-grade fever
   D. Elevated WBCs

17. The rupture of the ventricular free wall is a complication of an acute myocardial infarction (AMI). Which of the following would be the most likely presentation?

   A. Pericardial tamponade
   B. Congestive heart failure
   C. Atrial fibrillation
   D. Hypovolemic shock

18. Which of the following is a red flag that emergent intervention may be required?

   A. ST segment depression
   B. Elevated pro-brain natriuretic peptide (BNP) levels
   C. Elevated ST segments
   D. Narrowed QT interval

19. Antiplatelet therapy would be indicated in which of the following causes of myocardial infarction?

   A. Hypertensive crisis
   B. Severe anemia from blood loss
   C. Hypertrophic cardiomyopathy
   D. Atherosclerotic plaque

13. A) The level of the isthmus

The most common site of injury is at the level of the isthmus. This part of the aorta is secured by the ligamentum arteriosum, which limits movement following a deceleration injury. The mechanism of injury is a sudden deceleration, either horizontal (motor vehicle crash [MVC]) or vertical (fall), in which the aorta continues to travel forward except at the level of the isthmus, causing a tear.

14. B) Tracheal injury

Tracheal injury may not be evident for up to 5 days after injury. It commonly presents with signs of persistent air leak and hemoptysis. Tension pneumothorax is life-threatening; air enters the pleural space and becomes trapped, building pressure and shifting one or more mediastinal structures. Diaphragmatic injury and flail chest frequently cause chest pain and dyspnea.

15. D) Development of collateral circulation

The narrowing of the coronary artery by atherosclerotic plaque occurs over time allowing for the time to develop collateral circulation. These collaterals provide blood flow distal to the occlusion of the coronary artery, improving perfusion and preventing ischemic injuries and infarction. Remodeling of myocardial muscle actually increases the risk of ischemic injury (due to the increase in muscle) and sudden cardiac death. Bradycardia does allow for a longer diastolic time to fill the coronary arteries but is not the reason the heart is protected from myocardial infarction. Ischemia actually increases myocardial wall stress due to noncompliance.

16. A) Chest pain worsens with inspiration

Patients experiencing anginal chest pain typically experience dyspnea and can present with low-grade fevers and leukocytosis due to the inflammation. Anginal chest pain does not typically worsen with inspiration, and the characteristics of the patient's chest pain are used to assist with differential diagnosis of chest pain.

17. A) Pericardial tamponade

If the ventricular free wall ruptures, blood enters the pericardial space causing signs of a pericardial tamponade. These signs include hypotension, jugular venous distention, and muffled heart sounds. Left ventricular failure would cause signs of congestive heart failure. Ventricular rupture would more likely cause pulseless electrical activity (PEA) than atrial fibrillation. It would not lose enough blood volume into the pericardial sac to cause hypovolemic shock. The patient may develop cardiogenic shock though.

18. C) Elevated ST segments

Elevated ST segment is the defining characteristic of an ST-segment elevation myocardial infarction (STEMI) and is considered an emergency. It is associated with transmural ischemia commonly associated with complete obstruction of the coronary artery. ST depression is a sign of non-ST-segment elevation myocardial infarction (NSTEMI) and is typically nontransmural ischemia. Elevated pro-BNP levels are commonly found in patients with congestive heart failure. Widened QT interval is a greater concern for ventricular tachycardia, not a narrowed QT interval.

19. D) Atherosclerotic plaque

Myocardial infarctions classified as "Type 2" result from normal stable coronary artery without disease, but MI is result of an increase in myocardial demand. Atherosclerosis with the risk of plaque rupture is the indication for antiplatelet therapy. Hypertensive crisis, severe anemia, and hypertrophic cardiomyopathy cause an increased demand or decreased supply of oxygen to the myocardium without plaque and result in MI. Antiplatelet therapy will not benefit MI patients if not atherosclerotic disease.

20. A patient with presentation of heart failure (HF) is ordered an echocardiogram. The results found an ejection fraction (EF) of 51%. Which of the following is the most appropriate classification of the HF?

   A. Heart failure reduced ejection fraction (HFrEF)
   B. Heart failure preserved ejection fraction (HFpEF)
   C. Borderline HFpEF
   D. Systolic dysfunction HF

21. Which of the following is a recognized advantage for endovascular aneurysm repair (EVAR) of abdominal aortic aneurysm (AAA), compared to open surgical technique?

   A. Lowers risk of delayed rupture
   B. Long-term imaging is not required
   C. Decreased length of hospital stay
   D. Lowers risk of recurrence

22. Which of the following would be the least common mechanism of acute kidney injury (AKI) following abdominal aortic aneurysm (AAA) repair?

   A. Rhabdomyolysis
   B. Contrast-induce nephropathy (CIN)
   C. Renal microembolization
   D. Acute tubular necrosis (ATN)

23. Which of the following is an EKG finding that is found in patients with pericardial tamponade?

   A. Delta wave
   B. New-onset left bundle branch block (LBBB)
   C. Significant Q waves in all leads
   D. Electrical alternans

24. Which of the following is a neurological complication of chronic or acute hypertension?

   A. Posterior reversible encephalopathy syndrome (PRES)
   B. Migraine with an aura
   C. Vertebral artery stenosis
   D. Central venous thrombosis (CVT)

25. Which of the following is the most accurate statement about a transcatheter aortic valve replacement (TAVR)?

   A. Not used in patients with comorbidities
   B. Cardiopulmonary bypass is required
   C. Patients typically extubated in operating room (OR)
   D. High rate of restenosis

(See answers next page.)

20. B) HFpEF

HFpEF is when patients exhibit signs of HF but demonstrate EF of 50% or greater. This is commonly due to difficulty in the diastolic phase of the cardiac cycle. HFrEF is when patient exhibit signs of HF but demonstrate EF less than 40%. Borderline is EF between 41% and 49%. Systolic dysfunction is categorized as HFrEF.

21. C) Decreased length of hospital stay

There are advantages and disadvantages to the two approaches for repair of AAA. EVAR has a significantly decrease operative time, hospital stay, blood loss, and overall decrease in complications and mortality. An open technique with grafting of aorta permanently eliminates the aneurysm completely so long-term monitoring is not required and it has a lower risk of recurrence or rupture.

22. B) Rhabdomyolysis

The likely pathology for AKI following a repair of an AAA is CIN due to the amount of diagnostic procedures using contrast. Renal microembolization is a risk of endovascular repair of AAA during catheterization. ATN can be due to ischemia, a risk of AAA repair. Rhabdomyolysis is due to muscle breakdown and is not a typical risk of AKI in AAA patients.

23. D) Electrical alternans

The appearance of electrical alternans on the EKG is a sign indicative of the presence of pericardial tamponade. This is due to the heart "swinging" in the chest wall. Delta wave is present with Wolff–Parkinson–White (WPW) syndrome. A new-onset LBBB and significant Q waves in all leads are not signs of pericardial tamponade.

24. A) PRES

PRES is hypertensive encephalopathy and affects bilateral occipital lobes (posterior). Presentation is altered mental status, headache, and visual changes. It is typically reversible if BP is controlled. Migraines with an aura are not typically caused by hypertension. Vertebral artery stenosis is more likely to result in ischemic stroke in the posterior area but is not related to hypertensive crisis. CVT may result in ischemic or hemorrhagic strokes but is not a result of hypertension.

25. C) Patients typically extubated in OR

TAVR is most commonly used in patients with higher risk comorbidities because it is a less invasive technique to replace the aortic valve. Cardiopulmonary bypass is NOT required, and patients are typically extubated in the OR. TAVR has a lower rate of restenosis compared to balloon valvuloplasty.

BIBLIOGRAPHY

American College of Cardiology Foundation/American Heart Association. (2016). Guideline on the management of patients with lower extremity peripheral artery disease. *Circulation, 135*, 686–725.

American College of Cardiology Foundation/American Heart Association. (2017). Focused update of the 2013 ACCF/AHA Guideline for the management of heart failure. *Circulation, 136*, 137–161.

American Association of Critical-Care Nurses. (2009). AACN practice alert: ST segment monitoring. https://www.aacn.org/clinical-resources/practice-alerts

American College of Surgeons on Trauma. (2018). *Advanced trauma life support for physicians, students and instructor manual.* Chicago: American College of Surgeons.

Jneid, H., Addison, D., Bhat, D. L., Fonarow, G. C., Gokak, S., Grady, K. L., . . . Pancholy, S. (2017). 2017 AHA/ACC Clinical performance and quality measures for adults with ST-elevation and non-ST elevation myocardial infarction. Report from American College of Cardiology/AHA task force. *Journal of the American College of Cardiology, 70*, 2048–2090.

Kloos, J. (2015). Characteristics, complications, and treatment of acute pericarditis. *Critical Care Nursing Clinics, 27*(4), 483–497.

Mokashi, S. A., & Svensson, L. G. (2019). Guidelines for the management of thoracic aortic disease in 2017. *General Thoracic Cardiovascular Surgery, 67*, 59–65.

Unger, T., Borghi, C., Charchar, F., Khan, N. A., Poulter, N. R., Prabhakaran, D., . . . Schutte, A. E. (2020). International society of hypertension global guidelines. *Journal of Hypertension, 38*(6), 982–1004.

York, N., Kane, C., & Smith, C. (2018). Identification and management of pericardial tamponade. *Dimensions of Critical Care Nursing, 37*(3), 130–135.

Respiratory System Review

► LEARNING OBJECTIVES

In this chapter, you will review:

- Acute respiratory failure
- Acute respiratory distress syndrome (ARDS)
- Acute pulmonary embolism (PE)
- Chronic disorders (COPD exacerbations/severe asthma/status asthmaticus)
  - Chronic conditions (e.g., chronic obstructive pulmonary disease [COPD], asthma, bronchitis, emphysema)
  - Status asthmaticus
- Acute respiratory infections
- Pleural space abnormalities (e.g., pneumothorax, hemothorax, empyema, pleural effusions)
- Aspiration
- Pulmonary hypertension
- Thoracic trauma (e.g., fractured rib, lung contusion, tracheal perforation)
- Thoracic surgery
- Mechanical ventilation
- Failure to wean from mechanical ventilator
- Pulmonary fibrosis
- Respiratory monitoring devices
- Transfusion-related acute lung injury (TRALI)
- Testable nursing actions

● ACUTE RESPIRATORY FAILURE

Q What are the two characteristics of respiratory failure found on an arterial blood gas (ABG)?

A Hypercapnia and hypoxemia

Respiratory insufficiency occurs when the patient is struggling to breathe but still able to maintain gas exchange. Respiratory failure is difficulty breathing and the inadequacy of the respiratory system to support gas exchange. Respiratory failure is characterized by hypercapnia ($PaCO_2$ >45 mmHg) and hypoxemia (PaO_2 <55 mmHg).

HINT "Crossed blood gas" is an indicator of respiratory failure ($PaCO_2$ > PaO_2).

Q In normal conditions, what does the $PaCO_2$ directly vary with?

A Minute ventilation (MV)

MV is respiratory rate (RR) multiplied by tidal volume (TV). The $PaCO_2$ measures ventilation. In normal conditions, there is a direct inverse relationship between MV and $PaCO_2$. As the MV increases (rate or volume), the $PaCO_2$ decreases. Elevated $PaCO_2$ is the hallmark of hypercapnic respiratory failure.

HINT   Increasing $PaCO_2$ in asthma patients is an ominous sign of impending respiratory failure.

Q What is the most common cause of acute respiratory failure?

A Pulmonary infections

Pulmonary infections are the leading cause of acute respiratory failure, followed by pulmonary edema with heart failure (HF), sepsis with acute respiratory distress syndrome (ARDS), and chronic obstructive pulmonary disease (COPD) exacerbations.

HINT   Lungs can be adversely affected when managing other organ disorders resulting in lung toxicities.

▶ PATHOPHYSIOLOGY

Q What is a ventilation perfusion (VQ) mismatch in which there is perfusion without ventilation called?

A VQ shunt

A shunt occurs when the mixed venous blood from the right side of the heart enters the left side without being oxygenated. The primary problem is ventilation. The alveoli are not open and ventilating but are being perfused. A shunt is considered a low VQ state (Box 3.1).

HINT   Hypoxemia due to a shunt is not reversible with oxygen therapy alone.

Box 3.1 Common Causes of Shunts

Atelectasis Pneumothorax	Central airway obstruction Compressive atelectasis (pleural effusion)
ARDS	Chronic bronchitis
Pulmonary edema	Alveolar hemorrhage

ARDS, acute respiratory distress syndrome.

Q What is the compensatory mechanism in the lungs that occurs following onset of a VQ shunt?

A Pulmonary vasoconstriction

This hypoxic vasoconstriction reduces some of the blood flow to the areas of the lungs that are underventilated in an attempt to compensate.

HINT   This hypoxic response can result in pulmonary hypertension (PH) and right ventricular (RV) failure.

Q What is alveolar dead space?

A Ventilation without perfusion

Dead space is the opposite end of the spectrum from a shunt. In dead space, the alveoli are open and being ventilated but without perfusion. The VQ mismatch is related to decreased blood flow through the pulmonary capillaries. This is most commonly caused by a pulmonary embolism (PE). Dead space is a high VQ state (Box 3.2).

Box 3.2 Causes of Dead Space

Pulmonary embolism
Pulmonary hypertension (primary and secondary)
Emphysema/COPD

COPD, chronic obstructive pulmonary disease.

> **Q** What are two major conditions that lead to hypercapnic respiratory failure?
>
> **A** Hypoventilation and high dead space

Hypoventilation, or decrease in MV, leads to accumulation of CO_2. Alveolar ventilation decreases as dead space increases, resulting in hypercapnia even with a high MV. Air trapping from obstructive lung disease can also result in high dead space and hypercapnic respiratory failure (Box 3.3).

Box 3.3 Causes of Hypercapnic Respiratory Failure

Hypoventilation	High Dead Space
Respiratory muscle fatigue	COPD
Obesity (i.e., obstructive sleep apnea, obesity hypoventilation syndrome)	Pulmonary embolism
CNS depressants (i.e., opioid, benzodiazepines, alcohol)	Pulmonary hypertension
Spinal cord injury	Pulmonary fibrosis
Neuromuscular disorders (i.e., myasthenia gravis, Guillain–Barré)	
CNS disorders (i.e., stroke, traumatic brain injuries)	
Chest wall disorders (i.e., kyphosis)	

CNS, central nervous system; COPD, chronic obstructive pulmonary disease.

The pattern of increasing dead space can cause a downward spiral into respiratory failure in obstructive airway disease such as COPD (Figure 3.1).

HINT   Any cause of increased RR in obstructive airway diseases can cause rapid decline into respiratory failure.

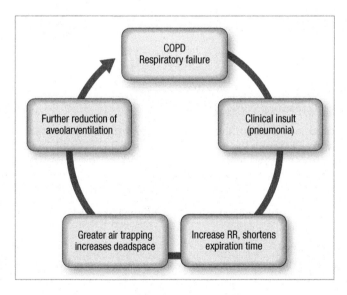

Figure 3.1 Respiratory failure due to dead space.
COPD, chronic obstructive pulmonary disease; RR, respiratory rate.

▶ SYMPTOMS/ASSESSMENT

> **Q** On the ABG, which component should be used to determine whether hypercapnia is acute or chronic?
>
> **A** pH

A patient with chronic respiratory failure with hypercapnia will have a high $PaCO_2$ but a normal pH due to metabolic compensation (elevated bicarbonate level). People with chronic respiratory failure appear to breathe comfortably, without dyspnea, with a low PaO_2.

HINT   A low pH in a COPD patient indicates "acute-on-chronic" respiratory failure.

> Q Which VQ mismatch results in uncoupling the relationship between MV and $PaCO_2$?
>
> A Dead space

Dead space may be recognized on an ABG by the uncoupling of the relationship between the MV and $PaCO_2$. The relationship may actually move in the opposite direction. An increase in MV does not result in a significant decrease in $PaCO_2$ and may actually have a high $PaCO_2$ with the increase in MV.

HINT   An increase in end-tidal CO_2 ($ETCO_2$; capnography) during normal ventilation may indicate the presence of dead space.

> Q What mental status change occurs with hypercapnic respiratory failure?
>
> A Decreased level of consciousness

Hypercapnia results in a decreased level of consciousness. Hypoxia causes agitation, confusion, and delirium initially (Box 3.4).

Box 3.4 Other Signs of Respiratory Failure

Increased WOB	Tachypnea
Use of accessory muscles	Inability to talk in complete sentences
Flushed appearance (hypercapnia)	Tachycardia/arrhythmias
Central cyanosis	Abdominal breathing

WOB, work of breathing.

▶ DIAGNOSIS

> Q Which lung volumes are most commonly measured using the spirometer?
>
> A TV and forced vital capacity (FVC)

TV is the volume moved in and out of the lungs during normal quiet breathing. FVC is the maximal amount of air forcibly expelled from the lungs following maximal inspiration. They are both measured by a spirometer. These tests are used to determine lung capacity during respiratory distress. A normal, spontaneous TV is 400 to 500 mL/breath and normal FVC is 3,700 to 4,800 mL (Table 3.1).

Table 3.1 Lung Volumes and Pulmonary Function Tests

Lung Volume Measurements	Description	Normal Findings
VC	Maximal breath in and maximal breath out (TLC − residual volume)	3,700–4,800 mL
Residual volume	Volume of air in lungs after maximal exhalation	1,200 mL
FRC	Volume of air in lungs after normal quiet exhalation	2,400 mL
TLC	Volume of air in lungs at maximal inspiration (VC + residual volume)	4.7–6.0 L
FEV1	Amount of air exhaled at the end of 1 second of forced exhalation after maximal inspiration	>80% of the predicted FEV1 (based on age, gender, ethnicity of patient)

(continued)

Table 3.1 Lung Volumes and Pulmonary Function Tests (*continued*)

Lung Volume Measurements	Description	Normal Findings
FEV1/FVC ratio	Ratio of FEV1 to the FVC	75%–80%
TV	Amount of air moved in and out during normal quiet breathing	400–500 mL
FVC	Maximal amount of air forcibly exhaled from the lungs following maximal inspiration	3,700–4,800 mL
PEFR	Highest forced expiratory flow (speed)	>80% predicted value (predicted PEFR based on height and gender)

fev1, forced expiratory volume in 1 second; frc, functional residual capacity; FVC, forced vital capacity; PEFR, peak expiratory flow rate; TLC, total lung capacity; tv, tidal volume; VC, vital capacity.

Q **If FEV1 is decreased, but the FVC is normal, resulting in a decreased FEV1/FVC ratio, is this a restrictive or obstructive disease?**

A **Obstructive disease**

An obstructive disease (i.e., asthma, COPD) will result in a decrease in FEV1 with typically normal FVC resulting in a decrease in the FEV1/FVC ratio. In a restrictive disease (i.e., pulmonary fibrosis), both FEV1 and FVC are decreased, which results in a normal FEV1/FVC ratio (Box 3.5).

HINT   FEV1/FVC is used to differentiate an obstructive from a restrictive disease process.

Box 3.5 Severity of Obstruction Determined by FEV1

FEV1 >80% predicted	Normal
FEV1 = 60%–79% predicted	Mild obstruction
FEV1 = 40%–59% predicted	Moderated obstruction
FEV1 <40% predicted	Severe obstruction

FEV1, forced expiratory volume in 1 second.

▶ MANAGEMENT

Q **What is the technique of applying positive pressure ventilation via a mask called?**

A **Noninvasive ventilation (NIV)**

NIV is the technique of supplying positive pressure ventilatory support to the airways through a mask attached to a patient's nose or mouth. It is used in an attempt to avoid artificial airways and the complications associated with them. Continuous positive airway pressure (CPAP) and bilevel positive airway pressure (BiPAP) are forms of NIV.

Q **Which patients are most likely to be successfully treated with NIV?**

A **COPD patients**

Patients who present with exacerbation of COPD or hypercapnic respiratory failure are most likely to benefit from NIV. The ideal patient is one in whom impending respiratory failure is present but in whom cooperation with a mask system is still possible. Early application has shown to be more effective. Respiratory failure resulting in reduction in functional residual capacity (FRC) can cause an increase in work of breathing (WOB), leading to respiratory muscle fatigue. Increasing the FiO_2 alone without assisting the ventilation may not treat the respiratory problem.

HINT   NIV has been found to "buy time" for reversible pulmonary issues (Box 3.6).

Box 3.6 Indications for NIV

COPD	Immunocompromised patient
Status asthmaticus Acute hypoxic respiratory failure	CHF Pulmonary edema
End of life (refusing intubation) or DNI	Cystic fibrosis
Compromised lung function during conscious sedation	Postoperative respiratory failure

COPD, chronic obstructive pulmonary disease; CHF, congestive heart failure; DNI, do not intubate; NIV, noninvasive ventilation.

Q Would NIV be a potential option for an upper gastrointestinal bleeding (GIB) patient with a compromised airway?

A No

NIV with a mask does not protect the airway and can increase risk of aspiration with vomiting. A compromised airway in an upper GIB would be an indication for intubation and mechanical ventilation.

HINT   NIV is not recommended for patients with altered mental status, swallowing abnormalities, or an inability to control secretions due to risk of aspiration (Box 3.7). Do not use NIV in rapidly deteriorating patients at risk for respiratory arrest. These patients should be intubated and placed on mechanical ventilation (Box 3.8).

Box 3.7 Contraindications for NIV

Cardiopulmonary arrest	Pneumocephalus
Hemodynamic instability	Cardiogenic shock
Apnea	Agitated or uncooperative patient
Vomiting	Decreased level of consciousness
GIB Facial trauma or surgery Burns facial region or inhalation injuries	Profuse secretions with need frequent suctioning

GIB, gastrointestinal bleeding; NIV, noninvasive ventilation.

Box 3.8 Advantages and Disadvantages of NIV

Advantage	Disadvantage
Avoid complications of endotracheal intubation (ventilator-acquired pneumonia, tracheal injury)	Does not provide airway protection or ready access for airway toiletry
Decreased length of stay	Increased risk of aspiration
Improved ability in communication	Facial skin abrasions/pressure injuries
Decreased need for sedation or analgesia	Decreased ability to clear secretions
Less antibiotic use	Gastric distension
Reduced need for prolonged mechanical ventilation	Aspiration gastric contents

NIV, noninvasive ventilation.

Q Is CPAP or BiPAP a time-cycled, pressure-targeted mode of NIV?

A BiPAP

BiPAP applies pressure during inspiration and expiration. It is a time-cycled, pressure-targeted mode of ventilation. The pressure provided during inspiration can assist with the work overload of the respiratory muscles, while the expiratory pressure can reduce the breath triggering resistance by the positive end-expiratory pressure (PEEP). CPAP raises the FRC, which may reduce the inspiratory work to breathe but does not provide ventilation.

HINT   BiPAP can further reduce the inspiratory workload over CPAP.

▶ COMPLICATIONS

Q In an awake patient with respiratory distress being placed on NIV, what should be restricted until the patient's tolerance increases and reverses acute ventilatory failure?

A Oral intake

Oral intake should be restricted during the initiation of NIV following acute ventilatory failure to prevent aspiration. Once the patient is tolerating NIV and the acute ventilatory failure is reversed, oral intake may be resumed unless there are other contraindications.

HINT   A nasal mask is better for oral intake because patients are able to take fluids without removing the mask, and there is a lower incidence of aspiration (Box 3.9).

Box 3.9 Complications of NIV

Claustrophobia	Skin breakdown
Aspiration	Gastric distention
Air leaks	

NIV, noninvasive ventilation.

⬤ ACUTE RESPIRATORY DISTRESS SYNDROME

Q What type of pulmonary edema occurs with ARDS?

A Noncardiogenic pulmonary edema

ARDS is defined as a noncardiac pulmonary edema characterized by an increase in capillary permeability with interstitial and alveolar edema of the lungs.

HINT   A patient with congestive heart failure (CHF) can be diagnosed with ARDS if the clinical condition cannot be fully explained by cardiac failure or fluid overload.

Q Is ARDS considered to be a primary or secondary lung disease?

A Secondary

ARDS is a secondary lung disease that develops as a result of a trauma or injury to the lung. The injury may be direct or indirect (through the bloodstream). ARDS is the pulmonary component of the generalized systemic inflammatory process affecting multiple organs and caused by circulating mediators in response to a major insult or injury.

HINT   ARDS is most commonly associated with sepsis/septic shock.

▶ PATHOPHYSIOLOGY

Q Is the excessive fluid in the lungs of an ARDS patient interstitial or intra-alveolar?

A Both interstitial and intra-alveolar

There is damage to the alveolar capillary endothelium resulting in an increase in capillary permeability leading to both interstitial and alveolar edema. The pathophysiology of ARDS centers on the processes of increased microvascular permeability, capillary endothelial damage, and neutrophil activation.

HINT This is what produces "white out" appearance on chest x-ray (CXR).

> **Q** What type of lung cells make up the alveolar–capillary membrane and are responsible for gas exchange?
>
> **A** Type I pneumocytes

The vascular endothelium and alveolar epithelium are made up of Type I pneumocytes and are responsible for integrity and gas exchange. Following injury, the Type I pneumocytes are damaged, which increases alveolar–capillary membrane permeability. The fluid in the lung is composed of sodium, water, and proteins that have crossed into the alveolar and interstitial compartments. Administration of albumin during a period of increased permeability may cause more protein extravasation in the lungs.

HINT Damage to the capillary–alveolar membrane results in initial hypoxemia and CXR changes.

> **Q** What do Type II pneumocytes produce in the lungs?
>
> **A** Surfactant

Damage to Type II pneumocytes results in a decrease and alteration in surfactant, leading to atelectasis, VQ mismatches, and further hypoxemia. Analysis of bronchial lavage after the development of ARDS found the surfactant to be low in phospholipids and proteins A and B, causing the surfactant to be ineffective.

HINT Disruption in the production of surfactant results in further hypoxemia and increased WOB.

> **Q** What role does a surfactant have in the lungs?
>
> **A** Decreases alveolar surface tension

A surfactant decreases surface tension in the alveoli, thus allowing the alveoli to inflate more readily and increase lung compliance. The surfactant "splints" alveoli open and allows for recruitment of alveoli, thus improving the FRC in the lungs. This correlates to WOB.

HINT Balloon analogy: Take a balloon that is already filled with air, empty some of the air out, and then blow it back up. It is easy because of the FRC or "splinting" of the balloon walls open with the remaining air. That is alveoli with a normal surfactant. Now take a new balloon and blow it up. It is much harder to inflate because of the surface tension within the balloon without air. This is alveoli without a normal functioning surfactant.

> **Q** What does the release of pro-inflammatory cytokines and activation of neutrophils cause in the pulmonary vasculature?
>
> **A** Pulmonary hypertension

Pro-inflammatory cytokines (i.e., tumor necrosis factor [TNF]) are released following a pulmonary injury. Pro-inflammatory cytokines recruit neutrophils into the lungs. Activation of the neutrophils in the lungs causes the release of toxic chemical mediators, further damaging the alveolar–capillary membrane, increasing capillary permeability, and causing pulmonary vasoconstriction leading to pulmonary edema. The resulting PH worsens hypoxemia and increases the workload of the right ventricle.

HINT Pulmonary vasoconstriction creates dead space, worsening the VQ mismatch.

> **Q** What is the chronic change that occurs in the lungs in ARDS patients?
>
> **A** Fibrosis

Fibrosis of the lung occurs during the proliferative phase. The repair component involves proliferation and altered function of endothelial cells, Type II pneumocyte cells, and interstitial matrix cells. Type I cells are destroyed and are replaced with Type II cells, which leads to fibrosis.

HINT The fibrosis contributes to a decrease in lung compliance of ARDS patients and long-term complications.

Q Which two lung volumes significantly decrease in ARDS?

A Vital capacity (VC) and FRC

There is a decrease in lung capacity and FRC due to the collapsed airways. There is a nonuniform collapse of the functional lung units.

HINT FRC correlates to WOB. As the FRC decreases, the WOB increases. PEEP applied to the ventilator will increase the FRC and lower the WOB and improve oxygenation (Box 3.10).

Box 3.10 Physiological Effects of ARDS

Decreased FRC	Dead space with pulmonary vasoconstriction
Decreased total lung capacity	Abnormal gas exchange
Hypoxemia due to alveolar shunt	

ARDS, acute respiratory distress syndrome; FRC, functional residual capacity.

HINT The primary VQ mismatch is an alveolar shunt due to the decreased ability to ventilate.

▶ SYMPTOMS/ASSESSMENT

Q What are the initial symptoms in a patient during the early stages of ARDS?

A Hypoxemia, tachypnea, and dyspnea

The symptoms usually have a quick onset, within hours to days after the initial injury or insult to the lungs. The initial presentation is hypoxemia with tachypnea and dyspnea. CXR changes may also be an early sign of ARDS and can occur within 4 to 24 hours of the initial insult (Box 3.11).

HINT A cardinal sign of ARDS is hypoxemia refractory to supplemental oxygen.

Box 3.11 Early Signs of ARDS

Use of accessory muscles	Course crackles
Shallow, rapid breathing	Restlessness
Respiratory alkalosis	Increased work of breathing

ARDS, acute respiratory distress syndrome.

Q What is the primary issue with ventilating a patient in the later stages of ARDS?

A Decreased lung compliance

The lung is considered a "baby lung," with only about one-third of the lung being ventilated during the later stages of ARDS. The lung is filled with fluid, and alveoli would have collapsed, signaling the onset of pulmonary fibrosis. The characteristic problem associated with ventilating ARDS patients is decreased lung compliance (Box 3.12).

HINT Peak inspiratory and plateau pressures increase on the ventilator due to decrease in lung compliance.

Box 3.12 Symptoms of ARDS at Later Stages

Increase PIP	Tachycardia
Course crackles and rhonchi bilateral	Severe hypoxemia
Metabolic acidosis due to elevated lactate levels	Pallor and cyanosis
Respiratory acidosis due to hypercarbia	Bilateral pulmonary infiltrates
Use of accessory muscles and nasal flaring	Increased work of breathing

ARDS, acute respiratory distress syndrome; PIP, peak inspiratory pressure.

▶ DIAGNOSIS

Q **What are the primary CXR criteria used to diagnose ARDS?**

A **Bilateral fluffy infiltrates**

ARDS is a bilateral lung disease characterized by pulmonary infiltrates. It is commonly seen as "white out on CXR." A CT scan may also be used to determine the presence of bilateral fluffy infiltrates (Box 3.13).

Box 3.13 Berlin Definition of ARDS

Acute onset	Within 7 days of a defined event
Impaired oxygenation	Abnormal PaO_2/FiO_2 ratio (PF ratio <200)
Bilateral fluffy infiltrates	CXR or CT scan
Not fully explained by cardiac failure or fluid overload	

ARDS, acute respiratory distress syndrome; CXR, chest x-ray; PF ratio, PaO_2/FiO_2 ratio.

Q **Severe ARDS is defined by what PaO_2/FiO_2 ratio?**

A **Less than 100**

The Berlin definition of ARDS includes categories of severity based on the PaO_2/FiO_2 ratio (also called the PF ratio). To calculate, use the PaO_2 from the blood gas and divide by the FiO_2 the patient was on when the blood gas was drawn. The normal PF ratio is >350.

HINT Remember, when calculating the PF ratio, use the decimal point (40% is 0.40; Table 3.2).

Table 3.2 Severity of ARDS

Severity of ARDS	PaO_2/FiO_2 Ratio
Mild	200–300
Moderate	100–200
Severe	<100

ARDS, acute respiratory distress syndrome.

For example:
If a patient's PaO_2 is 80 on 50% FiO_2,
$80 \div 0.50 = 160$

HINT A normal PaO_2 is only normal on room air. If on a higher FiO_2, a normal PaO_2 (80–100 mmHg) may actually be abnormal. PF ratio calculation is used to determine severity of impaired oxygenation.

Q **What is the most common indirect injury to the lungs that can result in the development of ARDS?**

A **Sepsis**

The development of respiratory failure following a clinical injury to the lungs, either directly or indirectly, leads to the diagnosis of ARDS. An indirect injury is usually the result of an inflammatory reaction to a certain disease or clinical state. Direct injury to the alveoli or lung parenchyma results in a loss of integrity of the alveolar–capillary membrane, leading to ARDS (Boxes 3.14 and 3.15).

Box 3.14 Indirect Lung Injury

Sepsis/septic shock	DKA
Pancreatitis	Drug or alcohol overdose
Massive trauma	Cardiopulmonary bypass
Multiple blood transfusions	Amniotic fluid embolus
Prolonged severe shock	Tissue necrosis

DKA, diabetic ketoacidosis.

Box 3.15 Direct Lung Injury

Excessive fluid resuscitation	Pneumonitis
Inhalation injuries (smoke or toxic gases)	Drug inhalation
Oxygen toxicity	Pulmonary contusions
Aspiration	Pneumonia
Near drowning	Pulmonary embolism

▶ MANAGEMENT

Q Is the current management of ARDS aimed at reversing permeability abnormalities or maintaining ventilation and organ perfusion?

A Maintaining ventilation and organ perfusion

The goal in managing an ARDS patient is to maintain acceptable gas exchange with minimal complications. Maintaining gas exchange and an aerobic metabolism will limit the hypoperfusion and organ dysfunction. When determining the appropriate ventilatory technique, the goal of oxygenation must be carefully weighed against the potential for further injury to the lungs.

HINT Positive pressure ventilation can cause further injury to lungs, and nonconventional modes of ventilation may be used to limit injury.

Q What is trauma to the lungs caused by repeated cycles of recruitment and derecruitment called?

A Atelectrauma

Atelectrauma is the injury caused by repeated cycles of recruitment and derecruitment of the alveoli. Damage to conducting airways may be secondary to the cyclical collapse and reopening of the terminal airways with shear stress. A high-pressure alarm sounding on the ventilator of an ARDS patient may indicate pneumothorax from barotrauma.

HINT Lung recruitment with PEEP can limit the injury of atelectrauma (Table 3.3).

Table 3.3 Ventilatory Complications in ARDS Patients

Complication	Description	Prevention
Barotrauma	High ventilatory pressures cause air to mitigate out of alveoli into the extrapulmonary space	Maintain PIP <40 cm H_2O PLP <30 cm H_2O
Atelectrauma	Hearing effect caused by repeated cyclic recruitment and derecruitment of alveoli	Utilize lung recruitment techniques to maintain alveoli open; PEEP

(continued)

Table 3.3 Ventilatory Complications in ARDS Patients (*continued*)

Complication	Description	Prevention
Volutrauma	Caused by overdistention and stretch-type injury with greater inflammatory response in lungs	Use small TVs for ventilating; recommended 6 mL/kg TV
Biotrauma	Release local mediators in lung and associated with large TV	Use small TVs, avoid overdistension on alveoli
Oxygen toxicity	Causes endothelial damage, decrease in surfactant, thickening of alveoli membrane, decreased macrophage activity	Maintain oxygenation on FiO$_2$ <60%

PEEP, positive end-expiratory pressure; PIP, peak inspiratory pressure; PLP, plateau pressure; TV, tidal volume.

Q What is the recommended TV for a patient with ARDS?

A 4 to 6 mL/kg

ARDS patients have been found to benefit from small TVs with lower plateau pressures (PLPs) with improved outcomes. The recommendation is TV of 4 to 6 mL/kg with PLP less than 30 to 35 cm H$_2$O. The high inspiratory pressure required to deliver traditional TVs (8–10 mL/kg) to the remaining normal lung tissue causes significant overdistension, barotrauma, and diffuse alveolar damage. Low TVs have also been associated with less release of intra-alveolar cytokines.

HINT   Use ideal body weight (in kilogram), not actual body weight, to calculate TV (Box 3.16).

Box 3.16 Goals of Ventilation

Oxygenation	Maintain >88%–90%
FiO$_2$	<60%–70%
PIP	< 40–45 cm H$_2$O
PLP	< 30 cm H$_2$O
TV	6 mL/kg ideal body weight
RR	Up to 35 bpm (MV 7–9 L/min)

bpm, breaths per minute; MV, minute ventilation; PIP, peak inspiratory pressure; PLP, plateau pressure; RR, respiratory rate; TV, tidal volume.

Q Which lung volume does PEEP increase when ventilating a patient with ARDS?

A FRC

FRC is the volume in the lungs at the end of expiration. PEEP is used to increase FRC of acutely injured lungs, resulting in an increased alveolar size, holding the alveoli open, and recruitment of collapsed alveoli. This increases the surface area for gas exchange and decreases shunting.

HINT   Monitor hemodynamics closely because PEEP can have a paradoxical effect on oxygen delivery by reducing venous return and cardiac output (CO).

Q What is that point on a compliance curve below which the alveoli will collapse?

A Lower inflection point

A compliance curve in the lungs has two inflection points. The lower inflection point is the critical opening pressure of most alveoli that are available for recruitment. It is the minimal pressure required to begin to open the alveoli, below which the alveoli will collapse. The upper inflection point is the maximal pressure beyond which no more alveoli will be recruited and overdistention occurs.

HINT   The pressure–volume curve is a method used to determine the amount of PEEP required to maximally recruit and maintain lung volumes without overdistention.

Q   What is the ventilatory technique that is used to reduce a patent's ventilatory support to a minimally acceptable PaO$_2$ while allowing PaCO$_2$ to rise?

A   Permissive hypercapnia

To achieve the low plateau and peak inspiratory pressures recommended, TVs may be very low with resulting elevations in the PaCO$_2$. Manipulation of the ventilator settings to lower the PaCO$_2$ may increase risk of barotrauma, volutrauma, and/or atelectrauma. This strategy is a deliberate hypoventilation in an effort to reduce pulmonary overdistention and high pressures within the noncollapsed portion of the lung (Box 3.17).

HINT   Ventilator changes usually made to correct hypercapnia include increasing the RR and/or TV.

Box 3.17 Permissive Hypercapnia Management

No upper limit of PaCO$_2$
Allow pH to decrease to at least 7.20 before treatment
If <7.20, sodium bicarbonate or THAM may be administered

Q   What clinical condition would be contraindicated in performing permissive hypercapnia?

A   Increased intracranial pressure (ICP)

Permissive hypercapnia is contraindicated in neurological patients with increased ICP. Hypercapnia causes cerebral vasodilation with an increase in cerebral blood volume, thus increasing ICP. Other conditions that may also be contraindicated are active coronary artery disease (hypercapnia causes a negative inotropic effect), arrhythmias, hypovolemia, and GIB.

Q   Which mode of ventilation is used to control peak inspiratory pressures?

A   Pressure-controlled ventilation (PCV)

PCV sets an upper pressure limit on the ventilator (pressure control) that determines the end of the inspiratory cycle and inspiratory volume. The TV varies per breath, depending upon the compliance of the airway and lungs. This method of ventilation is used to limit excessive airway pressures and improve mean airway pressure. Inverse inspiratory to expiratory ration (I:E) ratios may be used in this mode of ventilation.

HINT   The flow waveform used to deliver a breath in PCV is a decelerating waveform (volume control uses a square waveform).

Q   What change in the ventilator settings can be made to increase TV in PCV?

A   Increasing pressure limit

The inspiratory volume stops being delivered at a preset inspiratory pressure. Within a static period of lung compliance and airway resistance, an increase in the set pressure limit will increase the TV delivered. It allows a greater airway pressure to be reached before the end of inspiration.

HINT   Remember, airway resistance and lung compliance affect the amount of inspiratory volume delivered per breath in pressure-controlled ventilation.

Q   Which mode of ventilation not only uses a pressure limit but also allows spontaneous breathing throughout the cycle?

A   Airway pressure release ventilation (APRV)

APRV is a pressure-limited, time-cycled mode of ventilation used to manage ARDS patients. It allows for spontaneous breathing throughout the respiratory cycle. APRV is considered a lung-protective mode of ventilation that allows for the recruitment of alveoli and splints alveoli open to prevent injury from derecruitment. The proposed advantage is the ability to maintain a higher mean airway pressure while the peak alveolar pressure remains lower and allows for spontaneous breathing.

HINT   This mode of ventilation is also called bilevel, biphasic, and bi-vent.

> **Q** In the APRV mode of ventilation, is the majority of the time in the higher pressure (P high) or lower pressure (P low)?
>
> **A** Higher pressure (P high)

A baseline high pressure (called P high) and a low pressure (called P low) are set. Mandatory breaths of the ventilator are delivered by releasing the high pressure briefly to the low pressure, which allows the lungs to partially deflate, then quickly return to the high pressure. The amount of time spent at the high pressure is about 80% to 95% of the cycle. Other parameters set in this mode are T high and T low. T high is the time spent in the high pressure, and T low is the amount of time in the low pressure.

HINT   Remember, spontaneous breathing occurs throughout this cycle, increasing MV.

> **Q** What occurs when the expiratory time is limited in modes such as APRV or inverse I:E ratio with pressure control?
>
> **A** Auto-PEEP

When using the inverse I:E ratio, the expiratory time is shorter than the inspiratory time, allowing a residual amount of air to remain in the lungs, called intentional auto-PEEP. In APRV, the release time from high P to low P is much shorter than the equilibrium time in high P, causing air trapping or intentional auto-PEEP. Auto-PEEP is used to prevent derecruitment of alveoli and is optimally above the level of the lower inflection point.

HINT   Auto-PEEP occurs by restricting expiratory flow time. Monitoring of the amount of auto-PEEP is necessary when using these modes of ventilation.

> **Q** What ventilator settings can be changed to improve oxygenation in the APRV mode besides FiO_2?
>
> **A** Prolong T high or increase P high

Prolonging the time at the higher pressure (T high) or increasing the high pressure (P high) can improve oxygenation. These changes will increase the mean airway pressure and recruit more alveoli. Hypercapnia is an expected consequence of APRV ventilation, and permissive hypercapnia is typically used in combination with the APRV. If severe, reduce the $PaCO_2$ by reducing the T high (this increases the frequency of releases).

HINT   Pressure support can be added to APRV to improve spontaneous breaths.

> **Q** What is the method of weaning the ventilator in APRV mode?
>
> **A** Decrease P high and prolong T high

By decreasing the P high, there is less pressure splinting the alveoli, and lengthening the T high decreases the frequency of release allowing for more of the breaths to be spontaneous breaths over mechanical. The goal is for most or all of the MV to be from spontaneous breaths (Box 3.18).

HINT   APRV can be changed to CPAP once the spontaneous breaths are adequate to complete the weaning process.

Box 3.18 Advantages and Disadvantages of APRV

Advantage	Disadvantage
Spontaneous breaths, better ventilation for dependent regions of lungs	Potential overstretching of alveoli

(continued)

Box 3.18 Advantages and Disadvantages of APRV (*continued*)

Advantage	Disadvantage
Relatively comfortable form of ventilation and is well tolerated	Lack of ability to spontaneously breathe in this mode of ventilation
Less sedation	Increased ICP due to increase in mean airway pressures
Greater mean airway pressure	Increase in bronchopleural fistulas (worsening of air leaks)
Improved venous return and cardiac output	Patient maintains the work of breathing
Lower peak pressures	

APRV, airway pressure release ventilation.

Q What is the method of delivering the MV in high-frequency oscillatory ventilation (HFOV)?

A High frequencies and low TV

High-frequency ventilation is the use of higher than normal frequencies of ventilation with very small TVs. An oscillator ventilator provides a continuous flow in the circuit and oscillates or moves the air back and forth with a piston. In theory, HFOV minimizes alveolar overdistension and recruitment–derecruitment injury. It has the unique benefit that both inspiration and expiration are active.

HINT HFOV may be described as CPAP with a "wriggle."

Q In HFOV, how is the frequency of ventilation measured?

A Hertz (Hz)

The frequency is measured in hertz on an oscillator ventilator. The piston-driven diaphragm delivers the small TVs at frequencies between 3 and 15 Hz. Lowering the frequency will increase TVs and CO_2 elimination. The power is also set, which means the piston pressure swings generating the TV. Increasing the power will increase CO_2 elimination by increasing the TV.

HINT 15 Hz is equal to 15 breaths per second.

Q In HFOV mode of ventilation, oxygenation is dependent on what settings?

A Mean positive airway pressure (mPaw) and FiO_2

The mPaw and FiO_2 can be titrated to improve oxygenation. Improvement in VQ matching and oxygenation is found to correlate well with high mPaw. The mPaw is set in this mode of ventilation. The initial setting is typically 5 cm H_2O pressure above the mPaw in a conventional ventilator.

HINT Usually when the mPaw has been titrated down to less than 24 cm H_2O pressure and FiO_2 is 40% to 50%, the patient is ready to return to a conventional ventilator.

Q In transpulmonary pressure-guided ventilation, where is the catheter place, which is used to determine optimal PEEP levels?

A Esophageal

Transpulmonary pressure-guided ventilation uses an esophageal balloon catheter to estimate pleural pressures and titrate PEEP based upon the lung and chest wall mechanics.

HINT This method targets the end alveolar pressure to prevent atelectrauma.

Q A patient with ARDS demonstrating problems with maintaining saturations can be placed in what position?

A Prone

Lung infiltrates and damaged lung units in ARDS are not uniformly distributed. CT scans have found that dependent portions of the lungs are more affected, and less dependent areas remain normal with normal compliance. The prone position can improve oxygenation by improving ventilation perfusion ratios in the dependent regions. The use of the intermittent prone position can improve oxygenation. It is recommended in refractory hypoxemic patients (Boxes 3.19 and 3.20).

Box 3.19 Risks of Prone Position

Inadvertent dislodgement of the endotracheal tube	Initial worsening in respiratory status
Inadvertent dislodgement of lines or tubes	Facial edema
Development of pressure ulcerations	Hemodynamic instability

Box 3.20 Other Experimental Therapies

	NO or prostacyclin
Surfactant	Perflourocarbons ("liquid ventilation")

NO, nitric oxide.

▶ COMPLICATIONS

Q What is the first pharmacological intervention for ventilator dyssynchrony ("bucking the ventilator")?

A Sedation

Sedation is the first step to improve ventilator–patient synchrony. Neuromuscular blocking agents (NMBAs) can be used but are considered to be the last resort. If the patient continues to "fight" the ventilator, and ventilatory pressures remain elevated with sedation and analgesics alone, then adding an NMBA would be appropriate.

HINT Ensure adequate sedation and pain management before initiating NMBA.

Q How are NMBAs monitored?

A Peripheral nerve stimulation using the train-of-four (TOF)

Patients receiving NMBAs should be monitored with both observation and TOF. The peripheral nerve stimulator is used to assess neuromuscular blockade, and the most common stimulation is called TOF. Frequently used sites for peripheral nerve stimulation include the ulnar and facial nerves. Count the number of twitches. If stimulating the ulnar nerve, observe the thumb and the facial nerve, watch the muscle above the eyebrow.

HINT The goal for adjusting NMBA is typically to achieve one or two twitches (Table 3.4); 0/4 twitches indicate the need to lower the infusion rate to prevent prolonged paralysis.

Table 3.4 Train of Four Twitches

Number of Twitches	Amount of Blockade
4/4	0%–75% receptors blocked
3/4	At least 75% receptors blocked
2/4	80% receptors blocked
1/4	90% receptors blocked
0/4	100% receptors blocked

TOF, train of four.

Q What is the long-term complication of using NMBAs?

A Critical illness polyneuropathy or myopathy

Prolonged immobilization may contribute to the development of critical illness polyneuropathy and myopathy. The use of NMBA has been associated with long-term skeletal muscle weakness (Box 3.21). Long-term complications are more likely associated with neuromuscular, neurocognitive, and psychological rather than pulmonary dysfunction (Box 3.22).

HINT   A combination of NMBA and steroids may significantly increase the risk of skeletal muscle weaknesses.

Box 3.21 Acute Complications of ARDS

Cardiac dysrhythmias	Sepsis
Acute renal failure	Injury to lung with positive pressure ventilation
Thrombocytopenia	Chronic lung changes
Gastrointestinal bleed	

ARDS, acute respiratory distress syndrome.

Box 3.22 Long-Term Complications of ARDS

Neuromuscular	Neurocognitive	Psychological
Critical illness polyneuropathy Myopathy	Memory deficits Attention deficits Decreased ability to concentrate Alteration in higher cognitive functioning	Depression Anxiety Posttraumatic stress disorder (PTSD)

ARDS, acute respiratory distress syndrome; PTSD, posttraumatic stress disorder.

● ACUTE PULMONARY EMBOLISM

Q What is the most common site of origin for thrombus in a PE?

A Leg veins

A PE is defined as a partial or complete obstruction of a branch in the pulmonary arterial system. The most common site of origin is the leg or pelvic thrombosis. Deep vein thrombosis (DVT) and PE are caused by the same underlying physiological event, and the combination is called venous thromboembolism (VTE). The actual frequencies of VTEs are underestimated, and an unknown cause of death in the hospital may actually be a PE diagnosed on autopsy (Box 3.23).

Box 3.23 Origins of Thromboemboli

Leg veins (popliteal and calf)	Upper extremities
Pelvic	Right atrium (atrial fibrillation, tricuspid valve)
Inferior vena cava (iliac and femoral veins)	Right ventricle (myocardial contusion, right ventricular dysfunction)
Superior vena cava	Renal and hepatic veins

HINT   Peripherally inserted central catheter (PICC) lines are a common cause of an upper extremity DVT. Assessing and monitoring for DVTs after placement of PICC lines is recommended.

Q Which has a greater risk of embolization, DVT in the calf or popliteal veins?

A Popliteal veins

Calf DVTs involve the distal veins (i.e., peroneal, anterior tibial, posterior tibial), whereas the popliteal is a proximal vein. The proximal veins are more likely to extend or become an embolus. Distal DVTs may not require anticoagulation therapy.

HINT Femoral vein is at a greater risk of embolism due to proximity.

Q What is the highest risk for the development of a DVT?

A Immobilization

Critically ill patients are at high risk for the development of VTE. The majority of the patients are immobilized for long periods of time following their acute injury or disease process. Proactive nursing involves getting patients out of bed and ambulating as early as possible, based upon the stability of the patient (Box 3.24).

HINT Well's criteria are recommended for risk stratification of patients for likelihood of DVT.

Box 3.24 Risk Factors for VTE

Immobilization
  Bed rest
  Prolonged sitting position (traveling)
  Casts
  Paralysis
	Trauma
	  Major trauma
	  Orthopedic trauma
	  Spinal cord injury
	  Chronic venous insufficiency

Surgeries
  Orthopedic
  Vascular
  Major general surgery
  Laparoscopic surgery
	Heart failure
	Central venous lines (PICC lines)
	Malignancy
	Pregnancy
	Oral contraceptives and estrogen replacement
	Obesity

Hypercoagulable predisposition Dehydration	Increasing age

PICC, peripherally inserted central catheter; VTE, venous thromboembolism.

HINT Hypercoagulable states may be inherited or acquired.

▶ PATHOPHYSIOLOGY

Q What is the primary determinant of the severity of the PE?

A Size of the embolus

The hemodynamic consequence of a PE is determined by the size of the embolus and the amount of lung obstruction. Emboli range in severity from two to three pulmonary segments to 15 to 16 segments that are underperfused. Sudden death is caused by obstruction of the pulmonary trunk and/or both main pulmonary arteries. This is called a "saddle embolus."

HINT Comorbidities and the degree of pulmonary vasoconstriction also affect the outcomes.

Q With hemodynamically significant PE, what is the consequence of increased pulmonary resistance?

A RV failure

A sudden increase in pulmonary artery pressure due to a partial or complete obstruction and pulmonary vasoconstriction can cause RV dysfunction. RV failure causes the interventricular septal wall to deviate toward the left, resulting in a smaller left ventricular (LV) chamber. The pulmonary obstruction and RV failure cause less blood to flow to the LV, thus causing a decrease in CO.

HINT Symptoms of RV failure indicate a significant obstruction in the pulmonary vasculature and potential for hemodynamic instability.

▶ SYMPTOMS/ASSESSMENT

Q What is the most common initial presentation of a patient with a PE?

A Sudden-onset dyspnea

Sudden onset of dyspnea, tachypnea, and hypoxemia should raise the clinical suspicion of a PE. Symptoms of a PE are neither sensitive nor specific and require the clinician to consider the risk factors along with the presentation to recognize the PE (Boxes 3.25 and 3.26).

HINT   A PE can mimic other high-acuity disorders such as acute myocardial infarction.

Box 3.25 Symptoms of PE

Dyspnea	Hemoptysis
Tachypnea	Cough
Hypoxemia	Crackles
Chest pain	Feelings of "impending doom"

PE, pulmonary embolism.

Box 3.26 Other Associated Signs of PE

Palpitations	Tachycardia
Low-grade fever	Systolic murmur
Development of S_3 or S_4	Crackles
Syncope	Wheezing
Diaphoresis	New-onset atrial fibrillation

PE, pulmonary embolism.

▶ DIAGNOSIS

Q What 12-lead EKG finding is classic for PE with RV dysfunction?

A $S_1Q_3T_3$

The $S_1Q_3T_3$ is the EKG manifestation of acute pressure and volume overload of the RV. An S wave in lead I signifies a complete or more often incomplete right bundle branch block (RBBB). Lead III will have a Q wave, slight ST elevation, and an inverted T wave. These findings are due to the pressure and volume overload in the right ventricle, which causes repolarization abnormalities in leads correlating to the RV.

Q What laboratory test may be used to assist with the diagnosis of PE?

A D-dimer

The fibrin fragment D-dimer is produced by the degradation of fibrin by plasmin (proteolytic enzyme that breaks down clots). If the D-dimer is negative, the possibility of a PE is very low. An elevated D-dimer though only determines the need for further diagnostic evaluation. Elevated serum troponin and BNP levels may occur in moderate or large PE. Elevated levels of troponin and BNP can correlate with an increased risk of death.

HINT   Immediate postoperative patients will have elevated D-dimer, so a D-dimer test is not able to exclude PE in these patients.

> **Q** On a CXR, what is the presence of dilated pulmonary vessels with sharp cut-offs called?
>
> **A** Westermark sign

A CXR is typically obtained to exclude other pulmonary and cardiac abnormalities. It is not used to diagnose a PE exclusively. A late sign that can sometimes be found on a CXR is a Westermark sign, which is the dilation of the pulmonary vessels with a sharp cut-off. Atelectasis, small pleural effusion, and elevated diaphragm may also be found, but are nonspecific for a PE.

HINT   Hamptom's hump is another finding in PE, which is a wedged-shaped opacity at costophrenic angle indicating pulmonary infarction.

> **Q** Which test can be performed to diagnose a DVT?
>
> **A** Ultrasound

Compression ultrasound of the proximal leg veins or whole-leg ultrasonography may be performed to screen for a DVT in lower extremities. The presence of a known DVT in addition to clinical symptoms of a PE increases the likelihood of a positive PE diagnosis.

HINT   May have false-negative findings in obese patients and require further testing (i.e., CT venography).

> **Q** Which diagnostic test is recommended in a suspected high-risk PE hemodynamically unstable patient?
>
> **A** CT arteriogram (CTA)

A CTA is recommended to visualize the pulmonary arteries to confirm the diagnosis of PE in a high-risk patient suspected of PE. It is more accurate than a VQ scan and is replacing VQ scans and pulmonary angiograms as the gold standard for diagnosing PE. VQ scans may be used instead of CTA in patients with renal failure or known allergy to contrast.

HINT   If the patient is too unstable to transport for a CTA, then a bedside echocardiogram may be used (Box 3.27).

Box 3.27 Findings on Echocardiogram of PE

Abnormal right ventricular wall motion (hypokinesis)	Increased pulmonary artery pressure
Right ventricular dilation	Inferior vena cava congestion
Paradoxical septal motion	Dilated pulmonary artery
Tricuspid valve insufficiency	

PE, pulmonary embolism.

HINT   Transesophageal echocardiogram can confirm the diagnosis PE by showing emboli in main pulmonary artery.

▶ MANAGEMENT

> **Q** What is the pharmacological therapy recommended for preventing VTE in a high-risk patient?
>
> **A** Anticoagulation therapy

Heparin (unfractionated or low molecular), fondaparinux, or factor Xa inhibitors may be used to prevent a VTE in a high-risk patient as long as the patient is not at high risk for bleeding. Intermittent pneumatic compression devices (mechanical devices) may be used in patients with high bleeding risk instead of anticoagulation therapy.

HINT   All critically ill patients are considered at a high risk for VTE and should have some type of prophylaxis, including both mechanical and anticoagulation if not contraindicated.

> **Q** What is the pharmacological management recommended for a known DVT in the proximal leg veins or PE and no cancer?
>
> **A** Direct oral anticoagulants (DOACs)

The 2016 American College of Clinical Pharmacy (ACCP) guidelines recommend use of DOACs, which include dabigatran, rivaroxaban, apixaban, or edoxaban over vitamin K antagonists (VKA) for leg DVT or PE. Heparin (unfractionated or low molecular) is recommended as the initial treatment for a leg DVT or PE if administering dabigatran or edoxaban and overlapped if using VKA for 5 days or until the international normalized ratio (INR) is above 2.0 for longer than 24 hours. If not using DOACs, VKA (i.e., Warfarin) is recommended over LMWH.

HINT   If the patient is at high risk for bleeding (i.e., postoperative patient), an inferior vena cava filter may be placed instead of anticoagulation therapy.

> **Q** Which of the anticoagulation therapies used in treating a PE is recommended if severe renal failure is present?
>
> **A** Unfractionated heparin

Unfractionated heparin is recommended in renal-failure patients over low-molecular-weight heparin (LMWH) or Arixtra (fondaparinux). The therapeutic goal is 1.5 to 2.5 times the normal activated partial thromboplastin time (aPTT value). The recommended length of therapy with anticoagulants is a minimum of 5 days in combination with warfarin; then, warfarin is administered for 3 to 6 months.

HINT   Fondaparinux or argatroban (direct thrombin inhibitor) is the drug that may be used if the patient has developed heparin-induced thrombocytopenia (HIT) Type II.

> **Q** What would be the indication for administering a systemic thrombolytic to a patient diagnosed with a PE?
>
> **A** Persistent hypotension

A patient persistently hemodynamically unstable (blood pressure [BP] < 90 mmHg) may be treated with systemic thrombolytic therapy. It is not recommended in patients hemodynamically stable. The thrombolytic recommended is tissue plasminogen activator (tPA) due to its short infusion time. The infusion should be administered over 2 hours through a venous catheter. Heparin may be stopped during the infusion and restarted after the aPTT is less than 80 seconds. Thrombolytic therapy has shown improved pulmonary artery pressures, oxygenation, and RV performance but has a higher risk for bleeding. It is not recommended in stable patients with a PE.

HINT   In cardiac arrest caused by suspected PE, recommend administering thrombolytics even during resuscitation.

▶ COMPLICATIONS

> **Q** Obstruction in the pulmonary artery can lead to what major complication of the lung tissue?
>
> **A** Pulmonary infarction

Obstruction of the pulmonary artery causes a loss of blood flow distal to the balloon and may result in a pulmonary infarction. This commonly presents with dyspnea and hemoptysis (Box 3.28).

Box 3.28 Symptoms of Pulmonary Infarction

Dyspnea	Pleural effusions
Hemoptysis	Decreased excursion of affected hemothorax
Pleuritic pain	Pleural friction rubs

> **Q** Sudden-onset dyspnea associated with hypotension and an S_3 gallop would indicate which complication of a PE?
>
> **A** RV failure

RV failure caused by PH can result in a decreased CO and hypotension. The presence of RV involvement with a PE increases the risk of mortality. Elevated cardiac troponin and brain natriuretic peptides (BNP) are also predictors of risk of complications and mortality in a PE.

HINT An S_3 gallop typically indicates the presence of heart failure (HF) and is the clue in this question (Box 3.29).

Box 3.29 Symptoms of Right Ventricular Failure

Sudden unexplained dyspnea	Cyanosis
Jugular distention	Systolic murmur (tricuspid regurgitation)
S_3 gallop	New or complete RBBB
Hypotension	

RBBB, right bundle branch block.

> **Q** What is the development of leg ulcer in the affected leg of a known DVT called?
>
> **A** Post-thrombotic syndrome (PTS)

PTS develops in about 50% of the patients with a DVT in the lower extremity. The clot results in venous hypertension, which leads to PTS. The symptoms include chronic leg pain, redness, swelling, and venous ulcerations.

HINT PTS is the term that replaced postphlebitic syndrome.

> **Q** What long-term complication can result in elevated pulmonary artery pressures?
>
> **A** Chronic thromboembolic pulmonary hypertension (CTPH)

CTPH is defined as pulmonary artery (PA) pressures greater than 25 mmHg that persist for longer than 6 months after PE is diagnosed. Symptoms may not be present initially ("honeymoon period") even though PH exists. It is usually recognized when the patient presents later with dyspnea, hypoxemia, and RV dysfunction. Surgical management of choice for symptomatic CTPH is vascular disobliteration with pulmonary endarterectomy. Medical management is similar to primary PH (Box 3.30).

HINT Fibrinolytic therapy has been found to reduce the incidence of CTPH.

Box 3.30 Other Complications of PE

Sudden cardiac death	Atrial or ventricular arrhythmias
Shock	Pleural effusions
Pulseless electrical activity (PEA)	Severe hypoxemia

PE, pulmonary embolism; PEA, pulseless electrical activity.

CHRONIC DISORDERS (COPD EXACERBATIONS/ SEVERE ASTHMA/STATUS ASTHMATICUS)

> **Q** What is the most common cause of acute respiratory failure in a COPD patient?
>
> **A** Pulmonary infection

COPD is defined as symptoms of airflow obstruction in the absence of an alternative explanation for symptoms that is not fully reversible. Airflow obstruction is defined as postbronchodilator FEV1 – FVC ratio less than 0.70. Frequently, pulmonary infections (i.e., pneumonia, infectious bronchitis) are the cause of acute exacerbation and admission into the ICU for ventilatory support. These infections can be bacterial or viral infections. Other precipitating factors include CHF, PE, pollution, and worsening of chronic airflow.

HINT   Bacterial infections are the most common cause of pulmonary infections in COPD patients.

Q What is the most common factor that contributes to airway hyperresponsiveness in asthma patients?

A Environmental allergens

Exposure to environmental allergens is one of the most common factors contributing to bronchial hyperresponsiveness in asthma. Environmental allergens include cockroach allergens, dust mite allergens, pet allergens, mold spores, sulfur dioxide, ozone, and tobacco smoke (Box 3.31).

Box 3.31 Factors That Contribute to Airway Hyperreactivity

Environmental allergens	Examples: cockroaches, dust mites, pets, mold spores, fungi
Viral respiratory infections	Examples: history of viral pneumonia, rhinovirus
Environmental pollutants	Examples: smoke (tobacco or wood), dust, air pollution
Irritants	Examples: household sprays, paint fumes
Occupational exposure	Examples: coal mining, farmers, painters, plastic manufacture
Latex allergies	
Exercise induced	
GERD	
Chronic sinusitis	
Stress or emotional induced	
Aspirin or NSAID hypersensitivity	
Obesity	
Cold induced	
Nocturnal Asthma	

GERD, gastroesophogeal reflux disease; NSAID, nonsteroidal anti-inflammatory drug.

▶ PATHOPHYSIOLOGY

Q What is the underlying cause of the increased WOB that occurs in acute exacerbation of COPD?

A Greater limitations in airway flow

COPD exacerbation is associated with increased limitations of airway flow, air trapping, and reduction of chest wall and lung compliance leading to an increased WOB. The increased pressure required for airflow may overload the respiratory muscles decreasing MV and worsening hypercapnia. Air trapping generates auto-PEEP, resulting in the patient requiring greater negative inspiratory pressures to initiate a breath and worsen the VQ mismatch and WOB.

HINT   Use of accessory inspiratory muscles indicates an increasing severity of exacerbation (Figure 3.2).

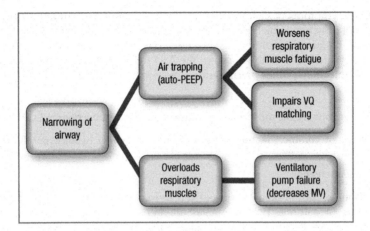

Figure 3.2 Airway obstruction in exacerbation of COPD and severe asthma.

COPD, chronic obstructive pulmonary disease; PEEP, positive end-expiratory pressure; VQ, ventilation perfusion; MV, minute ventilation.

Q What are three physiologic changes found in severe asthma that contribute to airway obstruction?

A Bronchoconstriction, airway inflammation, and mucus plugs

Bronchoconstriction is a result of an immune-mediated response to an allergen. Airway edema is a response to the bronchoconstriction and may be present within 6 to 24 hours. Mucus plugs are exudate composed of cellular debris and eosinophils. Chronic asthmatics may also have some airway remodeling due to the effects of long-term inflammation.

HINT The obstruction to airflow is both into the lung (during inspiration) as well as out of the lung (during expiration).

Q Is the hypoxemia associated with asthma a shunt, a dead space, or both a shunt and a dead space?

A Both

Bronchospasm and inflammation are not uniform throughout. Some alveoli are underventilated in relation to perfusion (shunt), whereas others are overinflated in relation to perfusion (dead space). Hypoxic pulmonary vasoconstriction occurs due to VQ mismatch and will worsen the mismatch.

HINT This also increases the afterload (resistance) of the right ventricle, which interferes with the filling of the left ventricle.

▶ SYMPTOMS/ASSESSMENT

Q What is a clinical sign of diaphragmatic fatigue that may indicate imminent ventilatory failure?

A Paradoxical breathing

Paradoxical breathing occurs when the diaphragm becomes fatigued and is no longer the primary muscle of the inspiratory effort. Normally, the diaphragm drops during inspiration pushing the abdominal wall outward. In paradoxical breathing, the fatigued diaphragm rises and the abdominal wall sinks inward.

HINT Another sign of impending respiratory failure is respiratory alternans (cyclic alternation between abdominal and thoracic breathing).

Q What typically brings a patient to the hospital in an exacerbation of COPD?

A Increased dyspnea

The presentation of exacerbated COPD involves a worsening or a change in the person's typical symptoms. The decrease in airflow experienced with the exacerbation results in increased dyspnea and typically results in the person seeking medical attention (Box 3.32).

Box 3.32 Other Signs of an Acute Exacerbation of COPD

Coughing is more severe or frequent	Increased wheezing and rhonchi
Increase in sputum production	More predominant use of accessory muscles
Sputum color changes from whitish to yellow-green	Orthopnea
Purulent sputum with streaks of blood	Paroxysmal nocturnal dyspnea

COPD, chronic obstructive pulmonary disease.

Q What clinical sign indicates a life-threatening presentation of an acute asthma attack?

A Speaking in incomplete sentences

The current classification of severity of asthma describes a subset of severe acute asthmatic patients who present with a life-threatening attack. These patients are more likely to be admitted to the ICU for management. The clinical sign used to differentiate severity is the degree of dyspnea. Assessing a patient's ability to talk is an objective assessment of dyspnea. An inability to talk accompanied by diaphoresis indicates a more severe episode of asthma, which may be life threatening. Other signs include a decreased level of consciousness or apnea (Box 3.33).

HINT Dyspnea that interferes with conversation indicates a more severe asthma.

Box 3.33 Signs of Exacerbation of Asthma

Wheezing (expiratory and inspiratory)	Anxiety
Cough	Tachypnea
Chest tightness or pain	Tachycardia
Dyspnea	Supraclavical and intercostal retractions
Diaphoresis	Nasal flaring and abdominal breathing
Hypoxemia	

Q In the early presentation of acute severe asthma, is the patient hypercarbic or hypocarbic?

A Hypocarbic

In the early stages of an acute asthmatic crisis, the patient will hyperventilate. This increase in MV lowers the CO_2 levels. The patient may have hypoxemia with hypocarbia due to the greater diffusion of CO_2 than O_2 across the pulmonary bed. Respiratory alkalosis will be present initially. As the airway obstruction increases and the patient's ventilatory effort fatigues, the patient will start to retain CO_2 and develop hypercarbia and respiratory acidosis.

HINT Normalization of the CO_2 (called "pseudonormalization") and the development of hypercapnia may be ominous signs indicating respiratory failure.

Q What is it called when the systolic BP decreases during inspiration due to large changes in intrapleural pressures?

A Pulsus paradoxus

Pulsus paradoxus is defined as a systolic decrease of more than 10 mmHg during inspiration. It can indicate the presence of an obstructed airway disease. During periods of limited airflow and air trapping with asthmatic patients, there is an increase in negative pressure in the intrapleural space during inspiration. This increase in negative pressure increases venous return and filling of the RV. The septal wall displaces toward the LV, limiting the filling of the LV and decreases the stroke volume during inspiration. Arterial waveforms will demonstrate a decrease in waveform amplitude during inspiration.

HINT Pulsus paradoxus is not a good indicator of the severity of acute asthma.

Q Can hypercapnia be detected by monitoring oxygen saturations with a pulse oximetry?

A No

Pulse oximetry is recommended while managing acute exacerbation of asthma, but it does not monitor changes in CO_2 levels. Hypercapnia is a sign of worsening of asthma with a potential need for intubation. Saturations of less than 92% (regardless of the FiO_2) are associated with an increased chance of hypercarbia and indicate the need to obtain an ABG.

HINT May use $ETCO_2$ (capnography) monitoring while managing acute exacerbation of asthma to monitor trends of CO_2.

▶ DIAGNOSIS

Q What finding on the ABG is used to determine whether there is an acute worsening of COPD?

A Respiratory acidosis

Patients who present with chronic respiratory acidosis will have a fully compensated blood gas with a normal pH. $PaCO_2$ and bicarbonate levels will be high. If the patient has an "acute on chronic" respiratory acidosis, the pH will be below the normal range. $PaCO_2$ and bicarbonate levels will also be high, but now they are only partially compensated due to an acute increase in CO_2.

HINT Life-threatening acute respiratory failure in COPD patients are identified with pH <7.25 and change in mental status.

Q What test is needed to establish the diagnosis of asthma?

A Spirometry

A pulmonary function test (PFT; spirometry) is used before and after the patient inhales a short-acting bronchodilator. This determines the presence of airflow obstruction, its severity, and whether it is reversible with short-term management (Box 3.34).

Box 3.34 PFTs With Spirometry

FEV1	FVC
FEV6	FEV1/FVC (FEV1 to FVC ratio)

FEV1, forced expiratory volume in 1 second; FEV6, forced expiratory volume in 6 seconds; FVC, forced vital capacity; PFTs, pulmonary function tests.

▶ MANAGEMENT

Q What would be the priority of care in a COPD patient with a saturation of 87% on room air?

A Administer oxygen

Oxygen should be administered to maintain the oxygen saturation of more than 90% to 92% and PaO_2 of 60 to 65 mmHg. Withholding oxygen during severe hypoxemia can increase complications and mortality.

HINT Higher levels of oxygen will increase dead space and $PaCO_2$ levels, so use the lowest FiO_2 to accomplish goals. The use of nonselective β-adrenergic agonists (i.e., theophylline) is not recommended due to frequently associated cardiac comorbidities of COPD patients (Box 3.35).

Box 3.35 Other Medications Used to Manage Acute Exacerbation COPD

Corticosteroids	Bronchodilators (i.e., Albuterol)
Antibiotics	Anticholinergics (i.e., Ipratropium)

COPD, chronic obstructive pulmonary disease.

Q Between acute exacerbation of COPD and severe asthma, which would more likely require antibiotics?

A COPD

Antibiotics may be useful in COPD patients presenting with pulmonary infections or who show changes in sputum production, color, or amount, even in the absence of pneumonia.

HINT   Antibiotics are not usually recommended in acute asthma.

Q What can be used as a first-line intervention for patients with acute exacerbation of COPD to provide short-term rest of their respiratory muscles?

A NIV

NIV through a nasal or face mask might provide time to manage the acute pulmonary infection and prevent the need for intubation. This allows the respiratory muscles a "rest period" while the underlying pathology that caused the exacerbation is being treated. It decreases WOB and increases alveolar ventilation (Box 3.36).

HINT   The decision to discontinue NIV and intubate is clinical. It involves monitoring hypercapnia/respiratory acidosis and assessing for fatigue or discomfort during NIV. The clinical benefit of NIV in COPD patients will typically be seen within the first few hours. Absence of improvement may be an indication for intubation.

Box 3.36 Potential Physiological Benefit of NIV in COPD

Increased TV	Improved oxygenation
Decreased RR	Better ventilation and gas exchange (lowering $PaCO_2$)
Decreased HR	Lower air trapping (decrease auto-PEEP)

COPD, chronic obstructive pulmonary disease; HR, heart rate; PEEP, positive end-expiratory pressure; RR, respiratory rate; TV, tidal volume.

Q A patient with COPD is intubated and mechanically ventilated. His initial $PaCO_2$ is 58 mmHg. Should the $PaCO_2$ be normalized while the patient is being mechanically ventilated?

A No

Normalization of $PaCO_2$ while on mechanical ventilation will cause difficulties with weaning from the ventilator in the future. Correcting the respiratory acidosis causes metabolic alkalosis (due to high compensatory bicarbonate levels), and the kidneys will "dump" the bicarbonate in the urine. During weaning, the patient will begin to retain CO_2 and develop uncorrected respiratory acidosis.

Q What is the most common PFT used to determine airway responsiveness to interventions during asthma treatment?

A FEV1/FVC ratio

FEV1 is the forced expiratory volume in 1 second and is expressed as a percentage of predicted value or the proportion of FVC.

HINT   The initial assessment goal is to determine the severity of the attack and follow-up assessments are to determine control of the asthma or responsiveness of the patient to interventions.

Q What is the first-line pharmacological agent used to manage acute exacerbation of asthma?

A Short-acting beta-agonists

Inhaled beta-agonists are used to relieve bronchoconstriction. The use of short-acting, $beta_2$-selective agonists is preferred due to fewer cardiovascular side effects. Repeat doses of the beta-agonist can be administered at 15- to 30-minute intervals until an adequate response is obtained. Steroids should also be administered to all acute asthma patients to manage the airway inflammation. Oxygen should be administered to maintain saturations of more than 94% to 98%.

HINT The earlier the steroids are given in an acute attack, the better the outcome.

> **Q** What is the electrolyte abnormality commonly associated with the administration of a beta-agonist?
>
> **A** Hypokalemia

Beta-agonist drugs cause a shift of potassium from the intravascular to the intracellular space. This lowers the plasma potassium levels. Patients being treated with frequent intervals of beta-agonists need to have K^+ levels drawn and closely monitored for complications of hypokalemia.

HINT A treatment for hyperkalemia is nebulized beta-agonist agents to drive the K^+ back into the cells.

> **Q** What nebulized drug can be added to beta-agonist while managing severe or life-threatening asthma?
>
> **A** Ipratropium bromide

Ipratropium bromide, an anticholinergic drug, can produce greater bronchodilation in a shorter time than a beta-agonist alone. It may not be needed in mild to moderate asthma, but it has been found to improve outcomes in severe and life-threatening attacks. Intravenous (IV) magnesium may also be considered as adjunctive therapy with a beta-agonist.

HINT Mg^+ levels need to be monitored if a magnesium infusion is administered to manage the asthma. Symptoms of hypermagnesemia can be muscle weakness and respiratory failure.

▶ COMPLICATIONS

> **Q** A patient remains unresponsive to short-acting bronchodilator therapy. A CXR is ordered. What is the potential complication?
>
> **A** Pneumothorax

A routine CXR is not recommended in the treatment of exacerbation of asthma. If the patient is unresponsive to interventions with short-acting bronchodilators, a CXR may be used to diagnose the presence of a pneumothorax. The increase in negative pressure for inspiration may cause barotrauma and the development of pneumothorax.

> **Q** What is a risk factor that predicts mortality from bronchial asthma?
>
> **A** Previous asthma that required intubation

Severe, near-fatal asthmatic episode requiring intubation is a single predictor of death from future bronchial asthma. Intubation is thought to contribute to a decreased sensation of dyspnea and can be fatal by not seeking medical assistance until too late.

HINT Chronicity of asthma disease or psychiatric illness can also contribute to the blunting of the dyspneic sensation and predict greater mortality.

● ACUTE RESPIRATORY INFECTIONS

> **Q** How long after intubation in which pneumonia develops would the infection be called a ventilator-acquired pneumonia (VAP)?
>
> **A** After 48 hours

VAP is defined as a pneumonia that develops more than 48 hours after endotracheal intubation that was not already present or incubating prior to intubation. VAP is considered a subset of hospital-acquired pneumonia (HAP) or nosocomial pneumonia. Community-acquired pneumonia (CAP) is defined as pneumonia that develops in a nonhospitalized patient or within 48 hours of hospitalization.

HINT   If the patient's clinical symptoms of pneumonia occur before 48 hours, it is not considered to be associated with intubation and mechanical ventilation.

▶ PATHOPHYSIOLOGY

Q What is the greatest risk of HAP?

A Endotracheal intubation

Endotracheal intubation and mechanical ventilation significantly increase the risk of pneumonia. The endotracheal tube (ETT) provides a direct access to oral secretions colonized by bacteria into the lungs. The ETT cuff is not completely occlusive, and secretions can pool above the cuff and leak into the lower airways.

HINT   Bacteria lining the ETT (biofilm) can become dislodged and embolized distal into the lungs from instillation of saline into the tube, suctioning, or repositioning the tube (Box 3.37).

Box 3.37 Risks of an ETT for VAP

Secretions pool in the subglottic region	Stimulates increase in sputum production
Compromises cough	Injuries to tracheal epithelium
Prevents mucociliary clearance	Bacteria aggregates on the tubing (biofilm)

ETT, endotracheal tube; VAP, ventilator-acquired pneumonia.

Q Which patient position can lower the risk of aspiration and VAP?

A Head of bed (HOB) elevated 30 to 45 degrees

Supine position with the HOB flat can increase the risk of aspiration. A recommendation is to keep the patient's HOB elevated at 30 to 45 degrees to prevent VAP, especially during enteral feeding (Box 3.38).

Box 3.38 Risk of VAP

Unintentional extubations/reintubations	Oropharyngeal bacterial colonization
Enteral feeding	Contaminated ventilator circuit
Elevated gastric pH (i.e., H_2 receptor blockers)	Naso-orogastric tubes
Bronchoscopy	Cross-contamination by healthcare providers
Altered mentation	Sedation or paralytic agents in mechanically ventilated patients
Endotracheal cuff pressure less than 20 cm of H_2O	Sinusitis

VAP, ventilator-acquired pneumonia.

▶ SYMPTOMS/ASSESSMENT

Q A patient has been on the ventilator for 72 hours. What CXR change would increase the suspicion of a VAP?

A New or progressive infiltrates

The occurrence of new or progressive infiltrates on CXR should increase suspicion of an HAP/VAP. A complete blood count (CBC) should be performed and the patient assessed for other signs of pneumonia. The diagnosis of VAP is determined by the CXR changes and one or more of the clinical findings of VAP/HAP, indicating that the infiltrate is infectious (Box 3.39).

HINT   Infiltrates may be caused by other pathologies in the lung (i.e., atelectasis).

Box 3.39 Clinical Findings of HAP/VAP

Fever >100.4°F (38°C)	Decrease oxygenation
Purulent secretions	Unexplained hemodynamic instability
Leukocytosis or leukopenia	

HAP, hospital-acquired pneumonia; VAP, ventilator-acquired pneumonia.

▶ DIAGNOSIS

Q Which route of obtaining sputum for a culture is the best to diagnose pneumonia and determine the causative agent?

A Bronchoalveolar lavage (BAL)

A BAL or protected specimen brush (PSB) can be obtained either by bronchoscopy or blindly without a bronchoscopy (distal airway sample). It is considered a quantitative culture that isolates fewer microorganisms growing above the threshold and allows more specific determination of the causative microorganism. A qualitative culture can be obtained by suctioning the ETT, but this sample grows a greater number of bacteria from the upper airway and may not reflect the lower airway. Fiberoptic bronchoscopy with transbronchial biopsy may be useful to detect pathogens such as *mycobacterium*.

HINT Diagnosis of VAP is based on clinical criteria, including the CXR findings and clinical findings.

Q What other pulmonary infection may present with clinical findings but without the new or progressive infiltrate on CXR?

A Ventilator-associated tracheobronchitis (VAT)

VAT is characterized by clinical findings of pulmonary infections (i.e., purulent secretions, fever, leukocytosis) without evidence of pneumonia on CXR (pulmonary infiltrates). VAT is a bacterial infection of the tracheobronchial tree following intubation.

HINT Diagnosis and treatment are similar to VAP.

▶ MANAGEMENT

Q What is a nursing intervention that has been found to lower the incidence of VAP?

A Oral care

Oral decontamination with tooth brushing (includes gums, teeth, and tongue) and rinsing of the oral cavity to remove plaque and bacteria lowers the incidence of VAP. The use of oral antimicrobials, such as chlorhexidine, has been found to lower bacterial colonization in the oral cavity. Meticulous handwashing, routine turning of patients, and aspiration prevention are also correct for nursing interventions in the prevention of VAP (Box 3.40).

Box 3.40 Prevention of HAP/VAP

Proper handwashing	Subglottic suctioning
Oral decontamination	Selective decontamination of digestive tract
Frequent turning of patient	Daily interruption from sedation
Keep HOB elevated 30 to 45 degrees	Avoid unintentional extubations and reintubations
Prevention of aspiration	Silver-coated ETT
Maintain adequate cuff pressures	Prevention of stress-related mucosal disease
Wean and extubate as soon as possible	Prevention of VTE
Avoid saline lavages	

ETT, endotracheal tube; HAP, hospital-acquired pneumonia; HOB, head of bed; VAP, ventilator-acquired pneumonia; VTE, venous thromboembolism.

3. RESPIRATORY SYSTEM REVIEW

HINT   Avoid the use of saline lavage when suctioning the ETT. It increases the risk of VAP and has not been found effective in preventing mucus plugs.

Q VAP caused by a multidrug-resistant (MDR) pathogen would most likely occur as an early or late infection?

A Late infection

Typically, MDR pathogens are found to cause infections, including VAP, in patients with longer than 5 days hospitalization. An early presentation of VAP is most commonly caused by pathogens more susceptible to antibiotics. Late presentation is commonly associated with MDR and is more difficult to manage. Antibiotics are the treatment of VAP and may be administered aerosolized in combination with IV.

HINT   Initiation of appropriate antibiotics prior to culture results depend on the length of hospitalization and other risk factors for MDR pathogens.

▶ COMPLICATIONS

See Box 3.41.

Box 3.41 Complications

Longer ICU and hospitalized days
Greater mortality
Greater costs

● PLEURAL SPACE ABNORMALITIES

Q Which of the air-leak syndromes is considered the most life-threatening?

A Tension pneumothorax

An air leak is defined as any extrusion of air from normal gas-filled cavities, including lungs, tracheobronchial tree, sinuses, and gastrointestinal (GI) tract. Of all the air-leak syndromes, a pneumothorax is considered to be the most serious complication and a tension pneumothorax is the most life-threatening. If a patient presents with or develops subcutaneous emphysema and/or pneumomediastinum, a pneumothorax should be ruled out.

HINT   Pneumopericardium can also be life-threatening but is less common than a pneumothorax (Box 3.42). Subcutaneous emphysema and pneumomediastinum are not life threatening except in rare cases and must be observed.

Box 3.42 Air-Leak Syndromes

Pneumothorax	Pneumopericardium
Pneumomediastinum	Subcutaneous emphysema
Pneumoperitoneum	

Q A pneumothorax can develop due to which ventilatory complication?

A Barotrauma

Positive pressure ventilation can result in barotrauma and air-leak syndromes. The patient can develop a pneumothorax, pneumomediastinum, or pneumoperitoneum following institution of positive pressure ventilation with high pressures. A pneumothorax is caused by the pressure gradient between the interstitium and the alveoli reaching a critical point followed by rupture of alveoli. Air then enters the interstitial space and pleural space (Box 3.43).

HINT   High risk for pneumothorax in mechanically ventilated patients include high levels of PEEP and large TVs.

Box 3.43 Other Causes of Pneumothorax

Iatrogenic	Traumatic	Spontaneous	Underlying Lung Pathology
Subclavian central-line placement	Barotrauma	Subpleural blebs	Asthma
Transthoracic needle biopsy	Penetrating chest trauma	Smokers	COPD
Lung resection	Blunt chest trauma	Valsalva maneuver	ARDS
Cardiopulmonary resuscitation	Tracheo-bronchial rupture	Coughing	Lung cancer
Misplaced tracheostomy tube			Sarcoidosis
			Cystic fibrosis
			Pulmonary infections

ARDS, acute respiratory distress syndrome; COPD, chronic obstructive pulmonary disease.

▶ PATHOPHYSIOLOGY

Q What may keep the lung from collapsing in a patient with chronic lung disease following pneumothorax?

A Adhesions

Adhesions can develop between the parietal and visceral layers of the pleural space in chronic lung disease patients. When a pneumothorax occurs, it may be a very localized, loculated area of the pleural space. Typically, pneumothoraces are widespread throughout the pleural space and result in the collapse of the lung.

HINT   A patient may require more than one chest tube to drain the different locations of loculated air.

▶ SYMPTOMS/ASSESSMENT

Q What are the two most common initial symptoms of a pneumothorax in an awake patient?

A Chest pain and dyspnea

A sudden-onset pleuritic chest pain and severe dyspnea are most commonly the initial symptoms of a patient who is awake and is developing pneumothorax.

HINT   The patient will typically also experience significant hypoxemia with a respiratory alkalosis (Box 3.44).

Box 3.44 Symptoms of Pneumothorax

Dyspnea	Absent or diminished breath sounds and affected lung
Pleuritic chest pain	Asymmetrical chest wall movement
Hypoxemia	Subcutaneous emphysema
Respiratory alkalosis	Tracheal deviation (away from affected side)
Tachypnea	Hypotension
Tachycardia	

> **Q** What change on the ventilator could be a sign of a new pneumothorax on a ventilated patient?
>
> **A** Acute increase in PIP

A sudden increase in the PIP on a ventilated patient can be an indication of a new pneumothorax. It is commonly associated with a sudden decrease in oxygen saturation and tachycardia. A CXR should be obtained and further assessment performed.

HINT The increase in PIP may be the initial symptom of a pneumothorax in ventilated patients not awake or unable to communicate.

▶ DIAGNOSIS

> **Q** Which diagnostic radiographic procedure is best to determine the size of the pneumothorax?
>
> **A** CT and ultrasonography

An anterior-posterior (AP) or posterior-anterior (PA) CXR generally underestimates the size of the pneumothorax. The PA view of a pneumothorax measuring 2 cm may actually be almost half of the hemithorax. Ultrasonography is more accurate for determining the size of the pneumothorax and is able to identify small collections of air. A CT scan is considered the gold standard to verify a pneumothorax if the diagnosis is doubted.

HINT CXR remains the first diagnostic test of choice to be obtained with a suspicion of a pneumothorax.

▶ MANAGEMENT

> **Q** If the pneumothorax is smaller than 2 cm and the patient is asymptomatic, what is the primary treatment?
>
> **A** Administer 100% FiO_2

A small pneumothorax (<2 cm on a chest radiograph) on an asymptomatic patient is usually observed closely for signs of hypoxemia or respiratory distress. Administering oxygen at 100% FiO_2 will assist with increasing the absorption of air more rapidly. Serial CXRs will be required to monitor the resolution of the pneumothorax.

HINT If the patient is on positive pressure ventilation (a CPAP or mechanical ventilator), then chest tube placement would be required. Positive pressure ventilation can increase the size of the pneumothorax.

> **Q** Your patient has a chest tube for a pneumothorax that was inserted 24 hours ago. Upon earlier assessment, you noted intermittent bubbling. While the radiology technician was obtaining a CXR, the chest drainage system was broken. What would be the best nursing action to manage the chest tube system?
>
> **A** Place chest tube in water

Because the chest tube was recently placed and had intermittent bubbling, this is an indication that the pneumothorax has not been resolved yet. Clamping this tube is not a good option since a tension pneumothorax can occur, which is life-threatening. The patient is in the unit, so a sterile cup of saline is readily available to put into the tube to make a water seal. Leaving the tube open until a new drainage system is prepared and then placing it back to suction would also be an option in this situation.

HINT If a chest tube is clamped, the patient needs to remain under close observation. On any sign of hemodynamic instability, the tube should be quickly unclamped.

> **Q** A patient inadvertently dislodged his chest tube when turning in the bed. The last CXR showed complete resolution of the pneumothorax. What would be the best nursing intervention at this time?
>
> **A** Cover with Vaseline gauze and an occlusive dressing

The pneumothorax has resolved based on the most recent CXR. Covering the incision with Vaseline gauze and an occlusive dressing will prevent air from reentering the pleural space. If the pneumothorax was unresolved based on CXR and clinical assessment, a three-sided dressing would be indicated to prevent a tension pneumothorax. The taping of the dressing on three sides only allows the air to exit, but it cannot reenter into the pleural space (one-way valve).

HINT   Continue to monitor the patient closely for deterioration, indicating a pneumothorax or tension pneumothorax.

▶ COMPLICATIONS

> **Q** What can be injected into the pleural space to treat a recurring pneumothorax?
>
> **A** Talc

The instillation of talc or bleomycin through the chest drainage tube can be used to treat recurring pneumothoraces or a continuous air leak. This is called medical pleurodesis. There is also a surgical pleurodesis in which the parietal pleura is abraded. These techniques produce fibrosis and scarring to allow the visceral layer to adhere to the chest wall, preventing further pneumothoraces.

> **Q** What could be the cause of a significant air leak and loss of delivered TV on a ventilated patient after chest tube insertion?
>
> **A** Bronchopleural fistula

A bronchopleural fistula is a communication between the pleural space and the bronchial tree. It presents as a persistent air leak or failure to reinflate the lung after chest tube placement. Management requires a lower TV, RR, PEEP level, and lower pressures to allow the fistula to heal. This may require accepting a lower oxygenation and permissive hypercapnia. Refractory cases may require surgical repair (Box 3.45).

HINT   Assess exhaled TV on the ventilator. It should be within 100 mL of the preset TV. More than 100 mL indicates a loss of delivered TV.

Box 3.45 Causes of Bronchopleural Fistula

Chest trauma	Complications with mechanical ventilation
Chest tube inadvertently placed into lung parenchyma	Complication with diagnostic or therapeutic thoracic interventions

⬤ ASPIRATION

> **Q** What type of aspiration is the most common in a critically ill patient?
>
> **A** Microaspirations

Small volume (microaspirations) is the most common form of aspiration in critically ill patients. Small aspirations of contaminated oropharyngeal secretions and gastric contents frequently occur in intubated critically ill patients and play a major role in VAP.

HINT   Oral decontamination will lower the risk of pneumonia with the aspirations.

▶ PATHOPHYSIOLOGY

> **Q** What is the intervention most likely to contribute to aspirations in a critically ill patient?
>
> **A** Tube-feeding infusion

Tube feeding has been found to increase the risk of both large-volume aspirations and small-volume microaspirations in more than 50% of the patients receiving tube feeds (Box 3.46).

Box 3.46 Risk Factors for Aspiration

Mechanically ventilated	Sedation
Decreased level of consciousness	Tube feeding
Presence of a feeding tube	No PEEP with mechanical ventilation
Abnormal gag or swallow reflex	

PEEP, positive end-expiratory pressure.

▶ SYMPTOMS/ASSESSMENT

Q What should be assessed after extubation following a prolonged intubation prior to feeding the patient?

A Swallow evaluation

Intubation, especially prolonged, may affect the ability of the patient to swallow after extubation. Performing a swallow evaluation prior to feeding the patient is recommended. If the patient is found to have a swallowing abnormality, then obtaining a consultation with a speech therapist for a complete dysphagia evaluation is recommended to lower the risk of aspiration.

HINT High-risk patients for dysphagia may have silent aspirations and should still have a speech consultation for swallow evaluation.

Q Which complication is a concern of checking residuals when tube feeding enteral nutrition (EN)?

A Incomplete calories

The practice of checking residuals and holding EN for high residuals can result in inadequate nutrition and calories. Recent studies indicate not monitoring residuals does not increase risk of VAP or HAP. Small-bore feeding tubes are more likely to collapse during aspiration and are not as reliable for checking residuals. Clinical assessment of tolerance to tube feeding should be used to determine proper response to large residuals (Box 3.47).

HINT Frequent stopping or holding EN for any reason can result in inadequate nutrition and should be avoided as much as possible.

Box 3.47 Signs of Intolerance With Tube Feeds

Large gastric residuals	Vomiting or regurgitation
Abdominal pain	No abnormal bowel sounds
Distended abdomen	Nausea
No flatus or stool passage	

▶ DIAGNOSIS

Q What measurement may be used to diagnose microaspiration of gastric contents?

A Pepsin

Quantitative pepsin in tracheal secretions is accurate in diagnosing microaspirations of gastric contents. Methylene blue has been used but requires a bronchoscopy to diagnose aspiration of blue dye, which is not always visible with suctioning. Dye in the enteral feed has been found to have side effects of diarrhea, gastric bacterial colonization, and systemic absorption with death.

HINT Glucose testing is not recommended as a method for testing for tube-feed aspirates.

▶ MANAGEMENT

> **Q What degree of the HOB elevation is recommended to prevent aspiration?**
>
> **A 30 to 45 degrees**

A sustained supine position (0 degree) has been shown to increase gastroesophageal reflux and increased risk of aspiration. To prevent aspiration elevating the HOB to a semirecumbent position of 30 to 45 degrees is recommended in high-risk patients. If unable to elevate the backrest, one may use the reverse Trendelenburg position to elevate the head unless contraindicated (Box 3.48).

HINT High-risk patients include those mechanically ventilated and/or with a feeding tube in place.

Box 3.48 Prevention of Aspiration

Maintain HOB elevated to 30 to 45 degrees	Assess swallowing ability
Avoid oversedation	Maintain endotracheal cuff at the appropriate level
Assure correct placement of feeding tube	Subglottic suctioning
Avoid bolus feeding	Postpyloric feeding

> **Q What is the recommendation for minimal ETT cuff pressure?**
>
> **A 20 cm H_2O**

The ETT cuff pressure needs to be within a particular range to maintain preset TVs and reduce the risk for aspiration secretions that accumulate above the cuff. A range of 20 to 30 cm H_2O is recommended. Less than 20 cm H_2O is inadequate to protect from aspiration. Hypopharyngeal suctioning prior to deflating the cuff is used to minimize aspiration of secretions.

HINT The addition of supraglottic suctioning can assist in the prevention of aspiration of pooled secretions.

▶ COMPLICATIONS

> **Q What complication is of the highest risk following aspirations?**
>
> **A Pneumonia**

Microaspirations and large-volume aspirations are associated with VAP and HAP.

▶ PULMONARY HYPERTENSION

> **Q Which ventricle is affected the most in pulmonary arterial hypertension (PAH)?**
>
> **A Right ventricle**

PAH is a syndrome that results from restricted blood flow through the pulmonary arterial bed, increasing pulmonary vascular resistance (PVR) and resulting in RV failure (Box 3.49).

Box 3.49 Causes of PAH

Idiopathic PAH	Connective tissue disease
Familial PAH	Drugs and toxins
HIV	Portal hypertension

PAH, pulmonary arterial hypertension.

Q Is elevated PVR caused by LV failure called pulmonary venous hypertension (PVH) or PAH?

A PVH

PVH is a subcategory of PH. PH is defined as abnormally high pulmonary vascular pressure. It affects both precapillary and postcapillary pressures (arterial and venous side pulmonary circulation) (Box 3.50).

Box 3.50 Causes of PH

Left ventricular failure	Chronic obstructive pulmonary disease
Left-sided valvular heart disease	Pulmonary fibrosis
Pulmonary embolism	Sarcoidosis

HINT PAH, primary pulmonary hypertension, primarily involves the pulmonary arteries, whereas PVH is a secondary PH caused by left-sided failure.

Q What hemodynamic findings define PAH?

A Mean pulmonary artery pressure (mPAP) more than 25 mmHg and pulmonary artery occlusive pressure (PAOP) less than 15 mmHg

mPAP is elevated, but the left atrial or left ventricular end diastolic pressure (LVEDP) remains relatively normal. PH caused by left-sided failure or pulmonary diseases would elevate the PAOP in addition to the mPAP.

HINT PAH is a primary PH that results in right-HF.

▶ PATHOPHYSIOLOGY

Q What are the pathological changes that occur within the pulmonary artery resulting in increase in resistance?

A Vascular remodeling

Vascular remodeling produced by excessive cell proliferation affects the small pulmonary arteries. The vascular changes can include intimal hyperplasia, medial hypertrophy, and adventitial proliferation (Box 3.51). Pulmonary artery vasoconstriction can contribute to the PH.

Box 3.51 Physiology of PAH

Excessive cell proliferation within pulmonary vasculature
Vasomotor dysregulation (pulmonary vasoconstriction)
Inflammation

PAH, pulmonary arterial hypertension.

Q Which connective tissue disease are common causes of PAH?

A Scleroderma and lupus

Scleroderma and lupus are connective tissue diseases that commonly result in PAH due to the vascular wall changes of collagen (Box 3.52).

HINT Portal hypertension can cause hepatopulmonary syndrome resulting in PAH.

Box 3.52 Causes of PAH

Idiopathic
Hereditary
Drug or toxin induced
Connective tissue disease
Portal hypertension
Congenital heart disease

PAH, pulmonary arterial hypertension.

▶ SYMPTOMS/ASSESSMENT

Q What are common symptoms of patients presenting with PAH?

A Dyspnea, chest pain, and syncope

Primary symptoms of PH include dyspnea, chest pain, and syncope. Symptoms may also include history of fatigue and peripheral edema. Assessment for signs of RV failure should be performed to determine the degree of RV involvement (Box 3.53).

Box 3.53 Symptoms of PAH

Dyspnea	Murmurs/extra heart sounds
Fatigue	Increased jugular distention
Chest pain	Hepatomegaly/splenomegaly
Syncope	Ascites
Cyanosis	Crackles
Clubbing of fingers	Lead II large p wave or rSR' pattern on 12-lead

PAH, pulmonary arterial hypertension.

Q What type of murmur is most likely to develop with severe PH?

A Systolic murmur

Development of a new-onset tricuspid regurgitation can occur following the onset of PH. The murmur is heard during systole because of the valve's incompetency to maintain intactness. Pulmonary regurgitation can also occur and presents with a diastolic murmur.

HINT   The presence of right ventricle S_4 can also indicate RV HF (Box 3.54).

Box 3.54 Heart Sounds With PH

Early systolic click	Sudden interruption in the opening of the pulmonic valve due to high arterial pressure
Midsystolic ejection murmur	Turbulent flow through the pulmonic valve
Right ventricular S_3 and S_4	Volume overload in the right ventricle due to heart failure or noncompliance of the ventricle
Holosystolic murmur	Tricuspid regurgitation
Accentuated pulmonary component S_2	High arterial pressure closed the pulmonic valve with greater force
Diastolic murmur	Pulmonic regurgitation

PH, pulmonary hypertension.

▶ DIAGNOSIS

> **Q What diagnostic test is frequently used to identify PH with RV involvement?**
>
> **A Echocardiogram**

An echocardiogram is used to screen for PH and right-sided involvement (right ventricle and atrium). Suspicion of PH is based on presenting symptoms and history. In order to treat effectively, the underlying associated disease or cause should be identified.

HINT   Etiology dictates treatment of the PH. For example, etiology of CHF causing PH requires treatment aimed at improving HF.

> **Q What is considered the confirmative diagnosis for PAH?**
>
> **A Right heart catheterization (RHC)**

RHC can confirm the hemodynamic measurements that verify the diagnosis of PAH. Other diagnostics include history and physical, CXR, and echocardiogram.

HINT   Echocardiogram can assist with identifying right atrial and ventricular enlargement and tricuspid regurgitation (Box 3.55).

Box 3.55 Findings of RHC Indicative of PAH

Transpulmonary gradient (PA mean − PAOP) is high	Normal to low PAOP
Elevated PVR	Increased "A" and "V" waves

PAOP, pulmonary artery occlusive pressure; PVR, pulmonary vascular resistance

> **Q Which of the hemodynamic parameters is the best diagnostic reading to differentiate between primary PAH and secondary PH?**
>
> **A PVR**

PVR may be more important than the mean PAP because it reflects influence of the transpulmonary gradient and is only elevated if vascular obstruction occurs on the precapillary side. It is useful to obtain whether the mean PAP is elevated.

HINT   PAH caused by pulmonary vascular pathology will elevate both PVR and mPAP, whereas PH caused by other disorders, including left-sided failure, will elevate the mPAP but not the PVR.

▶ MEDICAL MANAGEMENT

> **Q What is the primary contraindication for testing vasoreactivity in patients with PAH?**
>
> **A Hemodynamic instability**

Administration of a vasodilator is used to test vasoreactivity to consider potential patients for long-term calcium channel blocker therapy. Patients with hemodynamic instability and overt RV failure should not be tested with a vasodilator. A positive responder to the administration of a vasodilator includes a decrease in mPAP by at least 10 mmHg or absolute reduction less than 40 mmHg without a decrease in CO. The vasodilators frequently used to test vasoreactivity include inhaled nitric oxide, epoprostenol, or adenosine.

HINT   Close hemodynamic monitoring should be performed during testing with a vasodilator to determine reactivity in PAH.

Q Which of the calcium channel blockers is not indicated in managing PAH even with good reactivity testing?

A Verapamil

Calcium channel blockers are frequently used to vasodilate the pulmonary arteries and lower the pulmonary artery vascular resistance. Verapamil causes a decrease in myocardial contractility and can worsen RV failure in PAH patients.

Q What medical management is recommended for all patients with idiopathic PAH?

A Warfarin

Anticoagulation therapy with warfarin is recommended for all patients with idiopathic PAH. Calcium channel blockers are indicated in those patients found to be responsive to vasodilator therapy. Diuretics may be used if there are signs of acute right-side HF. Calcium channel blockers are used only in PAH patients shown to have positive reactiveness to vasodilator therapy. Phosphodiesterase (PDE)-5 inhibitors have improved exercise tolerance and hemodynamics.

HINT INR goal for patients on warfarin for PAH is 1.5 to 2.5.

Q Which drug has been found to increase survival in PAH?

A Epoprostenol

Epoprostenol, a prostanoid, is the preferred treatment for critically ill patients and has been found to improve survival. Prostanoids are vasodilators with antiproliferative effects. PAH causes a reduction in prostacyclin synthase, thus resulting in lower levels of prostacyclin.

HINT Epoprostenol may be administered as a continuous infusion through a long-term catheter (Table 3.5). Treprostinil administered SC may cause pain and erythema at the sites of injection. IV route has possibly been associated with a higher risk of catheter sepsis (Box 3.56).

Table 3.5 Routes of Prostanoids

Prostanoid	Route of Administration
Epoprostenol	Continuous IV
Treprostinil	SC or continuous IV
Iloprost	Aerosolized devices

IV, intravenous.

Box 3.56 Common Side Effects of Epoprostenol

Headache	Diarrhea
Jaw pain	Nausea
Flushing	Musculoskeletal pain

Q What laboratory value needs to be monitored monthly and indefinitely when on endothelin receptor antagonists?

A Liver function tests (LFTs) and hemoglobin and hematocrit (H&H)

Endothelin receptor antagonist (Bosentan, Sitaxsentan) is administered orally. The significant side effect is elevated liver enzymes. It also requires close monitoring of liver enzymes monthly and hematocrit every 3 months. Endothelin-1 is a vasoconstrictor that contributes to PAH. This class is used to inhibit or block endothelin-1 resulting in vasodilation. Other drugs that may be used to treat PAH include PDE-5 inhibitors (Sildenafil).

HINT Due to the different mechanism of action, a combination of drugs is usually used to medically manage PAH.

▶ SURGICAL MANAGEMENT

> **Q** What surgical procedure can be performed in patients experiencing worsening of symptoms on multiple medications for PAH?
>
> **A** Atrial septostomy

Atrial septostomy creates a right-to-left shunt that decreases right heart filling pressures and improves right heart function. This procedure increases LV filling and improves CO. It will cause a greater systemic hypoxia, but the goal is for the increase in CO to improve systemic oxygen delivery.

> **Q** What is the potential surgical option for end-stage pulmonary disease?
>
> **A** Lung transplant

Lung transplant is an option in select patients with worsening of symptoms despite maximal pharmacological treatments. The transplant may include single lung, double lung, or heart/lung transplant. The decision is made on the severity of the decompensated HF. Extracorporeal membrane oxygenation (ECMO) is also gaining popularity with unstable patients with end-stage pulmonary disease refractory to adequate oxygenation while on mechanical ventilation.

HINT   RV assist device may be used as a "bridge" for transplantation.

> **Q** Following a large PE, a patient can develop chronic PH. What surgical intervention can be used to lower the PVR in such a patient?
>
> **A** Pulmonary thromboendarterectomy

The diagnosis of chronic PH following a PE is perfusion scanning and, potentially, pulmonary angiogram. If PH develops and the patient is an acceptable surgical risk, removal of the fiber strands and material from the pulmonary artery with pulmonary thromboendarterectomy can lower the PVR.

▶ COMPLICATIONS

> **Q** What is the most common cause of death in a patient with PAH?
>
> **A** RV failure

RV failure is a common complication of PAH. The initial response of the RV when pumping against the high resistance is to develop hypertrophy. This compensatory mechanism can reduce wall stress and improve CO. Second, the RV begins to dilate, and less blood flows to the LV. Prolongation of RV contraction encroaches on the LV filling. The effect is a decrease in LV filling and CO causing cardiovascular collapse. Atrial arrhythmias are caused by RV failure and include paroxysmal atrial tachycardia, atrial flutter, and atrial fibrillation.

HINT   Increased RV tension may lead to RV ischemia and acute myocardial infarction.

▶ THORACIC TRAUMA

> **Q** What is the most common mechanism of injury for a pulmonary contusion (PC)?
>
> **A** Blunt trauma

The most common mechanism of injury for PC is a blunt, high-impact trauma to the chest producing a compression–decompression effect. The most common cause is a motor vehicle collision. Thoracic trauma is more commonly caused by blunt mechanism compared to penetrating.

HINT   PC can also be caused by penetrating trauma with high-velocity missiles to the chest.

▶ PATHOPHYSIOLOGY

> **Q** What is the physiological change in the lungs following a high-impact blunt trauma to the chest?
>
> **A** Disruption of alveolar–capillary integrity

The disruption of the alveolar–capillary integrity results in hemorrhage and edema in both the interstitial and intra-alveolar spaces in the lungs. Reflexive increase in bronchial mucus secretions result in early development of atelectasis and ventilation/perfusion defects. The combination of atelectasis, blood and fluid, and interstitial edema produces a decrease in pulmonary compliance and an increase in airway pressures.

HINT Injury to the thoracic cavity can disrupt respiration and/or circulation and are the common causes of death.

> **Q** What is the most common site of injury for tracheobronchial tear following blunt trauma?
>
> **A** Bifurcation mainstem bronchus

The most common site of injury is at the bifurcation of the mainstem bronchus, approximately 1 inch from the carina. The injury may not be evident for up to 5 days after the injury.

▶ SYMPTOMS/ASSESSMENT

> **Q** Following blunt trauma to the chest, a patient develops productive cough. What would you expect the sputum to look like?
>
> **A** Blood streaked (hemoptysis)

Hemoptysis may occur after a blunt injury to the chest wall due to the rupture of the alveolar–capillary membranes. The blunt force causes damage to the pulmonary vasculature, allowing blood to enter the alveoli and interstitium. This causes a "bruise" in the lung tissue and manifests as blood-tinged or blood-streaked sputum (Box 3.57).

Box 3.57 Symptoms of PC

Dyspnea	Wheezing over affective area
Tachypnea	Labored respirations
Chest pain	Tachycardia
Hemoptysis	Pallor or cyanosis
Crackles or rhonchi	Hypoxemia

PC, pulmonary contusion.

HINT The onset of symptoms with PC occurs within 6 to 48 hours following the injury.

> **Q** A nurse finds subcutaneous air when assessing a patient 24 hours after a blunt trauma to the chest. The patient also demonstrates noisy breathing. What is the most likely cause of these findings?
>
> **A** Tracheobronchial tear

Tracheobronchial tears may not be recognized immediately following the trauma but can present 24 to 48 hours later. The typical presentation is pneumothorax or unresolved pneumothorax and subcutaneous air (Box 3.58).

Box 3.58 Symptoms of Tracheobronchial Tear

Noisy breathing	Progressive mediastinal emphysema
Hemoptysis	Pneumothorax
Cough	Air leak in chest
Subcutaneous air	

> **Q What is the most common physical symptom of a flail chest following blunt chest trauma?**
>
> **A Paradoxical movement flail segment**

Flail chest results from multiple consecutive rib fractures (three or more ribs in two or more locations). A common sign is paradoxical chest wall movement, which leads to respiratory compromise.

▶ DIAGNOSIS

> **Q The extended fast (e-fast) exam is used in thoracic trauma to identify what potential injury?**
>
> **A Pneumothorax**

Fast is the ultrasonic technique for identifying abdominal injuries. Adding thoracic views are used to assess for pneumothorax.

> **Q What CXR changes occur with a PC?**
>
> **A Diffuse infiltrates**

The infiltrates are diffuse and do not conform to segments or lobes of the lung. Findings on CXR may not appear until 4 to 6 hours after injury and up to 48 hours later.

HINT   CXR findings are similar to those found in ARDS.

> **Q Which radiograph is the most sensitive in determining the extent of the PC?**
>
> **A CT**

A CT scan is highly sensitive to findings of PC and the volume of lung involvement. CT scanning may be used to determine the clinical outcomes. PC involving more than 18% of the lung is considered a significant injury, associated with poorer outcomes.

HINT   Occult PC is defined as changes seen on initial CT but not visible on CXR. This has a good prognosis.

> **Q What is a finding on CXR that may indicate tracheobronchial injury?**
>
> **A Pneumomediastinum**

A tracheobronchial tear results in air introduced into the mediastinum. The air can be recognized on CXR if the tear is below the level of the carina.

> **Q What test is considered to be the definitive diagnosis for a tracheobronchial tear?**
>
> **A Bronchoscopy**

Bronchoscopy can be used to visualize the actual tear, whereas CXR only identifies mediastinal air or pleural effusions.

HINT   Esophageal injuries may occur with tracheobronchial injuries due to close proximity. An esophagoscopy is used to identify an esophageal injury.

▶ MANAGEMENT

> **Q What is the recommended management of pneumothorax or hemothorax?**
>
> **A Placement chest tube**

Thoracostomy tube is placed for pneumothoraces or hemothoraces. The size of the tube depends upon the pathology, air or blood.

HINT   Occult pneumothorax is a pneumothorax seen on CT scan but not CXR. And may just be observed

> **Q** What emergency management of a hemodynamically unstable trauma patient may affect PC outcomes?
>
> **A** Volume overload

Too much volume used in resuscitation can worsen the PC, increasing lung fluid, and worsening hypoxia. Adequate resuscitation to improve blood flow to the organs is important, but over-resuscitation can cause pulmonary complications (Box 3.59).

Box 3.59 Overall Management of PC

Good pulmonary toiletry
Avoid volume overload
Adequate ventilation

pc, **pulmonary contusion.**

HINT Current research does not support the use of corticosteroids or antibiotics when treating PC.

> **Q** What mode of ventilation may benefit a patient with severe unilateral lung injury following a blunt chest trauma?
>
> **A** Independent lung ventilation (ILV)

If the PC involves a single lung, the lung compliance becomes unequal. This results in asymmetrical ventilation. Airflow will take the path of least resistance, causing an overinflation of the noninjured lung and underinflation of the injured lung. ILV uses a double-lumen ETT allowing for separate ventilation of each lung (Box 3.60).

HINT Ventilator management is similar to that used for patients with ARDS.

Box 3.60 Ventilator Modes for PC

PEEP	Pressure release ventilation
Pressure controlled ventilation	Independent lung ventilation
High-frequency oscillator/jet ventilation	

PC, pulmonary contusion; PEEP, positive end-expiratory pressure.

▶ COMPLICATIONS

> **Q** What is a major complication of a severe PC?
>
> **A** Acute respiratory distress syndrome (ARDS)

ARDS is a complication of a severe PC. An injury to the alveolar capillary membrane causes noncardiogenic pulmonary edema, which is one criterion for the diagnosis of ARDS.

HINT VAP can also be a complication of PC.

> **Q** What is a life-threatening complication of tracheobronchial injury?
>
> **A** Tension pneumothorax

Air can be introduced into the mediastinum and pleural space. A tension pneumothorax can occur due to air being forced into the pleural space and unable to leave, developing tension.

HINT Assess for tension pneumothorax by palpating trachea to determine if midline. A deviated trachea indicates a tension pneumothorax.

MECHANICAL VENTILATION

Q **Which measured pressure is considered to be equal to the alveolar pressure?**

A **Plateau pressure (P_{plat})**

Plateau pressure is obtained after inspiration and before exhalation by delaying the expiration on the ventilator. This equalizes the pressures in the alveoli to the mouth and correlates to the pressure within the alveoli (alveolar pressure).

HINT Plateau pressures are measured by holding inspiratory time.

Q **Which measured pressure, when elevated, causes barotrauma to the lungs?**

A **PIP**

PIP is the amount of pressure required by the ventilator to deliver the set TV. This is the highest pressure recorded at the end of inspiration. Pressures that are too high may cause barotraumas. Pressures greater than 35 to 40 may be damaging to the lungs (Table 3.6).

Table 3.6 Measurement Compliances in Lungs

Calculated Compliance	Measures	Causes of Decreased Compliance	Calculation

Dynamic compliance	Measurement of the total compliance (lung and chest wall)	■ Bronchoconstriction
		■ Increase in airway resistance
		  ● Secretions
		  ● Mucus plug
		■ Flail chest
		■ Muscle tension
			TV ÷ PIP − PEEP
			Normal 100 mL/cm H_2O

Static compliance	Measurement of the lung compliance reflects changes within the alveoli	■ Air trapping ■ Pulmonary edema ■ Atelectasis ■ Pneumonia ■ Pneumothorax/hemothorax ■ Loss of surfactant ■ Abdominal distension	TV + P_{plat} − PEEP Normal 70–100 mL/cm H_2O Goal >50 mL/cm H_2O

PEEP, positive end-expiratory pressure; PIP, peak inspiratory pressure; TV, tidal volume.

HINT Static compliance takes resistance airway and compliance of the chest wall out of the equation and looks only at the alveoli.

Q **Which measured pressure may improve oxygenation when increased?**

A **mPaw**

Paw is the sum of the amount and duration of pressure applied to the chest on the intrathoracic structures. A lower mean pressure will have less negative cardiovascular effects. But an increase in Paw may increase oxygenation.

Q **Auto-PEEP occurs when the I:E ratio does not allow what to occur?**

A **Adequate expiratory time**

After a breath is delivered, if the next breath is delivered before all the air leaves the lungs, it causes "stacking of breaths" or auto-PEEP. If breaths continue to be delivered without adequately allowing the complete exhalation of air, the end-expiratory pressure and volumes increase and can result in a lung injury called barotrauma. Auto-PEEP is not set on the ventilator, but it has an additive effect in increasing end-expiratory pressure with the actual set PEEP.

HINT   Total PEEP = set PEEP + auto-PEEP.

Q How is auto-PEEP typically measured on the ventilator?

A Occlusion of expiratory time

It is measured by temporarily occluding the expiratory circuit in the ventilator, which equalizes pressures in the lungs and ventilator circuit.

HINT   This measurement is most accurate if the patient is sedated or paralyzed.

Q What is the best method to manage auto-PEEP?

A Decrease breaths per minute

The best method to decrease the inspiratory time is to decrease the total breaths per minute. This allows for greater exhalation times. A lowering of the TV may also be used but is not as efficient as changing the ventilatory rate. Increasing the inspiratory flow rate is not effective at lowering total inspiratory time unless inappropriately set in the beginning.

HINT   Many patients are breathing over the set RR and may require sedation or NMBAs to lower the total ventilatory rate.

Q What is the adverse effect of auto-PEEP on ventilation?

A Increases WOB

The inspiratory effort of the patient must not just equal the sensitivity setting on a demand ventilator but must now overcome the level of auto-PEEP to initiate the airflow into the lungs. This increases WOB.

HINT   Decrease WOB by setting the PEEP level slightly below the total PEEP level to decrease the amount of inspiratory effort needed to trigger the ventilator breath.

FAILURE TO WEAN FROM MECHANICAL VENTILATOR

Q What is the primary point when clinicians suspect that a patient may be ready to wean?

A Disease process improved

One of the clinical changes that indicate the timing to begin weaning is the adequate treatment of the disease process that caused the respiratory failure. The decision to attempt weaning and discontinue the ventilator is also based on the patient being hemodynamically stable, awake, and meeting the minimal ventilator dependency criterion (Box 3.61).

HINT   Shortening the weaning process is an important goal to prevent VAP and other ventilation complications.

Box 3.61 Minimal Ventilator Dependency

FiO_2 <40%	PaO_2 >60
PEEP <8 cm H_2O	No vasopressors
PF ratio >200 mmHg	No continuous sedation
Arterial saturation >90%	

PEEP, positive end-expiratory pressure; PF ratio, PaO_2/FiO_2 ratio.

Q What are the most common techniques used to perform a spontaneous breathing test (SBT)?

A T-Bar (or flow-by), CPAP, and pressure support ventilation (PSV)

A T-bar SBT involves taking the patient off the ventilator, whereas CPAP and PSV modes can be performed while the patient remains on the ventilator. A CPAP of 5 cm H_2O is frequently used for weaning. Higher CPAP levels defeat the purpose of spontaneous breathing.

HINT Close observation of the patient during SBT is needed to recognize respiratory fatigue or failure.

Q What is the rapid shallow breathing index (RSBI) used to determine readiness for extubation?

A RR/TV

The RSBI is used to predict successful weaning from a ventilator. RSBI can be calculated after 5 to 10 minutes of initiation of a weaning trial (Box 3.62).

Box 3.62 RSBI Scores

≤80 predicts successful weaning
80–100 predicts weaning may or may not be successful
≥100 predicts weaning unsuccessful

RSBI, rapid shallow breathing index.

Q During an SBT, which is used to wean patients, what is the primary cause for an increase in airway resistance?

A ETT

The ETT has a smaller diameter than the patient's own airway. This narrowing of the upper airway increases the airway resistance and WOB.

HINT CPAP and/or PSV can be used during spontaneous breathing trials to overcome the resistance of the ETT.

Q Which of the weaning parameters most closely correlates with inspiratory muscle strength?

A Negative inspiratory pressure (NIP)

NIP is also known as negative inspiratory force (NIF). The NIP is the maximal inspiratory pressure and is used to assess muscle strength. An NIP value of less than −20 to −25 cm H_2O is predictive for successful weaning.

HINT Remember, spontaneous inspiration is a negative pressure. A greater negativity of the NIP correlates to a stronger inspiratory effort (Box 3.63).

Box 3.63 Weaning Parameters

RR <35 bpm	VC >10 mL/kg
NIP <−20 to −25 cm H_2O	RR/VT <105 bpm/L
TV >5 mL/kg	

NIP, negative inspiratory pressure; RR, respiratory rate; TV, tidal volume; VC, vital capacity; VT, ventricular tachycardia.

Q What is the most common arrhythmia associated with failure of weaning from the ventilator?

A Sinus tachycardia

Sinus tachycardia is the most common arrhythmia caused by a failure to wean from the ventilator. Failure of weaning includes the failure of SBT or reintubation within 48 hours after extubation (Box 3.64).

Box 3.64 Signs of Failed Weaning

Objective Signs	Subjective Signs
Tachypnea (>35 bpm)	Anxiety
Tachycardia (increase >20)	Dyspnea
Hypertension (increase >20)	Increased WOB
Hypotension	
Hypoxemia ■ PaO_2 <50 mmHg ■ SaO_2 <90%	
Acidosis	
New arrhythmias	
Agitation	
Diaphoresis	
RSBI >100	
Depressed mental status	
Increased use of accessory muscles	

RSBI, rapid shallow breathing index; WOB, work of breathing.

> **Q Immediately following extubation, a patient develops audible wheezing and increased difficulty in breathing. What would be the most likely cause?**
>
> **A Laryngospasm**

Laryngospasm is a prolonged protective reflex of the vocal cords. It is seen immediately post extubation and is due to airway irritation, presence of a foreign body, or secretions (saliva, blood, vomitus). It may also be associated with emergence anesthesia, airway trauma, or a difficult intubation. There are certain factors that increase the risk of laryngospasm and include the history of smoking, COPD, airway irritability, and asthma.

HINT Inability to speak indicates a complete airway obstruction (Box 3.65).

Box 3.65 Symptoms of Laryngospasm

High-pitched inspiratory stridor	Wheezing
Anxiety	Chest and abdominal paradoxical movement
Tracheal tug	Tachypnea

> **Q What is the initial management of laryngospasm?**
>
> **A Apply oxygen 100% FiO_2**

If stridor develops or if the patient begins to exhibit other signs of laryngospasm, place the patient in a lateral position unless contraindicated to promote drainage of secretions. Apply supplemental oxygen using 100% FiO_2 and humidification. Administer racemic epinephrine to decrease the edema and consider the administration of succinylcholine at a low dose in an attempt to relax the laryngeal muscles. Severe cases may require intubation and positive ventilation.

> **Q Prior to extubation, what intervention can be performed to assess for airway edema?**
>
> **A Deflate the cuff to assess for an air leak**

Prior to extubation, assess for the presence of airway edema by deflating the cuff and ensuring an audible air leak is heard around the deflated cuff. If no audible air leak is present, this indicates airway swelling, and extubation should be delayed. Management of airway edema following extubation is similar to laryngospasm with the addition of steroid treatments.

HINT   Prevention of airway swelling includes limiting the amount of trauma to the airway such as limiting ETT movement and prevention of coughing or "bucking" of the ventilator.

 PULMONARY FIBROSIS

▶ PATHOPHYSIOLOGY

Q What is a diagnosed interstitial lung disease or fibrosis of an unknown cause called?

A Idiopathic pulmonary fibrosis (IPF)

Unexplained symptomatic or asymptomatic patients with patterns of bilateral fibrosis on CXR of CT scan are classified as IPF. This is a form of chronic, progressive, fibrosing interstitial disease occurring primarily in adults and limited to lungs.

HINT   Age is typically greater than 60 years old.

Q What is the underlying damage to the lungs in IPF?

A Inflammation, edema, and/or fibrosis

Damage to the lung parenchyma includes the mechanisms of inflammation, edema, and/or fibrosis. It results in dilation of bronchi, alveolar remodeling, and bibasilar parenchymal fibrosis.

HINT   May have periods of pulmonary function stability interspersed with acute deterioration of lung function.

▶ SYMPTOMS/ASSESSMENTS

Q What are the hallmark characteristic symptoms of IPF?

A Progressive worsening of dyspnea and lung function

IPF should be considered in adult patients presenting with unexplained chronic exertional dyspnea, nonproductive cough, bibasilar inspiratory crackles, and/or digital clubbing.

HINT   Detailed history assessment frequently identifies an underlying cause for pulmonary fibrosis. The history assessment includes detailed medication use and environmental exposure at home, work, and other places (Box 3.66).

Box 3.66 Occupational and Environmental Factors

Silica dust
Asbestos fibers
Hard metal dusts
Coal dust
Grain dust
Bird and animal droppings

▶ DIAGNOSIS

Q Which radiographic study is recommended to diagnose IPF?

A Volumetric CT scan

The features of the volumetric CT scan characteristics of IPF include honeycombing, traction bronchiectasis, and appearance of ground-glass opacification. The chest CT scan, in combination with history and symptoms, is used to make the diagnosis of PF. Lung biopsy allows for specific identification of interstitial lung patterns but is not as commonly used due to risks.

HINT Testing for connective tissue disease which can cause pulmonary fibrosis (i.e., scleroderma) is recommended.

> **Q** Which PFT is frequently monitored to monitor lung function in pulmonary fibrosis?
>
> **A** VC

Disease progression is monitored through VC and 6-minute walk test. Pulmonary rehabilitation is recommended in the early stages to improve lung function.

HINT Supplemental oxygen may be required during exercise and long-term oxygen therapy at end-stage disease.

▶ MEDICAL MANAGEMENT

> **Q** Which class of medication is commonly used in patients with PF?
>
> **A** Antifibrotic agents

Nintedanib and pirfenidone are two of the approved antifibrotic agents used to manage PF. The most frequent side effect of nintedanib is diarrhea. The most common side effects of pirfenidone are nausea and rash. Low-dose corticosteroids may be used and have been found to improve the cough in some of the IPF patients.

HINT These antifibrotic drugs have been found to slow the progression but do not cure PF.

> **Q** What would be considered to be the most important lifestyle change recommended in patients with diagnosis of PF?
>
> **A** Cessation of smoking

Smoking cessation counseling should be provided to patients with the diagnosis of PF. Other areas of patient education and recommendations include receiving vaccinations (influenza, pneumococcal, Tetanus–diphtheria–pertussis, and zoster).

HINT Encourage them to have minimal exposure to airborne lung irritants or pollution.

▶ SURGICAL MANAGEMENT

> **Q** What is the surgical treatment considered as the pulmonary fibrosis progresses?
>
> **A** Lung transplant

Early referral for lung transplant is recommended due to the variation in presentation and progression of the disease process. Frequency of acute exacerbations is also considered in evaluating for transplant.

▶ COMPLICATIONS

> **Q** Which vascular complication is commonly associated with PF?
>
> **A** Pulmonary hypertension

The thickening and scarring of the alveoli can compress the capillaries resulting in higher pressures required to perfuse the lungs. This results in the development of PH.

HINT Overtime, PH can contribute to development of HF, cor pulmonale.

RESPIRATORY MONITORING DEVICES

Q What is the technique used to continuously measure exhaled CO_2?

A Capnography

Capnography is the continuous measurement of $ETCO_2$. Capnography is used to verify ETT placement, confirming that the tube is in the trachea. $ETCO_2$ can determine changes in pulmonary circulation and respiratory status before pulse oximetry. Substantial hypercarbia must occur before the patient demonstrates hypoxemia.

Q Which VQ mismatch demonstrates a greater discrepancy between $PaCO_2$ and $ETCO_2$?

A Dead space

The difference between $PaCO_2$ and $ETCO_2$ increases as dead space volume increases.

HINT   An acute discrepancy in arterial and $ETCO_2$ with sudden-onset dyspnea increases the suspicion of a PE.

Q What affects the accuracy of the capnography?

A High breathing rates

High breathing rates can exceed capnography capabilities and may decrease the accuracy of the readings. Increased airway resistance may also affect the accuracy of the reading.

Q A patient is admitted with carbon monoxide poisoning. The pulse oximetry reading is 99% to 100% saturation, but the ABG sent to the lab revealed an 86% saturation. Which of the two is more accurate in this situation?

A ABG saturation

Carbon monoxide diffuses faster, binds to hemoglobin, and forms carboxyhemoglobin in the blood. This reduces the oxygen-carrying capacity of the hemoglobin, resulting in hypoxia. The pulse oximetry measures bound hemoglobin, whether bound with oxygen or any other substance, whereas an ABG analyzed in the laboratory can differentiate between oxygen and carbon monoxide.

HINT   This discrepancy also occurs with Nipride (nitroprusside) toxicity due to cyanide poisoning.

1. Which of the following diagnostic studies is the most reliable method of distinguishing acute respiratory distress syndrome (ARDS) from cardiogenic pulmonary edema?

   A. Chest x-ray (CXR)
   B. Bronchoalveolar lavage
   C. Pulmonary artery occlusion pressure (PAOP) measurement
   D. PaO_2/FiO_2 ratio

2. Which of the following statements by an ICU nurse would indicate that she understands the concept of airway pressure release ventilation (APRV)?

   A. We will need to keep this patient heavily sedated because it is an uncomfortable way of breathing
   B. If the patient is unable to breathe spontaneously, the benefits of APRV are lost
   C. If the patient is fighting the ventilator, administration of a paralytic agent is indicated in APRV mode
   D. This mode of ventilation results in more respiratory muscle atrophy and a longer weaning process

3. Which of the following methods used to obtain a sputum sample is the most accurate for the diagnosis of pneumonia?

   A. Suction endotracheal tube
   B. Expectorant
   C. Bronchoalveolar lavage (BAL)
   D. Nasotracheal aspirate

4. A postpneumonectomy patient is admitted to the ICU. Her left lung was removed and she is currently on a ventilator. Which of the following orders would the ICU nurse expect to have regarding the positioning of this patient?

   A. Turn Q 2 hours
   B. Do not turn patient onto right side
   C. Turn patient prone
   D. Maintain supine only

5. A patient has a traumatic brain injury from a motor vehicle collision 10 days prior. Her Glasgow Coma Scale (GCS) is 10 and she is being mechanically ventilated. She had a tracheostomy and percutaneous endoscopic gastrostomy (PEG) tube placed yesterday. While moving her from the chair to the bed, the tracheostomy tube is accidentally dislodged. What would be the best nursing intervention in this situation?

   A. Assess ventilation, assist with bag-valve-mask (BVM) as needed while covering the stoma, and call the physician
   B. Reinsert the tracheostomy tube immediately
   C. Insert a tracheostomy tube that is one size smaller than the original
   D. Stat page anesthesia to intubate the patient

1. B) Bronchoalveolar lavage

Although rarely used, bronchoalveolar lavage is the most reliable method for differentiating ARDS from cardiogenic edema. Fluid rich in proteins would indicate increased capillary permeability. Patients with high PAOP pressure may still develop ARDS, so this is not considered a reliable method to rule out ARDS. CXR that is characteristic of ARDS is bilateral fluffy infiltrates, but there is variability in the CXR appearance and thus differentiation may not always be possible. Both ARDS and cardiogenic pulmonary edema can present with an abnormal PaO_2/FiO_2 ratio.

2. B) If the patient is unable to breathe spontaneously, the benefits of APRV are lost

APRV uses prolonged periods of spontaneous breathing at high-end-expiratory pressure, interrupted by brief periods of pressure release. The benefits of this mode of ventilation are alveolar recruitment and improved oxygenation, but it relies on spontaneous breathing. Oversedation or paralysis will eliminate this benefit and require other modes of ventilation.

3. C) BAL

Collecting sputum from BAL allows the sample to be contained without contamination of the upper airways. Samples obtained via the other three methods are contaminated from upper airway and/or oral secretions.

4. B) Do not turn patient onto right side

Following a pneumonectomy, the patient may be turned, but typically the surgical lung should be down. This is to protect the remaining lung from injury if the bronchial stump leaks or ruptures. The prone position is not indicated for this patient; she should be turned but not onto her right side.

5. A) Assess ventilation, assist with BVM as needed while covering the stoma, and call the physician

If an artificial airway is accidentally dislodged, initially assess to determine adequacy of breathing. This tracheostomy stoma is only 1 day old and has not matured yet. Attempting to replace or insert a tracheostomy tube into the stoma can result in inadvertent placement into a false tract. If breathing is inadequate, you may cover the stoma and bag with a BVM system. Notify the physician stat for evaluation and possible replacement of the tracheostomy tube. The patient may not need to be intubated.

6. Which of the following findings is seen in patients with primary pulmonary hypertension?

   A. Elevated pulmonary artery occlusion pressure (PAOP) and pulmonary artery diastolic (PAD) pressure
   B. Elevated pulmonary artery (PA) pressures regardless of PAOP
   C. Normal PAOP and elevated PAD
   D. Elevated PAD and decreased central venous pressure (CVP)

7. In an acute asthma episode, which of the following interventions would be the most appropriate to thin secretions and prevent a mucus plug?

   A. Administer a mucolytic agent
   B. Maintain adequate hydration with intravenous (IV) fluids
   C. Provide continuous lateral rotation therapy (CLRT)
   D. Administer a beta-2 selective agonist

8. What is the most common reason for admission and mechanical ventilation in a patient with an admitting diagnosis of chronic obstructive pulmonary disease (COPD)?

   A. Pneumonia
   B. Pulmonary edema
   C. Bronchospasms
   D. Atelectasis

9. A patient is admitted with acute respiratory failure and a history of obesity hypoventilation syndrome. Which of the following is the best initial intervention for this patient?

   A. Immediate intubation
   B. Tracheostomy
   C. Noninvasive ventilation (NIV) with bilevel positive airway pressure (BiPAP)
   D. 2-L nasal cannula

10. A mechanically ventilated patient with acute respiratory failure is noted to have hypercapnia and difficulty with weaning. Which of the following is the most likely cause of the hypercapnia?

    A. Overfeeding the patient
    B. Acute renal failure
    C. Intrapulmonary shunt
    D. High tidal volumes

11. Which of the following would best explain the benefit of pressure-controlled ventilation (PCV)?

    A. Lower alveolar pressure
    B. Higher tidal volumes
    C. Able to use less positive end-expiratory pressure (PEEP)
    D. Uses a square waveform for air delivery

12. While caring for a mechanically ventilated patient in the ICU, the nurse notes a sudden increase in end-tidal CO_2. What should the ICU nurse suspect as the cause?

    A. Acute respiratory distress syndrome (ARDS)
    B. Pulmonary embolism
    C. Atelectasis
    D. Ventilator-associated pneumonia

(See answers next page.)

6. C) Normal PAOP and elevated PAD

In primary pulmonary hypertension, the pressures in the PA are high, including the PAD pressure. It does not affect the PAOP, so that value is normal. The diagnosis is that the PAD pressure is greater than the PAOP by 4 mmHg or more. If both the PAD and PAOP are elevated and are within 4 mmHg of each other, it is considered secondary pulmonary hypertension. The CVP is typically elevated as well, due to the greater resistance in the pulmonary arteries.

7. B) Maintain adequate hydration with IV fluids

IV hydration is the best method to thin secretions and prevent airway obstruction by a mucus plug. A mucolytic agent can thin secretions, but it is not indicated in acute asthma. Lateral rotation can improve pulmonary function, but it does not thin secretions. Beta agonists are administered in asthma patients to bronchodilate (which may facilitate expelling of mucus), but they do not thin secretions.

8. A) Pneumonia

Most of the acute exacerbations of COPD, especially those severe enough to require mechanical ventilation, are due to pulmonary infections (pneumonia). PE can also prompt a COPD exacerbation requiring ventilation. Pulmonary edema, bronchospasms, and atelectasis are not typically associated with acute exacerbations of COPD.

9. C) NIV with BiPAP

NIV with BiPAP is recommended as an initial intervention for patients with obesity hypoventilation syndrome who are admitted with acute respiratory distress/failure. It is also used as a routine therapy to reduce the severity of hypercapnia. Intubation and tracheostomy may be required after other interventions have failed but are not initial interventions. Respiratory failure requires more than just administering a 2-L nasal cannula.

10. A) Overfeeding the patient

Nutrition-associated hypercapnia can occur in mechanically ventilated patients. Overfeeding with high calories, especially carbohydrates, causes an overproduction of CO_2. Mechanical ventilation typically prevents removal of excess CO_2, resulting in hypercapnia. Acute renal failure causes metabolic acidosis and would more likely result in hypocapnia. Dead space ventilation, not intrapulmonary shunts, can cause hypercarbia. High tidal volumes would cause hypocarbia.

11. A) Lower alveolar pressure

PCV sets a pressure limit, not a tidal volume, when delivering air. The biggest advantage of PCV is the ability to control alveolar pressure, which is most closely related to the risk of alveolar overdistention and injury. It typically ventilates with lower tidal volumes, especially in noncompliant lungs. PEEP is still used to improve oxygenation. It delivers the breath using a decelerating waveform.

12. B) Pulmonary embolism

PE causes dead space ventilation, which causes an increase in exhaled end tidal CO_2 and an increase in $PaCO_2$-$PetCO_2$ gradient. The other three answers result in intrapulmonary shunts and are not causes of a sudden increase in $PetCO_2$.

13. Which of the following is an indication for use of rapid sequence intubation (RSI)?

   A. Cardiac arrest patient
   B. Awake patient
   C. Unconscious patient
   D. Only postoperative patient

14. A patient is improving from her pneumonia and is undergoing weaning parameters. Which of the following parameters would indicate that the patient is ready for weaning?

   A. Vital capacity (VC) 8 mL/kg
   B. Maximal inspiratory pressure (MIP) 5
   C. Respiratory rate (RR)/tidal volume (TV) ratio 85
   D. VT 3 mL/kg

15. A patient in the ICU with a diagnosis of meningitis has been on bed rest. The patient suddenly becomes short of breath, and a pulmonary embolism (PE) is suspected. Which of the following lab results may assist with the diagnosis of a PE?

   A. D-dimer
   B. B-type natriuretic peptide (BNP)
   C. Troponin I
   D. Factor Xa

16. What is considered to be the biggest advantage of high-frequency oscillatory ventilation (HFOV) in acute respiratory distress syndrome (ARDS) patients?

   A. Improved cardiac output
   B. Uses a conventional ventilator
   C. Improves complete volume exhalation
   D. Creates high mean airway pressure

17. What is a bedside test that may be used on a ventilated patient to estimate the intrapulmonary shunt fraction?

   A. End-tidal CO_2 (EtCO$_2$)
   B. Forced vital capacity (FVC)
   C. PaO_2/FiO_2 ratio (PF ratio)
   D. FVC/forced expiratory volume in 1 second (FEV1) ratio

18. A patient is 3 days post–motor vehicle collision. He has blunt chest trauma with an admitting diagnosis of multiple rib fractures, pneumothorax, and potential pulmonary contusions. You note an intermittent air leak in the chest tube system, and the chest x-ray (CXR) shows an unresolved pneumothorax. He now has diffuse subcutaneous air across his chest. What is the most likely diagnosis?

   A. Pulmonary contusion
   B. Bronchial perforation
   C. Flail chest
   D. Improperly placed chest tube

13. B) Awake patient

RSI is used for awake patients who need to be intubated. It involves the administration of a drug to produce unconsciousness, followed by the administration of a short-acting paralytic to facilitate the intubation. In cardiac arrest patients and unconscious patients, RSI is not indicated. RSI can be used on both medical and surgical patients who are awake.

14. C) RR/VT ratio 85

RR/VT ratio (also called "rapid shallow breathing index") is considered one of the more predictive weaning parameters. A RR/VT ratio of <105 bpm/L is predictive of successful weaning. Spontaneous VT of 4–6 mL/kg, VC >10 mL/kg, and a MIP of −15 to −30 are considered predictive of successful weaning.

15. A) D-dimer

The D-dimer is used to measure fibrin degradation products. An elevated D-dimer indicates the presence of blood clots and is used in nonsurgical patients to assist with the diagnosis of PE. BNP and troponin levels may also be elevated in PE, but are not typically used to assist with this diagnosis at this time. Factor Xa is a study to assess anticoagulated state and is not used to diagnose a PE.

16. D) Creates high mean airway pressure

The oscillations create a higher mean airway pressure, which improves gas exchange. The use of smaller volumes and more rapid rates also lowers the incidence of overdistention and volutrauma. A special ventilator is required to perform HFOV. Complete exhalation may not occur due to the rapid rate, resulting in air trapping and intrinsic positive end-expiratory pressure (PEEP).

17. C) PF ratio

The PF ratio is an indirect estimate of a shunt fraction. A PF ratio of <200 correlates to a >20% intrapulmonary shunt. FVC and the FVC/FEV1 ratio are used to measure obstructive airway disease. $EtCO_2$ can be used to identify alveolar dead space.

18. B) Bronchial perforation

Tracheal and bronchial perforations may have a delayed presentation and typically present with an unresolved pneumothorax and the presence of an air-leak syndrome (including subcutaneous air). The patient may have pulmonary contusions and flail chest, but the symptoms presented in this scenario do not indicate this. An improperly placed chest tube is not likely to cause these symptoms, and can be identified on CXR.

19. You are precepting a new ICU nurse. While caring for a patient with acute respiratory distress syndrome (ARDS), the physician orders that the patient be turned to a prone position. Which would be the most correct explanation to the orientee?

A. The prone position will lower the risk of skin breakdown due to prolonged immobility
B. Placing ARDS patients prone has been found to improve oxygenation
C. We will have to turn the patient every 1 to 2 hours
D. Turning ARDS patients prone is done to move the fluid in the lungs toward the anterior chest for better suctioning

20. Which of the following cells are responsible for the production of surfactant?

A. Kupffer cells
B. Glial cells
C. Type I pneumocyte cells
D. Type II pneumocyte cells

21. What is the purpose of the shorter low-pressure period of time in airway pressure release ventilation (APRV)?

A. Remove carbon dioxide
B. Improve oxygenation
C. Recruit alveoli
D. Prevent pressure trauma to lungs

22. Which of the following patients suspected of a pulmonary embolism would be most appropriate for ventilation perfusion (VQ) scan instead of CT angiogram (CTA) chest?

A. Heart failure
B. Hypertensive patient
C. Renal failure
D. Hepatic failure

23. Which of the following tools is designed to stratify the risk of patients for deep vein thrombosis (DVT)?

A. Atherosclerotic cardiovascular disease (ASCVD) risk
B. Well's criteria
C. Ranson's criteria
D. CHADS$_2$

24. Which of the following presentation of an asthmatic episode would have the highest risk of being hospitalized in critical care?

A. Sudden, acute exacerbation
B. Episode during exercise
C. Triggered by an allergen
D. Slow onset exacerbation

25. Which of the following thoracic traumatic injuries would most likely produce hypotension?

A. Pulmonary contusion
B. Cardiac tamponade
C. Tracheobronchial rupture
D. Rib fractures

19. B) Placing ARDS patients prone has been found to improve oxygenation
Turning an ARDS patient with bilateral lung disease prone has been shown to improve oxygenation. The frequency of turning has not been well established and is not currently recommended every 1 to 2 hours. It is not performed to prevent skin breakdown or to assist with suctioning.

20. D) Type II pneumocyte cells
Type II pneumocyte cells are responsible for the production of surfactant. Type I pneumocyte cells form the alveolar capillary membrane. Glial cells are brain cells and Kupffer cells are in the liver.

21. A) Remove carbon dioxide
The longer high-pressure phase of APRV is used to recruit alveoli and improve oxygenation. The shorter, low-pressure time period is used to allow for improved exhalation of CO_2. The low-pressure phase of APRV is not used to prevent trauma to the lungs.

22. C) Renal failure
Patients with renal insufficiency or kidney injury should avoid large doses of contrast, which are used with CTA. In these cases, VQ scans are preferred to CTA even if not as accurate. Heart failure, hypertensive and hepatic failure patients do not have as much risk for renal injury with contrast so CTA is preferred.

23. B) Well's criteria
Well's criteria are used to stratify risks of patients for DVT. Risk stratification is for low, moderate, and high risk of a DVT. ASCVD is a tool used to calculate the risk for cardiovascular disease. Ranson's criteria are used to predict the severity of pancreatitis. $CHADS_2$ score is used to determine risk of embolic stroke in patients with AF.

24. D) Slow onset exacerbation
Slow onset of exacerbation with a worsening of peak expiratory flow rates that occurs over days is associated with a higher severity and more likely to require mechanical ventilation. Due to the subacute onset and length of development, more edema and mucus plugging are present in airways. It also tends to reflect noncompliance or inadequate disease control over time. Acute, sudden onset exacerbation is usually due to mass exposure to allergens, but patient presents rapidly to emergency treatment. Exercise-induced asthma is not at higher risks for severity.

25. B) Cardiac tamponade
Cardiac tamponade and tension pneumothorax are two injuries in the thoracic cavity that result more frequently in hypotension or circulatory involvement. Pulmonary contusion, tracheobronchial rupture, and rib fractures present with respiratory dysfunction.

BIBLIOGRAPHY

American Association of Colleges of Pharmacy. (2016). Antithrombotic therapy for VTE disease: CHEST guidelines and expert report. *Chest, 149*(2), 315–392.

American College of Cardiology Foundation/American Heart Association. (2009). Expert consensus document on pulmonary hypertension. *Circulation, 119*, 2250–2294.

Modrykamien, A., Chat-Burn, R. L., & Ashton, R. W. (2011). Airway pressure release ventilation: An alternative mode of mechanical ventilation in acute respiratory distress syndrome. *Cleveland Clinical Journal of Medicine, 78*(2), 101–110.

Papazian, L., Aubron, C., Brochard, L., Chiche, J.-D., Combes, A., Dreyfuss, D., … Faure, H. (2019). Formal guidelines: Management of acute respiratory distress Syndrome. *Annals of Intensive care, 9*, 69.

Endocrine System Review

4

◯ DIABETIC KETOACIDOSIS/HYPERGLYCEMIC HYPEROSMOLAR STATE (HHS)/ACUTE HYPOGLYCEMIA

Q An insulin-dependent patient is more likely to have which of these diabetic complications: diabetic ketoacidosis (DKA) or hyperglycemic hyperosmolar state (HHS)?

A DKA

Clinically, diabetics are not referred to as type 1 or 2 diabetes. In the past, the thought was that type 1 diabetics required insulin and type 2 diabetics did not; this has changed because clinically many type 2 diabetics require insulin. Patients are now more commonly defined as insulin-dependent diabetes mellitus (IDDM) or noninsulin-dependent diabetes mellitus (NIDDM). Insulin-dependent diabetics are more likely to develop DKA, whereas noninsulin-dependent diabetics develop HHS. Increasing number of noninsulin-dependent diabetics present with DKA. HHS is hyperglycemia with hyperosmolar states but without ketonemia and ketoacidosis. HHS may occur over days to weeks, whereas DKA tends to have a shorter time to symptoms.

HINT Noninsulin-dependent diabetics still produce some insulin (although inadequate for glucose control) allowing for control of the ketone bodies.

Q Of the two complications of diabetes, DKA and HHS, which has a higher mortality?

A HHS

DKA and HHS are both life-threatening complications of diabetes mellitus, but HHS has greater mortality. HHS may persist for several days without significant symptoms resulting in higher glucose and osmolality levels. HHS causes hyperglycemia and hyperosmolar states similar to DKA but without the increase in ketones, which causes nausea and vomiting in DKA patients and initiates seeking medical care. Symptoms of HHS are less severe, which can result in the delay of treatment.

HINT   The serum osmolality correlates to mortality. Other predictors include the extremes of age, coma, and hypotension.

> **Q What is the most common precipitating factor for the development of DKA or HHS?**
>
> **A Infection**

The most common cause for the development of life-threatening complications of diabetes is infection. Another common cause of DKA is new-onset insulin dependence or noncompliance with use of insulin (Box 4.1).

HINT   Sudden onset of insulinopenia in noninsulin-dependent diabetic may improve with aggressive insulin replacement within several months.

Box 4.1 Precipitating Factors

Infection	Treatment errors (inadequate insulin or noncompliance)
New-onset diabetes	Abdominal disorders
Stroke	Stress induced
Trauma	Emotional factors
Drug induced	Acute coronary syndrome

▶ PATHOPHYSIOLOGY

> **Q The basic underlying physiology of DKA is a decrease in insulin and an increase in which hormones?**
>
> **A Counterregulatory hormones**

The combination of a decrease in insulin and an increase in counterregulatory hormones causes an increase in glucose production and impaired utilization in the peripheral tissue cells. Stress response in critical illness is a result of the release of counterregulatory hormones.

HINT   The role of counterregulatory hormones is opposite to that of insulin (Box 4.2).

Box 4.2 Counterregulatory Hormones

Glucagon	Growth hormone
Catecholamines	Cortisol

> **Q Is insulin an anabolic or a catabolic hormone?**
>
> **A Anabolic hormone**

Insulin, being an anabolic hormone, synthesizes or builds proteins from amino acids and triglycerides from free fatty acids. It allows for the utilization of glucose in the peripheral tissues and controls glucose levels in the serum. Without the suppressive effects of insulin and the catabolic effects of the counterregulatory hormones, a patient will develop proteolysis and lipolysis. As muscles break down, they release amino acids and the adipose tissues release fatty acids.

HINT   Anabolic hormones build, whereas catabolic hormones break things down (Box 4.3). A decrease in insulin allows K^+ to leave the cells and enter the serum, resulting in an initial increase in K^+ levels.

Box 4.3 Actions of Insulin

Promotes	Inhibits
Glycogen synthesis in muscle and liver	Glucagon
Peripheral use of glucose by muscle	Lipolysis of triglycerides in adipose tissue
Uptake of amino acids by muscle and liver	Mobilization of stored fatty acids
Protein synthesis (builds amino acids to proteins)	Proteolysis
Synthesis of free fatty acids from glucose	Hepatic glucose production
Conversion of free fatty acids to triglycerides	Fatty acid oxidation
Movement of extracellular K^+, PO_4^+, Mg^+ into cells	

Q As the glucose levels increase in both DKA and HHS, what happens to the serum osmolality levels?

A Elevates

Glucose is a component of serum osmolality. Hyperglycemia increases osmolality in a progressive manner. Every 100 mg/dL increase in glucose will increase serum osmolality by 5.5 mOsm/kg. The increase in osmolality causes fluid shifts from the intracellular to extracellular spaces, resulting in cellular dehydration.

HINT Fluid resuscitation includes administering "free water" after vascular resuscitation to replace the cellular losses. Free water losses are typically about 6 L.

Q What is the primary cause of hypovolemia in DKA and HHS patients?

A Hyperglycemic osmotic diuresis

Hyperglycemia stimulates the renal excretion of glucose when it exceeds the resorptive capacity of the proximal tubules. Glycosuria occurs with serum glucose levels of 170 to 200 mg/dL. Osmotic diuresis causes hypovolemia and primary losses of Na^+, Cl^-, K^+, Ca^{++}, PO_4^+, and Mg^+.

HINT Even though the initial K^+ values do not reflect the extent of potassium deficit, there is an overall depletion of K^+. Potassium losses average 400 to 600 mEq/L, which is a combined loss of intracellular and extracellular K^+ (Figure 4.1).

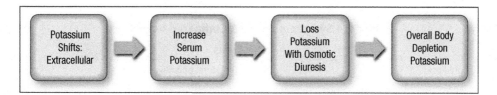

Figure 4.1 Effects of potassium on DKA and HHS.

HINT Patients with initial hypokalemia have a severe depletion and require cardiac monitoring for arrhythmias.

Q What causes the increase in ketones in patients with DKA?

A Lipolysis

The breakdown of adipose tissue (lipolysis) to free fatty acids results in oxidation by the ketogenic pathway to ketone bodies (β-hydroxybutyrate and acetoacetate). Ketones uncontrolled by the insulin feedback loop will result in ketonemia and ketoacidosis (ketones are strong acids). Ketones are excreted by kidneys (ketonuria) and neutralized by bicarbonate, causing a greater metabolic acidosis. HHS results in a decrease in insulin, causing inadequate utilization of glucose, but patients with this syndrome may make enough insulin to prevent lipolysis and control the production of ketone bodies.

HINT Remember, both DKA and HHS have hyperglycemia and hyperosmolality, but only DKA develops elevated ketones with the development of ketoacidosis.

> **Q What is the primary compensatory mechanism for ketoacidosis?**
>
> **A Kussmaul's respiration**

The primary compensatory mechanism for ketoacidosis is Kussmaul's respiration. Increased minute ventilation (respiratory rate and depth of ventilation) will "blow off" carbon dioxide, which decreases ketones through the respiratory tract. Ketones are also neutralized by bicarbonate, buffered by potassium, and excreted by kidneys. Usually, as a ketoacid is added a bicarbonate will decrease in a 1:1 ratio.

HINT A DKA patient's breath develops a fruity or musty odor because of the ketones (acetone breath).

▶ SYMPTOMS/ASSESSMENT

> **Q What are the classical two "Ps" that patients with both DKA and HHS may present with in their recent history?**
>
> **A Polyuria and polydipsia**

Both DKA and HHS develop a hyperglycemic, hyperosmolar state with osmotic diuresis resulting in increased urine output (polyuria) and dehydration. Polyuria can cause polydipsia (increased thirst).

> **Q What is the triad of symptoms of DKA?**
>
> **A Hyperglycemia, acidosis, and ketonemia**

Both DKA and HHS result in hyperglycemia and hyperosmolar states, but only DKA presents with elevated ketones and metabolic acidosis caused by the ketones.

> **Q Which is more likely to present in a coma: DKA or HHS?**
>
> **A HHS**

The level of consciousness (LOC) can range from being alert to a decrease in LOC or coma. HHS patients are more likely to develop a decrease in LOC or progress to a coma because they have less abdominal pain (Box 4.4).

Box 4.4 Symptoms of DKA Compared to HHS

DKA	HHS
Polyuria, polydipsia	Polyuria, polydipsia
Abdominal pain	Dehydration
Nausea and vomiting	Decreased level of consciousness or coma
Anorexia	Normal ventilation
Hypotension (vasodilation)	
Tachycardia	
Dehydration	
Hypothermia	
Decreased level of consciousness	
Kussmaul's respiration	
Acetone breath	
Ketonemia, ketonuria	

DKA, diabetic ketoacidosis; HHS, hyperglycemic hyperosmolar nonketotic state.

▶ DIAGNOSIS

Q What level of serum bicarbonate meets the criteria for DKA?

A Less than 18 mEq/L

The American Diabetes Association (ADA) has set criteria to define DKA. These include acidosis with a serum bicarbonate level of less than 18 mEq/L (Box 4.5).

Box 4.5 ADA Criteria for DKA

Blood glucose > 250 mg/dL	Anion gap > 10 mEq/L
pH < 7.30	Ketone presence in serum
Bicarbonate < 18 mEq/L	

DKA, diabetic ketoacidosis.

Q Which patient is more likely to have a higher glucose level: one with DKA or one with HHS?

A HHS

The higher serum glucose concentration is due to underrecognition of the hyperglycemia because of lack of ketones. Serum glucose can get extremely high before the person becomes symptomatic, which usually presents as a decrease in LOC. HHS is typically associated with blood glucose level greater than 600 mg/dL and low to normal ketones.

HINT   Remember that ketones are what cause the patient to feel "bad."

Q What is a normal anion gap?

A Less than 10 mEq/L

DKA develops a high-anion gap metabolic acidosis (>10 mEq/L). To calculate, subtract major anions from the cations. Omission of K^+ in the daily calculation is acceptable clinically because the number is so low that it has little effect on clinical decisions (Box 4.6).

HINT   Ketoacids are unmeasured anions and therefore elevate the anion gap.

Box 4.6 Calculation of Normal Anion Gap

$$(Na^+) - (Cl + CO_2)$$

Q What is an osmolar gap?

A Difference between calculated and measured osmolality

Osmolar gap is used to identify presence of certain substances, such as ketones. A normal osmolar gap is <10 mmOsm/L. A high gap (>15 mmOsm/L) indicates presence of ketones in a DKA patient (Box 4.7).

Box 4.7 Calculation of Osmolality

$$2(Na^+ + K^+) + glucose/18 + BUN/2.8$$

HINT   Anion and osmolar gaps are used to guide treatment of ketoacidosis.

Q What does the serum β-OHB lab test measure?

A Ketone beta-hydroxybutyrate

Serum β-OHB test is used in DKA to measure one of the ketones that will elevate with ketoacidosis, beta-hydroxybutyrate. A level >3.8 mmol/L has been found to be a sensitive indicator for presence of ketones and may be used to diagnose DKA.

HINT   Alcoholic ketoacidosis can also significantly elevate β-OHB levels but seldom presents with hyperglycemia.

Q Why is the initial serum potassium normal to high when the overall body potassium is depleted?

A Potassium shifts

Despite the initial potassium level being normal to elevated, the overall body potassium is depleted. Potassium continually shifts from the intracellular to the extracellular space due to lack of insulin, acidosis, and hyperosmolality. When fluids and insulin are initiated, potassium concentrations may fall quickly because of shifts back into the cells, resulting in hypokalemia and arrhythmias. During fluid resuscitation, serum potassium should be measured frequently (minimum of every 4 hours).

HINT   Presence of hypokalemia initially is a significant finding and requires potassium replacement prior to insulin replacement.

Q In hyperglycemic emergencies (DKA and HHS), is the patient hypernatremic or hyponatremic?

A Hyponatremic

Hyponatremia is usually associated with hypo-osmolality. Severe hyperglycemia causes hyperosmolality with concurrent hyponatremia (called translocational hyponatremia). The altered Na^+ level does not reflect the change in total body water (TBW). The hyperosmolar state (due to the added glucose) causes fluid shift from the intracellular space to the extracellular space. Sodium and chloride are severely lost during osmotic diuresis in an attempt to maintain normal osmolality.

HINT   The hint in the question will be hyponatremia in the presence of hemoconcentration.

Correcting or calculating the sodium level is recommended when replacing fluid and sodium during the management of hyperglycemia to provide a more accurate sodium level (Box 4.8).

Box 4.8 Calculated Serum Sodium

For each 100 mg/dL of glucose over 100 mg/dL, add 2.4 mEq to Na^+ value

Q The depletion of which three electrolytes is usually masked by initial hemoconcentration?

A Phosphorous, calcium, and magnesium

The hemoconcentration that occurs with hyperglycemic, hyperosmolar serum of diabetic emergencies masks the depletion of electrolytes. Once hypovolemia is corrected, the depletion becomes apparent (Boxes 4.9 and 4.10).

HINT   Initial lab results may appear to have normal electrolytes. Frequent metabolic profiles are required during fluid and insulin replacement.

Box 4.9 Laboratory Values for DKA

Leukocytosis (hemoconcentration)	Urine ketones positive
Plasma glucose > 250 mg/dL (typically between 250 and 800 mg/dL)	Increased hematocrit (hemoconcentrated)
Serum osmolality elevated but usually < 320	Hyponatremia
Glycosuria	Elevated amylase and lipase
Metabolic acidosis pH < 7.30	Hypophosphatemia
Low bicarbonate < 18 mEq/L	Hypocalcemia
Anion gap elevated > 10 mEq/L	Hypomagnesemia
Positive serum ketones > 5 mEq/L	Osmolar gap > 10

DKA, diabetic ketoacidosis.

Box 4.10 Laboratory Values for HHS

Leukocytosis (hemoconcentration)	Slight elevation in urine ketones
Anion gap normal to variable (due to lactic acidosis)	Increased hematocrit (hemoconcentrated)
Plasma glucose > 600 mg/dL (typically between 900 and 1100 mg/dL)	Hyponatremia Hypophosphatemia
Serum osmolality ≥ 320	Hypomagnesemia
Glycosuria	
Normal pH (unless lactic acidosis)	
Normal anion gap	

HHS, hyperglycemic hyperosmolar nonketotic state.

Q **What laboratory test can be used to determine whether the DKA is a result of an acute process or progressive, undiagnosed diabetes?**

A **Hemoglobin A1$_c$ test**

The hemoglobin A1$_c$ test measures the percentage of hemoglobin to which glucose molecules have become attached (glycosylated). As plasma glucose levels rise, more hemoglobin molecules become glycosylated. Red blood cells (RBCs) are replaced after about 4 months so the amount of glycosylated hemoglobin at any one time reflects the average plasma glucose level over the last 2 to 3 months. Normal levels of plasma glucose produce an A1$_c$ value of about 5% or less.

HINT   A 1% change in an A1$_c$ value reflects a change of about 30 mg/dL in average plasma glucose.

▶ MANAGEMENT

Q **Which intravenous (IV) fluid is recommended initially to resuscitate patients with DKA and HHS?**

A **Normal saline (0.9% NaCl)**

The initial resuscitation of fluid is aimed at replacing the intravascular losses and restoring renal perfusion. Normal saline may be infused at a rate of 1 L/hr in the first 1 to 2 hours and adjusted to 15 to 20 mL/kg over the first several hours. About 50% of the fluid deficit should be replaced within the first 8 to 12 hours and the remaining fluid within the following 12 to 16 hours, as tolerated (Box 4.11). If patient is hypotensive, aggressive fluid resuscitation is required.

HINT   Fluid replacement must be done with caution in patients with renal or cardiac impairment and requires close monitoring. Serum glucose levels will begin to decrease with volume replacement alone.

Box 4.11 Average Fluid Deficit

DKA	HHS
5–9 L	9–12 L

DKA, diabetic ketoacidosis; HHS, hyperglycemic hyperosmolar nonketotic state.

Q **What value should be used to determine when to administer 0.45% sodium chloride (NaCl) versus 0.9% NaCl after the initial fluid replacement?**

A **Corrected calculated serum sodium**

After initial fluid replacement with 0.9% NaCl, corrected sodium is used to guide the type of fluid in the remaining resuscitation. If the corrected sodium is normal or elevated, 0.45% NaCl is recommended. If it is low, then 0.9% NaCl is continued.

HINT   Note 0.45% NaCl is "free water," which is used to replace extravascular fluid losses (Figure 4.2).

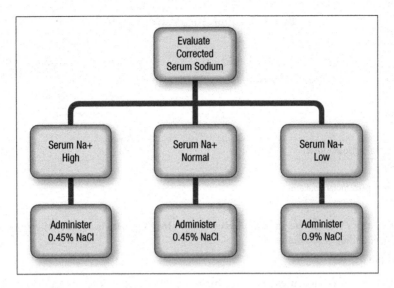

Figure 4.2 Guide for determining type of intravenous fluids.

Q At what rate should glucose be lowered per hour?

A Between 50 and 75 mg/dL

A low-dose continuous infusion of regular insulin is administered with the goal of decreasing blood glucose levels by 50 to 75 mg/dL/hour. The rate of insulin infusion can be started at a dose of 0.1 U/kg/hour and is adjusted to maintain this steady rate of decline in glucose levels. An initial bolus of insulin may be administered prior to the initiation of the infusion.

HINT   Do not bring the blood glucose levels down too rapidly. A blood glucose level of 600 mg/dL may require 8 hours to lower.

Q What level of blood glucose would indicate the need to add glucose into the infusion?

A 250 to 300 mg/dL

When the serum glucose reaches 250 mg/dL in DKA and 250 to 300 mg/dL in HHS, the insulin infusion may be decreased and glucose may be added to the IV fluids to prevent hypoglycemia until acidosis in DKA is resolved. This is done to avoid severe hypoglycemia as a result of fluid resuscitation and insulin administration. Intravenous administration of serum glucose is recommended unless the DKA is considered to be mild, in which case it may be administered subcutaneously.

HINT   Insulin and glucose infusion may be continued in HHS until an increase in mental awareness is achieved.

Q What is the primary treatment of ketoacidosis in DKA?

A Insulin therapy

Insulin is the primary treatment of ketoacidosis. Sodium bicarbonate is not recommended unless the pH remains less than 7.0 after initial fluid replacement. The correction of ketones usually takes longer than glucose so the insulin infusion will continue until the metabolic acidosis and anion gap are normalized. Venous pH may also be monitored frequently to evaluate for continued or improving acidosis. Bicarbonate therapy is not indicated unless pH is extremely low (usually < 6.9).

HINT   Adding glucose to the IV fluids will prevent hypoglycemia during correction of ketones.

> **Q** What potassium levels must be established before insulin may be administered?
>
> **A** Greater than 3.3 mEq/L

Insulin administration should be delayed until potassium levels are greater than 3.3 mEq/L to prevent complications of arrhythmias, cardiac arrest, and respiratory weakness. Adding 20 to 30 mEq of potassium to the 1 liter of IV infusion fluids may be sufficient to maintain normal potassium levels.

HINT   Remember, insulin drives potassium back into the cells, thus causing a drop in serum potassium levels. Potassium levels should also be monitored every 4 hours.

> **Q** Once DKA is resolved, what is the recommended change for the insulin routine?
>
> **A** Initiate subcutaneous route

Once DKA has resolved, continue IV infusion of insulin and supplement with subcutaneous regular insulin as needed every 4 hours. Once the patient starts taking food by mouth, changing the insulin regimen to intermediate or long-acting insulin in addition to short-acting insulin may be indicated. Continuing the IV infusion for several hours after subcutaneous injections have been initiated is important to continue to maintain adequate plasma insulin levels (Box 4.12).

Box 4.12 Criteria for Resolution of DKA

Glucose < 200 mg/dL
Bicarbonate > 18 mEq/L
Venous pH > 7.3

HINT   Abrupt discontinuation of intravenous insulin may result in rebound hyperglycemia because of erratic absorption through the subcutaneous route.

▶ COMPLICATIONS

> **Q** If the osmolality decreases too rapidly, what life-threatening complication can occur?
>
> **A** Cerebral edema

Correction of osmolality by reducing blood glucose and sodium that is too rapid quickly results in interstitial fluid shifts. Cerebral edema is a rare complication but is usually fatal. Neurological deterioration may be rapid, with a decrease in LOC, pupillary changes, and seizures.

HINT   Frequent glucose monitoring is needed to prevent rapid reduction of blood glucose and potentially fatal complications.

> **Q** What is the most common complication of DKA and HHS?
>
> **A** Hypoglycemia

The most common complication of DKA and HHS is hypoglycemia from overzealous treatment with insulin and not adding glucose into the fluids during resuscitation.

HINT   Remember, glucose needs to be added to the fluids when the blood glucose reaches 250 to 300 mg/dL to avoid hypoglycemia.

> **Q** Use of 0.9% NaCl in fluid resuscitation of patients with DKA/HHS may cause what complication?
>
> **A** Hyperchloremic acidosis

Use of large amounts of 0.9% NaCl and electrolyte replacements can result in hyperchloremic acidosis. Chloride replaces ketoanions lost as sodium and potassium salts during osmotic diuresis, resulting in transient hyperchloremic acidosis (Box 4.13).

HINT Hyperchloremic acidosis is a nonanion gap metabolic acidosis compared to ketoacidosis, which produces an anion gap.

Box 4.13 Complications of DKA/HHS

Hypoglycemia	Refractory shock
Rebound hyperglycemia	ARDS
Cerebral edema	Electrolyte abnormalities
Hypokalemia	Seizures
Arrhythmias	Mucormycosis
Acute kidney injury	Hyperchloremic acidosis

ARDS, acute respiratory distress syndrome.

DIABETES INSIPIDUS/SYNDROME OF INAPPROPRIATE ANTIDIURETIC HORMONE/ CEREBRAL SALT WASTING SYNDROME

Q Do patients with SIADH have an increase or a decrease in the antidiuretic hormone (ADH)?

A Increase

Patients with SIADH have too much ADH and will conserve water. DI patients do not have enough ADH and will lose water. The negative feedback that normally controls the ADH release does not function, and water imbalances occur (Box 4.14).

Box 4.14 Water Imbalances

DI	SIADH	CSWS
Not enough ADH	Too much ADH	No effect on ADH

ADH, antidiuretic hormone; CSWS, cerebral salt wasting syndrome; DI, diabetes insipidus; SIADH, syndrome of inappropriate ADH.

Q Overall, what type of patient is most likely to develop water abnormalities such as DI, SIADH, or CSWS?

A A patient with a neurological disorder

Neurological disorders are most likely to involve water abnormalities because of abnormal levels of ADH. This disorder is a neuroendocrine abnormality that involves the hypothalamic–pituitary axis. DI can be neurogenic or nephrogenic. In nephrogenic DI, ADH is produced and released into the circulation normally, but the kidneys do not respond appropriately to the ADH by conserving water (Boxes 4.15 and 4.16). DI occurring in neurological patients is commonly called central neurogenic DI.

HINT In oat cell carcinoma, there is an ectopic production of ADH from the malignant tissue and can cause SIADH.

Box 4.15 Common Causes of DI/SIADH/CSWS

Traumatic brain injury	Intracranial hypertension
Postcraniotomy	Subarachnoid hemorrhage
Primary brain tumors	Ischemic strokes
Meningitis/encephalitis	Hemorrhagic strokes

Box 4.16 Nonneurological Causes of SIADH

Bronchogenic carcinoma	Lung abscess
Oat cell carcinoma of lungs	Positive pressure ventilation
Pneumonia	Certain medications (i.e., SSRIs)
Pain	Nausea

SSRIs, Selective serotonin uptake inhibitors.

Q Which of the ADH abnormalities occurs following brain death?

A Diabetes Insipidus

ADH is synthesized, stored, and released from the brain. Following brain death, the brain does not produce or release ADH and will develop DI.

HINT   Desmopressin (DDAVP) is commonly administered to organ donor patients due to the DI.

▶ PATHOPHYSIOLOGY

Q What area of the brain is responsible for the production of ADH?

A Hypothalamus

The hypothalamus synthesizes ADH, which is then stored in the posterior pituitary in the brain and is responsible for water balance. ADH works on the distal convoluted tubules and collecting ducts in the kidneys. ADH is also called "vasopressin" and increases the reabsorption of water.

HINT   Thinking of "anti" can get confusing when taking the test so when you read ADH, think "water-saving hormone" (Figure 4.3).

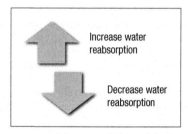

Figure 4.3 Effects of the ADH.

Q What is the primary role of ADH in the body?

A Maintain osmolality and blood volume

ADH is controlled by osmoreceptors and baroreceptors. Osmoreceptors are sensitive to changes in serum osmolality, and baroreceptors are affected by changes in pressure or blood volume. For example, as the osmolality increases, ADH is released to conserve water and lower the osmolality (Box 4.17).

Box 4.17 ADH Regulation

Increases ADH Release	Decreases ADH Release
Increases serum osmolality	Decreases serum osmolality
Decreases circulating blood volume	Increases circulating blood volume
Hypotension	Hypertension

ADH, antidiuretic hormone.

HINT   Positive pressure ventilation can also stimulate the release of ADH and increase water reabsorption in ventilated patients.

Q   What is the cause of hyponatremia in CSWS?

A   Renal loss of Na⁺

The hyponatremia of CSWS is a true loss of sodium through the renal system. There is a loss of sodium and fluid, resulting in hypovolemia (volume-contracted) and hyponatremia. It is a release of brain natriuretic peptides (BNP) from the brain resulting in diuresis of sodium. It is not associated with an abnormal ADH level as are SIADH or DI. It is commonly found in SAH patients.

HINT   SIADH is dilutional hyponatremia, whereas CSWS constitutes a true loss of Na⁺.

▶ SYMPTOMS/ASSESSMENT

Q   What is the initial clinical sign of DI?

A   Diuresis

DI is associated with an abnormally polyuria, typically more than 250 mL/hr. If the patient is awake and able to take oral fluids, he will have an increase in thirst and fluid intake (polydipsia). This large diuresis will lead to hypovolemia and hemoconcentration.

HINT   Both DI and Diuresis begin with a "D." So, remember DI causes diuresis.

Q   Which of the three water abnormality disorders (DI, SIADH, or CSWS) produces hypernatremia?

A   DI

In DI, there is a loss of fluid that results in total body depletion of water, causing hemoconcentration. The total body sodium is relatively normal, but the serum sodium will be increased due to the hemoconcentration.

HINT   The other two water abnormalities, SIADH and CSWS, result in hyponatremia.

Q   In DI, is the urine diluted or concentrated?

A   Diluted

Because of high urine output and the kidneys' inability to conserve water, the urine is diluted. This is measured by urine osmolality and urine specific gravity.

HINT   Remember the 3Ds: DI, Diuresis, and Diluted urine (Box 4.18).

Box 4.18 Symptoms of DI

Polyuria	Decreased urine osmolality
Polydipsia	Decreased urine specific gravity
Thirst	Low urine sodium
Hypernatremia	Weight loss (prolonged or chronic)
Hypokalemia	Signs of dehydration
Hypomagnesemia	Hypotension
Increased serum osmolality	Tachycardia

Q   What is typically the first sign of SIADH?

A   Hyponatremia

In SIADH, the abnormally high levels of ADH cause renal reabsorption and retention of water. This water retention results in hemodilution and lowers the serum sodium levels. TBW increases but total body sodium is normal. This results in a dilution of hyponatremia. A decrease in urine output occurs but may not be initially recognized as SIADH.

HINT   The 24-hour intake/output records will show a positive fluid balance. It is considered hypervolemic hyponatremia (Box 4.19).

Box 4.19 SIADH Symptoms

Decreased urine output (400–500 mL/24 hours)	Increased urine specific gravity Increased urine sodium
Hyponatremia	Generalized weight gain
Decreased serum osmolality Increased urine osmolality	

Q **SIADH patients are at risk for neurological complications, including altered mentation and seizures. Which electrolyte abnormality causes this complication?**

A **Hyponatremia**

Hyponatremia and fluid overload (water intoxication) can cause neurological complications (Box 4.20).

Box 4.20 Symptoms of Hyponatremia and Water Intoxication

Headache	Confusion
Nausea and vomiting	Lethargy progresses to coma
Muscle twitching	Seizures
Fatigue	

Q **What causes the clinical signs of CSWS: volume overload or volume depletion?**

A **Volume depletion**

In CSWS, there is a loss of sodium and water by the kidneys. This leads to a hypovolemic state as well as hyponatremia. The symptoms of CSWS are due to this combination (Box 4.21).

HINT   This is considered a hypovolemic hyponatremia.

HINT   The primary difference between SIADH and CSWS is fluid status.

Box 4.21 Symptoms of CSWS

Orthostatic hypotension	Dry mucus membranes
Tachycardia	Lethargy
Dehydration	Decreased level of consciousness
Weight loss	Seizures

▶ DIAGNOSIS

See Boxes 4.22, 4.23, and 4.24.

Box 4.22 Diagnosis of DI

Urine output > 250 mL/hour	Serum Na$^+$ > 145 mEq/L
Urine specific gravity < 1.005	Urine Na$^+$ normal to low (< 20 mEq/L)
Urine osmolality < 300 mOsm/kg	BUN is elevated
Serum osmolality > 295 mOsm/L	

BUN, blood urea nitrogen.

Box 4.23 Diagnosis of SIADH

Urine output < 20–30 mL/hour	Serum osmolality < 275 mOsm/L
Urine sodium > 25 mEq/L	Serum Na$^+$ < 135 mEq/L
Urine osmolality > the serum osmolality	Urine Na$^+$ high (>25 mEq/L)

Box 4.24 Diagnosis of CSWS

Hyponatremia	Increased BUN
Serum osmolality < 275 mOsm/L	Increased hematocrit
Elevated urine osmolality	Increased urine specific gravity
Urine sodium > 25 mEq/L	

BUN, blood urea nitrogen.

▶ MANAGEMENT

Q What is the primary fluid management goal when treating a patient with DI?

A Fluid replacement

An awake and alert patient taking oral fluids may increase intake to replace the losses in DI. Patients with impaired mental status or those unable to receive oral fluids will need IV fluids to replace these losses. The volume and rate of IV fluid replacement can be calculated using the mL per mL replacement rule or by calculating the free water deficit (FWD). For example, if maintenance fluid was at 60 mL/hour and at 10:00, the urine output was 300 mL; at 11:00 IV fluid rate should be 300 plus 60 mL for a total of 360 mL/hour. If water loss occurs over a greater time period, then replacement may need to be corrected at a slower rate. The calculation of the FWD determines the total amount to be replaced. The first half of the calculated deficit is replaced within the first 12 hours and the second half is replaced over the next 24 to 48 hours (Box 4.25).

Box 4.25 Free Water Deficit (FWD) Calculation

$$[0.6 \times \text{Total body weight}] \times [(\text{Measured } [Na^+]/140) - 1]$$

Q What is the primary medical management of DI?

A Replace ADH

In DI, the patient does not have enough of ADH, so replacement is the primary medical management. Exogenous replacement of ADH can be with either DDAVP or vasopressin (aqueous Pitressin).

HINT Disorders that are deficient in a hormone is managed by replacing the hormone.

Q What is the fluid goal recommended for SIADH?

A Fluid restrictions

The treatment of SIADH is to restrict fluids because the underlying cause of the hyponatremia is volume overload (dilutional hyponatremia). Diuretics may also be used in combination with the fluid restrictions. In the case of symptomatic hyponatremia, therapy may include replacing the sodium carefully with a hypertonic 3% NaCl or salt tablets. Chronic management of SIADH includes medications to either suppress ADH activity (demeclocycline hydrochloride) or to inhibit renal response to ADH (lithium carbonate).

HINT Fluid restrictions and diuresis are usually enough when managing SIADH acutely.

> **Q What is the fluid recommendation to manage CSWS?**
>
> **A Administer fluids**

Management of CSWS requires fluid replacement because of renal losses of fluid. Replacement fluid is 0.9% NaCl with the addition of hypertonic 3% NaCl to correct the hyponatremia. Treatment may also include fludrocortisone acetate to increase absorption of sodium from the renal tubules.

HINT Fluid management of CSWS is opposite to that of SIADH.

> **Q What is a complication of administering hypertonic 3% NaCl too rapidly?**
>
> **A Central pontine myelinolysis (CPM)**

The administration of a hypertonic solution too rapidly can cause a rapid shift in serum osmolality to a hyperosmolar state. This results in irreversible demyelination of the neurons in the brain, particularly in the pons (Box 4.26).

HINT The pons is where all of the myelinated motor tracts cross to the opposite side and descend into the spinal cord.

Box 4.26 Symptoms of CPM

Confusion	Quadriplegia
Dysarthria	Pseudobulbar palsy
Gaze disturbances	

> **Q What is the maximal recommended rate of correction of sodium in a 24-hour period?**
>
> **A 10 mEq/L in 24 hours**

To prevent this complication, Na^+ should not be corrected at a rate exceeding 1.3 mEq/L/hour with a total correction of no more than 10 mEq/L in 24 hours. Assure serum sodium levels are obtained every 4 to 6 hours depending on whether the patient is symptomatic or not.

HINT Remember, give 3% NaCl in small amounts very slowly to correct sodium over a longer time (Box 4.27).

Box 4.27 Differentiating SIADH from CSWS

CSWS	SIADH
Serum sodium < 135 mEq/L	Serum sodium < 135 mEq/L
Decreased extracellular fluid volume	Increased extracellular fluid volume
Increased hct	Normal hct
Increased albumin levels	Normal albumin levels
Normal or Increased K^+	Normal K^+
Normal or decreased plasma uric acid	Decreased plasma uric acid
Increased BUN/creatinine	Decreased BUN
Signs of dehydration	Urine Na^+ > 25 mEq/L
	Serum osmolality < 280 mOsm/kg
	Urine osmolality > serum osmolality
	Concentrated urine
	Signs of hypervolemia

BUN, blood urea nitrogen; CSWS, cerebral salt wasting syndrome; hct, hematocrit; SIADH, syndrome of inappropriate ADH.

▶ COMPLICATIONS

See Box 4.28.

Box 4.28 Complications of DI/SIADH/CSWS

Hypo- or hypernatremia	Central pontine myelinolysis
Volume overload or dehydration	Acute renal failure

CPM, central pontine myelinolysis.

⬤) ADRENAL INSUFFICIENCY

Q Which portion of the adrenal gland produces the hormones?

A Cortex

The adrenal gland is composed of the cortex and medulla. The cortex is responsible for the production of hormones such as androgens, estrogens, glucocorticoids, mineralocorticoids, and aldosterone.

HINT The medulla portion of the adrenal gland produces catecholamines.

Q Which structure in the brain controls the release of cortisol from the adrenal gland?

A Hypothalamus

Cortisol is secreted from the cortex of the adrenal gland but the secretion is controlled by the hypothalamus. This is called the hypothalamic-pituitary-adrenal (HPA) axis. (Figure 4.4).

HINT Adrenal gland is key organ to deal with stress. Stress releases the catecholamines and stimulates HPA axis.

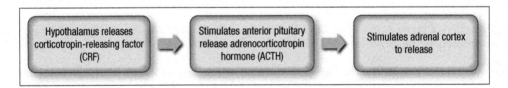

Figure 4.4 Physiology Adrenal System

▶ PATHOPHYSIOLOGY

Q When are cortisol levels normally found to be higher bloodstream?

A Early morning

Cortisol levels are normally found to be the highest during the time of awakening and falls during the day. The lowest levels are found in the evening/night. This contributes to the circadian rhythm.

HINT Disease processes, including plaque rupture, may be influenced by the circadian rhythm.

Q An adrenal tumor is found to be the cause of a patient's adrenal insufficiency. Is this considered a primary or secondary cause?

A Primary

Adrenal insufficiency can be a result of either a primary or secondary cause (Box 4.29). Adrenal tumors are classified as a primary cause. A significant number of primary causes are related to autoimmune disorders. Absolute or relative adrenal insufficiency can occur in critical illness and sepsis.

HINT   A secondary cause is most commonly attributed to the sudden withdrawal of corticoid therapy.

HINT   St. John's Wort can cause an increase in cortisol clearance resulting in adrenal insufficiency and should be stopped at least 2 weeks prior to surgery.

Box 4.29 Causes of Adrenal Insufficiency

Primary	Secondary
Adrenal tumors	Withdrawal from corticosteroid therapy
AIDS associated	Pituitary tumors
Infections (including fungal) of adrenal gland	Traumatic brain injury
Idiopathic (probably immune)	Post radiation pituitary region
Hemorrhage into adrenal glands	Rare genetic syndromes
Septic shock	
Critical illness	

▶ SYMPTOMS/ASSESSMENTS

Q What is the most common hemodynamic symptom of adrenal insufficiency?

A Hypotension

Presentation of cardiovascular collapse and fever are common in the critical illness associated with adrenal insufficiency. It is accompanied by fever and tachycardia (Box 4.30).

HINT   The electrolyte abnormalities associated with adrenal insufficiency are hyponatremia and hyperkalemia.

Box 4.30 Symptoms of Adrenal Insufficiency

Fever
Hypotension
Hyponatremia/hyperkalemia/hypercalcemia/hypoglycemia
Elevated eosinophils with neutropenia
Weakness/fatigue/apathy
Anorexia/weight loss
Skin hyperpigmentation
Nausea, vomiting, and abdominal pain
Mild acidosis

▶ DIAGNOSIS

Q Which laboratory test is usually ordered to determine the location of involvement and responsiveness of the adrenal gland in adrenal insufficiency?

A Adrenocorticotropin hormone (ACTH) stimulation test

Adrenal insufficiency can be caused by problems in the hypothalamus or adrenal gland. The ACTH test can help determine the responsiveness of the adrenal gland to stimulation. It can also be used to assist with determining the underlying cause by locating the abnormality to be in the hypothalamus or adrenal gland (Figure 4.5).

HINT ACTH testing is not currently recommended in sepsis/septic shock patients.

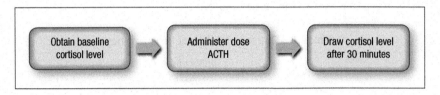

Figure 4.5 Adrenal Stimulation Test

Q What is the most commonly ordered laboratory test used to determine adrenal abnormalities?

A Random serum cortisol level

Random serum cortisol levels obtained on admission can be used to determine the presence of or rule out adrenal insufficiency.

▶ MANAGEMENT

Q What is the primary medical management of adrenal insufficiency?

A Steroid replacement

Administration of steroids to replace the cortisol deficiency is the primary medical management. It typically involves administration of hydrocortisone. Other treatments include IV hydration with isotonic solution and managing the underlying cause.

HINT If patient is experiencing cardiovascular complications and electrolyte abnormalities, it might be reasonable to administer fluorohydrocortisone (synthetic mineralocorticoid).

Q What is the indication for administration of corticosteroids in patients with sepsis?

A Inadequate response to vasoconstrictors

When patients in sepsis/septic shock are on vasoconstrictors but continue to be hypotensive, corticosteroid administration is an option for treatment. This refractory hypotension is due to critical-illness-caused adrenal insufficiency. Replacement of steroid level can improve responsiveness to vasoconstrictors.

⬤ HYPER- AND HYPOTHYROIDISM

The hypothalamic-pituitary-thyroid axis is a controlled loop feedback system. Thyrotropin-releasing hormone (TRH) is produced in the hypothalamus, which stimulates the anterior pituitary to secrete thyroid-stimulating hormone (TSH). The TSH stimulates the release of the thyroid hormone from the thyroid gland. The thyroid gland releases prohormone thyroxine (T4), which is converted in the peripheral to active hormone triiodothyronine (T3).

▶ PATHOPHYSIOLOGY

Q What is a common trigger for patients with Grave's disease to progress to thyroid storm?

A Infections

Patients with a history of Grave's disease have a tendency toward hyperthyroidism. The onset of an infection with fever can trigger the release of thyroid hormones resulting in a thyroid crisis.

HINT This is called "thyrotoxicosis" and is considered a "thyroid storm."

Q In a critically ill patient, does the thyroid hormone typically increase or decrease?

A Decrease

It has been noted that the thyroid hormone very rapidly decreases following acute stress such as major surgeries, trauma, and in critically ill patients. The thyroid hormones have been found to decrease based upon the severity of the disease process.

HINT It may be difficult to distinguish between critically induced decrease in thyroid hormone versus hypothyroidism.

Q What is the syndrome which occurs in untreated prolonged hypothyroidism?

A Myxedema coma

Myxedema coma is severe hypothyroidism that presents with unresponsive or severe altered mentation.

▶ SYMPTOMS/ASSESSMENT

Q What is the most common cardiac arrhythmia found in thyrotoxicosis?

A Supraventricular tachycardia (SVT)

Hyperthyroidism causes an increase in metabolism and an increase in response of the different body systems. SVT is a common symptom of thyrotoxicosis. It is due to an increase in sensitivity to catecholamines. (Box 4.31)

HINT Atrial fibrillation (AF) is another tachyarrhythmia found in hyperthyroidism.

Box 4.31 Signs of Hyperthyroidism

Peripheral vasodilation
Palmar erythema
Rosy complexion
Hyperthermia
Tachycardia (SVT, AF)
Hypertension
Tachypnea
Muscle wasting
Increased GI motility/diarrhea
Restlessness, short attention span

AF, atrial fibrillation; SVT, supraventricular tachycardia.

HINT Hyperthyroidism presents with increased metabolism or heat production; everything speeds up. Hypothyroidism has a decreased metabolism; everything slows down (Box 4.32).

Box 4.32 Signs of Hypothyroidism

Altered mentation to coma
Cool, clammy skin
Hypothermia
Nonpitting edema
Depressed respiratory drive with hypercapnia
Bradycardia
Hypotension

▶ DIAGNOSIS

Q What laboratory tests are used to identify thyroid abnormalities?

A TSH, T3, T4

TSH levels are low, with normal to elevated free T4 and T3 levels in hyperthyroidism. Hypothyroidism will elevate TSH but with low T3 and T4.

HINT Laboratory findings may assist with the definitive diagnosis but diagnosis is primarily clinical.

▶ MEDICAL MANAGEMENT

Q Which medication is used in hyperthyroidism to lower thyroid levels?

A Propylthiouracil (PTU)

PTU prevents thyroidal synthesis and release of thyroid hormone. It is typically used with corticosteroids and beta-adrenergic receptor blocking agents to control heart rate and blood pressure (BP). Antihypertensives and antiepileptics may be required.

HINT PTU can temporarily lower the WBC and may place the patient at higher risk for infections. Another medication is methimazole (Tapazole), which is used to lower thyroid hormone levels.

Q Which drug toxicity can actually induce thyrotoxicosis?

A Amiodarone

Amiodarone toxicity may induce thyrotoxic crisis.

HINT Treatment remains similar to other causes of thyrotoxicosis.

Q What medication is commonly ordered with thyroid replacement therapy in myxedema patients?

A Corticosteroids

Initial dosing with T3 or T4 can cause temporary adrenal insufficiency that occurs with the restoration of thyroid hormone.

HINT Initiate glucosteroids before beginning thyroid replacements.

Q While cooling a patient in a thyroid storm, what is important to prevent?

A Shivering

Shivering can increase body temperature and cardiac demands by increasing metabolism in a patient with an already increased metabolism. Cooling is typically accomplished with acetaminophen or external cooling devices.

HINT   Controlling the rapidity of the decreasing temperature and administering medications to prevent shivering should be a part of the protocol in managing thyroid storm.

▶ SURGICAL MANAGEMENT

Q   What surgical procedure can potentially be used in hyperthyroidism?

A   Thyroid resection

Surgical resection of the thyroid gland may be considered if the patient remains hemodynamically unstable despite medical management.

HINT   One of the possible complications of the surgery is vocal cord paralysis.

▶ COMPLICATIONS

Q   What is the most common complication of a thyroid storm that is most likely to cause death?

A   Cardiac arrhythmias

Supraventricular tachycardia and ventricular tachycardia can result in death in hyperthyroidism.

Q   What cardiac arrhythmia is potential complication of myxedema coma that can result in death?

A   Torsades de pointes

Hypothyroidism can prolong the Q-T interval increasing the risk of Torsades de pointes.

HINT   Recommend monitoring of Q-T intervals in critically ill patients.

Q   Which neurological complication can commonly occur in both thyrotoxicosis and myxedema coma?

A   Seizures

Myxedema coma does not always present with comatose state but can present with seizures. Hyperthyroidism causes an increase in metabolism, and seizures are prominent in these patients.

HINT   Phenytoin is not recommended in seizures caused by hypothyroidism because it decreases thyroid levels.

1. In which part of the brain is the antidiuretic hormone (ADH) produced and stored?

   A. Hypothalamus and posterior pituitary
   B. Thalamus and hypothalamus
   C. Anterior pituitary and amygdala
   D. Hippocampus and posterior pituitary

2. While correcting ketones in a patient with diabetic ketoacidosis (DKA), which of the following should be monitored to determine the resolution of the ketoacidosis?

   A. Bicarbonate level
   B. Base deficit
   C. Anion gap
   D. Serum pH

3. A patient with diabetic ketoacidosis (DKA) is noted to have a low sodium level on the morning labs. Which electrolyte abnormality must be taken into account when determining treatment for the hyponatremia?

   A. Glucose
   B. Calcium
   C. Potassium
   D. Phosphate

4. Which of the following interventions is considered to be the first-line treatment for a patient with a hyperglycemic emergency?

   A. Insulin replacement
   B. Fluid administration
   C. Administration of sodium bicarbonate
   D. Replacement of magnesium losses

5. Which of the following situations would indicate the need to withhold insulin initially when treating hyperglycemia in a diabetic patient?

   A. Metabolic acidosis
   B. Hypokalemia
   C. Allergy to soy
   D. Inability to obtain intravenous (IV)

6. Which of the following is used as differentiation between cerebral salt wasting syndrome (CSWS) and the syndrome of inappropriate antidiuretic hormone secretion (SIADH)?

   A. Sodium level
   B. Underlying disease process
   C. Fluid volume status
   D. Urine sodium

1. A) Hypothalamus and posterior pituitary

ADH is produced in the hypothalamus and stored in the posterior pituitary. Injury or swelling in these areas can result in central diabetes insipidus (DI) or syndrome of inappropriate antidiuretic hormone secretion (SIADH).

2. C) Anion gap

Anion gap is used to determine the correction of ketoacidosis. The serum bicarbonate level and pH are not reliable measurements of acid-base balance in DKA patients, because the isotonic saline being used to manage dehydration causes a hyperchloremic acidosis that prevents the bicarbonate from increasing. The base deficit may be used to determine adequate fluid resuscitation and return to normal perfusion.

3. A) Glucose

Dehydration is universal in DKA, but this might not be reflected in plasma sodium because hyperglycemia has a dilutional effect on sodium. The plasma sodium concentration decreases by 1.6 mEq/L for every 100 mg/dL increase in plasma glucose concentration.

4. B) Fluid administration

Fluid administration is considered the first-line treatment in managing hyperglycemic emergencies (diabetic ketoacidosis, DKA; hyperosmolar hyperglycemic syndrome, HHS). Fluid is used to correct the significant water depletion that occurs with severe hyperglycemia and establishes reperfusion of the kidneys. The administration of fluid begins to correct the hyperglycemia and can decrease serum glucose concentrations by up to 50 mg/dL. Insulin replacement should be initiated after initial fluid resuscitation is given. Sodium bicarbonate is not usually recommended in the management of DKA or HHS. Electrolyte replacement is a component of treatment, but fluids are still initiated before magnesium replacement.

5. B) Hypokalemia

Hypokalemia should be corrected prior to the administration of insulin due to the shift of potassium intracellular. Potassium levels should be corrected before insulin is started. Most diabetic ketoacidosis (DKA) or hyperosmolar hyperglycemic syndrome (HHS) patients have normal, or even elevated, initial potassium levels, and potassium is replaced during the administration of insulin.

6. C) Fluid volume status

Patients with CSWS are hypovolemic, whereas patients with SIADH are euvolemic to hypervolemic. They both have hyponatremia and high urine sodium levels. Both can be the result of a neurological injury.

7. Which of the following combinations is a "hallmark" for the recognition of the syndrome of inappropriate antidiuretic hormone secretion (SIADH)?

   A. Hyponatremia and dilute urine
   B. Hypernatremia and dilute urine
   C. Hypernatremia and increased urine sodium
   D. Hyponatremia and concentrated urine

8. Which of the following is considered a "hallmark" of diabetes insipidus (DI)?

   A. It is found only in neurologically injured patients
   B. It is an acute process without risk of chronic involvement
   C. It presents with a dilute urine in combination with hypertonic serum
   D. It involves loss of sodium in the urine with osmotic diuresis

9. Noninsulin-dependent diabetics can present with diabetic ketoacidosis (DKA). These patients are identified as having which of the following?

   A. Hyperglycemic hyperosmolar nonketotic coma
   B. Hypoglycemia
   C. Ketosis-prone diabetes
   D. Gestational diabetes

10. Which of the following is considered a counterregulatory hormone?

   A. Melatonin
   B. Thyroid stimulating hormone
   C. Glucagon
   D. Adrenocorticotropin hormone (ACTH)

11. Which of the following complications can significantly increase metabolic acidosis in patients being treated for diabetic ketoacidosis (DKA)?

   A. Acute kidney injury (AKI)
   B. Altered mentation
   C. Hypokalemia
   D. Hypoglycemia

12. An elevated Beta-hydroxybutyrate in the presence of hyperglycemia can be used to diagnose which of the following disorders?

   A. Cushing's syndrome
   B. Diabetic ketoacidosis (DKA)
   C. Hypoparathyroidism
   D. Hashimoto's thyroiditis

13. Which of the following medications may have side effect of hyponatremia, which is caused by syndrome of inappropriate antidiuretic hormone secretion (SIADH)?

   A. Tolvaptan
   B. Demeclocycline
   C. Selective serotonin uptake inhibitors (SSRIs)
   D. Lithium

(See answers next page.)   **177**

7. D) Hyponatremia and concentrated urine

SIADH is an inappropriate release of antidiuretic hormone (ADH), resulting in the reabsorption of water in the kidney. This results in hypotonic serum and hyponatremia while having concentrated urine and high urine sodium levels. Hypernatremia is a result of diabetes insipidus (DI).

8. C) It presents with a dilute urine in combination with hypertonic serum

The hallmark of DI is a dilute urine and hemoconcentrated serum. This is a result of a decrease in antidiuretic hormone (ADH) and the resulting diuresis. The excessive loss of water, even during a period of fluid restriction, is diagnostic of DI. DI can be neurogenic (central DI) or nephrogenic (caused by the kidneys not responding to ADH). DI can be acute or chronic. The diuresis is due to loss of water, not sodium. This causes the increase in serum osmolality. Cerebral salt wasting syndrome (CSWS) causes a loss of sodium in urine with an osmotic diuresis.

9. C) Ketosis-prone diabetes

Noninsulin-dependent diabetics will typically present with hyperglycemia hyperosmolar syndrome which is without the elevated ketones. So, if a noninsulin diabetic presents with diabetic ketoacidosis (DKA) (elevated ketones), it is called "ketosis-prone diabetes." DKA has hyperglycemia not hypoglycemia. Gestational diabetes occurs during pregnancy.

10. C) Glucagon

Glucagon is a counterregulatory hormone as well as cortisol, growth hormone, and adrenaline. Melatonin, thyroid stimulating hormone, and ACTH are not considered counterregulatory hormones.

11. A) AKI

A compensatory mechanism in ketoacidosis is the excretion of ketones by the kidneys. AKI with decreased urine output will not be able to compensate for the high ketones, and ketoacidosis will worsen. Patients in DKA are prone to AKI due to hypoperfusion. Altered mentation, hypokalemia, and hypoglycemia are all potential complications of DKA or the treatment of DKA but will not increase ketones.

12. B) DKA

β-OHB is a serum test used to measure the ketone beta-hydroxybutyrate. The presence of both hyperglycemia and elevated β-OHB levels indicate DKA. Cushing's syndrome will elevate glucose but not β-OHB levels. Neither hypoparathyroidism nor Hashimoto's thyroiditis can cause hyperglycemia and elevated serum β-OHB levels.

13. C) SSRI

Medication-induced SIADH can occur with several classes of medications, including SSRIs. The hyponatremia of SIADH can be reversed by discontinuation of the medication. Tolvaptan is a novel diuretic that is used to treat acute SIADH. Demeclocycline and lithium have been used to manage chronic SIADH, not cause the water abnormality.

14. Which of the electrolyte abnormalities is most commonly found in patients presenting with acute adrenal insufficiency?

   A. Hypocalcemia
   B. Hypokalemia
   C. Hyponatremia
   D. Hyperphosphatemia

15. A septic patient in the ICU is hypotensive despite vasoconstrictors being administered. Which of the following medications may be administered to stabilize this patient's hemodynamic status?

   A. ACE inhibitors
   B. Decadron
   C. Dobutamine
   D. Isuprel

14. C) Hyponatremia

Acute adrenal insufficiency can result in cardiovascular collapse. Commonly associated electrolyte abnormalities include hyponatremia and hyperkalemia. This is primarily the result of the release of mineralocorticosteroids. Hypercalcemia and hypophosphatemia are also commonly associated with adrenal insufficiency.

15. B) Decadron

Sepsis and critical illness can cause adrenal insufficiency with presentation similar to Addison's disease and refractory hypotension. The replacement of the steroid with Decadron allows the body to become more responsive to the vasoconstrictors. ACE inhibitors would be contraindicated because of the decrease in BP. Dobutamine and Isuprel have inotropic effects but are not considered vasoconstrictors and will not significantly improve this patient's BP.

BIBLIOGRAPHY

American Diabetes Association. (2019). Standards of medical care in diabetes update. *Diabetes Care*, *42*(Suppl. 1), S1–S194.

Baldeweg, S., Bali, S., Gleeson, H., Levy, M., Prentice, M., Wass, J., … the Society of Endocrinology Clinical Committee. (2018). Society of endocrinology clinical guidance: Inpatient management of cranial diabetes insipidus. *Endocrinology Connection*, *7*(7), G8–G11.

Garrahy, A., Moran, C., & Thompson, C. (2019). Diagnosis and management of central diabetes insipidus in adult. *Clinical Endocrinology*, *18*(23).

Kreider, K. (2018). Update in the management of diabetic ketoacidosis. *Journal of Nurse Practioners*, *14*(8), 591–597.

Hematology and Immunology System Review

5

> ▶ **LEARNING OBJECTIVES**
>
> In this chapter, you will review:
> - ■ Coagulopathies
>   - ○ Disseminated intravascular coagulation (DIC)
>   - ○ Heparin-induced thrombocytopenia (HIT)
>   - ○ Idiopathic thrombocytopenia purpura (ITP)
> - ■ Anemia
> - ■ Transfusion reactions
> - ■ Immune deficiencies
> - ■ Leukopenia
> - ■ Oncologic complications (Tumor lysis syndrome, plural effusion)
> - ■ Thrombocytopenia

● COAGULOPATHIES

▶ DISSEMINATED INTRAVASCULAR COAGULATION (DIC)

> **Q** What type of coagulopathy is disseminated intravascular coagulation (DIC)?
>
> **A** Consumptive

DIC is an acquired syndrome characterized by intravascular activation of coagulation factors. It can originate from and cause damage to microvasculature, which, if sufficiently severe, can cause organ dysfunction and bleeding. The bleeding is caused by the consumption of the clotting factors as well as the activation of the fibrinolytic system. DIC is called a consumptive coagulopathy because the platelets and clotting factors are consumed in the microvascular circulation. Platelets become activated and aggravate, progressively causing thrombocytopenia.

HINT DIC begins as a clotting problem but manifests itself as a bleeding disorder.

> **Q** What is the most common cause of death in disseminated intravascular coagulation (DIC) patients?
>
> **A** Multisystem organ failure (MSOF)

Occlusion in the microcirculation by the thrombi may manifest as multisystem organ failure. The deposits of fibrin and clots in the microcirculation result in ischemia to organs, skin, and limbs.

HINT Microvascular thrombosis and fibrin deposits together contribute to MSOF

▶ PATHOPHYSIOLOGY

Q What is considered the "trigger" for increased clotting in microcirculation and activation of the coagulation system?

A Procoagulants

Procoagulants are factors that can increase clotting in microcirculation and initiate the release of tissue factor. Procoagulants include bacterial toxins, free hemoglobin, fragments of cancer or placental tissue, acidosis, and the release of tissue factor into the blood. Tissue factor (TF) is found on the surface of endothelial cells, macrophages, and monocytes and is not usually in contact with general circulation but can be exposed after vascular damage. Once activated, TF binds to coagulation factors, which then trigger the extrinsic pathway (via factor VII) and intrinsic pathway (initially via XII).

HINT The most common cause of DIC is sepsis. (Box 5.1).

Box 5.1 Clinical Conditions Associated With DIC

Sepsis and septic shock	Snake bites
Traumatic injuries/crush injuries	Obstetrical emergencies
Hypoxia	Amniotic fluid embolism
Acidosis	Intrauterine fetal demise
Burns	Eclampsia
Transplant rejections	Recreational drugs
Transfusion reactions	Cancerous tumors
Hemorrhagic pancreatitis	Rocky Mountain spotted fever
Pancreatitis	Malignancy
Liver disease	Vascular anomalies

DIC, disseminated intravascular coagulation.

Q What is the normal process for fibrinolysis following thrombin clot formation?

A Plasminogen converts to plasmin

Plasminogen circulates in an inactive form in the blood. Following fibrin clot formation, plasminogen is activated and converts to plasmin, a proteolytic enzyme. Plasmin lysis or dissolves the fibrin to restore blood flow through the vessel. In DIC, the process of clot formation and degradation is accelerated, and the complete process leads to consumption of circulating clotting factors.

HINT In DIC, there is suppression of the fibrinolysis system due to elevated plasminogen activator inhibitor-1.

Q What is the byproduct of a fibrin clot?

A Fibrin degradation products (FDPs)

Following fibrinolysis, the byproducts of fibrin breakdown are FDPs. As the body forms clots and breaks the clots down, it releases more FDPs, which work as an anticoagulant to prevent further clot formation. Other causes of anticoagulation effects in DIC include a reduction in antithrombin III and protein C.

HINT D-dimer test is used to measure FDPs.

▶ SYMPTOMS/ASSESSMENT

Q What is the most obvious sign of DIC?

A Bleeding

Overt bleeding may occur from old intravenous (IV) puncture sites or present as bruising, purpura, ecchymosis, and expanding hematoma. Bleeding can occur from mucous membranes, hemoptysis, hematuria, or the intracranial and gastrointestinal (GI) tracts.

HINT   Remember, bleeding is the first sign of DIC but the underlying cause of death MSOF.

> **Q** **What is the systemic finding of microvascular occlusion and organ dysfunction in disseminated intravascular coagulation (DIC)?**
>
> **A** **Elevated serum lactate levels**

The microvascular occlusion that occurs in DIC results in the conversion of aerobic to anaerobic metabolism with the elevation of lactate levels and metabolic acidosis.

HINT   Respiratory rates may increase to buffer the increase in H^+ ions by lowering the $PaCO_2$ levels.

▶ DIAGNOSIS

> **Q** **Which laboratory finding distinguishes a diagnosis of disseminated intravascular coagulation (DIC)?**
>
> **A** **Elevated D-dimer**

The D-dimer measures FDPs. The FDPs are byproducts of fibrin and will elevate when fibrin clots are formed and then lysed. DIC is the only coagulopathy that elevates FDPs because of the clotting. Multiple coagulopathies will produce elevated clotting times and thrombocytopenia, but DIC is the primary coagulopathy that forms clots and then consumes the clotting factors thereby in turn leading to bleeding complications. The decreasing platelet count is due to consumption of the platelets in an attempt to form clots. DIC diagnosis requires predisposition, clinical findings, and laboratory tests for accurate diagnosis.

HINT   Elevated D-dimer is not specific to DIC. There are many causes of elevated FDPs but D-dimer assists with the differential diagnosis in DIC (Box 5.2).

Box 5.2 Laboratory Findings of DIC

Prolonged PT and PTT	Thrombocytopenia
Decreased fibrinogen levels	Decreased antithrombin III
Increased D-dimer	Increased FDPs

DIC, disseminated intravascular coagulation; FDPs, fibrin degradation products; PT, prothrombin time; PTT, partial thromboplastin time.

> **Q** **What is the International Society for Thrombosis and Haemostasis (ISTH) scoring system used for?**
>
> **A** **Used guide treatment DIC**

ISTH score is calculated daily to guide treatment of DIC. It indicates an improvement or worsening of the patient's status.

HINT   This scoring is used only when the clinical presentation of the patient matches DIC.

▶ MANAGEMENT

> **Q** **What is the most accepted intervention in managing patients with disseminated intravascular coagulation (DIC)?**
>
> **A** **Treat the underlying cause**

The most accepted treatment of DIC is to identify the underlying cause and to treat or remove it. DIC is an acquired syndrome caused by another underlying disease process that works as a procoagulant. The best method of treating DIC is to remove the procoagulant material.

> **Q** When would transfusion of red blood cells (RBCs) and components be indicated in a disseminated intravascular coagulation (DIC) patient?
>
> **A** Active hemorrhage

Administration of blood and blood components in DIC patients has been controversial; however, during periods of active bleeding, acute decline in clotting factors, or deterioration in the clinical status, transfusion therapy is recommended.

HINT Administering clotting factors while the procoagulant is still active may "fuel the fire" and produce more clots (worsen ischemia) and FDPs (work as anticoagulants).

> **Q** What blood component may be indicated if fibrinogen levels are below 100 mg/dL and the patient is not responding to fresh frozen plasma (FFP)?
>
> **A** Cryoprecipitate

Cryoprecipitation is recommended for symptomatic bleeding patients with fibrinogen levels less than 100 mg/dL. It may be used when the patient does not respond to FFP in elevating fibrinogen levels. The disadvantage is that cryoprecipitate is rich in fibrinogen and can increase FDPs and coagulopathy if the patient is still clotting in the microcirculation.

HINT FFP is used in bleeding patients with prolonged bleeding times to replace clotting factors and fibrinogen.

> **Q** When would platelets most likely be transfused?
>
> **A** Active bleeding patient with platelets less than 50,000

Platelets may be transfused for symptomatic bleeding patients with platelet count less than 50,000 or less than 10,000 to 20,000 without signs of bleeding.

HINT Replacement therapy is only recommended if the patient is symptomatic; it is not used to treat laboratory abnormalities only.

> **Q** What is the physiological effect of heparin that in theory may benefit the patient in disseminated intravascular coagulation (DIC)?
>
> **A** Indirect thrombin inhibitor

The administration of heparin or low-molecular-weight heparin (LMWH) in treating DIC remains controversial. In theory, heparin interacts with antithrombin to inactivate factor X, thus preventing conversion of prothrombin to thrombin. This will alter the ability of the clot to become stable.

▶ COMPLICATIONS

> **Q** What are the two primary complications of disseminated intravascular coagulation (DIC) patients?
>
> **A** Bleeding and multisystem organ failure

The consumption of the platelets and clotting factors lead to abnormal bleeding. Clots forming in the microcirculation, due to the release of a procoagulant, cause obstruction and hypoperfusion of organs (Table 5.1).

Table 5.1 Symptoms of Multisystem Organ Failure (MSOF)

Organ Involved	Symptoms
Lungs	PaO_2/FiO_2 ratio <150, ARDS
Kidneys	Elevated creatinine, blood urea nitrogen (BUN), decreased urine output
Liver	Elevated liver enzymes
Brain	Altered level of consciousness
Gastrointestinal tract	Stress-related ulcerations

ARDS, acute respiratory distress syndrome; BUN, blood urea nitrogen.

▶ HEPARIN-INDUCED THROMBOCYTOPENIA (HIT)

Q What is the most common drug-related immune thrombocytopenia?

A HIT

HIT is a drug-related immune thrombocytopenia. There are two classifications of HIT. HIT type I is a nonimmune reaction to heparin that decreases the platelet count. It is a reversible form of HIT. Type II is a more serious, immune-related form of HIT. HIT with thromboembolic syndrome (HITTS) includes patients who develop thromboembolic complications.

HINT In HIT, more patients develop thrombocytopenia alone than thrombocytopenia with thromboembolic complications.

Q Which anticoagulation therapy, unfractionated heparin (UFH) or low molecular weight heparin, has a greater risk of developing heparin-induced thrombocytopenia (HIT)?

A Unfractionated heparin (UFH)

UFH has a greater incidence of HIT than LMWH. UFH has approximately 2% to 3% risk, whereas LMWH is less than 1%. There is a lower frequency if heparin is used primarily as a flush. HIT occurs more frequently in patients receiving higher doses of heparin than standard prophylaxis doses.

HINT Once HIT occurs, the patient should not receive either UFH or LMWH.

▶ PATHOPHYSIOLOGY

Q What antigen complex do the antibodies react with to cause platelet aggregation?

A Heparin-platelet factor 4 complex

Antibodies recognize complexes between heparin and platelet factor 4 (PF4). Heparin elicits a platelet-active antibody that specifically interacts with the GP IIb/IIIa receptors on the platelets. Following administration of heparin (antigen), heparin-platelet factor 4 stimulates the platelets and causes them to aggregate.

HINT Platelet aggregation leads to thrombotic events and consumption of platelets (thrombocytopenia).

▶ SYMPTOMS/ASSESSMENT

Q What is the most common timing for the presentation of heparin-induced thrombocytopenia (HIT) after heparin exposure?

A 5 to 10 days

This syndrome usually occurs within 5 to 10 days of heparin therapy. It may be present as early as 24 to 48 hours in patients with previous exposure to heparin within the past 100 days. The first day of immunizing heparin exposure is equal to day 0. Exposure to heparin within the previous 100 days indicates that antibodies may still be circulating and can cause abrupt thrombocytopenia after starting heparin.

HINT HIT is not generally associated with bleeding presentation.

Q Which type of onset is the least common for the presentation of heparin-induced thrombocytopenia (HIT)?

A Delayed onset

Delayed-onset HIT is uncommon. Symptoms occur 2 weeks after being exposed to heparin. It is typically associated with very high-titer anti-PF4/heparin antibodies and requires a high dose and prolonged alternative anticoagulation to control massive thrombin generation.

▶ DIAGNOSIS

> **Q** What finding is the most common reason for suspicion of heparin-induced thrombocytopenia (HIT)?
>
> **A** Decrease in platelet count greater than 50%

The hallmark sign is a significant decrease in platelet count (>50%) over a 24-hour period without any other known cause of thrombocytopenia within 5 to 10 days after starting heparin.

HINT Another sign is a thromboembolic event within 5 to 10 days after starting heparin.

> **Q** Which laboratory test has a high negative predictive value but may be positive in patients without HIT?
>
> **A** Anti-PF4/heparin antibody

The anti-PF4/heparin antibody test has a high negative predictive value; if it is negative, the patient has a very low possibility of having HIT. Not all positive anti-PF4/heparin antibodies are pathogenic and elevate due to exposure to heparin. The test is unable to clearly distinguish between pathogenic and nonpathogenic antibodies. Antigen assay (ELISA) is a quantitative test that increases in specificity relative to the magnitude of a positive test. Additional test of the serotonin release assay (SRA) can be used to rule out HIT.

HINT It is not recommended to routinely screen for the antibodies unless the patient exhibits clinical symptoms (Table 5.2).

Table 5.2 Four Ts Probability Scores

Four Ts	2 Points	1 Point	0 Point
Thrombocytopenia	Platelet count decrease >50% and platelet nadir ≥20,000	Platelet count decrease 30%–50% (>50% decrease resulting from surgery) or platelet nadir 10,000–19,000	Platelet count decrease <30% or platelet nadir <10,000
Timing of platelet count decrease	Clear onset between days 5 and 10 or platelet decrease within 1 day (heparin exposure within 30 days)	Consistent with immunization but unclear history; onset after day 10; <1 day (heparin exposure 1–3 months ago)	Platelet count decrease <4 days of recent exposure
Thrombosis or other sequelae	New thrombosis (confirmed); skin necrosis; acute systemic reaction post-IV UFH bolus	Progressive or recurrent thrombosis; non-necrotizing (erythematous) skin lesions; suspected thrombosis not yet proven	None
Other causes of thrombocytopenia	None apparent	Possible	Definite

High probability: 6–8 points (HIT is likely); intermediate probability: 4–5 points (HIT is possible); and low probability: ≤3 points (HIT is unlikely)

▶ MANAGEMENT

> **Q** Once the diagnosis of heparin-induced thrombocytopenia (HIT) is established, what is the priority of care?
>
> **A** Stop all heparin administration

Once this syndrome is suspected or diagnosed, heparin must not be given to the patient because of the potential life-threatening effects. All heparins need to be stopped, including LMWH, heparin catheter flushes, IV, or SC routes of heparin. High cross-reactivity occurs with LMWH once the patient develops the pathogenic antibody to heparin.

HINT Recommend placing a heparin allergy in the chart and post a sign at the bedside.

Q After stopping heparin, what intervention is recommended to prevent thromboembolic complications?

A Administer nonheparin anticoagulation therapy

Nonheparin anticoagulation should be initiated promptly to limit thrombosis complications. Upon discontinuation of heparin, platelet counts start to recover within 4 days but may take longer than 2 weeks in patients with high-titer HIT antibodies. Heparin is replaced with a direct thrombin inhibitor (DTI), Factor Xa inhibitor, or fondaparinux (Table 5.3).

Warfarin should not be initiated until after platelet counts recover, preferably greater than 150,000.

Table 5.3 Anticoagulants

Drug	Classification	Half-Life	Elimination
Arganova (Argatroban)	Synthetic DTI	45 min	Liver
Fondaparinux (Arixtra)	Pentasaccharide	17 hr	Renal
Xarelto (rivaroxaban)	Factor Xa Inhibitor	5–9 hours	Metabolic degradation and renal
Eliquis (apixaban)	Factor Xa inhibitor	12 hours	Renal

DTI, direct thrombin inhibitor.

Q What is the laboratory test recommended to monitor a direct thrombin inhibitor (DTI)?

A Activated partial thromboplastin time (aPTT)

Frequent aPTT monitoring is recommended when starting these patients on DTIs. aPTT may underestimate the bleeding time, and an ecarin clotting time may be required.

HINT Arganova (Argatroban) can erroneously elevate the PT/INR (prothrombin time/international normalized ratio), but it is not accurate for determining bleeding times.

Q Which anticoagulant is recommended for more long-term management of heparin-induced thrombocytopenia (HIT) after alternative anticoagulant is started?

A Warfarin (Coumadin)

American College of Chest Physician's guidelines recommend warfarin therapy in patients requiring more long-term management to prevent thrombosis. The initial effect of warfarin, however, is a transient procoagulation. It is not recommended to start warfarin therapy in acute HIT as long as thrombocytopenia persists due to the risk of warfarin-induced microthrombosis. Initiate warfarin after the alternative anticoagulation therapy and overlap with the DTIs. Discontinue DTI only after a 5-day overlap and when the platelet count is stable.

HINT Obtain an initial PT/INR as baseline before warfarin is started. After the desired overlap days and the goal INR is reached, withhold DTI for 48 hours and recheck PT/INR.

Q What other treatment may be used to manage heparin-induced thrombocytopenia (HIT) as an adjunct to anticoagulation therapy?

A Intravenous immunoglobulin (IVIG)

IVIG therapy interrupts platelet activation by HIT antibodies and results in a rapid increase in platelet counts. IVIG can be used in conjunction with nonheparin anticoagulation therapy.

HINT IVIG may be used to prevent acute HIT with re-exposure to heparin in antibody positive patients.

▶ COMPLICATIONS

Q What is the most common thromboembolic complication of heparin-induced thrombocytopenia (HIT)?

A Venous thromboembolisms (VTEs)

Approximately 50% to 75% of patients with HIT develop symptomatic thrombosis, which can occur even if platelet count remains greater than 150,000, but usually, the risk of thrombosis correlates with the magnitude of decrease in platelets. The thrombosis may occur 1 to 3 days before thrombocytopenia is recognized. Thromboembolic events are defined as thrombosis during therapy or worsening of thrombosis as confirmed by invasive or noninvasive diagnostic techniques.

HINT Thrombotic events can be venous and/or arterial. This may occur as a single event or multiple thromboses (Boxes 5.3 and 5.4).

Box 5.3 Venous Thrombotic Complications

VTE
Axillary vein thrombosis
Renal vein thrombosis
Adrenal vein thrombosis

VTE, venous thromboembolism.

Box 5.4 Arterial Thrombotic Complications

Limb ischemia/infarction
Mesenteric artery thrombosis
Stroke
Acute coronary syndrome (ACS)

▶ IDIOPATHIC THROMBOCYTOPENIA PURPURA (ITP)

Q What is the other name for idiopathic thrombocytopenia purpura (ITP)?

A Immune thrombocytopenia

ITP is an autoimmune disorder characterized by a decrease in platelet count and an increased risk of bleeding. The new term is recommended to emphasize the underlying immune pathophysiology. Primary ITP refers to occurrence without an underlying disease process, while secondary ITP refers to ITP associated with other disease processes (Box 5.5).

Box 5.5 Secondary ITP-Associated Disease Processes

HIV
HCV
Lymphoproliferative disorder
Systemic lupus erythematosus

HCV, hepatitis C virus.

HINT ITP is commonly chronic in adult patients (Table 5.4).

Table 5.4 Classification of ITP

Classification	Duration of Findings
Newly diagnosed	<3 months
Persistent	3–12 months
Chronic	>12 months

▶ PATHOPHYSIOLOGY

Q Does ITP involve humoral or cellular immunity?

A Both

ITP is a complex syndrome that involves both humoral and cellular immunity causing the destruction of the platelets and also a decrease in production. Autoantibodies are developed against the platelet membrane glycoprotein IIb/IIIa (humoral immunity). Patients with ITP also have CD4+ T cells that react to GP IIb/IIIa and produce antiplatelet antibodies (cellular immunity).

HINT Antibody-coated platelets are rapidly cleared by the spleen and liver, resulting in a decrease in platelets.

▶ SYMPTOMS/ASSESSMENT

Q What underlying physiological change causes the clinical findings of ITP?

A Thrombocytopenia

The clinical features of ITP are due to thrombocytopenia and microvascular bleeding. These signs include petechiae (microvascular hemorrhage) and purpura (bruising).

HINT ITP may just present with a low platelet count and no other features of thrombocytopenia (Box 5.6).

Box 5.6 Symptoms of Thrombocytopenia

Petechiae	Gum bleeding
Purpura	Fatigue
Epistaxis	

▶ DIAGNOSIS

Q What is the primary finding used in the diagnosis of ITP?

A Low platelet count

ITP is primarily a diagnosis of exclusion. It may or may not be associated with clinical findings of bleeding. Other causes of thrombocytopenia are ruled out before the diagnosis of ITP is made. A peripheral blood smear may be used to assist with the differential diagnosis. In some patients, a bone marrow aspirate may be used if there are abnormalities on blood smear.

Q What is the most common drug associated with drug-induced thrombocytopenia?

A Heparin

Other drugs that can cause an acute drop in platelets include antiepileptic agents, sulfonamides, interferon, and quinine. The decrease in platelet count within 5 to 10 days of initiating drug therapy should alert the practitioner of a potential, secondary, drug-induced thrombocytopenia.

> **Q** What is another cause of thrombocytopenia that causes acute anemia and fever?
>
> **A** Thrombotic thrombocytopenia purpura (TTP)

The presence of fragmented RBCs on a peripheral blood smear helps make the differential diagnosis of ITP and TTP. TTP complications include renal failure and neurological involvement.

HINT Plasmapheresis is the treatment of choice for TTP.

▶ MEDICAL MANAGEMENT

> **Q** What platelet level would platelets most likely be administered to prevent bleeding complications of thrombocytopenia?
>
> **A** 30,000

If the platelets are low, but the patient is asymptomatic, then the patient may not necessarily require platelet transfusion. If the count is less than 30,000, platelets may be administered to prevent spontaneous hemorrhage, which can occur with platelet counts less than 20,000.

> **Q** What drug therapy is considered the primary treatment for ITP?
>
> **A** Steroids

Oral corticosteroids are considered the initial treatment for ITP. This includes oral prednisone or high-dose dexamethasone (Decadron). IV administration of immunoglobulin is recommended in patients who do not respond to steroids or who demonstrate active bleeding. This therapy is typically successful at increasing the platelet count, but it may have a transient effect and require multiple infusions. IV immunoglobulins are usually well tolerated but may have significant side effects and the rare complication of anaphylaxis. Secondary ITP is treated by managing the underlying infection or disease process.

HINT Remember ITP is considered to be an autoimmune disorder. Steroids and immunosuppressants are typically first-line treatments for autoimmune disorders (Box 5.7).

Box 5.7 Side Effects of IV Immunoglobulin

Fever	Headache
Chills	Myalgias
Back pain	Arthralgias (joint pain)

> **Q** A second-line drug may be given if steroids are ineffective in managing ITP. What is this drug?
>
> **A** Rituximab (Rituxan)

Rituximab is a monoclonal antibody that targets B cells responsible for the production of antiplatelet antibodies. Side effects include infusion reactions and a rare complication of progressive multifocal leukoencephalopathy. Other drugs that have been used include thrombopoietin receptor agonists and immunosuppressants such as azathioprine (Imuran).

▶ SURGICAL MANAGEMENT

> **Q** If patients do not respond to medical management, what surgical procedure may be performed to manage ITP?
>
> **A** Splenectomy

A splenectomy may be performed if the patient is not responsive to medical management of ITP with primary and secondary pharmacological management. It still maintains the most durable, best response of the platelets in the long term.

HINT The spleen is responsible for removing the platelets from circulation. Following a splenectomy, the platelets will remain in circulation longer and increase the platelet count.

Q What vaccinations are recommended in a patient with splenectomy?

A Pneumococcal, *Hemophilus influenzae*, and meningococcal

Vaccinations may be administered 2 weeks prior to a planned splenectomy. Following the removal of the spleen, the patient is at a higher risk for certain systemic illnesses, including pneumococcal and meningococcal infections.

HINT Early antibiotic therapy is recommended in post-splenectomy patients, with fever and signs of systemic infections.

▶ COMPLICATIONS

Q What is the biggest risk associated with ITP?

A Intracerebral hemorrhage

Bleeding is the biggest complication of ITP, especially intracerebral bleeding. However, major bleeding is uncommon with ITP, and most complications are due to the pharmacological and surgical management of ITP.

● ANEMIA

Q Which of the following, liberal or restricted, blood transfusions in critically ill patients is recommended?

A Restrictive

Critically ill patients commonly experience episodes of anemia due to multifactorial causes, including frequent blood draws. Blood transfusions are associated with many complications. The potential risk versus benefit needs to be reviewed on individual basis.

HINT Transfusion trigger for blood administration is most commonly a Hgb 7.0.

▶ PATHOPHYSIOLOGY

Q What is the most common cause of anemia in critically ill patients?

A Loss of blood

Loss of blood may be due to frequent lab draws, bleeding from surgical sites, GI bleeding, trauma, or venous/arterial accesses. Other causes of anemia in critically ill include decreased production of RBCs, nutritional deficiency, and increased destruction. Certain disorders develop coagulation abnormalities such as sepsis syndrome and hepatic failure (Box 5.8).

HINT Daily labs can add up to 1 unit of blood per week.

Box 5.8 Causes of Anemia in Critical Care

Loss of Blood	Phlebotomy Bleeding from surgical site Trauma Venous or arterial accesses
Decreased Production (Suppression Bone Marrow)	Inflammation Drug induced Erythropoietin deficiency (renal failure)
Nutritional	Iron, folic acid and vitamin B deficiency
Increased Destruction (Hemolysis)	Toxins Drug Induced

▶ SYMPTOMS/ASSESSMENT

Q What are the clinical signs of severe anemia in critically ill patients?

A Signs of Organ Dysfunction

Anemia affects the oxygen carrying capacity and oxygen delivery to vital tissues and organs. Clinically, the symptoms are secondary due to decrease in oxygen delivery such as mental changes with brain hypoxia.

HINT Most reliable tool to recognize anemia in critically ill patients is monitoring of the Hgb/hct.

▶ DIAGNOSIS

Q Besides an actual blood loss, what could cause a decrease in hemoglobin level?

A Overhydration

Overhydration can cause a dilutional decrease in Hgb levels due to excessive intravascular volume. This is not an actual loss of blood. A patient that is dehydrated will demonstrate an increase in Hgb level.

HINT An important factor when evaluating the patient's Hgb is the hydration status.

Q Which component of the complete blood count (CBC) is used to evaluate the cause of the anemia?

A Erythrocyte Morphology and Reticulocyte counts

The RBC size is used to identify potential causes of anemia (Table 5.5). The mean corpuscular volume is the measurement of the size of the RBC. Reticulocyte count is used to evaluate the erythropoietic response of bone marrow to anemia.

HINT Acute inflammatory process can disrupt normal iron metabolism, resulting in iron deficiency anemia.

Table 5.5 Anemia Etiology

RBC Morphology	Potential Cause of Anemia
Macrocytic RBC	Vitamin B12 or folate deficiency Hyposplenism Liver disease
Microcytic RBC	Anemia of Chronic Disease Thalassemia Copper deficiency
Normocytic RBC	Renal failure

▶ MANAGEMENT

Q What therapy can be initiated in a stable ICU patient with anemia?

A Erythropoiesis-stimulating agents (ESAs)

ESAs can be utilized in hemodynamically stable patients to increase red blood cell mass and hemoglobin levels. If the underlying cause of the anemia is identified, treatment can be focused on managing the etiology (i.e., iron deficiency would be managed with iron replacement).

HINT Hemodynamically unstable ICU patients or significant acute blood loss would require blood transfusions.

Q During active blood loss, what can be done to reduce blood loss?

A Administer tranexamic acid

Tranexamic acid is a lysine analogue that functions as a antifibrinolytic agent, preventing blood clot from breaking down. This limits blood loss and lowers the requirement of blood transfusion. Other approaches used to decrease need for blood transfusions include red cell salvage, minimally invasive procedures, and hemostatic agents.

HINT A complication of tranexamic acid is venous thromboembolic events.

▶ COMPLICATIONS

Q What is a complication of severe anemia in a critically ill patient?

A Tissue hypoperfusion

Oxygen delivery is determined by Hgb level, oxygenation, and cardiac output. Severe anemia will decrease oxygen delivery to the tissues.

⬤ TRANSFUSION REACTIONS

Q One unit of blood transfused should be expected to increase the hematocrit by how much?

A 3% increase

One unit of blood should increase the patient's hemoglobin by 1.0 g/dL or hematocrit by 3%.

Q What is the most common reason for an acute hemolytic transfusion reaction (AHTR)?

A Administering incompatible blood

AHTRs are almost always due to an error with administering incompatible blood. The reaction is caused by the activation of a complement system by inherited immunoglobulin M (IgM) anti-A, or anti-B antibodies. The result is a massive intravascular hemolysis. The complications and causes of death include DIC and acute kidney injury (AKI).

HINT The first intervention is to stop the transfusion immediately (Box 5.9).

Box 5.9 Symptoms of AHTR

Fever	Hypotension
Chills	Hemoglobinemia
Pain at infusion site	Hemoglobinuria
Back/flank pain	

AHTR, acute hemolytic transfusion reaction.

> **Q** Following an acute hemolytic transfusion reaction (AHTR), what laboratory test would one expect to send?
>
> **A** Direct antiglobulin

Direct antiglobulin (Coomb's test) is used to detect antibodies or proteins that are bound to the transfused RBCs causing agglutination and hemolysis. Other laboratory tests include sending a new hemoglobin, type and crossmatch (T&C), and urine to assess hemoglobinuria.

HINT Do not throw away the blood bag; send it back to the blood lab to retype.

> **Q** What blood transfusion reaction can occur after the patient receives multiple units of antigen-specific uncross-matched blood?
>
> **A** Delayed hemolytic transfusion reactions (DHTRs)

This delayed hemolytic reaction occurs due to the production of antibodies (usually of IgG class) to RBC antigens to which they have been previously exposed (such as pregnancy, previous transfusions, etc.). The antigens may not have been recognized in the first type and crossmatch due to the low titers. The result is a decrease in hemoglobin over the following 5 to 10 days due to hemolysis.

HINT Any time large amounts of uncross-matched blood are administered, a new T&C is recommended to prevent DHTR.

> **Q** What is the most common type of reaction a patient will have to blood transfusions?
>
> **A** Febrile nonhemolytic transfusion reaction (FNHTR)

Fever is the most common type of reaction a patient will have to the administration of blood. Always respond and treat fever as the "worst-case scenario" and test for AHTR. Once ruled out, continue with the transfusion. FNHTR is a febrile reaction caused by the effects of cytokine interleukin (IL)-6, IL-8, and tumor necrosis factor (TNF), which are produced by the donor leukocyte store within the blood product.

HINT Treat with antipyretics.

> **Q** During the administration of packed red blood cells (PRBCs), the patient develops dyspnea, hypoxia, angioedema, and hypotension. What is the most likely cause?
>
> **A** Anaphylactic reaction

Anaphylactic transfusion reactions (ATRs) are due to the development of anti-IgA antibodies after a blood or blood product transfusion (PRBC, FFP, platelets, IV immunoglobulin). This occurs in patients who are IgA-deficient and is a rare reaction. The symptoms occur within minutes of initiating the transfusion.

HINT Stop the transfusion, administer epinephrine, antihistamine, and IV fluids.

> **Q** What is the transfusion reaction that can result in pulmonary failure and the development of acute respiratory distress syndrome (ARDS)?
>
> **A** Transfusion-related acute lung injury (TRALI)

TRALI is the most commonly reported cause of transfusion-related deaths. The theory behind TRALI is that it is a "two-hit" insult. The first hit is a stressful situation (such as trauma, sepsis, massive transfusion, cardiopulmonary bypass surgery), which causes the neutrophils to be "primed" and adhere to the pulmonary endothelial bed. The second hit is the actual transfusion of the blood. The transfused blood contains donor antibodies against neutrophil antigens, and these antibodies activate the "primed" neutrophils and monocytes, resulting in increased capillary permeability and noncardiogenic pulmonary edema.

HINT Manifestations of TRALI may occur within hours of the transfusion.

> **Q** An acute decrease in blood pressure after the initiation of a blood transfusion can be due to the patient being on which medication?
>
> **A** Angiotensin-converting enzyme (ACE) inhibitor

Acute hypotensive transfusion reactions present as a rapid and sudden decrease in blood pressure (BP) soon after the initiation of the transfusion. It is often a severe hypotension of systolic BP less than 70 mmHg. Bradykinin is metabolized by ACE. Inhibiting ACE elevates bradykinin, causing the hypotension.

HINT Immediately stop the transfusion. Do not administer that unit of blood and hold the ACE inhibitor.

 # IMMUNE DEFICIENCIES

▶ PATHOPHYSIOLOGY

> **Q** What is the most common cause of immune deficiencies in critically ill patients?
>
> **A** Secondary other disease processes

Primary immune deficiencies are characterized by failure of immune system that is not explained by infectious, neoplastic, or iatrogenic causes. Most immune deficiencies in critical care are secondary to other disease processes. (Box 5.10)

HINT Immunodeficiencies in critical ill patients are classified as primary or secondary.

Box 5.10 Common Causes of Secondary Immunosuppression

Primary immune deficiencies
Solid organ transplant recipients
HIV infections
Malignancy
Asplenia
Stem cell transplant recipients
Immunosuppression for autoimmune disease
HIV patients
Chemotherapy/radiation

> **Q** What is the leading cause of admission to the critical care unit in patients with cancer?
>
> **A** Sepsis

Sepsis is the leading cause of admission into ICU in patients with cancer. Immunosuppression is a result of the disease process, as well as treatment therapies for the cancer such as chemotherapy. Immune deficiency or immunosuppression causes the patients to be more susceptible to infections including infections from organisms, which may not normally cause issues.

HINT This is also true in all other immunosuppressed states.

▶ SYMPTOMS/ASSESSMENT

> **Q** What is a common sign of an infection that is NOT present in immunosuppressed patients with infections?
>
> **A** Leukocytosis

Patients who are immunosuppressed from disease processes or drug-induced immunosuppression are not able to elevate their WBCs during an infection, so they will not present with leukocytosis. Infections are dangerous in these patients because symptoms are not typically present.

HINT   Immunosuppressed patients frequently present with infections and sepsis.

> **Q What is typically an associated sign with a neutropenic sepsis?**
>
> **A Hypothermia**

Neutropenic or immunosuppression with sepsis used to be called "cold shock" because it is commonly associated with hypothermia. Subtle signs of impaired immune response in sepsis include hypothermia, altered mental status, and presence of frequent nosocomial infections.

▶ DIAGNOSIS

> **Q What overall laboratory test is used to assist in the diagnosis of autoimmune disorders?**
>
> **A Autoantibodies**

Autoantibodies are commonly used in identifying and diagnosing autoimmune disorders. The problem with autoantibodies is typically the frequent false positives and negatives. Insufficient serum levels of immunoglobulins (Igs) are frequently used to determine presence of immunosuppression.

▶ MANAGEMENT

> **Q What is a primary treatment used in patients with primary immunodeficiency?**
>
> **A IgG replacement**

IgG replacement therapy is a mainstay of treatment for primary immunodeficiencies. IVIG treatments have been found to lower the incidence of acute and chronic infections. They may be used during an acute crisis or long-term to manage the disease process. Treatment depends upon primary versus secondary and the underlying etiology of the immunosuppression.

HINT   Side effects of IVIG therapy are usually minor and do not usually require discontinuation of the infusion therapy.

▶ COMPLICATIONS

> **Q What is a common complication of leukopenia?**
>
> **A Infections**

Infections are common complications of leukopenia and immune-compromised patients. Infections leading to sepsis and septic shock typically bring these patients into the ICU. (Box 5.11)

HINT   Neutropenic sepsis has a high morbidity and mortality rate.

Box 5.11 Complication of Leukopenia or WBC dysfunction

Infections
Delayed wound healing
Pulmonary disorders/infections

> **Q Which organ is most frequently involved in an immunosuppressed patient?**
>
> **A Lungs**

Immunocompromised patients are prone to various infections and organ involvement (Box 5.12). The most frequent organ involved is the lungs.

HINT   Infections are frequently a result of opportunistic organisms such as candida.

Box 5.12 Organ Involvement in Immunocompromised Patients

GI Tract	Diverticular disease Ulceration GI mucosa GI infections GI malignancies Diarrhea Pancreatitis (less common)
Respiratory System	Pneumonia ARDS Pneumonitis
Central Nervous System	CNS infections Spinal infections/abscesses Encephalitis
Musculoskeletal/Skin	Skin infections Arthralgia Cellulitis/Abscess Osteomyelitis
Renal System	Urinary tract infection Acute and chronic renal failure

ARDS, acute respiratory distress syndrome; CNS, central nervous system; GI, gastrointestinal.

ONCOLOGIC COMPLICATIONS

▶ PATHOPHYSIOLOGY

Q What is the most common trigger of tumor lysis syndrome (TLS)?

A Chemotherapy

TLS is commonly triggered by chemotherapy and results in acute, rapid neoplastic cell lysis. The lysis of cells release intracellular products such as uric acid, phosphates, potassium, and calcium. It may also occur with radiation and biological therapies but not as common.

HINT This is most common in hematologic malignancies, especially acute leukemia.

Q Which type of cancer is most tumor lysis syndrome (TLS) most commonly associated with?

A Acute leukemia

Patients with acute leukemia and high WBC counts are one of the highest risk patients to develop TLS. Patients at highest risk are those with bulky, rapidly proliferating tumors that are sensitive to treatment.

Q What is the most common cause of hypercalcemia in oncology patients?

A Humoral causes

Humoral causes of hypercalcemia in oncology patients include increase parathyroid hormone and vitamin D3. Other causes include bone invasion and local osteolysis.

HINT Common cancers presenting with episodes of hypercalcemia include multiple myeloma and breast cancer.

Q What is the most common complication related to chemotherapy?

A Febrile neutropenia

Fungal and bacterial infections are common in patients receiving certain chemotherapy medications in which develop febrile neutropenia.

HINT Presentation is fever with an absolute neutrophil count of less than 500 cells/mm³.

▶ SYMPTOMS/ASSESSMENT

> **Q** What is a common presentation of tumor lysis syndrome (TLS) present with on admission to ICU?
>
> **A** Severe electrolyte abnormalities

TLS is a metabolic emergency that commonly presents with severe electrolyte abnormalities. Electrolyte abnormalities include azotemia, hyperkalemia, hyperphosphatemia, and hypocalcemia. The uric crystals result in acute kidney injury (AKI) due to mechanical obstruction in renal tubules. Clinical signs of hyperkalemia and hypocalcemia frequently are present.

HINT Symptoms usually present within 7 days of cancer treatment.

> **Q** What are the more common symptoms of pericardial effusions in cancer patients?
>
> **A** Dyspnea, chest pain, and palpitations

Malignant pericardial effusions can occur in certain types of cancer (i.e., lung, breath, and esophageal) and can also be attributed to the therapy such as radiation. Symptoms depend upon how quickly the fluid accumulates in the pericardial sac. Slow accumulation is more vague dyspnea, chest pain, and palpitations.

HINT Fast accumulation of pericardial fluid can present as cardiac tamponade with Beck's triad of symptoms.

> **Q** What is the hallmark sign of superior vena cava syndrome in cancer patients?
>
> **A** Facial swelling

Facial edema is the hallmark sign of superior vena cava syndrome (Box 5.13). This is caused by the compression or obstruction of superior vena cava and inability to drain blood from head and neck region.

HINT Most commonly associated with lung cancers.

Box 5.13 Signs of Superior Vena Cava Syndrome

Edema of face, neck, and chest
Cough
Dyspnea at rest
Hoarseness
Chest and shoulder pain
Discoloration of neck and upper extremities

▶ DIAGNOSIS

> **Q** What is considered diagnostic for TLS?
>
> **A** Histologic findings

The presence of uric acid in the distal renal tubules, renal pelvis, and ureters is diagnostic along with the clinical findings for TLS.

HINT Patients typically present with positive anion gap metabolic acidosis.

> **Q** What is a priority lab in a chemotherapy patient that prevents with fever and neutropenia?
>
> **A** Blood cultures

Patients with febrile neutropenia are prone to infections and should have blood cultures obtained to identify causative agent. Fever soon after receiving chemotherapy should alert the clinicians of the risk for the complication febrile neutropenia.

HINT Early initiation of antibiotics can improve outcomes in febrile neutropenia.

▶ MANAGEMENT

Q What is the commonly used medication to reduce uric acid and prevent acute kidney injury in patients with TLS?

A Allopurinol

Allopurinol is used to decrease the conversion of nucleic acid byproducts to uric acid. This can assist with prevention of urate nephropathy and oliguric renal failure.

HINT Adverse effects include mild to severe rash.

Q Which classification of drug is commonly used to prevent osteolytic activity in oncology patients prone to hypercalcemia?

A IV Bisphosphonate therapy

Frequently, oncology patients presenting with hypercalcemia are initially managed with aggressive IV hydration and Lasix. IV Bisphosphonates are used to manage hypercalcemia caused by osteolysis. It inhibits the osteoclastic activity.

HINT Patient presents with typical clinical signs of hypercalcemia such as weakness, anorexia, nausea and vomiting, and altered mentation.

▶ COMPLICATIONS

Q Which organ is most commonly damaged in tumor lysis syndrome (TLS)?

A Kidneys

Filtering of the substances released by the cellular rupture occurs in the kidneys. They are susceptible to precipitation of uric acid, calcium phosphate, and hypoxanthine leading to renal failure.

HINT The acute kidney injury, which occurs with TLS, presents as oliguric renal failure.

Q What is an overall complication found in immunotherapy agents for oncological patients?

A Immune-related adverse effects

Immunotherapy use is increasing and potential complications involve the immune system. Immunotherapy include vaccines, cytokines, adoptive cell therapy, or checkpoint inhibitors.

HINT Immune-related adverse effects range from vague, flu-like symptoms to more severe pneumonitis. (Box 5.14)

Box 5.14 Immune-Related Adverse Effects

Hypophysitis
Uveitis and orbital inflammation
Hypothyroidism
Pneumonitis
Adrenal insufficiency
Enterocolitis
Rash
Pancreatitis
Arthralgia

1. A patient who presents with a hemorrhagic stroke is found to have been taking warfarin for his atrial fibrillation and has an international normalized ratio (INR) of 3.8. Which of the following infusions would most rapidly lower the INR?

   A. Intravenous (IV) vitamin K
   B. Prothrombin complex concentrate (PCC)
   C. Desmopressin
   D. Fresh frozen plasma (FFP)

2. Which of the following interventions would be most appropriate following a diagnosis of heparin-induced thrombocytopenia (HIT)?

   A. Discontinue unfractionated heparin and monitor for venous thromboembolism (VTE)
   B. Discontinue the unfractionated heparin and anticoagulate with Argatroban
   C. Change unfractionated heparin to a low molecular weight heparin (LMWH)
   D. Discontinue all anticoagulation therapy and initiate antiplatelet therapy

3. Which of the following is the most accurate statement regarding DIC?

   A. No single diagnostic test for DIC
   B. Diagnosis can be made on clinical findings alone
   C. Diagnosis is only rule out of other coagulopathies
   D. Decreased fibrinogen is the only required finding to diagnose DIC

4. Which of the following is considered an adjunct to anticoagulation therapy in treating heparin-induced thrombocytopenias (HITs)?

   A. Antiplatelet medication
   B. Plasma concentrate complex (PCC)
   C. IVIG therapy
   D. Amicar (aminocaproic acid)

5. Which of the following is the most common presenting symptom of a patient with heparin-induced thrombocytopenia (HIT)?

   A. Purpura
   B. Elevated international normalized ratio (INR)
   C. Excessive bleeding
   D. Thrombocytopenia

6. Which of the following types of anemia can be caused by acute inflammation?

   A. Iron deficient anemia
   B. Thalassemia
   C. Copper deficiency
   D. Bone marrow suppression

1. B) Prothrombin complex concentrate (PCC)

A PCC can normalize the international normalized ratio (INR) rapidly with a small-volume infusion. This is accomplished in less than 30 minutes; vitamin K can takeup to 24 hours, and FFP may take several hours and have an incomplete reversal of the INR. Desmopressin may be administered to increase von Willebrand factor, but it does not reverse Coumadin overdose.

2. B) Discontinue the unfractionated heparin and anticoagulate with Argatroban

Following HIT, all heparins must be discontinued (including LMWH). Direct thrombin inhibitors, such as Argatroban, are started immediately to prevent thrombosis. Monitoring for VTE is insufficient, because the patient requires further anticoagulation therapy. Antiplatelet therapy is not recommended for preventing thrombosis in HIT.

3. A) No single diagnostic test for DIC

There is no single diagnostic test that will accurately diagnose DIC. The diagnosis is a combination underlying predisposition, clinical findings, and laboratory results. Diagnosis cannot be made on clinical findings alone or with a low fibrinogen finding alone.

4. C) IVIG therapy

IVIG has been found to interrupt the platelet activation by HIT antibodies and more rapid improvement in the platelet counts. Antiplatelet therapy is not recommended in HITs due to the thrombocytopenia. PCC and Amicar would increase the thrombosis risk in HITs and would be contraindicated.

5. D) Thrombocytopenia

A decrease in platelet count by greater than 50% within 24 hours is typically the identifying sign of heparin-induced thrombocytopenia (HIT). Thrombosis may precede thrombocytopenia in some people with HIT. Purpura and increased international normalized ratio (INR) are not signs of HIT. HIT is not commonly associated with bleeding as a presentation or complication.

6. A) Iron-deficient anemia

Acute inflammation can alter iron metabolism resulting in iron-deficient anemia. Thalassemia is an inherited disorder that produces abnormal Hgb. Copper deficiency is most commonly caused by lack of absorption in stomach due to bypass surgery. Bone marrow suppression may be a result of chemotherapy and certain medications but is not usually caused by acute inflammation.

7. Which of the following is the most common lab abnormality found in patients with Tumor Lysis Syndrome (TLS)?

   A. Hypoalbuminemia
   B. Hypokalemia
   C. Hypocalcemia
   D. Hypophosphatemia

8. Which of the following is the most common cause of the hyponatremia in lung cancers?

   A. Diabetes insipidus (DI)
   B. Cerebral salt wasting syndrome (CSWS)
   C. Elevated brain natriuretic protein (BNP) levels
   D. Syndrome of inappropriate antidiuretic hormone (SIADH)

9. A patient with acute leukemia has been undergoing treatment with chemotherapy. They present to the unit with arrhythmias induced by hyperkalemia and severe muscle spasms. Which of the following is the most likely cause for this presentation?

   A. Febrile neutropenia
   B. Tumor lysis syndrome
   C. Syndrome of inappropriate antidiuretic hormone (SIADH)
   D. Hyperviscosity syndrome

10. Which of the following is the hallmark sign of superior vena cava syndrome?

   A. Facial edema
   B. Altered mentation
   C. Bradycardia
   D. Hypotension

7. C) Hypocalcemia

Intracellular components and electrolytes are released when the neoplastic cells rupture leading to kidney injury. Common electrolyte abnormalities include hypocalcemia, hyperphosphatemia, and hyperkalemia. Albumin levels are not affected directly by TLS.

8. D) Syndrome of inappropriate antidiuretic hormone (SIADH)

SIADH is a common cause of hyponatremia in cancer patients. The low sodium is a result of hemodilution and is typically managed with fluid restriction and diuretics. Oat cell carcinoma of the lungs is a common non-neurological cause of SIADH. CSWS occurs when the kidneys cannot reabsorb sodium, resulting in an increased excretion of sodium. This is thought to be due to an increase BNP level and is not commonly found in lung cancer patients. DI results in hypernatremia.

9. B) Tumor lysis syndrome

TLS is the rupture of neoplastic cells and the release of intracellular contents in cancer patients, especially acute leukemia. Common electrolyte abnormalities include hyperkalemia and hypocalcemia, which explains the patient's presentation. Febrile neutropenia, SIADH, and hyperviscosity syndrome are all complications of cancer patients but would not present with hyperkalemia and muscle spasms.

10. A) Facial edema

Obstruction of the superior vena cava affects the drainage of the internal jugular and subclavian veins. This results in the backup of venous blood into the face and neck. Swelling of the face, neck, and chest are hallmark signs. Other signs include cough, dyspnea at rest, hoarseness, neck and shoulder pain, and discoloration of neck and upper extremities. It does not initially present with altered mentation or bradycardia and hypotension.

BIBLIOGRAPHY

Cuker, A., Arepally, G., Chong, B., Cines, D., Greinacher, A., Gruel, Y., … Santesso, N. (2018). American Society of Hematogology 2018 guidelines for management of venous thrmbosis: Heparin induced thrombocytopenia. *Blood Advances, 2*(22), 3360–3392.

Papageorgiou, G., Jourdi, G., Adjambri, E., Wlaborn, A., Patel, P., Fareed, J., … Gerotziafas, G. T. (2018). Dissiminated intravascular coagulation: An update on pathogenesis, diagnosis and therapeutic strategies. *Clinical and Aplied Thrombosis/Hemostasis, 24*(9 Suppl), 8S–28S.

Thakur, A., Ziahttps, Sous, M., & Trelles, D. (2020). Dissiminated Intravascular coagulation and malignancy: A case report and literatue review. *Case Reports in Oncological Medicine, 2020,* 9147105.

Gastrointestinal System Review

LEARNING OBJECTIVES

In this chapter, you will review:

- Pancreatitis
- Acute gastrointestinal (GI) hemorrhage
- Hepatic failure/coma
- Acute abdominal trauma
- Bowel infarctions/perforation/obstruction
- Malnutrition and malabsorption
- Abdominal compartment syndrome (ACS)
- Enteral and parenteral nutrition
- GI surgeries

PANCREATITIS

Q Which of the types of pancreatitis has the greatest morbidity and mortality?

A Hemorrhagic (necrotizing) pancreatitis

Pancreatitis is an inflammatory response with potential necrosis of pancreatic cells, resulting from premature activation of pancreatic digestive enzymes. It is caused by the escape of enzymes into surrounding pancreatic tissue, producing interstitial edema. Interstitial (edematous) pancreatitis is more self-limiting with lower acuity and better outcomes. Hemorrhagic (necrotizing) pancreatitis involves fat necrosis and hemorrhage within the pancreatic parenchyma. This form causes "auto-digestion" of the pancreas and is more severe with a higher mortality.

HINT On initial presentation, it may be difficult to determine the severity of pancreatitis.

▶ PATHOPHYSIOLOGY

Q Does the stimulation of the pancreas to release digestive enzymes occur with activation of the sympathetic or parasympathetic autonomic nervous system?

A Parasympathetic nervous system (PNS)

PNS is responsible for stimulation of the gastrointestinal (GI) system, including the pancreas, via the vagal nerve. The pancreas produces approximately 1,500 to 2,500 mL of fluid in 24 hours. Limiting pancreatic stimulation to decrease the production of digestive enzymes during periods of pancreatitis is a mainstay of treatment (Box 6.1).

HINT PNS is the "rest and feed" portion of the autonomic nervous system.

Box 6.1 Pancreatic Stimulation

PNS stimulation	Small bowel stimulation
Gastric distention	Release secretin and cholecystokinin

PNS, parasympathetic nervous system.

Q Which of the digestive enzymes produced from the pancreas breaks down protein?

A Trypsin

Trypsinogen is the precursor to trypsin, which is a proteolytic enzyme produced to break down or digest proteins. Normally, digestive enzymes remain inactivated until they are within the duodenum. Pancreatic injury can lead to the cleavage of trypsinogen to trypsin, causing autodigestion of the pancreas. The activated trypsin may also activate other digestive enzymes such as amylase and lipase, furthering pancreatic injury (Table 6.1).

HINT   Premature activation of digestive enzymes in the pancreas stimulates the release of neutrophils and macrophages, causing a local inflammation within the pancreas.

Table 6.1 Digestive Enzymes

Digestive Enzymes	Role
Trypsin	Protein to amino acids
Amylase	Carbohydrate to glucose
Lipase	Lipids to free fatty acids
Elastase	Elastin

Q What is the primary reason for injury to the pancreatic parenchyma in pancreatitis?

A Activation of digestive enzymes within the pancreas

Initial injury of the acinar cells causes the activation of the digestive enzymes, especially trypsin, within the pancreas, resulting in autodigestion of the pancreas. Hemorrhagic pancreatitis is characterized by a cycle in which release and activation of more digestive enzymes lead to further pancreatic necrosis.

HINT   The continual cycle of activation and necrosis in the pancreas is the reason for serial surgeries to debride the pancreas in hemorrhagic pancreatitis (Box 6.2).

Box 6.2 Three Stages of Hemorrhagic Pancreatitis

Stage I: Activation of digestive enzymes	Premature activation of trypsin within pancreatic acinar cells Once activated, activates other digestive enzymes Begin autodigestion of pancreas
Stage II: Intrapancreatic inflammation	Activates neutrophils and macrophages Releases proinflammatory cytokines Increases vascular permeability Promotes thrombosis and hemorrhage Leads to ischemia and necrosis
Stage III: Extrapancreatic inflammation	Systemic inflammatory response ARDS MSOF

ARDS, acute respiratory distress syndrome; MSOF, multisystem organ failure.

HINT   Requires abdominal CT scan to differentiate sterile and infected pancreatic necrotic tissue (Box 6.3).

Box 6.3 Necrotic Pancreatic Tissue

Sterile Pancreatic Necrosis	Infected Pancreatic Necrosis
Aseptic necrotic tissue	Presence of bacteria within necrotic tissue
Less severe	Greater severity and mortality
May involve organ failure but is less frequent	Greater incidence of multisystem organ failure

Q What are the two most common causes of pancreatitis in the United States?

A Alcoholism and gallstones

Chronic alcoholism may cause pancreatitis through several mechanisms. Alcohol increases pressure in the pancreatic ductal system, resulting in atony and edema of the sphincter of Oddi, permitting reflux of duodenal contents with activated enzymes. Alcohol-induced ductal hypertension is also associated with permeability changes in the duct, allowing enzymes to leak out to the surrounding tissues. Excessive alcohol use may lead to activation of proteolytic enzymes within the pancreas. Gallstones cause pancreatitis by obstruction of the ampulla of Vater (common bile duct), causing pressure to back up into the pancreatic duct (Boxes 6.4 and 6.5).

Box 6.4 Causes of Pancreatitis

Chronic alcoholism	Vasculitis
Binge drinking	Iatrogenic
Pancreatic tumors	Endoscopic retrograde cholangiopancreatography
Allergies	Liver biopsy
Metal toxicities	Cardiopulmonary bypass
Pancreatic trauma	Congenital

Drug induced
    Salicylates
    Thiazide diuretics
    Corticosteroids
    Estrogen contraceptive
	Autoimmune response
	Hypercalcemia

Box 6.5 Mechanism of Drug-Induced Pancreatitis

Pancreatic duct constriction	Accumulation of a toxic metabolite
Cytotoxic and metabolic effects	Hypersensitivity reactions

▶ SYMPTOMS/ASSESSMENT

Q What symptom is considered to be the hallmark of pancreatitis?

A Epigastric pain

Severe onset of acute epigastric pain accompanied by nausea and vomiting is the hallmark of pancreatitis. Pain is frequently described as severe, relentless, knife-like, and twisting deep in the midepigastrium region or periumbilical region. It may radiate to the back. The patient will take a knee-to-chest position to relieve the pain. Supine positions typically exacerbate the pain (Box 6.6).

HINT Onset of pain may be associated with heavy fatty meals (biliary) or binge drinking (alcohol-related).

Box 6.6 Symptoms of Pancreatitis

Epigastric pain	Grey Turner's sign
Low-grade fever	Cullen's sign
Nausea and vomiting	Fox's sign
Abdominal tenderness and guarding	Jaundice (biliary)
Hypotension	Steatorrhea (biliary)
Hypoactive or absent bowel sounds	

> **Q** What is the presence of ecchymosis along the flank in hemorrhagic pancreatitis called?
>
> **A** Grey Turner's sign

Hemorrhagic pancreatitis can cause tissue ecchymosis. When present along the flank area, the ecchymosis is in the retroperitoneal space and is called Grey Turner's sign. Cullen's sign is bruising in the periumbilical area due to ecchymosis in the intraperitoneal, and Fox's sign is bruising at the inguinal ligament.

HINT   Ecchymotic signs are not usually present on initial presentation.

▶ DIAGNOSIS

> **Q** Which two laboratory values are most frequently used to assist with the diagnosis of pancreatitis?
>
> **A** Amylase and lipase

Damaged acinar cells release digestive enzymes systemically. Among those frequently measured are amylase and lipase. Both amylase and lipase elevate rapidly (within 3–6 hours) following the onset of pancreatitis; lipase has a longer half-life, therefore it remains elevated longer (8–14 days). Neither is specific for pancreatitis and can be elevated in other disorders.

HINT   Degree of amylase or lipase elevation has no prognostic significance (Box 6.7).

Box 6.7 Other Causes of Elevated Amylase and Lipase

Perforated ulcer	Cholecystitis
Small bowel obstruction	Peritonitis
Acute kidney injury	Stomach tumors
Salivary glandular disease	

> **Q** Diagnosis of pancreatitis requires any two of three signs. What are the three diagnostic evaluations used to diagnose pancreatitis?
>
> **A** Pain, amylase, and CT scan

Diagnosis requires two of the three signs:

1. Abdominal pain characteristic of pancreatitis
2. Serum amylase and/or lipase more than three times the upper limit of normal
3. Characteristic findings of acute pancreatitis on CT scan

HINT   Elevation of amylase by three times or greater than normal is almost always the result of pancreatitis.

> **Q** Which radiographic test is the gold standard for diagnosing pancreatitis?
>
> **A** Abdominal CT scan with intravenous (IV) contrast

Abdominal CT scans can differentiate between interstitial and necrotizing pancreatitis reliably with IV contrast after 2 to 3 days; the degree of necrosis is also prognostic. Abdominal CT scans are used to estimate size of the pancreas, evaluate cystic lesions, and identify fluid collections. MRI is not as widely used but may have some advantages, including lack of nephrotoxicity of gadolinium and greater ability to differentiate necrosis from fluid. The use of MR cholangiopancreatography is increasingly used in evaluating pancreatitis.

HINT   Early CT scan (within 24 hours of illness onset) might underestimate the amount of necrosis but is an indicator that rules out other causes of abdominal pain.

Q Which radiographic study is the diagnostic test of choice to evaluate for gallstones?

A Abdominal ultrasound

The main role of abdominal ultrasound is to identify the presence of gallstones. It is not accurate for determining necrosis or inflammation of the pancreas. Endoscopic retrograde cholangiopancreatography (ERCP) is used to identify anomalies and evaluate the biliary tract for strictures or stones. It may be considered in recurrent episodes of pancreatitis.

Q Which laboratory value when elevated may be used to assist in determining the prognosis of pancreatitis?

A Hematocrit (hct)

A concentrated hct predicts the potential for complications of pancreatitis. It is an early marker for organ failure and pancreatic necrosis when elevated within 24 hours. Leaking of exudate (third spacing) results in the increase in hct and is defined as hct greater than 44% on admission (Box 6.8).

HINT   A significant decrease in hct following volume replacement indicates that elevated hct was concentrated.

Box 6.8 Abnormal Laboratory Findings in Pancreatitis

Concentrated hct	Hypocalcemia
Hyperamylasemia	Hyponatremia
Hyperlipasemia	Elevated liver enzymes
Leukocytosis	Hyperglycemia
Hypokalemia	Hyperlipidemia

hct, hematocrit.

Q What does the Ranson criteria determine in pancreatitis patients?

A Severity of pancreatitis

Ranson criteria are frequently used to determine the severity of pancreatitis and correlate to mortality. Ranson criteria comprise a total of 11 criteria, 5 of which are determined on admission and the remaining 6 during the first 48 hours. The Apache II score and CT-based severity index can also be used to determine severity.

HINT   Presence of three of five Ranson criteria on admission is considered severe pancreatitis (Box 6.9).

Box 6.9 Ranson Criteria

On Admission	During Initial 48 Hours
Age older than 55 years	Hematocrit decreases > 10%
WBC > 16,000/mL	Blood urea nitrogen increases of > 5 mg/dL
Glucose > 200 mg/dL	Base deficit > 4 mg/dL
	Fluid sequestration > 6 L

AST, aspirate aminotransferase; LDH, Lactate dehydrogenase; WBC, white blood cells.

▶ MEDICAL MANAGEMENT

> **Q** What is considered the most important component in the management of hemorrhagic pancreatitis?
>
> **A** Fluid resuscitation

Adequate fluid replacement is required to correct the severe fluid losses due to third spacing. Inadequate fluid replacement can cause intestinal ischemia with translocation of bacteria into the pancreas (infected necrosis) as well as distal organ hypoperfusion. Early resuscitation reduces the incidence of systemic inflammatory response syndrome (SIRS) and multisystem organ failure (MSOF). The target for fluid resuscitation is to correct concentrated hematocrit (hct) and maintain adequate urine output. Administration of supplemental oxygen or intubation with mechanical ventilation in patients with compromised respiration is necessary. Pain control is also an important aspect of medically managing pancreatitis.

HINT   Lactated Ringer's solution may be recommended to prevent hyperchloremic acidosis, which occurs with large volumes of 0.9% NaCl administration.

> **Q** What is the purpose of nothing by mouth (NPO) status in the patient with pancreatitis?
>
> **A** "Rest" pancreas

Allowing the pancreas to "rest" and not release digestive enzymes will interrupt the progression of the pancreatic injury from autodigestion. The use of octreotide (Somatostatin, Sandostatin) has been used to decrease production of gastrin and cholecystokinin and to reduce secretions of the pancreas (Box 6.10).

HINT   Enteral feeding, including distal feeding through a nasojejunal tube, may have fewer complications than parenteral nutrition.

Box 6.10 Interventions to Decrease Pancreatic Stimulation

NG tube to low wall suction	Octreotide
NPO	Total parenteral nutrition or enteral feeding
Proton pump inhibitors	

NG, nasogastric; NPO, nothing by mouth.

▶ SURGICAL MANAGEMENT

> **Q** What is the primary surgical treatment for an infected necrosis of the pancreas?
>
> **A** Surgical debridement

Infected necrosis of the pancreas typically requires some route of surgical debridement and may require multiple surgeries to completely debride the necrotic areas of the pancreas. Sterile necrosis usually does not require surgical debridement and may be managed medically for 2 to 3 weeks (Box 6.11).

HINT   Debridement of sterile necrosis can result in development of infected necrosis.

Box 6.11 Types of Surgical Debridement

Necrosectomy with closed continuous irrigation via indwelling catheter	Percutaneous placement of drainage catheter
Necrosectomy and open packing	Minimally invasive retroperitoneal necrosectomy
Necrosectomy with closed drainage without irrigation CT-guided needle aspiration	Laparoscopic necrosectomy

HINT   Postoperative bleeding can be a life-threatening complication of pancreatic debridement procedures.

▶ COMPLICATIONS

Q What is a fluid collection walled off by a rim of fibrous granulation tissue called?

A Pseudocyst

A pseudocyst is a collection of "sterile" fluid that is lined or walled off by a fibrous layer. If the fluid is infected and walled off by well-defined granulated tissue, it is called a pancreatic abscess. Pseudocysts can resolve spontaneously, but they also have the potential of becoming infected, bleeding, or rupturing (Box 6.12).

HINT Pain management is a high priority in patients who develop pseudocysts.

Box 6.12 Complications of Pancreatitis

Pancreatic Complications	Systemic Complications
Pancreatic necrosis	ARDS
Pseudocyst	Sepsis/systemic inflammatory response syndrome
Pancreatic abscess	Abdominal compartment syndrome
Fistula or pancreatic duct leak	MSOF
	Disseminated intravascular coagulation

ARDS, acute respiratory distress syndrome; MSOF, multisystem organ failure.

● ACUTE GI HEMORRHAGE

Q What is the landmark that divides the intestines between an upper and lower gastrointestinal bleed (GIB)?

A Ligament of Treitz

An upper GIB (UGIB) is defined as bleeding occurring proximal to the ligament of Treitz. The ligament of Treitz is the suspensory muscle of the duodenum that connects the duodenum to the diaphragm.

HINT The ligament of Treitz is the anatomical landmark of the duodenojejunal junction.

▶ PATHOPHYSIOLOGY

Q What is it called when an upper GIB (UGIB) is caused by excessive retching and vomiting causing tear esophagogastric junction?

A Mallory–Weiss tear

A Mallory–Weiss tear is a tear in the mucosa at the esophageal gastric junction caused by forceful vomiting or retching. The vomiting can be due to the flu, food poisoning, or eating disorders but becomes bloody once the mucosa tears (Box 6.13).

Box 6.13 Causes of UGIB

Esophageal varices	Esophagitis
Peptic ulcer disease	Mallory–Weiss tear
Stress-related mucosal disease	Gastric/duodenal tumors
Diffuse gastritis	Angiodysplasia

> **Q**   Critically ill patients are at a greater risk for upper GIB (UGIB) due to the development of what GI complication?
>
> **A**   Stress-related mucosal disease (SRMD)

Ulcerations in the upper gastrointestinal (GI) tract (stomach and duodenum) can occur within hours of a severe injury or major surgery. GI ulcerations caused by critical illness have several different names but are commonly called SRMD. The ulcerations range from superficial to deep ulcerations at risk for perforation. The most common complication of SRMD is UGIB.

HINT   Brain-injured patients and patients with burns are the two patient populations with the highest incidence of SRMD (Box 6.14).

Box 6.14 Risk Factors of SRMD

Mechanical ventilation	Hypotension and shock states
Coagulopathy	Hepatic failure
Major or multiple trauma	Renal failure
Sepsis and multisystem organ failure	Administration of steroids

SRMD, stress-related mucosal disease.

> **Q**   What causes the loss of protective secretion of mucus that shields the gastrointestinal (GI) mucosa from the acids?
>
> **A**   Hypoperfusion

The development of stress-related mucosal disease (SRMD) is caused by multiple factors. The stomach is normally protected from the gastric acids by secretion of glycoprotein mucus that protects the mucosa and secretes bicarbonate to neutralize some of the acids. Hypotension or shock states cause vasoconstriction and shunts blood away from nonessential organs, such as the GI tract. Decreased gastric blood flow diminishes the amount of protective mucus secretions allowing acids to flow back into the mucosal layer, causing tissue injury.

HINT   There is also an increase in acid production during stress periods lowering the gastric pH.

> **Q**   What bacteria are frequently found colonizing the stomach and are associated with peptic ulcer disease?
>
> **A**   *Helicobacter pylori (H. pylori)*

Colonization of the stomach by *H. pylori* can result in chronic gastritis at the site of infection. Ulcers in the stomach and duodenum result when the consequences of inflammation allow stomach acid and the digestive enzyme pepsin to overwhelm the mechanisms that protect the stomach and duodenal mucous membrane.

HINT   *H. pylori* is more common in community-acquired UGIB and less often in SRMD.

> **Q**   What is the underlying physiology that causes esophageal varices?
>
> **A**   Portal hypertension

Portal hypertension is caused by fibrotic changes in the liver that collapse and distort the hepatic vasculature; therefore, blood backs up and increases portal venous pressure. Portal hypertension results in the development of collateral circulation that redirects the portal venous blood flow through vessels of lower resistance in the esophagus and stomach (varices). Collateral blood flow also occurs in the rectum, resulting in hemorrhoids and lower gastrointestinal (GI) bleeding (Box 6.15).

Box 6.15 Causes of Lower Gastrointestinal Bleed (LGIB)

Ulcerative colitis	Neoplasm
Mesenteric vascular ischemia	Hemorrhoids
Vascular ectasias	Angiodysplasia
Diverticulosis	

▶ SYMPTOMS/ASSESSMENT

Q What laboratory value is elevated in an upper gastrointestinal bleed (UGIB) but not in a lower gastrointestinal bleed (LGIB)?

A Blood urea nitrogen (BUN)

The BUN is elevated in UGIB because of greater absorption of protein in the stomach and duodenum (Box 6.16).

Box 6.16 Signs of Upper and Lower Gastrointestinal Bleeds

Upper Gastrointestinal Bleed	Lower Gastrointestinal Bleed
Hematemesis (coffee grounds or bloody)	No hematemesis
Melena stools (dark, tarry, odorous)	Bloody stools
Elevated blood urea nitrogen (normal creatinine)	Normal BUN
Decreased hemoglobin and hematocrit	Decreased hemoglobin and hematocrit

BUN, blood urea nitrogen.

Q What assessment tool can be used to determine the need for an intervention for an upper gastrointestinal bleeding (UGIB)?

A Blatchford score

The Blatchford score is a tool used to assess UGIB patients to determine the likelihood that the patient will require an intervention. The higher score is more likely to require endoscopy and transfusions (Table 6.2).

Table 6.2 Blatchford Score

Admission Risk Marker	Score Component Value
BUN	
≥6.5 and <8.0	2
≥8.0 and <10.0	3
≥10.0 and <25.0	4
≥25	6
Hemoglobin (g/L) for men	
≥12.0 and <13.0	1
≥10.0 <12.0	3
<10.0	6
Hemoglobin (g/L) for women	
≥10.0 and <12.0	1
<10.0	6
Systolic blood pressure (mmHg)	
100–109	1
90–99	2
<90	3
Other markers	
Pulse ≥ 100 (per minute)	1
Presentation with melena	1
Presentation with syncope	2
Hepatic disease	2
Cardiac failure	2

Scores of 6 or more are associated with a greater than 50% risk of needing an intervention.

▶ DIAGNOSIS

> **Q** What is the most common diagnostic intervention for an upper gastrointestinal bleeding (UGIB)?
>
> **A** Endoscopy

An endoscopy is used to localize site of bleeding, determine the cause of the bleed, and allow the estimation of blood loss.

> **Q** What is the recommended diagnostic procedure to diagnose a lower gastrointestinal bleeding (LGIB)?
>
> **A** Colonoscopy

A colonoscopy is the recommended diagnostic procedure to identify a LGIB. Blood in the terminal ileocecal valve indicates the bleeding source is the small bowel. The small bowel can be visualized with push enteroscopy, double-balloon enteroscopy, and video capsule endoscopy. A more rapid bleed may use mesenteric angiography or CT angiography to localize the source. A slow bleed may be found with nuclear scintigraphy that involves nuclear tagging of the red blood cells (RBCs).

HINT A full colonoscopy is recommended because of potential bleeding in the right colon.

▶ MEDICAL MANAGEMENT

> **Q** Which two risk factors have the greatest incidence for stress-related mucosal disorder (SRMD) and require prophylactic interventions?
>
> **A** Mechanical ventilation and coagulopathy

Respiratory failure requiring mechanical ventilation and coagulopathy are the two risk factors for SRMD that are commonly documented as requiring gastrointestinal (GI) prophylaxis. Mechanical ventilation may decrease splanchnic blood flow by lowering mean arterial pressure (MAP) and increasing vascular resistance of the GI tract. It can also initiate a proinflammatory response.

HINT The greater the number of risk factors, the higher the risk of GI bleeding and, therefore, the greater the need for prophylaxis.

> **Q** Of the drugs used for gastrointestinal (GI) prophylaxis, which class of drug has a greater risk for development of thrombocytopenia?
>
> **A** H_2-receptor antagonists

GI prophylaxis can include antacids, H_2-receptor antagonists, sucralfate, and proton pump inhibitors. Of these drugs, H_2-receptor antagonists can cause thrombocytopenia as a side effect. Another proposed complication of H_2-receptor antagonists and antacids is a higher incidence of nosocomial pneumonias. The change of the pH from acidic to alkaline causes an overgrowth of bacteria in the stomach that can be aspirated into the lungs.

HINT Proton pump inhibitors have been associated with a higher incidence of diarrhea and may have an association with *Clostridium difficile* (*C. diff*).

> **Q** What is a potential contraindication for placement of a gastric tube following onset of vomiting blood?
>
> **A** Esophageal varices

Placement of a gastric tube can damage the enlarged, tortuous varices in the esophagus, resulting in greater blood loss. Endoscopy prior to placement of a gastric tube is recommended to identify the source of bleeding and rule out esophageal varices. Gastric tubes have been used to lavage the stomach with saline or water to cause cooling. Cooling decreases peptic acid activity in the stomach, decreases gastric mucosal blood flow, and gastrointestinal (GI) motility.

HINT   If a clot was present on ulcer bed, lavaging the gastric tube may dislodge the clot and worsen blood loss.

Q   **What drug therapy is used to manage upper gastrointestinal bleeding (UGIB) caused by varices?**

A   **Octreotide or Terlipressin**

Octreotide administered as a continuous infusion in patients with variceal bleeds can lower the rate of hemorrhage. The effects of octreotide may include a decrease in portal hypertension and splanchnic blood flow. Terlipressin is an analog of vasopressin and produces vasoconstriction, thus reducing pressure in the portal vein. Terlipressin has minimal coronary vasoconstriction compared to vasopressin with reduced risks of causing coronary artery syndrome.

HINT   Vasopressin (Pitressin), administered as an IV infusion to manage UGIB, requires administration of nitroglycerin to protect from coronary vasoconstriction.

Q   **What is the role of lactulose in managing an upper gastrointestinal bleeding (UGIB) patient?**

A   **Prevents absorption of ammonia**

Lactulose and magnesium citrate are frequently given to patients with UGIB to prevent absorption of ammonia that is released in the bowel with blood degradation. Lactulose is metabolized by the enteric bacteria in the colon, resulting in the acidification of the stool, thus preventing ammonia from converting to an absorbable form. So, less ammonia is absorbed into the bloodstream, lowering the risk of encephalopathy.

HINT   Magnesium citrate is used to purge the bowel of blood and fecal matter.

▶ SURGICAL MANAGEMENT

Q   **What would be an indication for surgical management of an upper gastrointestinal bleeding (UGIB) caused by stress-related mucosal disorder (SRMD)?**

A   **Active bleeding in a hemodynamically unstable patient**

Endoscopy therapy is the intervention of choice initially, but if the patient has ongoing bleeding and is hemodynamically unstable or required more than 6 units of packed red blood cells (PRBCs) in the past 48 hours, surgical management may be required.

Q   **What is the endoscopic treatment of varices?**

A   **Sclerotherapy or band ligation**

Sclerotherapy involves the injection of a sclerosing agent in and around the varices causing localized constrictive edema, induced thrombosis, and sclerosis of the vein, with minimal damage to the esophageal mucosa and muscle. This may be accomplished with vasoconstrictors, sclerosing agents, tissue adhesives, or saline. Band ligation can also be performed on the varices and in some studies has been shown to improve outcomes. Endoscopic band ligation is varices that are ligated and strangulated with small rubber bands. Ischemic necrosis of the mucosa within 24 hours, displacement of the bands in 3 to 7 days, and complete healing in 21 days are seen.

   If endoscopic therapy fails to control bleeding, a second attempt is recommended before surgical management of varices.

HINT   Indications for endoscopy intervention include actively bleeding ulcers and visible vessels in ulcer beds or varices.

Q   **What is the most common surgical procedure to treat bleeding gastric ulcers not amendable by endoscopic interventions?**

A   **Antrectomy**

The removal of the antrum portion of the stomach that has the ulcer and produces acids will control hemorrhage and decrease risk of future development of gastric ulcers. The remaining portion of the stomach is anastomosed either to the duodenum (called Billroth I) or to the jejunum (called Billroth II). Truncal, selective, or highly selective vagotomy are other surgical options for treatment of peptic ulcer disease for acid suppression (Table 6.3).

HINT   Acid-reduction surgeries are less common because of the use of acid-suppressing proton pump inhibitors.

Table 6.3 Types of Gastric Ulcer Surgeries

Type of Gastric Ulcer	Location of Ulcer	Surgical Management
Type I	Lesser curvature of stomach	Wedge resection
Type II	Lesser curvature of stomach and duodenum	Truncal vagotomy or antrectomy
Type III	Prepyloric	Truncal vagotomy or antrectomy
Type IV	Lesser curve near cardiac and esophagogastric junction	Distal gastrectomy and Roux-en-Y reconstruction
Type V	Diffuse ulcers	Removal of the area of ulcer

Q What is a less invasive procedure used to control hemorrhage of a gastric ulcer?

A Angiography with embolization

Angiography with embolization of bleeding vessels is another option to control hemorrhage of an actively bleeding ulcer. This involves embolization of the vessel within the ulcer bed with coils, gel foam, or polyvinyl alcohol.

HINT   Patient may remain on proton pump inhibitor therapy for continual acid suppression.

Q What is a less invasive option for management of varices if endoscopy and variceal ligation are ineffective?

A Transjugular intrahepatic portosystemic shunts (TIPS)

In a TIPS procedure a shunt is placed between the portal and hepatic veins through a catheter in a nonsurgical procedure. The stent redirects some of the portal blood directly into the hepatic vein, thus decreasing portal pressure and decompression of varices.

HINT   Postprocedure management includes assessing for hemorrhage and management of pain (Box 6.17).

Box 6.17 Complications of TIPS Procedure

Pain Hemorrhage	Inadvertent puncture of bile ducts, hepatic arteries, and hepatic capsule
Infection at site or stent	New-onset encephalopathy
Allergic reaction to dye	Shunt occlusion or stenosis
Airway and respiratory compromise (conscious sedation)	Recurrent UGIB

UGIB, upper gastrointestinal bleeding.

Q A splenorenal shunt placed for variceal bleeding reroutes which vein away from the portal vein to bypass the liver?

A Splenic vein

The splenic vein flows into the portal vein providing a portion of the blood that goes through the liver. A shunt is used to surgically manage portal hypertension by decreasing the volume of blood in the portal vein and diverting it around the liver. Splenorenal shunt involves the splenic vein shunt anastomoses to the left renal vein. Other shunts include portacaval shunt (portal vein anastomoses to inferior vena cava) and mesocaval shunt (superior mesenteric vein anastomoses to inferior vena cava). Patients who are transplant candidates are best treated with orthotopic liver transplantation.

HINT Look at the name of the shunt to determine which vein is removed from the portal vein and where it is reconnected. The first part of the word indicates the vein that is being removed (splenic), and the second part of the word indicates where it has been anastomosed (renal vein).

Q What is the nonshunt surgery to prevent recurrent variceal hemorrhaging?

A Esophagogastric devascularization

Esophagogastric devascularization is an effective nonshunt surgery to prevent recurrent bleeding from esophageal varices. This procedure may also be used in patients with ascites or splenic thrombosis, who are contraindicated for a shunt procedure. This involves ligation of venous branches entering the distal esophagus and proximal stomach. It combines this with highly selective vagotomy and pyloroplasty.

Q What procedure is used to control lower gastrointestinal bleedings (LGIBs) with hemodynamic instability?

A Angiography

Angiography is used to determine the location of the hemorrhaging in LGIB patients who are hemodynamically unstable and unable to undergo colonoscopy. It may also be used if the colonoscopy has been unable to localize the bleeding source. Embolization and intra-arterial vasopressin may be used to control hemorrhage. Surgery for an LGIB is not performed often because of complications and higher risk of mortality. Surgical management includes subtotal colectomy.

HINT Patients who have undergone visceral embolization should be monitored for bowel ischemia for several days.

▶ COMPLICATIONS

Q A patient suddenly develops hypotension and complains of severe midsternal to midabdominal pain following an endoscopy. What potential endoscopy complications would be the most likely cause?

A Esophageal perforation

Iatrogenic perforation accounts for more than half of all esophageal perforations. Prompt recognition and treatment are required to prevent contamination of visceral spaces. Esophageal perforation is life-threatening (Box 6.18).

HINT Treatment of perforation of the esophagus during endoscopy is the placement of clips.

Box 6.18 Complications of Endoscopy

Esophageal perforation	Esophageal strictures
Esophageal hemorrhage	Bacteremia/sepsis
Aspiration	Myocardial infarction

Q Following a splenorenal shunt, what is the neurological complication that may occur?

A Hepatic encephalopathy

The splenic vein is removed from the portal circulation and anastomosed to the renal artery that directly flows into the inferior vena cava. The amount of blood shunted around the liver correlates to the incidence of encephalopathy. The liver detoxifies the blood and makes ammonia water soluble to be removed by the kidneys. When blood is shunted around the liver, it results in the accumulation of ammonia and development of hepatic encephalopathy. Another complication of selective distal splenorenal shunt is ascites formation due to extensive retroperitoneal dissection.

HINT   The greater amount of blood being bypassed around the liver, the greater the risk of encephalopathy.

HEPATIC FAILURE/COMA

Q How is acute liver failure (ALF) differentiated from chronic liver failure?

A Length of time from onset of signs

ALF is defined as the onset of hepatic encephalopathy and coagulopathy within 26 weeks of jaundice in a patient without preexisting liver disease. ALF can be a result of primary liver failure or secondary failure due to multisystem organ failure (MSOF).

HINT   Patients with chronic liver failure typically have one or more complications.

▶ PATHOPHYSIOLOGY

Q What is the most common cause of acute liver failure (ALF)?

A Acetaminophen

Acetaminophen is a substance-induced ALF and is currently the most common cause of ALF. It can be due to intentional or unintentional overdose. Accumulation of high levels of acetaminophen unintentionally occurs as a result of consuming multiple products containing acetaminophen. Unintended overdoses typically are not recognized until symptoms of liver failure develop (Box 6.19).

HINT   The recommended dosing should not exceed 4,000 mg in a 24-hour period. The 24-hour dose may be lower (3,000 mg) in geriatric and alcohol-abuse patients.

Box 6.19 Causes of ALF

Infectious	Substance-Induced	Other Disease Processes
Viral hepatitis (A to G)	Acetaminophen	Wilson disease
Coxsackie viruses	Alcohol	Fatty liver in pregnancy
Echoviruses	Carbon tetrachloride	Reye's syndrome
Adenoviruses	Wild mushrooms	Autoimmune hepatitis
	Parenteral hyperalimentation	Budd–Chiari syndrome
	Blood transfusion reaction	

ALF, acute liver failure.

Q What is the physiological change that occurs with viral hepatitis resulting in liver failure?

A Hepatocyte necrosis

There are three major pathological changes that can occur within the liver that result in liver failure. These include necrosis of the hepatocytes, cirrhosis (widespread replacement of hepatocytes with fibrous tissue), and lesions within hepatocytes without necrosis (Box 6.20).

Box 6.20 Major Physiological Changes in Liver Failure

Hepatocyte Necrosis	Cirrhosis	Non-necrotic Lesions
Viral hepatitis	Cardiac (right heart failure)	Starvation
Drug-induced hepatitis	Biliary	Obesity
Hyperthermia	Alcohol ingestion	Alcohol ingestion
Blood transfusion reaction		Diabetes mellitus
Alcohol ingestion		Reye's syndrome
		Hyperalimentation

▶ SYMPTOMS/ASSESSMENT

Q What is the primary cause of the development of hepatic encephalopathy?

A Elevated ammonia levels

Liver failure patients are unable to convert ammonia (by-product of protein) to urea for renal excretion. Hepatic encephalopathy is a clinical disorder characterized by impaired mentation, neuromuscular disturbances, and altered level of consciousness. It is due to elevated ammonia levels, which interfere with normal cerebral metabolism and the amount of energy produced by brain cells.

HINT The quantitative level of ammonia does not correlate with the grade of hepatic encephalopathy or prognosis (Table 6.4).

Table 6.4 Grades of Hepatic Encephalopathy

Grade of Encephalopathy	Symptoms
Grade I	Slight personality and behavioral changes Impaired mentation Reversal of sleep/wake patterns
Grade II	Mental confusion Asterixis (liver flap) Deterioration of handwriting
Grade III	Progressive confusion Decreased LOC but arousable Combative
Grade IV	Unresponsive

LOC, level of consciousness.

Q What is the presence of spider angiomas across the face and chest in liver failure patients caused by?

A Elevated estrogen

The liver detoxifies substances by converting substances from a fat-soluble to a water-soluble state, which allows the kidneys to excrete the substance. Substances include sex hormones, ammonia, mineralocorticoids (aldosterone), glucocorticoids (cortisol), and numerous drugs.

HINT Drugs are typically metabolized (made water soluble) in the liver and excreted by the kidneys (Table 6.5).

Table 6.5 Symptoms of Liver Failure

Normal Liver Function	Symptoms of Liver Failure
Liver produces bile composed of bile salts to emulsify fats	Steatorrhea (fatty, clay-colored stools) Malnutrition (inability to absorb fats) Decreased absorption of fat-soluble vitamins
Synthesizes proteins (albumin)	Hypoalbuminemia Third-spacing Ascites
Stores Vitamin B	Vitamin B deficiency Anemia (folic acid deficiency) Peripheral nerve degeneration Nystagmus Paresthesia of feet
Absorption of Vitamin K Produces coagulation factors Removes activated clotting factors from blood	Coagulopathy Thrombocytopenia Elevated PT
Conjugates bilirubin (makes it water soluble for kidneys to remove)	Jaundice Dark, foamy urine Elevated bilirubin levels Pruritus (elevated bile salts deposited in skin)
Detoxifies substances	Elevated estrogen Spider angiomas Gynecomastia Testicular atrophy Impotence in males Elevated ammonia Hepatic encephalopathy Elevated aldosterone and ADH Increased circulating blood volume Palmar erythema Sodium and water retention Loss of potassium through kidneys Increased ascites and edema Elevated cortisol Moon face Striae Truncal obesity

ADH, antidiuretic hormone; PT, prothrombin time.

HINT Liver function tests (LFTs) may elevate before clinical signs of liver dysfunction occur.

▶ DIAGNOSIS

> **Q** Which of the liver enzymes is the most specific for liver injury?
>
> **A** Alanine aminotransferase (ALT)

Enzymes are present within the liver cells (hepatocytes), when damaged, are released in serum. The aminotransferase enzymes are the most sensitive and widely used. ALT is also known as serum glutamic pyruvic transaminase (SGPT). It is typically found only with liver injury and is the most specific for liver damage. Aspirate aminotransferase (AST), also known as serum glutamic oxaloacetic transaminase (SGOT), is also used in diagnosing liver injury but is less specific. AST can elevate with myocardial injury and sepsis. The ratio of AST to ALT is sometimes used to differentiate between causes of liver diseases.

HINT Names have changed: ALT = SGPT and AST = SGOT.

Q **Which liver enzyme will increase with biliary duct obstructions?**

A **Alkaline phosphatase (ALP)**

ALP is the enzyme that lines the biliary ducts of the liver. Elevation of ALP occurs with biliary duct obstructions as well as intrahepatic cholestasis and infiltrative disease of the liver (Table 6.6).

Table 6.6 Liver Enzymes

Liver Enzyme	Normal Levels
AST	5–60 U/L
ALT	10–40 U/L
ALP	44–147 IU/L
Albumin	3.9–5.0 g/dL
Total bilirubin	0.2–1.2 mg/dL

ALP, alkaline phosphate; ALT, alanine aminotransferase; AST, aspirate aminotransferase

Normal levels vary based on source or laboratory.

HINT Level of liver enzymes does not always correlate to the actual extent of liver damage or prognosis. For example, acute viral hepatitis A may develop really high AST/ALT but has full recovery, whereas chronic hepatitis C frequently has only a slight elevation of liver enzymes but has advanced damage and scarring of liver (Box 6.21, Table 6.7).

Box 6.21 Liver Enzyme Elevation With Hepatic Injury

Highest Level Elevations of LFTs	Mild to Moderate Elevations of LFTs
Hepatitis B and C	Normal variation
Acetaminophen overdose	Chronic hepatitis C
Alcohol–acetaminophen syndrome	Fatty liver due to: Obesity Diabetes mellitus
Prolonged hypoperfusion	Biliary obstruction
Active cirrhosis	
Primary or metastatic cancer	
Alcoholic induced	
Reye's syndrome	

LFTs, liver function tests.

Table 6.7 Specific LFT Findings

Acute Viral Hepatitis	Complete Biliary Obstruction	Cirrhosis	Liver Metastasis
AST 14 × nml	AST 3 × nml	AST 2 × nml	AST 1–2 × nml
ALT 17 × nml	ALT 4 × nml	ALT 1–2 × nml	ALT 1–2 × nml
ALP 1–2 × nml	ALP 4–14 × nml	ALP 1–2 × nml	ALP 10–20 × nml

ALP, alkaline phosphate; ALT, alanine aminotransferase; AST, aspartate aminotransferase; nml, normal.

Q **If the patient's total bilirubin is elevated but the direct bilirubin is normal, is the abnormality in the liver or bile ducts?**

A **Liver**

If the total bilirubin is elevated, then looking at the direct and indirect bilirubin can assist with determining where the injury is located. If direct bilirubin (conjugated bilirubin) is normal, then the problem is excess of unconjugated bilirubin (indirect bilirubin). The problem is within the liver, such as the effects of viral hepatitis or due to hemolysis. If direct bilirubin is elevated, the liver is conjugating the bilirubin normally but is not able to excrete it. Bile duct obstruction by gallstones or cancer should be suspected.

HINT   Conjugated bilirubin is water-soluble and goes "directly" to the kidneys for excretion. So the laboratory value of direct bilirubin measures conjugated bilirubin (or after the liver pass).

▶ MEDICAL MANAGEMENT

Q A patient presents with an acute overdose of acetaminophen. What is the antidote used to reverse the hepatic involvement?

A N-acetylcysteine (NAC)

If a known toxin causes the acute liver failure (ALF), acute management should include known antidotes to the toxin. For acetaminophen overdoses, intravenous NAC is the antidote recommended. In managing symptoms of ALF, including encephalopathy and coagulopathy, NAC is administered until reversal of symptoms (resolution of encephalopathy, international normalized ratio [INR] is less than 1.5, and liver enzymes are declining).

HINT   Treat the underlying cause if possible. For example, steroids are used to treat autoimmune hepatitis, lamivudine is used for hepatitis B patients, and acyclovir is used for herpes simplex.

▶ SURGICAL MANAGEMENT

Q What set of criteria is commonly used to determine the prognosis of acute liver failure (ALF) and potential candidate for liver transplant?

A King's College Criteria

This is a prognostic tool that is used for patients who present with ALF and is used to determine potential candidates for liver transplantation in ALF (Box 6.22).

Box 6.22 King's College Criteria Predicting Poor Outcome in ALF

Acetaminophen Induced	Nonacetaminophen Induced
pH < 7.3 after fluid resuscitation or arterial lactate > 3.5 at 4 hours or arterial lactate > 3 at 12 hours or all of the following:	INR > 6.5 or any three of the following:
INR > 6.5	Age younger than 10 or older than 40 years
Serum creatinine > 3.4 mg/dL	Time from onset of jaundice to the development of coma of more than 7 days
Grade 3 or 4 hepatic encephalopathy	PT > 50 seconds (INR > 3.5) Serum bilirubin > 17.5 g/dL

INR, international normalized ratio; PT, prothrombin time.

▶ COMPLICATIONS

Q What role does the liver play in preventing infections and bacteremia?

A Filters blood

The normal function of the liver is to filter the blood. Kupfer cells line the sinusoids to remove bacteria from the blood, especially from the gastrointestinal (GI) tract. Virtually no bacteria reach systemic circulation, but in liver failure, Kupfer cells have limited ability for phagocytosis and bacteria reach systemic circulation. This causes the patient to be prone to infection, bacteremia, and overwhelming sepsis.

HINT   Minimize invasive lines and administer antibiotics with signs of sepsis or SIRS.

> **Q What is the most common cause of death in liver failure?**
>
> **A Hepatorenal syndrome**

Hepatorenal syndrome is progressive renal failure that is associated with acute or chronic liver disease. It is the leading cause of death in hepatic failure. There are no anatomical or histological changes, and the syndrome is believed to be caused by decreased renal perfusion. Management includes the treatment of the underlying hepatic failure and fluid resuscitation (Box 6.23).

Box 6.23 Symptoms of Hepatorenal Syndrome

Oliguria	Increased urine osmolality
Hyponatremia	Elevated blood urea nitrogen and creatinine

> **Q What is the acute complication of hepatic encephalopathy and elevated ammonia levels?**
>
> **A Increased intracranial pressure (ICP)**

An increased ICP can lead to long-term neurological deficits and is a cause of death in acute liver failure (ALF). The mechanism of cerebral edema is not totally understood but may be due to the conversion of ammonia to glutamine by the astrocytes in the brain. Management includes treating the cerebral edema and managing ammonia levels with lactulose.

HINT   Highest incidence is a rapid presentation of ALF from jaundice to encephalopathy in fewer than 4 weeks.

> **Q Which drug is primarily used in the management of the coagulopathy in acute liver failure (ALF)?**
>
> **A Vitamin K**

The coagulopathy of ALF is caused by a combination of vitamin K deficiency, abnormal clotting cascades, and platelet dysfunction. Clinically significant bleeding is relatively uncommon, and management typically includes empirical administration of vitamin K. Fresh frozen plasma (FFP) should only be used to reverse coagulopathy in a patient with clinically significant bleeding. Cryoprecipitate may be used in a patient with low fibrinogen levels. Another drug for hepatic coagulopathy is vasopressin.

HINT   To prevent complication of GI bleeding, GI prophylaxis is important with either H_2-receptor antagonists or proton pump inhibitors.

ACUTE ABDOMINAL TRAUMA

> **Q What type of abdominal organs are more likely to be injured in a blunt mechanism?**
>
> **A Solid organs**

Common organs injured by blunt mechanism include the solid organs such as the spleen, liver, and pancreas. Hollow organs, like the stomach, collapse with blunt mechanism. Other abdominal organs frequently injured include the small bowel, especially the duodenum. The duodenal injury occurs with a sudden deceleration mechanism due to ligament of Treitz securing the duodenum, while the small bowel is relatively mobile, resulting in a tear (Box 6.24).

Box 6.24 Mechanism of Injury of Blunt Abdominal Trauma

Entrapment of organ between vertebral column and impacting force	Change in organ position
Sudden increase in uniform pressure	Puncture from bone fractures

> **Q** Which two abdominal organs are most commonly injured in penetrating injuries to the abdomen?
>
> **A** Bowel and liver

Bowel is at a greater risk of injury with penetrating injury because of the quantity of bowel present in the abdomen. The liver is one of the most commonly injured organs in the abdomen because of the liver's size and location. The spleen and liver are commonly injured in blunt mechanism.

> **Q** Which abdominal organs are commonly damaged by a lap belt?
>
> **A** Colon and bladder

Mechanism of injury includes crush injury or sudden decompression of an air-filled bowel or urine-filled bladder with the lap belt. Colon and bladder injuries are commonly associated with pelvic fractures.

▶ PATHOPHYSIOLOGY

> **Q** Are the kidneys located in the peritoneal or retroperitoneal space?
>
> **A** Retroperitoneal space

The abdominal cavity is divided into peritoneal and retroperitoneal space. Certain diagnostic tests are able to locate injuries in the peritoneal cavity better than the retroperitoneal space. Organs in the retroperitoneal space that sustain an injury are more likely to be missed due to the greater difficulty in diagnosis (Box 6.25).

Box 6.25 Peritoneal and Retroperitoneal Organs

Peritoneal Space	Retroperitoneal Space
Stomach	Duodenum
Small bowel	Ascending colon
Liver	Descending colon
Spleen	Kidneys
Gallbladder	Part of the bladder
Transverse colon	Pancreas
Sigmoid colon	Major vessels
Upper one-third of rectum	
Part of bladder	
Uterus	

> **Q** What is the most common cause of death following liver injury in abdominal trauma?
>
> **A** Hemorrhage

The liver is very vascular as both the portal vein and hepatic artery bring blood into the liver. It is the most common cause of hemorrhagic shock in abdominal trauma (both penetrating and blunt), followed by the spleen and kidneys.

HINT   Initially "damage" control is frequently performed intraoperatively to control bleeding, followed by a return trip to the operating room later to actually repair the liver injury.

> **Q** Which part of the bladder, when ruptured, would result in intraabdominal injury (peritonitis)?
>
> **A** Dome of the bladder

Bladder rupture results from a blunt trauma to the lower abdomen when the bladder is full. The dome is the weakest point of the bladder and is the most common site of rupture. The dome of the bladder is covered by the peritoneum, so rupture of the dome causes urine to enter the intraperitoneal space.

HINT   Extraperitoneal bladder ruptures are usually associated with pelvic fractures.

▶ SYMPTOMS/ASSESSMENT

Q What is the most common finding for stomach injuries following penetrating trauma to the abdomen?

A Bloody gastric aspirate

The most common sign of stomach injury is blood in the gastric aspirate. Other findings include rapid-onset epigastric pain, tenderness, and signs of peritonitis due to release of gastric contents, and free air on abdominal x-ray.

HINT Blunt trauma may result in blood in gastric aspirate without stomach injuries, if facial trauma or oral-cavity injury resulted in swallowing of blood.

Q Why does a duodenal tear not cause immediate peritonitis, as seen often with gastric injuries?

A Alkaline fluid in duodenum

The fluid in the stomach is acidic and, when spilled into the peritoneal cavity, causes a rapid, severe peritonitis. Gastric injuries typically present with abdominal pain, abdominal tenderness, or a "board-like" abdomen. Duodenal tears, however, may have minimal signs of peritonitis with mild irritation or tenderness of the abdomen initially. This is because the fluid in the duodenum and small bowel is alkaline, which causes less irritation. Symptoms of peritonitis occur later as a result of infection in the peritoneum.

HINT Duodenal injuries may be missed due to the delayed presentation of peritonitis because it is a retroperitoneal organ (Box 6.26).

Box 6.26 Symptoms of Delayed Peritonitis With Duodenal Injuries

Fever	Increased bilirubin and amylase
Leukocytosis	High intestinal obstruction
Third spacing with hypovolemia	Jaundice

Q What is pain in the neck area because of irritation of the phrenic nerve following splenic injury called?

A Saegesser's sign

Following splenic injury, pain occurs as generalized abdominal pain that is localized in the left upper quadrant and can refer to the neck region (Saegesser's sign) or to the left shoulder or scapula (Kehr's sign). Splenic injuries can cause life-threatening hemorrhage with signs of shock.

▶ DIAGNOSIS

Q What may be found on a chest x-ray (CXR) or kidneys, ureters, and bladder (KUB) x-ray that would be an indication for surgery?

A Free air or foreign bodies

An upright CXR and left lateral decubitus are used to identify free air (ruptured hollow organ) or presence of foreign bodies. Supine abdominal x-ray can identify retroperitoneal free air, gross organ injury, presence of blood, or foreign objects in the abdominal cavity.

Q What is the diagnostic focused abdominal sonography trauma (FAST) test that is used to evaluate blunt abdominal trauma?

A Ultrasonography of the abdomen

FAST is ultrasonography that can be used to evaluate the abdomen following blunt trauma. It can detect the presence of free intraperitoneal or pericardial fluid. Ultrasound can estimate the amount of blood in the abdomen, thus preventing unnecessary laparotomies, and can identify candidates for observation. It is not as reliable for the retroperitoneal space.

HINT Greater than 1,000 mL of fluid (blood) in the peritoneum requires immediate surgical intervention.

Q Which diagnostic test is the gold standard to evaluate the abdomen following a blunt trauma?

A Abdominal CT scan

Abdominal CT scans are able to view both the retroperitoneal cavity as well as intra-abdominal injuries. Abdominal CT scans able to identify the organs involved and grade the severity of injury. This allows for the ability to observe some patients with less severe injuries instead of performing an exploratory laparotomy (Box 6.36).

HINT Unstable patients require evaluation in the emergency department and may not be able to be transported to CT scan (Table 6.8).

Table 6.8 Diagnostic Evaluation of Blunt Abdominal Trauma

Diagnostic Test	Advantages	Disadvantages
KUB or CXR	Performed in the ED Free air indicates hollow organ rupture without having to perform further workup	Unable to identify severity of organ injuries or fluid in the abdomen
Ultrasound	Performed in the ED High sensitivity to detect intra-abdominal fluid	Not accurate in obese patients, ileus, emphysema Unable to differentiate blood, bile, urine, or ascites Decreased accuracy of retroperitoneal injuries
CT scan	View retroperitoneal space Identify organs injured Grade severity of organ injury Determine patients for observation instead of surgery	Transport patient out of the ED May miss mesenteric, bowel, or diaphragm injuries More expensive
DPL	Performed in the emergency department	Unable to identify retroperitoneal injuries Inability to determine type or severity of injury False-negative results False-positive results Potential bowel or bladder perforation

CXR, chest x-ray; DPL, diagnostic peritoneal lavage; KUB, kidney, ureters, and bladder.

Q Would a patient with pelvic injuries more likely have a false-positive or a false-negative result with a diagnostic peritoneal lavage (DPL)?

A False-positive result

Patients with pelvic injuries may receive a positive DPL due to blood from the pelvic region being found in the peritoneum. False-positive and false-negative results can occur with a DPL. For example, multiple previous abdominal surgeries resulting in adhesions can sequester the blood and cause a false-negative result.

HINT A false-positive result occurs when a DPL is positive, indicating surgery, when an injury was not present, whereas a false-negative result means the DPL was negative but an injury was present.

Q What should be placed prior to performing a diagnostic peritoneal lavage (DPL)?

A Foley catheter

Bladder or bowel perforation can occur with the placement of the peritoneal catheter to perform the DPL. A Foley catheter should be inserted prior to placement of the catheter to empty the bladder and lower the risk of unintentional perforation (Boxes 6.27 and 6.28).

Box 6.27 Relative Contraindications for DPL

Advanced pregnancy	Morbid obesity
Pelvic injuries	Advanced cirrhosis
History of previous abdominal surgeries	Coagulopathy

DPL, diagnostic peritoneal lavage.

Box 6.28 Positive Findings in DPL

Aspiration > 10 mL of blood	Hematocrit > 2%
>100,000 RBCs	Presence of bile, bacteria, or fecal material
>500 WBCs	Elevated amylase

DPL, diagnostic peritoneal lavage.

▶ MEDICAL MANAGEMENT

Q What is a medical option for a hemodynamically stable blunt abdominal trauma patient with a splenic injury Grade II?

A Observation

The American Association for the Surgery of Trauma (AAST) developed a grading system for organ injury based on the CT scan to determine potential success for a nonoperative approach. Hemodynamically stable patients with low-grade injuries of the spleen or liver without any other evidence of intraabdominal injuries may be observed without initial surgery. Another nonsurgical method is embolization of the spleen or liver (Tables 6.9 and 6.10).

Table 6.9 Grading Liver Injuries

Grade	Description of Injuries
Grade I	Subcapsular hematoma < 10% surface area Capsular tear < 1-cm depth
Grade II	Subcapsular hematoma with 10%–50% surface area Intraparenchymal hematoma < 10-cm diameter Capsular tear 1- to 3-cm depth, < 10-cm length
Grade III	Subcapsular hematoma > 50% surface area, or ruptured with active bleeding Intraparenchymal hematoma > 10-cm diameter Capsular tear > 3-cm depth
Grade IV	Ruptured intraparenchymal with active bleeding Parenchymal disruption involving 25%–75% of hepatic lobes
Grade V	Parenchymal disruption involving > 75% of hepatic lobes Vascular: Juxtahepatic venous injuries (inferior vena cava [IVC], major hepatic vein)
Grade VI	Vascular: Hepatic avulsion

Reprinted with permission, *The Journal of Trauma*, 1995; 38(3), 323–324.

Table 6.10 Grading Spleen Injuries

Grade	Description of Injuries
Grade I	Capsular tear, < 1 cm parenchymal
Grade II	Capsular tear, 1- to 3-cm depth, which does not involve a trabecular vessel
Grade III	Laceration > 3-cm parenchymal depth involving trabecular vessels Ruptured subcapsular or parenchymal hematoma Intraparenchymal hematoma > 5 cm or expanding
Grade IV	Laceration involving segmental or hilar vessels producing major devascularization (>25% of spleen)
Grade V	Shattered spleen or hilar vascular injury, which devascularizes spleen

Reprinted with permission, *The Journal of Trauma*, 1995; 38(3), 323–324.

▶ SURGICAL MANAGEMENT

> **Q** What surgical procedure would a patient with ongoing blood loss from an unknown source following a blunt trauma require?
>
> **A** Exploratory laparotomy

Following a blunt trauma, the most common site to cause hemorrhagic shock is the abdomen. If a patient remains unstable and an immediate source of blood loss is unable to be located, the patient should undergo an exploratory laparotomy (Box 6.29).

Box 6.29 Indications for Exploratory Laparotomy

Penetrating trauma to abdomen	Ongoing blood loss from unknown source
Presence of free air on x-ray	Known significant injuries found with diagnostic studies
Eviscerated bowel or omentum	Positive peritoneal signs
Significant bleeding from NG tube or rectum	

NG, nasogastric.

> **Q** What is the priority in an emergency exploratory laparotomy performed on an abdominal trauma patient?
>
> **A** Control blood loss

The immediate priority in an exploratory laparotomy in a trauma patient is to find the source of blood loss and control the bleeding. The most common organs involved in significant blood loss are the liver, spleen, and kidneys. Typically, an unstable patient may require control of bleeding by either removing the organ (spleen or kidneys) or packing to tamponade the bleeding liver (Box 6.30).

Box 6.30 Exploratory Laparotomy Priority

First priority	Find source of blood loss and control bleeding
Second priority	Locate any colonic injuries to control fecal contamination
Third priority	Identify injured organs
Fourth priority	Repair injured organs

> **Q** What is "damage control" when managing a bleeding liver intraoperatively?
>
> **A** Temporary control of blood loss

Control of blood loss from the liver is frequently obtained by a technique called "damage control." If hemorrhage is severe, the liver may be packed with lap pads to tamponade the bleeding. Other techniques used in "damage control" include use of fibrin glue (sealant made from concentrated fibrinogen and thrombin) and/or selective hepatic artery or portal vein ligation. Following packing of the liver, a temporary closure is used to cover the abdomen and a planned reoperation to control bleeding and repair the liver is performed. The packing may be kept in place for 48 to 72 hours while the patient is being maintained in the ICU (Box 6.31).

HINT Assess for uncontrolled hemorrhage, monitor coagulation studies, administer FFP, and warm the patient to reverse the coagulopathy.

Box 6.31 Surgical Interventions of Abdominal Organ Injuries

Stomach	Debridement of devitalized tissue Closure with sutures Partial gastrectomy NG tube postoperative for decompression
Duodenum and small bowel	Debridement of devitalized tissue Bowel resection and anastomosis NG tube and/or duodenal tube for decompression
Pancreas	Suture and drain if minor injury Debridement of pancreas if major injury Occurs over several days Placement of drains around pancreatic bed
Liver	Control bleeding ("damage control") Debridement of devitalized tissue Minor injuries may be sutured, topical agents applied or electrocautery performed Placement of drains around hepatic bed Drain bile ducts
Spleen	Minor injury repaired Major injury may require splenectomy Surgery if separated from blood supply or macerated
Colon	Primary closure Resection with primary anastomosis Primary closure with proximal colostomy Delayed closure Colostomy (double-barrel loop colostomy)

NG, nasogastric.

HINT Postoperative management and complications of stomach injuries are the same as for postoperative gastrectomy patients.

Q What is a common laboratory finding following a splenectomy?

A Elevated platelets and white blood cells (WBCs)

Following a splenectomy, the platelet count typically is elevated (thrombocytosis) and can cause thrombotic evens such as an acute myocardial infarction, mesenteric vein thrombosis, and venous thromboembolism (VTE). The incidence of thrombocytosis will peak between 9 and 10 days postoperatively. Platelet counts typically return to normal within weeks to several months post splenectomy. Leukocytosis can also be seen following splenectomy.

HINT Prophylaxis for VTE is recommended post splenectomy.

▶ COMPLICATIONS

Q Which combination of organs injured following abdominal trauma will have the highest rate of postoperative sepsis?

A Liver and colon

When injured, the colon will leak or spill fecal material into the peritoneum. The liver is very vascular and susceptible to bleeding. Abscess formation is due to foreign body fragments, necrotic tissue, blood, or bile remaining at the site of injury. The combination of blood and fluid with fecal contamination in the peritoneum increases the risk of peritonitis and sepsis.

HINT Postop fluid collections or abscesses can be drained by CT-guided placement of a catheter.

> **Q** Following a splenectomy to control hemorrhaging, what needs to be given to the patient prior to discharge?
>
> **A** Pneumococcal vaccination

A complication of a splenectomy is overwhelming postsplenectomy sepsis (OPSS), which can occur as a result of the loss of some immune responses that will increase the mortality rate. The majority of OPSS occurs within 1 year post-splenectomy but can occur several years later. *Streptococcus pneumoniae* (pneumococcus), *Haemophilus influenzae* type B, and *Neisseria meningitidis* are organisms that cause OPSS. Infections are associated with mortality as high as 50% to 80% following a splenectomy.

HINT Pneumovax vaccination is required before discharge (Box 6.32).

Box 6.32 Complications of Abdominal Organ Injuries

Stomach	Breakdown of anastomosis Abscesses Fistulas Alkalosis Hypokalemia Peritonitis
Duodenum and small bowel	Breakdown of anastomosis Peritonitis Abscess Wound dehiscence Bowel ischemia Fistula formation Bowel obstruction Abdominal compartment syndrome
Pancreas	Hemorrhage Signs of peritonitis Fluid and electrolyte imbalance Pseudocyst Abscess Fistulas Sepsis ARDS Necrosis due to autodigestion
Liver	Hemorrhage Sepsis ARDS DIC Abdominal abscess Hematobilia (free communication between biliary tree and vascular system) Hepatorenal syndrome Jaundice Bile peritonitis
Spleen	Hemorrhage Overwhelming postsplenectomy sepsis
Colon	Fistulas Abscesses Peritonitis Sepsis Bowel obstruction Incisional infection

ARDS, acute respiratory distress syndrome; DIC, disseminated intravascular coagulopathy.

HINT   Duodenal fistulas cause acidosis secondary to loss of bicarbonate from pancreatic juices, whereas jejunal fistulas produce low volumes of neutral pH fluid with little change in acid–base balance (Box 6.33).

Box 6.33 Late Complications From Abdominal Trauma

Peptic ulcers	Fistulas
Intestinal obstruction from adhesions	Chronic abscess
Hernia	Cholelithiasis and cholecystitis

BOWEL INFARCTIONS/PERFORATION/OBSTRUCTION

Q What does bowel ischemia related to venous obstruction result in: thrombosis or embolism?

A Thrombosis

Acute mesenteric ischemia is a syndrome of inadequate blood flow through the mesenteric vessels resulting in infarction, necrosis, and death. Bowel ischemia can be caused by either arterial or venous system abnormalities. Occlusive venous disease is due to thrombosis, whereas arterial disease may be caused by thrombosis or embolism. Arterial disease that is not caused by occlusion of blood flow that results in hypoperfusion is also possible (Box 6.34).

Box 6.34 Acute Mesenteric Ischemia

Nonocclusive mesenteric ischemia (NOMI)

Occlusive mesenteric arterial ischemia (OMAI)
  Acute mesenteric arterial embolism
  Acute mesenteric arterial thrombosis

MVT

MVT, mesenteric venous thrombosis; NOMI, nonocclusive mesenteric ischemia; OMAI, occlusive mesenteric arterial ischemia.

Q What is a complication following abdominal surgery that can cause a bowel obstruction?

A Adhesions

Acute bowel obstruction occurs when the forward flow of intestinal contents is interrupted and can occur anywhere in the intestines. The obstruction is classified as either small- or large-bowel obstructions. The three most common causes of bowel obstruction are intra-abdominal adhesions, malignancy, and abdominal hernias.

HINT   Bowel obstructions may be complete or partial.

▶ PATHOPHYSIOLOGY

Q What artery supplies blood to the jejunum?

A Superior mesenteric artery

The arteries that supply the GI viscera branch off the anterior portion of the descending aorta. The most clinically important is the territory of the superior mesenteric artery, which affects the small and large intestines. The esophagus and stomach are not commonly affected by local ischemia versus a global ischemia (Box 6.35).

Box 6.35 Arterial Supply of the Gastrointestinal (GI) System

Celiac Artery	Superior Mesenteric Artery	Inferior Mesenteric Artery
Esophagus	Inferior portion duodenum	Left one-third of transverse colon
Stomach	Jejunum	Descending colon
Superior portion duodenum	Ileum	Sigmoid colon
Liver	Cecum	Rectum
Spleen	Appendix	Upper portion anal canal
	Ascending colon	
	Right two-thirds of transverse colon	

Q What is a common cause in an ICU patient for nonocclusive arterial bowel infarction?

A Hypotension

Arterial disease is divided into occlusive and nonocclusive ischemia. Occlusive bowel ischemia is typically caused by an obstruction to flow due to either an embolism or thrombosis, whereas nonocclusive ischemia is decreased blood flow through the mesenteric vessels. Critically ill patients frequently experience periods of shock and hypotension. Blood may be shunted away from the gastrointestinal (GI) system, causing hypoperfusion to the bowel.

HINT Vasoactive drugs may also cause nonocclusive bowel infarctions (Box 6.36).

Box 6.36 Causes of Acute Arterial Mesenteric Ischemia

Nonocclusive Arterial Mesenteric Ischemia	Occlusive Arterial Mesenteric Thrombosis	Occlusive Arterial Mesenteric Embolism
Hypotension	Atherosclerotic disease	Cardiac emboli Atrial fibrillation Septic emboli
Vasopressor drugs	Aortic aneurysm	Fragments of atheromatous plaque
Ergotamine	Aortic dissection	
Sympathomimetic drugs cocaine	Arteritis	
Digitalis	Dehydration	

Q What disease state most commonly causes mesenteric venous ischemia due to venous congestion?

A Hepatic failure

Venous congestion occurs in portal hypertension from hepatic failure. Portal hypertension can cause venous blood to back up into mesenteric vessels, causing venous stasis and thrombosis (Box 6.37).

Box 6.37 Causes of Mesenteric Venous Ischemia

Hypercoagulable state	Abdominal compartment syndrome
Tumor causing venous obstruction	Venous trauma
Intraabdominal infection	Decompression sickness
Venous congestion	

Q What happens proximal to bowel obstruction?

A Dilation of bowel

Proximal to the bowel obstruction, the intestinal lumen dilates due to accumulation of secretions, ingested food and fluid, bowel contents, and gas. There is little to no movement of bowel contents or flatus distal. This results in an increased intraluminal pressure. Distal bowel collapses and alters the normal secretory or absorptive function of the bowel.

HINT   Fluid and electrolyte abnormalities commonly occur with bowel obstruction.

Q What is a major concern in bowel obstructions that affects management and mortality?

A Vascular compromise

Bowel dilation and obstruction increase intraluminal pressures. When pressures exceed venous pressures, the bowel becomes edematous and swollen. This leads to compromised arterial flow and bowel ischemia. Bowel obstruction can occur with or without vascular compromise.

HINT   Presence of vascular compromise to the bowel determines the need for surgery instead of medical management (Box 6.38).

Box 6.38 Causes of Bowel Obstruction

Intraabdominal adhesions	Intraabdominal abscess
Malignancy	Foreign bodies
Abdominal hernia	Diverticulosis
Inflammatory bowel disease	Fecal impaction
Intestinal intussusception	Crohn's disease
Volvulus	Parasitic infestation

Q What is it called when there is a complete twist of the intestine?

A Volvulus

Volvulus is the complete twisting of a loop of intestine around the mesenteric attachment. It is a malposition or malrotation of the intestines. It can cause bowel obstruction and bowel ischemia. In the elderly population, it most commonly occurs at the sigmoid colon.

HINT   Intussusception occurs when the intestine is invaginated into another section of the intestines, resulting in obstruction.

▶ SYMPTOMS/ASSESSMENT

Q Bloody diarrhea is most likely to be the presentation of bowel infarction, bowel obstruction, or bowel perforation?

A Bowel infarction

All of the above can present with severe abdominal pain, nausea and vomiting, and diarrhea. Infarctions are more likely to develop bloody diarrhea than obstructions or perforation. In small-bowel infarctions, bleeding from the rectum may be seen as a late sign caused by tissue necrosis. Colonic infarctions may involve bloody diarrhea but not necessarily to the point of significant blood loss. Bowel obstructions, if complete, will not allow passing of stool, but partial obstructions may present with diarrhea.

HINT   Colonic infarctions have more severe abdominal pain than small-bowel infarctions. Small-bowel ischemia may be very nonspecific until signs of peritonitis appear (Box 6.39)

Box 6.39 Symptoms of Bowel Infarction

Small-Bowel Infarction	Colonic Infarction
Abdominal pain	Severe abdominal cramping
Increased peristalsis	Diarrhea
Vomiting	Bloody diarrhea
Diarrhea	Ileus
Blood from rectum	Signs of sepsis
Signs of peritonitis	
Signs of sepsis	

HINT Abdominal pain is frequently described as a constant, diffuse, nonlocalized, colicky type of pain.

Q During abdominal auscultation in early bowel obstruction, what would you expect to occur with bowel sounds?

A Bowel sounds should be hyperactive and high pitched

Early obstruction typically results in hyperactive, high-pitched bowel sounds. The colon may develop loud borborygmi due to increased peristalsis. Late obstruction may present with minimal bowel sounds due to hypotonia.

HINT Emesis may be odorous and frequently has a feculent odor due to intestinal stasis and the effect of bacteria on abdominal contents (Box 6.40).

Box 6.40 Symptoms of Bowel Obstruction

Colicky abdominal pain	Cessation of flatus and stool
Nausea and vomiting	Signs of dehydration
Abdominal distention	High-pitched bowel sounds
Palpable abdominal mass	

▶ DIAGNOSIS

Q What is the most confirmative diagnosis for small-bowel infarction?

A Exploratory laparotomy

Plain radiographs are not useful in the diagnosis of acute mesenteric ischemia. A diagnostic finding is intramural or intravascular air, but this is a late sign of intestinal infarction. A CT scan may identify a thickening of the bowel wall, characteristic "thumb printing" caused by submucosa necrosis, and intramural or intravascular air may also be seen. Other diagnostics include MRI, MRA, and ultrasonography. Frequently, the confirmation of the diagnosis is an exploratory laparotomy.

HINT Angiography is beneficial for occlusive arterial disease but has been shown to be less effective with nonobstructive or venous thrombosis disease.

Q What electrolyte is typically found elevated in patients with mesenteric ischemia?

A Phosphate

Phosphate is somewhat sensitive to mesenteric ischemia and infarctions and will increase in the first 4 hours. Hematocrit initially is elevated due to third spacing and hemoconcentration but will decrease with gastrointestinal (GI) bleeding. Amylase levels may be elevated but are nonspecific (Box 6.41).

Box 6.41 Laboratory Findings of Mesenteric Ischemia

Hyperphosphatemia	Moderately elevated amylase
Elevated hematocrit initially	Elevated lactase
Leukocytosis	Metabolic acidosis
Elevated D-dimer	

Q Does bowel obstruction with emesis result in metabolic acidosis or metabolic alkalosis?

A Metabolic alkalosis

Obstruction in the bowel leads to high intraluminal pressures and commonly presents with emesis. Gastric acids, potassium, chloride, and hydrogen ions are lost with emesis. The kidneys reabsorb bicarbonate and further lose chloride, contributing to metabolic alkalosis. The loss of fluids from the stomach and kidneys also contribute to hypovolemia and dehydration. Hypochloremic metabolic alkalosis is a combination of a loss of acids and reabsorption of bicarbonate.

HINT If a patient with a bowel obstruction presents with metabolic acidosis, suspect bowel ischemia. Lactate levels will be elevated due to anaerobic metabolism (Box 6.42).

Box 6.42 Abnormal Laboratory Findings in Bowel Obstruction

Hypokalemia	Increase in bicarbonate
Hypochloremia	Elevated blood urea nitrogen

hct, hematocrit; Hgb, hemoglobin.

Q Which radiographic diagnostic test is used most frequently to diagnose bowel obstruction?

A Plain abdominal radiograph

A plain abdominal radiograph is used to determine the presence of dilated loops of small bowel or dilated colon with decompressed small bowel. Early obstruction or high duodenal or jejunal obstruction may not appear on a plain radiograph and require abdominal CT scan. An advantage of abdominal CT scan over plain radiograph is the ability to identify the location of a cause of the obstruction. Other diagnostic examinations include ultrasonography, MRI, and contrast fluoroscopy.

HINT CT scans are not as valuable for partial obstructions, and the patient may require fluoroscopy.

MEDICAL MANAGEMENT

Q What is the initial treatment of patients with bowel ischemia and bowel obstruction?

A Fluids and antibiotics

The initial management includes fluid resuscitation, correction of electrolyte and other metabolic abnormalities, and initiation of antibiotic therapy. Antibiotics are administered to prevent or treat infections caused by bowel infarction and necrosis. Antibiotics used for bowel obstruction prevent bacterial overgrowth and translocation of bacteria causing septicemia.

HINT Antibiotics should cover gram-negative organisms and anaerobes.

Q What other treatment may be used to conservatively manage a high-grade bowel obstruction?

A Decompression of the intestines

Conservative management includes fluid and electrolyte management as well as a nasogastric tube to suction for decompression. Other drugs may include probiotics, oral magnesium hydroxide, and simethicone.

HINT Patient will have NPO status to "rest" bowel while aggressively replacing fluid intravenously.

> **Q** What is the treatment for patients with acute mesenteric venous thrombosis (MVT)?
>
> **A** Anticoagulation therapy

Heparin may be used in the acute care setting as an anticoagulant to treat the venous thrombosis. If no bowel necrosis exists, anticoagulation therapy is used to treat without surgical intervention. Warfarin is commonly used for long-term management of MVT.

HINT Venous thrombosis anywhere in the vasculature is managed with anticoagulation therapy.

▶ SURGICAL MANAGEMENT

> **Q** Nonocclusive arterial mesenteric ischemia is initially managed with which minimally invasive procedure?
>
> **A** Angiography with papaverine infusion

Angiography with papaverine infusion may be used in all forms of arterial mesenteric ischemia, but in nonocclusive ischemia it is the only treatment except bowel resection. Papaverine infusion through a catheter placed in an angiosuite will relieve vasospasms in the occluded arterial vessel. Thrombolytic infusion may be used for embolic mesenteric ischemia in patients without peritonitis or bowel infarction.

HINT Signs of peritonitis indicate the need to stop infusion of thrombolytics for embolic mesenteric ischemia and prepare patient for surgery.

> **Q** What complication indicates the need for surgery in all types of mesenteric ischemic disease?
>
> **A** Bowel necrosis

Bowel necrosis presents as peritonitis and is an indication for surgery and bowel resection in all types of mesenteric ischemia. Signs of peritonitis include fever, leukocytosis, abdominal pain, and a "board-like" abdomen. Thrombotic mesenteric occlusion may undergo emergency revascularization surgery if the gut is not gangrenous. Transthoracic endarterectomy is an alternative when no vein is available for bypass.

> **Q** Which two complications of bowel obstruction would indicate the need for immediate abdominal surgery?
>
> **A** Bowel ischemia and perforation

Onset of peritonitis or unexplained sepsis with abdominal signs would indicate a complication of bowel obstruction or perforation and need for surgical management. Another indication for abdominal surgery is to manage the underlying cause of obstruction, such as hernia or adhesion.

HINT Abdominal tumors will need to be evaluated to determine whether surgery or palliative care is indicated.

▶ COMPLICATIONS

> **Q** Bowel obstruction and the resulting ischemia can cause what complication?
>
> **A** Bowel perforation

Following bowel obstruction, perforation can occur. Vascular compromise leads to ischemia and is the most common site of perforation. This typically occurs in the small bowel but can also occur in the colon or cecum with large dilation.

HINT Free air found in an upright KUB is diagnostic of bowel perforation.

MALNUTRITION AND MALABSORPTION

Q What is the malabsorption syndrome commonly associated with the ICU?

A Sepsis

Malabsorption is defined as intestinal absorption capacity of 85% or less. It is commonly associated with sepsis and multiple organ dysfunction or failure (such as acute renal failure). Malabsorption is the clinical sign of intestinal dysfunction or failure.

HINT   Malabsorption can contribute to translocation of bacteria and septicemia.

Q Hypercatabolism in critically ill patients can result in loss of what?

A Muscle mass

Hypercatabolism is recognized in critically ill patients to cause a cachectic state in which the person's muscle is used as an energy source. This results in a loss of muscle mass, including the respiratory muscles. Critically ill patients have a high metabolism rate and require an increase in caloric and nutrient requirements (Box 6.43).

Box 6.43 Risk for Malnutrition

Obese	Increased nutrient losses Malabsorption
Underweight	Short bowel syndrome
Recent weight loss	Fistula
Inadequate digestion	Draining wounds
Recent GI surgeries	Renal dialysis, peritoneal dialysis
Alcohol or substance abuse	Severe diarrhea
NPO status	Corticosteroid therapy

Increased nutrient requirements
  Burns
  Trauma
  Sepsis
  Fever
  Surgery
  ESRD	

ESRD, end-stage renal disease; GI, gastrointestinal; NPO, nothing by mouth.

▶ PATHOPHYSIOLOGY

Q What function of the intestines, when altered in critical illness, can result in an ileus?

A Motility

A function of the intestine is coordinated intestinal transport or motility. A decreased motility results in an ileus, malnutrition, and increased risk of translocation of bacteria. Critically ill patients are at risk for altered intestinal activity due to a decrease in splanchnic blood flow (Box 6.44).

HINT   Adequate absorption in the intestines is important in critically ill patients for improvement.

Box 6.44 Functions of the Intestines

Motility	Mucosal immunological response
Coordinate exocrine digestive functions (pancreas, jejunum, liver)	Intestinal barrier function

> **Q** What is a common cause of intestinal disruption in the ICU?
>
> **A** Bowel rest

Complete bowel rest causes progressive atrophy, disruption, and degenerative changes of the intestinal mucosa. These changes can occur within a few days of assigning nothing by mouth (NPO) status. Parenteral nutrition does not prevent intestinal disruption. Translocation of bacteria can occur during bowel rest. Enteral nutrition can help prevent sepsis from bowel origin (gram-negative bacteria).

HINT   Early feeding can lower the incidence of bacteremia from translocation of bacteria.

> **Q** What is the amino acid required to replace the intestinal mucosa?
>
> **A** Glutamine

The bowel mucosa relies on nutrients from the bowel lumen. One important nutrient is an amino acid called "glutamine." Glutamine is a principal metabolic fuel for the intestinal epithelial cells. The entire lining of the GI tract mucosa is replaced every 2 to 8 days. The replacement of these cells is dependent on the nutrition of the patient. Food has a trophic effect on the GI mucosa.

HINT   Glutamine is the major fuel of the cells of the small intestine.

▶ SYMPTOMS/ASSESSMENT

> **Q** What is a symptom of protein malnutrition and cachectic state?
>
> **A** Muscle wasting

Wasting of muscle and subcutaneous fat are signs of protein malnutrition. The body begins to break down its own supply of protein and fat to meet the high caloric demands of critically ill patients.

HINT   The diaphragm is a muscle, so critically ill patients in cachectic states may have increased difficulty weaning from ventilators.

▶ DIAGNOSIS

> **Q** What hepatic protein is considered the best predictor of nutrition in critically ill patients?
>
> **A** Prealbumin

Prealbumin levels are used in assessing nutritional status in critically ill patients. They have been shown to predict outcomes and correlate to patient recovery. Prealbumin is the earliest indicator of protein malnutrition and is not as affected by liver disease as other proteins.

HINT   Prealbumin may allow earlier recognition and intervention for malnutrition. A prealbumin less than 15 mg/L requires nutritional consult (Table 6.11).

Table 6.11 Plasma Proteins

Plasma Proteins	Half-Life	Range
Albumin	20 days	3.30–4.8 g/L
Prealbumin	2 days	16–35 mg/L
Transferrin	10 days	0.16–0.36 g/L

HINT   These are called negative acute phase proteins.

▶ MEDICAL MANAGEMENT

> **Q** Which two drugs are commonly used as prokinetics to improve tolerance to feeding?
>
> **A** Erythromycin and metoclopramide

Prokinetic therapy is used in patients with feed intolerance and gastroparesis. The two drugs used as first-line therapy as a prokinetic include erythromycin and metoclopramide. Erythromycin is a dopamine agonist, and metoclopramide is a promotility agent. Metoclopramide has been found most effective in improving gastric emptying. Erythromycin has been found effective in both gastric emptying and improving tolerance to feeding but may cause an increase in bacterial resistance. A combination of both erythromycin and metoclopramide may be more effective with less tachyphylaxis.

HINT Prolongation of QT interval is a potential complication of erythromycin and metoclopramide administration.

▶ COMPLICATIONS

> **Q** What is the pulmonary complication of total parenteral nutrition (TPN) with overfeeding?
>
> **A** Elevated $PaCO_2$

Overfeeding can impair pulmonary function. Too much caloric intake from lipids or carbohydrates alone can result in an increased production of carbon dioxide (CO_2). This can cause difficulty in weaning patients from ventilators due to hyperventilation. Avoid overfeeding by monitoring caloric intake and using balanced lipids and carbohydrates to supply the calories (Box 6.45).

Box 6.45 Complications of Total Parenteral Nutrition

Catheter-related sepsis

Central-line complications
  Air embolus
  Pneumothorax
  Central venous thrombosis
  Catheter occlusion

Hypoglycemia or hyperglycemia
Gram-negative sepsis
Elevated $PaCO_2$

● ABDOMINAL COMPARTMENT SYNDROME (ACS)

> **Q** When pressure within an anatomical compartment increases to the point of compression and tissue perfusion compromise, what is it called?
>
> **A** Compartment syndrome

Compartment syndrome can occur in the extremities, as well as in intracranial, thoracic, and abdominal areas. Compression results in altered cellular oxygenation and initiates a cycle of progressive cellular injury, with edema and hypoperfusion leading to anaerobic metabolism, metabolic acidosis, and cellular death.

> **Q** When the pressure increases in the abdominal cavity to the extent of causing organ dysfunction/failure, what is it now known as?
>
> **A** Abdominal compartment syndrome (ACS)

This syndrome was initially recognized and managed in abdominal trauma patients, but it is now known to occur in any critically ill patient (also medical patients without abdominal conditions). ACS results in multiple complications, including acute respiratory distress; acute renal failure; dehiscence of abdominal wound and evisceration of bowel, bowel ischemia, sepsis, and multiple system organ failure (MSOF). Intraabdominal pressure (IAP) is a compartment pressure that is monitored and measured and is defined as a steady-state pressure concealed within the abdominal cavity (Box 6.46).

Box 6.46 Factors That Influence IAP

Abdominal organ volume	Grossly swollen bowel (occupies several times original volume) Excessive crystalloid resuscitation
Presence of space-occupying substances (blood, ascites, tumor, free air)	Bleeding, leakage of abdominal contents, bowel edema Blood or blood clots
Abdominal wall compliance	Mechanical ventilation PEEP Increased BMI

BMI, body mass index; PEEP, positive end expiratory pressure.

Q What is the primary injury that occurs in abdominal compartment syndrome (ACS)?

A Trauma or ischemic insult

The "primary" injury occurs due to the direct trauma or ischemic insult. The "secondary" injury occurs due to cytokine release and systemic inflammatory response. The inflammatory response results in an increase in capillary permeability and edema. The goal of treatment is to manage or prevent the secondary injuries. Recurrent ACS is a "second hit" phenomenon in which ACS redevelops following initial medical or surgical treatment of either primary or secondary ACS.

HINT Chronic ACS occurs in the presence of cirrhosis and ascites, often end-stage disease.

Q How does ACS cause respiratory distress and pulmonary complications?

A Upward displacement of the diaphragm

When the intraabdominal pressure (IAP) increases, the abdominal organs displace the diaphragm upward, resulting in respiratory distress and pulmonary complications. The abdominal pressure is also displaced on the bladder and kidneys, resulting in renal dysfunction and elevation of bladder pressures. The elevated IAP can also cause elevation in thoracic and cerebral pressures. An increase in thoracic pressures affects the venous return and cardiac output.

HINT The increase in ACS causes a decrease in venous return from the cerebral circulation. This can cause an increased ICP (Box 6.47).

Box 6.47 Organ Involvement in ACS

Acute kidney injury	Gastrointestinal
Cardiovascular	Altered blood flow to gut, liver, pancreas Bowel ischemia/infarction
Decreased venous return Increased afterload	Eyes
Pulmonary	Rupture of retinal capillaries
Decreased lung compliance	Decreased central vision (Valsalva retinopathy)
Increased peak inspiratory pressure	Surgical wound
Decreased tidal volume	Abdominal wound dehiscence
Neurological Increased intracranial pressure	

> **Q** Which patient population is at the greatest risk for development of abdominal compartment syndrome (ACS)?
>
> **A** Abdominal trauma

Abdominal trauma and abdominal surgeries are the most common causes of ACS, and patients with abdominal injury were the first who were recognized to have complications from increased intraabdominal pressure (IAP). Since there is an increased awareness of ACS, multiple patient populations, including medical patients, have been found to have ACS (Box 6.48).

Box 6.48 Causes of ACS

Abdominal trauma	Liver failure with ascites/liver transplant
Abdominal surgery	Multiple blood transfusions (>10 U blood/24-hour period)
Damage-control laparotomy	Pneumonia/pneumonitis
Ischemic bowel	Mechanical ventilation/PEEP
Abdominal infections/abscesses/masses	Hypothermia (core temperature < 33°C)
Gastroparesis/gastric distention/ileus	Coagulopathy (platelets < 55,000, or PT > 15 sed. Or PTT > 2 × normal or INR > 1.5)
Major burns (with or without abdominal eschar)/trauma	Kidney transplant
Bacteremia/sepsis	Rupture of aortic aneurysms
Massive fluid resuscitation (> 5 L/24 hr)	Pelvic fracture
Acute hemorrhagic pancreatitis	

ACS, abdominal compartment syndrome; INR, international normalized ratio; PEEP, positive end expiratory pressure; PT, prothrombin time; PTT, partial thromboplastin time.

> **Q** What is frequently monitored to determine elevated intraabdominal pressure (IAP) and abdominal compartment syndrome (ACS)?
>
> **A** Bladder pressure

Aggressive monitoring of IAP and assessing for the development of ACS is important to prevent complications and mortality. Monitoring is performed with bladder pressure readings to determine IAP. Clinical examination and assessment of abdominal girth have been found to be poor indicators of ACS. The frequency of monitoring depends on the patient. Some resources recommend monitoring every 4 to 6 hours until IAP remains less than 12 mmHg for at least 24 hours in the absence of organ dysfunction in high-risk patients.

HINT Obtain readings at end-expiration with the zero reference level at the iliac crest midaxillary line.

> **Q** What pressure is considered elevated in abdominal compartment syndrome (ACS)?
>
> **A** Greater than 12 mmHg

An elevated intraabdominal pressure (IAP) is defined as greater than or equal to 12 mmHg. End-organ damage is observed with IAP as low as 10-cm H_2O pressure. It is graded based on the degree of elevation of pressures (Table 6.12).

HINT Morbidly obese patients often also range from 9 to 14 mmHg.

Table 6.12 Grading of IAP

Grade	Intraabdominal Pressure
I	12–15 mmHg
II	16–20 mmHg
III	21–25 mmHg
IV	>25 mmHg

IAP, intraabdominal pressure.

> **Q** What is the equation for calculating abdominal perfusion pressure (APP)?
>
> **A** MAP – IAP = APP

The mean arterial pressure (MAP) minus the intraabdominal pressure (IAP) is used to calculate the perfusion pressure of the abdomen. Resuscitative therapy is titrated to maintain an adequate APP and has been found to correlate better with survival than maintenance of any particular IAP. Normotensive or hypertensive patients may have outcomes better than patients who are hypotensive.

HINT APP is similar to cerebral perfusion pressure (CPP). The MAP is the "driving force," and the IAP is the "opposing force."

> **Q** A patient "fighting" the ventilator can demonstrate elevated intraabdominal pressure (IAP). What drugs can be used to lower IAP in this particular patient?
>
> **A** Sedation and neuromuscular blocking agents

Medical management can assist with lowering IAP. The goal of the medical intervention is to reduce IAP and optimize abdominal perfusion pressure (APP), maintaining APPs higher than 60. Increased resistance during ventilation caused by a patient "fighting" the ventilator can increase IAP. Providing sedation and neuromuscular blocking agents if sedation is not adequate can lower the resistance and the IAP (Box 6.49).

Box 6.49 Medical Interventions for ACS

Avoid excessive fluid resuscitation	Administer albumin or hypertonic solutions
Administer diuretics	NG tube to low-wall suction to decompress stomach
Perform continuous venovenous ultrafiltration	Rectal tube to decompress colon
Administer prokinetic agents (i.e., Metoclopramide) Minimize or discontinue enteral feeding Provide adequate sedation and analgesics Administer neuromuscular blocking agents	Remove constrictive abdominal dressings Maintain head-of-bed elevation > 30° (reverse Trendelenburg position to "unfold the abdomen") Avoid prone position Vasopressors to increase mean arterial pressure

ACS, abdominal compartment syndrome; NG, nasogastric.

HINT A goal in managing ACS is a negative fluid balance within 3 days of injury.

> **Q** What is the most common surgical procedure used to manage abdominal compartment syndrome (ACS)?
>
> **A** Decompressive laparotomy

An excessively high intraabdominal pressure (IAP) or progressive ACS or refractory ACS typically requires a decompressive laparotomy. Many surgeons now leave high-risk patients' abdomens open following surgery to prevent elevated IAP and ACS. After the patient's abdominal pressure decreases and the visceral edema recedes, the abdomen can be closed.

HINT Open abdomens commonly require sedation and even neuromuscular blocking agents to prevent injury (Box 6.50).

Box 6.50 Complications of an Open Abdomen

Serous fluid losses	Bowel perforation
Infection/peritonitis	Bleeding
Enterocutaneous fistulas	Inability to close wound edges later
Ventral hernia	Hypothermia
Increased abdominal scarring	Ileus

> **Q** What type of dressing can be used on an open abdomen that draws fluid away from the abdominal cavity?
>
> **A** Negative pressure wound dressing

Negative pressure systems control the abdominal contents with an open abdomen, manage third-space fluids, and facilitate wound closure. Vacuum-assisted fascial closure (VAFC) systems provide constant tension on the abdominal wound edges, facilitating the ability to successfully perform a late fascial closure. The open abdomen can also be covered with a temporary closure to maintain and protect the viscera.

ENTERAL AND PARENTERAL NUTRITION

> **Q** Does enteral or parenteral nutrition have a greater incidence of gram-negative septicemia?
>
> **A** Parenteral

Prolonged exclusive use of total parenteral nutrition (TPN) can cause intestinal atrophy, loss of small-bowel integrity that results in increased permeability and a decrease in absorptive capacity. Enteral feeding enhances cell renewal, decreases epithelial cell death, and increases expression of collagen. Enteral nutrition (EN) also has a trophic effect on the gastrointestinal (GI) mucosa and is recommended over parenteral nutrition.

HINT Even "trickle" or low infusion rates of enteral feeding has a lower incidence of septicemia than NPO or parenteral nutrition (Box 6.51).

Box 6.51 Prevention of Infections With Total Parenteral Nutrition

Maintain sterile set up
Change tubing every 24 hours

Use dedicated line total parenteral nutrition
    No medication administration in this line
    Exception: lipid infusions

IV site care sterile technique
Treat hyperglycemia

IV, intravenous.

HINT Monitor blood glucose levels every 6 hours, and if lipids are administered, measure serum triglyceride levels.

> **Q** What is the goal for initiating enteral feeding in an ICU patient?
>
> **A** Within 24 to 48 hours of injury

Timing of enteral feeding is critical in an ICU patient. If the patient is adequately resuscitated, then enteral nutrition (EN) is started within 24 to 48 hours following injury or admission to the ICU. Early EN has been found to reduce infectious complications and decreased length of stay (LOS). It may blunt the hypermetabolic response and modulate the inflammatory reaction of critically ill patients. EN has been found to preserve gut mucosa.

HINT A contraindication to early enteral feeding is complete bowel obstruction.

> **Q** When signs of enteral feeding intolerance occur, what alternative nutrition may be recommended?
>
> **A** Combination of enteral and parenteral

Patients with enteral feeding can develop signs of enteral feeding intolerance. When this occurs, an alternative treatment is to decrease the enteral feeding rate and add parenteral nutrition to assure adequate calories and nutrition.

HINT Two common signs of enteral feeding intolerance include high gastric residuals and severe diarrhea.

> **Q** What is the recommended method for determining correct placement of an oro- or nasogastric tube for the purpose of enteral feeding?
>
> **A** Kidney, ureters, and bladder (KUB)

Routine for assessing correct placement of a gastric tube has been auscultation of air bolus. If the purpose of the gastric tube is administration of enteral nutrition (EN), a KUB radiographic study should be performed to assure correct placement before initiation of feeding or administering medications. Dislodgment of the feeding tube with reinsertion should have the tube reverified for correct placement with radiographic KUB.

HINT Air auscultation alone may miss adverse placement of the gastric tube in the lungs. A KUB is more definitive ability in determining the location of the feeding tube.

> **Q** What is the best method to prevent obstruction of the enteral feeding tube?
>
> **A** Frequent flushes

Frequent flushes used to irrigate the feeding tube are the best method for prevention of tube occlusion. Current recommendation is 20 to 30 mL of warm water flushed every 4 hours during continuous feeding and before and after medication administration. Tube occlusion may occur due to a stagnant enteral feeding formula and improperly crushed medications. Liquid medications or elixirs should be used if possible to avoid occlusion with pill fragments.

HINT Use pancreatic enzymes to remove the obstruction in the feeding tube.

> **Q** What is the best method to prevent aspiration during enteral nutrition (EN)?
>
> **A** Elevate the head of the bed (HOB)

Elevation of HOB 30 degrees to 45 degrees can decrease the risk of reflux (if not contraindicated). Coloring the feeding formula with dye has also been used in the past but is currently not recommended. Risks are higher using the blue dye than is the perceived benefit. The presence of blue dye in the tracheal aspirate is not a sensitive indicator of aspiration. Stop tube feedings 10 to 15 minutes prior to turning or flattening the HOB. See Box 6.52.

HINT Current studies show that the risk of aspiration with feeding in the duodenum is the same as gastric feeding. The time and effort needed to advance into the duodenum may not be justified and delays initiation of nutrition.

Box 6.52 Signs of Enteral Feeding Intolerance

Absent bowel sounds	Diarrhea
Gastric distension/bloating	Constipation
Cramping	High gastric residuals
Nausea/vomiting	

> **Q** What type of enteral formula should be used in patients who develop noninfectious diarrhea with tube feeding?
>
> **A** Fiber-enriched formula

Fiber-enriched formulas of enteral feeding or bulking agents, such as Metamucil, may be used to manage diarrhea and normalize stools. Certain medications may increase the likelihood of diarrhea, and alternatives should be considered if possible. Prevent bacterial contamination of delivery sets with meticulous hand washing prior to set-up and handling of the enteral formula. Limit time of formula hanging at room temperature to 8 hours and rinse bag in between. Change administration sets every 24 hours.

| **Q In a malnourished patient, what should be monitored due to the risk of refeeding syndrome?** |
| **A Electrolytes** |

Malnourished patients are at risk for the development of refeeding syndrome, causing sudden fluid shifts and electrolyte imbalances. This can be life-threatening. Glucose, sodium, chloride, potassium, magnesium, and phosphorous should be monitored routinely. Diabetics or those with risk for glucose intolerance may require insulin during enteral feeding (Box 6.53).

Box 6.53 Risk Factors of Refeeding Syndrome

Chronic alcoholism	Eating disorders
Acute weight loss post weight-loss surgery	Long-term use of antacids (binds phosphate)
Postoperative	Long-term use of diuretics
Elderly	Obesity
Chronic malnutrition	Little or no nutritional intake for 7–10 days

HINT   The hallmark of refeeding syndrome is hypophosphatemia.

| **Q What is the drug interaction that occurs with phenytoin and enteral feeding?** |
| **A Decreases absorption of phenytoin** |

Administration of phenytoin with enteral feeds lowers the absorption and peak serum levels of phenytoin. It may be necessary to increase dosing to maintain therapeutic serum concentrations. If the continuous tube feeding is discontinued, the dosage needs to be adjusted down and levels followed closely.

HINT   Hold tube feeding 1 to 2 hours before and after administration of phenytoin to improve absorption.

1. Which of the following diagnostic studies is considered to be the gold standard in diagnosing acute pancreatitis?

   A. Endoscopic retrograde cholangiopancreatography (ERCP)
   B. Abdominal CT scan
   C. Ultrasonography
   D. Angiogram

2. Which of the following monitoring techniques is used to measure intra-abdominal pressures (IAPs) in patients with abdominal compartment syndrome?

   A. Bladder pressure monitoring
   B. Abdominal circumference measurements
   C. Umbilical catheter
   D. Bispectral index (BIS) monitoring

3. Following a gastrectomy, the patient develops delirium and pulls his nasogastric (NG) tube out during an agitated state. Which of the following nursing interventions would be most appropriate?

   A. Reinsert the NG tube immediately
   B. Sedate the patient and then reinsert the NG tube
   C. Call the physician and inform her of the unintentional removal of the NG tube
   D. Prepare the patient for surgical replacement of the NG tube

4. The use of gastric acid-suppressing drugs for stress ulcer prophylaxis is associated with which complication?

   A. Metabolic acidosis
   B. Sepsis
   C. *H. pylori*
   D. Nosocomial pneumonia

5. A patient presents with a variceal upper gastrointestinal bleed. Which of the following would the ICU nurse expect to be ordered to lower the risk of hepatic encephalopathy?

   A. Sodium bicarbonate
   B. Lactulose
   C. Albumin
   D. DDAVP

6. Which of the following is the cause of esophageal varices in liver failure?

   A. Translocation of bacteria
   B. Stress response of critical illness
   C. Abdominal compartment syndrome
   D. Portal hypertension

1. B) Abdominal CT scan
An abdominal CT scan is the most reliable way to diagnose acute pancreatitis, as it can differentiate between the two types of pancreatitis (edematous and hemorrhagic). ERCP and ultrasound are used to diagnose acute biliary pancreatitis. An angiogram is not considered a standard evaluation of the pancreas.

2. A) Bladder pressure monitoring
Bladder pressures are used to measure intra-abdominal pressures and to monitor for abdominal compartment syndrome (ACS). Abdominal circumference measurements are not a reliable method to determine the presence of ACS. A BIS monitor is used to measure levels of sedation. Umbilical catheters are not used in adults.

3. C) Call the physician and inform her of the unintentional removal of the NG tube
Following a gastrectomy, the NG tube should not be manipulated. If the tube is discontinued unintentionally, call the physician and inform her of the incident. The NG tube should not be replaced, even with sedation, due to potential for damage of the anastomosis. The patient should not require a return to the operating room (OR) unless complications occur.

4. D) Nosocomial pneumonia
Gastric acid-suppressing agents, such as H2 receptor blockers and proton pump inhibitors, are associated with higher incidence of nosocomial pneumonia due to the change in the gastric acidity that allows overgrowth of bacteria. *H. pylori* is a bacterium commonly associated with peptic ulcer disease. It does not cause sepsis or metabolic acidosis.

5. B) Lactulose
Lactulose will reduce the amount of ammonia absorption in the bowel and promote osmotic diarrhea. Sodium bicarbonate is not indicated in gastrointestinal (GI) bleed patients. Albumin is administered to prevent hepatorenal syndrome. DDAVP may be used with coagulopathy in patients with liver failure but does not affect the ammonia levels.

6. D. Portal hypertension
Portal hypertension occurs as a result of a liver derangement such as cirrhosis. The liver causes a higher pressure in the portal vein, resulting in backflow of blood into the variceal veins in the esophagus and the development of varices. Stress response of critical illness causes gastric ulcerations. Abdominal compartment syndrome can cause respiratory and renal complications. Translocation of bacteria can result in septicemia and sepsis.

7. Acalculous cholecystitis is more common in critically ill patients. Which of the following is MOST likely to contribute to the development of this abdominal infection?

    A. Use of multiple antibiotics
    B. Prolonged use of total parenteral nutrition (TPN)
    C. Translocation of bacteria
    D. Loss of normal flora in the gastrointestinal (GI) tract

8. Liver disease produces hepatic encephalopathy. In which stage of the encephalopathy is asterixis usually present?

    A. Stage 1
    B. Stage 2
    C. Stage 3
    D. Stage 4

9. A patient with chronic liver failure is in the ICU with ascites. Which of the following interventions is commonly used for initial management?

    A. Large-volume paracentesis
    B. Administration of diuretic therapy
    C. Increased sodium intake
    D. Decompressive abdominal surgery

10. Which of the following medications can cause acute pancreatitis?

    A. Salicylates
    B. Loop diuretics
    C. Acetaminophen
    D. Acetylcholinesterase inhibitors

11. Which of the following bacteria is most commonly found in patients with peptic ulcer disease?

    A. Methicillin-resistant staphylococcus aureus (MRSA)
    B. *Helicobacter pylori*
    C. Actinobacteria
    D. *Streptococcus pneumoniae*

12. Which of the following medications is used to absorb ammonia to lower the risk of hepatic encephalopathy?

    A. Calcium gluconate
    B. Octreotide
    C. Lactulose
    D. Oral antibiotics

13. A patient returns from an endoscopy. He suddenly complains of severe midsternal pain and becomes hypotensive. Which of the following would be the most likely complication?

    A. Aspiration pneumonia
    B. Bacteremia
    C. Myocardial infarction
    D. Esophageal perforation

7. B) Prolonged use of TPN

Prolonged use of TPN to rest the bowel predisposes patients to acalculous cholecystitis by promoting cholestasis. The use of multiple antibiotics, loss of normal flora in the GI tract, and translocation of bacteria are all associated with bacteremia and multiple drug-resistant bacteria.

8. B) Stage 2

Stage 2 is characterized by lethargy and disorientation, and asterixis is usually present. Asterixis is clonic movements that occur with wrist extension. Stage 1 may sometimes begin development of asterixis, but this is not common. In stage 3, the patient becomes less responsive and asterixis may disappear. Stage 4 is a coma.

9. B) Administration of diuretic therapy

The formation of ascites in chronic liver disease is a result of sodium retention. Administering diuretic therapy (spironolactone and furosemide) can facilitate the loss of urinary sodium and water. The sodium in the diet would be decreased, not increased. Large-volume paracentesis is usually indicated only if respiratory compromise accompanies the ascites. Decompressive surgery is more commonly used for acute causes of abdominal compartment syndrome.

10. A) Salicylates

Salicylates can cause acute pancreatitis. Thiazide diuretics, not loop diuretics, have been associated with risks of pancreatitis. Acetaminophen is associated with hepatic failure, not pancreatitis. Acetylcholinesterase inhibitors are not commonly associated with pancreatitis.

11. B) *Helicobacter pylori*

Colonization of the stomach by *H. pylori* can result in chronic gastritis at the site of infection. This can contribute to peptic ulcer disease. MRSA, Actinobacteria, and *S. pneumoniae* are not associated with gastric ulcers.

12. C) Lactulose

Lactulose and magnesium citrate are frequently given to patients with upper gastrointestinal bleeding (UGIB) to prevent absorption of ammonia that is released in the bowel with blood degradation. Lactulose is metabolized by the enteric bacteria in the colon, resulting in the acidification of the stool, thus preventing ammonia from converting to an absorbable form. Octreotide may be used in gastrointestinal (GI) bleeds to decrease portal hypertension. Oral antibiotics may be used to decontaminate the gut but do not bind to ammonia. Calcium gluconate does not bind ammonia.

13. D) Esophageal perforation

Esophageal perforation is life-threatening and presents with pain located midsternal to mid abdomen and shock symptoms. Aspiration pneumonia is a risk of endoscopy but will present with greater respiratory symptoms. Bacteremia can cause the new-onset hypotension but is not associated with the midsternal pain. Myocardial infarction has chest pain but is not typically described as severe midsternal pain, more of a heaviness in the chest.

14. A patient attempted suicide with an overdose of acetaminophen. Which of the following would be the priority of care in this situation?

    A. Administer N-acetylcysteine (NAC)

    B. Determine eligibility for liver transplant

    C. Induce vomiting with ipecac

    D. Initiate suicide precautions

15. Which abdominal organ is most likely affected by superior mesenteric occlusion?

    A. Stomach

    B. Intestines

    C. Liver

    D. Esophagus

14. A) Administer antidote NAC

If a known toxin causes the acute liver failure (ALF), acute management should include known antidotes to the toxin. For acetaminophen overdoses, intravenous NAC is the antidote recommended. Suicide precautions are also important but administering the antidote will prevent further liver injury. Inducing vomiting with ipecac is not recommended due to high risks of aspiration. Manage the current situation with the antidote, if the liver is severely damaged, discussion of liver transplant may be required later.

15. B) Intestines

The arteries that supply the gastrointestinal (GI) viscera branch off the anterior portion of the descending aorta. The most clinically important is the territory of the superior mesenteric artery, which affects the small and large intestines. The esophagus and stomach are not commonly affected by local ischemia versus a global ischemia

BIBLIOGRAPHY

Bouzatt, P., Vladenaire, G., Gauss, T., Charbit, J., Arvieux, C., Balandraud, P., … Weiss, E. (2020). Early management of acute abdominal trauma. *Anesthesia and Critical Care Medicine, 39*(2), 269–277.

Laet, I., Malbrain, M., & Waele, J. (2020). A clinicians guide to management of intra-abdominal compartment syndrome in critically ill patients. *Critical Care, 24,* 97.

Moore, S., Dumas, R., & Sims, C. (2017). Necrotizing pancreatitis: Advances in management. *Clinics in Surgery, 2,* 1437.

Reintam Blaser, A., Regli, A., De Keulenaer, B, Kimball, E. J., Starkopf, L., Davis, W. A., … Incidence, risk factors, and outcomes of intra-abdominal (IROI) Study Investigators. (2019). Incidence, risk factors, and outcomes of intra-abdominal hypertension in critically ill patients-a prospective multicenter study (IROI Study). *Critical Care Medicine, 47,* 535–542.

Renal and Genitourinary System Review

7

> ▶ **LEARNING OBJECTIVES**
>
> In this chapter, you will review:
> - ▪ Acute kidney injury (AKI)
> - ▪ Chronic kidney disease (CKD)
> - ▪ Contrast-induced nephropathy
> - ▪ Rhabdomyolysis
> - ▪ Life-threatening electrolyte imbalances
> - ▪ Infections
> - ▪ Acute genitourinary trauma

● ACUTE KIDNEY INJURY AND CHRONIC KIDNEY DISEASE

Q What urine output (UO) is considered a criterion for an acute kidney injury (AKI)?

A Less than 0.5 mL/kg/hr for six consecutive hours

AKI is an abrupt or rapid decline in renal function and is defined by the serum creatinine (SCr) increase and decrease in UO. This definition is from the Acute Kidney Injury Network (AKIN). A decrease in UO may occur before an increase in creatinine levels. (Box 7.1).

HINT Remember, a low UO is based on less than 0.5 mL/kg/hour instead of less than 30 mL/hour, which is frequently used at the bedside.

Box 7.1 Criteria for Acute Kidney Injury

Serum creatinine rises by ≥0.3 mg/dL within 48 hours *or*
Serum creatinine rises ≥1.5-fold from reference value (if known) *or*
Urine output is <0.5 mL/kg/hour for more than six consecutive hours

Q Acute Kidney Injury Network (AKIN) devised the RIFLE staging system for AKI. What does the "R" in RIFLE mean?

A Risk

Earlier recognition of renal involvement can improve outcomes. The RIFLE criteria are used to identify early changes in renal function to allow for early interventions. RIFLE categorizes AKI into three grades of increasing severity using SCr or glomerular filtration rate (GFR) and UO criteria. Risk of AKI is considered if SCr increases by more than 1.5 or GFR decreases by more than 25%, or UO is less than 0.5 mL/kg/hr for 6 hours.

HINT The "I" stands for injury, and the "L" in RIFLE is the "loss" that is persistent in complete loss of renal function for longer than 4 weeks. The "E" is "end stage" or complete loss of renal function for longer than 3 months (Figure 7.1).

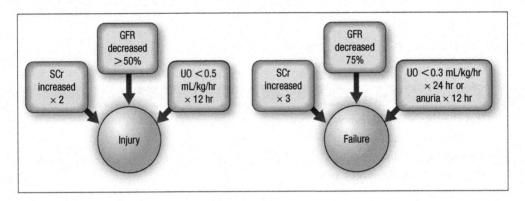

Figure 7.1 RIFLE staging.

> **Q Chronic kidney disease (CKD) is defined as a GFR of less than what?**
>
> **A Less than 60 mL/minute**

CKD is defined as a GFR less than 60 mL/min for 6 months or longer (Box 7.2).

Box 7.2 Chronic Kidney Disease Criteria

GFR >90 but disease diagnosed
GFR 60–89, mild
GFR 30–59, moderate
GFR 15–29, severe
GFR <15, end-stage renal disease

> **Q What are the three categories of acute renal failure (ARF)?**
>
> **A Prerenal, intrarenal, or postrenal failure**

Prerenal, intrarenal, and postrenal failures are terms used to describe the underlying causes of ARF. Prerenal failure is hypoperfusion without actual kidney damage. Intrarenal failure is kidney injury that includes reversible and irreversible injury. Postrenal failure occurs "after the kidneys" caused by obstruction to outflow. Postrenal failure results in kidney injury (Box 7.3).

Box 7.3 Causes of Prerenal, Intrarenal, and Postrenal Failure

Prerenal Failure	Intrarenal Failure	Postrenal Failure

Shock
  Sepsis
  Cardiogenic
  Hypovolemic
  Anaphylaxis
	Ischemia
	  Prerenal etiology
		Urinary tract obstructions
		  Blood clots
		  Benign prostatic hypertrophy
		  Urethral strictures
		  Tumor
		  Urinary stones

Trauma	Immune/infections	Urinary tract infections

(continued)

Box 7.3 Causes of Prerenal, Intrarenal, and Postrenal Failure (*continued*)

Prerenal Failure	Intrarenal Failure	Postrenal Failure

Congestive heart failure	Nephrotoxicity
	    Aminoglycosides
	    Nonsteroidal anti-inflammatory
	        agents (NSAIDs)
	    Radiographic contrast dye
	    Antibiotics
	    Myoglobin
		Neuropathy
		    Spinal cord-injured patient

Hepatorenal syndrome	Glomerulonephritis
	    Systemic lupus erythematosus
	    Postinfections
	    Good pasture syndrome
		Trauma
		    Bilateral ureteral injuries
		    Bladder rupture
		    Urethral injury

Medication induced
    NSAIDs
    Angiotensin converting enzyme
        inhibitors/angiotensin
        receptor-blocking agents
    Vasoconstrictors
	Medication induced
	    NSAIDs
	    Amphotericin B
	    Radiocontrast agents
	    Antiretrovirals
		Medication induced
		    Anticholinergic drugs

Diuretics (excessive diuresis)		
Abdominal compartment syndrome		

HINT The same mechanism can cause prerenal and intrarenal failure. In prerenal AKI, the kidneys are not injured and can still function, whereas intrarenal failure kidneys are injured and can no longer function appropriately.

▶ PATHOPHYSIOLOGY

Q What electrolyte is reabsorbed by the renal system in response to hypoperfusion?

A Sodium

Prerenal AKI is caused by renal hypoperfusion. Because the kidneys are not damaged, they respond appropriately to aldosterone and reabsorb sodium, followed by water. This is a compensatory mechanism for volume depletion.

HINT Renin-angiotensin system (RAS) triggers the release of renin during a hypoperfused state. This results in release of aldosterone and reabsorption of sodium.

Q Nonsteroidal anti-inflammatory drugs (NSAIDs) affect renal perfusion by blocking which substance in the body?

A Prostaglandins

Prostaglandins are partially responsible for vasodilating afferent arterioles. Prostaglandins play a role in renal perfusion during periods of hypoperfusion. NSAIDs block the prostaglandins, resulting in a decrease in GFR and renal blood flow, exacerbating hypoperfusion of kidneys during periods of decreased blood flow. Drugs that affect the vasodilation of the afferent or vasoconstriction of the efferent arterioles can result in prerenal failure.

HINT Vasodilation of afferent (toward glomerulus) and vasoconstriction of efferent (away from glomerulus) will increase GFR. There is more flow going in and less flow coming out. NSAIDs affect the inability to vasodilate afferent.

> **Q** Do angiotensin converting enzyme (ACE) inhibitors and angiotensin receptor-blocking agents (ARBs) affect the afferent or efferent arterioles?
>
> **A** Efferent

ACE inhibitors and ARBs prevent efferent vasoconstriction by inhibiting angiotensin II vasoconstriction and the kidneys' ability to maintain an adequate perfusion.

HINT Angiotensin II is a potent vasoconstrictor.

> **Q** Acute tubular necrosis (ATN) is a common problem causing intrarenal failure. This affects which part of the kidneys?
>
> **A** Renal tubules

Renal tubules are responsible for dilution and concentration of urine. ATN is characterized by the failure to maximally dilute or concentrate the urine. This is called isosthenuria. ATN is associated with prolonged prerenal insult or a direct nephrotoxin (Table 7.1).

> **Q** In postrenal failure, upper urinary tract obstruction can cause AKI. What must happen for this to occur?
>
> **A** Bilateral obstruction

The upper urinary tract involves the ureters and renal pelvis. For AKI to occur, both ureters need to be involved in the obstruction, otherwise only one kidney is affected. The lower tract involves the bladder and urethra. Obstruction at any level in the lower tract can cause AKI. Obstruction of the flow of urine results in backing up into the renal parenchyma, leading to hydronephrosis. If not treated immediately, it can cause CKD due to elevated tubule pressure.

HINT The upper urinary tract has two ureters that drain to one bladder out through one urethra. For AKI to occur in the upper tract, both ureters must be obstructed (unless only one functioning kidney).

▶ SYMPTOMS/ASSESSMENT

> **Q** Which of the renal failure categories is more likely to result in anuria?
>
> **A** Postrenal failure

Obstruction to outflow is the most likely cause of a sudden cessation of urine rather than development of oliguria. There is an initial increase in intratubular pressure that decreases the filtration-driving force, and reabsorption of urine occurs. Once the pressure gradient equalizes, the depressed GFR depends on renal efferent vasoconstriction, which results in anuria.

HINT Postrenal failure may also present with sudden anuria with intermittent periods of polyuria.

> **Q** AKI causes electrolyte abnormalities. Which two electrolytes significantly elevate following renal injury?
>
> **A** Potassium and phosphate

Hyperkalemia and hyperphosphatemia occur with AKI and CKD due to the inability of the kidney to remove excess potassium and phosphates. Intrarenal failure results in a loss of sodium in combination with dilutional sodium (Box 7.4).

HINT Early in prerenal failure, potassium may be low because the kidney responds to aldosterone by conserving sodium and water. If the kidney reabsorbs sodium, then potassium is lost in urine.

Box 7.4 Electrolyte Abnormalities in Kidney Injury

Hyperkalemia	Hyponatremia
Hyperphosphatemia	Normal to elevate magnesium
Hypocalcemia	

Table 7.1 Five Types of Intrarenal Failure

	Tubular Injury	Interstitial Injury	Glomerular Injury	Vascular Injury	Intratubular Obstruction
Site of injury	Renal tubules	Kidney interstitium	Glomerular nephrons	Renal artery	Renal tubules
Mechanism of injury	Prolonged ischemia or nephrotoxins	Inflammatory infiltrates and edema within interstitium	Immunological mechanism triggers inflammation and proliferation	Major renal artery obstruction or severe abdominal aortic disease	Precipitation of proteins or crystals within tubule lumen causing obstruction
Clinical presentation	Failure to maximally dilute or concentrate urine	Fever, rash, eosinophilia	Fever, malaise, arthralgia	Microangiopathic anemia, thrombocytopenia	
Urine characteristics	"Muddy brown" sediment (casts)		Severe proteinuria and erythrocyte casts		
Treatment	Steroid		Corticosteroids and cyclophosphamide		

HINT Remember, phosphorous and calcium have an inverse relationship. As phosphate levels increase, the calcium levels decrease (inverse relationship).

> **Q** Acute kidney injury results in metabolic acidosis or alkalosis?
>
> **A** Metabolic acidosis

Metabolic acidosis occurs as a result of accumulation of excessive acidic substances in the blood as well as the renal tubules' inability to secrete H+ ions and reabsorb bicarbonate.

HINT Another abnormality caused by AKI is anemia due to the decrease in production of erythropoietin.

▶ DIAGNOSIS

> **Q** A fractional excretion of sodium (FENa) less than 1% indicates which of the categories of AKI, pre-, intra-, or postrenal failure?
>
> **A** Prerenal failure

A FENa measures the ratio of sodium excreted (urine sodium × volume) to sodium filtered (serum sodium × GFR). The ratio is used in determining whether the kidneys can function by conserving sodium during periods of hypoperfusion. Loop diuretics can increase sodium excretion, making FENa less useful in diagnostics.

HINT Exception to prerenal cause is in myoglobinuria, which will have a FEN less than 1% but is classified as intrarenal failure.

Urine sodium levels are also used to determine the ability of the kidneys to reabsorb sodium. In prerenal failure, the renal tubules still function, so they readily reabsorb Na$^+$. This gives a low urine sodium concentration (<20–40 mEq/L). In intrarenal failure, the renal tubules are unable to reabsorb Na$^+$, so the urine concentration will be elevated (>40 mEq/L). Elderly patients may have an obligatory loss of sodium in the urine.

HINT Glomerulonephritis is an intrarenal failure that maintains the ability to reabsorb sodium, because renal tubules remain intact.

> **Q** A patient with AKI has a blood urea nitrogen (BUN) of 40 and a SCr of 3.8. Based on this BUN:Creatinine ratio, would this be prerenal or intrarenal failure?
>
> **A** Intrarenal failure

The BUN:Creatinine ratio is also used to determine the category of AKI. A normal BUN:Creatinine ratio is 10:1 up to a 15:1 ratio. An abnormal ratio of greater than 20:1 indicates prerenal failure. The kidneys increase reabsorption of urea because of the slow renal tubular flow rates, but creatinine is not reabsorbed in the renal tubules and will increase out of proportion to the BUN. An elevated creatinine and BUN that remain within a normal ratio indicates intrarenal or postrenal failure (Table 7.2).

Table 7.2 Summary for Differentiation of Renal Failure

Lab Test	Prerenal	Intrarenal	Postrenal
Urine Na+	<10–20	>20–40	>20–40
Urine osmolality	>500	<350–400	<350–400
Urine specific gravity	>1.015	~1.010	~1.010
Urine sediment	No cells, casts	RBC, WBC, casts	RBC, no casts
Blood urea nitrogen:creatinine	>20:1	10:1	10:1
Fractional excretion of sodium	<1%	>1%	Variable

RBC, red blood cell; WBC, white blood cell.

HINT   BUN and creatinine are typically elevated in all AKI, but the ratio is what is used to assist in determination of categories of AKI. Liver impairment affects BUN levels but not the SCr (Box 7.5).

Box 7.5 Factors Affecting SCr

Greater muscle mass increases SCr	Men: Greater SCr levels than women
Old age lowers SCr	Inadequate protein diet decreases SCr
African Americans: Higher SCr	Neuromuscular disease increases SCr

Q What are the two urine tests that are used to determine the ability of the kidneys to concentrate the urine?

A Urine osmolality and urine specific gravity

One of the functions of the kidneys is to concentrate the urine. Urine osmolality and urine specific gravity are indicators of the kidneys' ability to concentrate urine. If the kidneys are hypoperfused, the renin–angiotensin system (RAS) is initiated and aldosterone is released. This leads the kidneys to reabsorb sodium and water, thus concentrating the urine. In prerenal failure the kidneys are still able to concentrate urine, but in intrarenal failure they are unable to concentrate urine.

HINT   In AKI, urine laboratory tests are required to determine whether the urine is concentrated or dilute. Urine in renal failure is typically dark amber and appears to be concentrated even when dilute.

Q What laboratory test is used to determine the GFR?

A Creatinine clearance

GFR is the volume of blood filtered by the glomerulus in 1 minute. Creatinine clearance is a calculated number that provides information about the GFR. Normal rate of creatinine clearance is 85 to 135 mL/min (normal GFR). Men have a higher normal GFR than women. In postrenal failure, the urine sodium is abnormally elevated in chronic kidney injury and usually low in AKI.

HINT   Above the age of 40 years, creatinine clearance decreases by 1 mL/min per year.

Q What is the gold standard for diagnosing upper urinary tract obstruction in postrenal failure?

A Ultrasound

Ultrasound is the gold standard for diagnosing upper urinary tract obstruction but can be less reliable in a volume-depleted situation. It is recommended that the ultrasound be repeated after successful fluid resuscitation.

HINT   Placement of a urinary catheter or irrigation of the present catheter may assist with the diagnosis of a lower urinary tract obstruction.

▶ MANAGEMENT

Q What is the primary treatment in prerenal failure?

A Reestablish perfusion to the kidneys

The primary management of prerenal failure is to treat the underlying cause of the hypoperfusion. For example, if the patient is hypovolemic then administer fluid replacement.

HINT   Buffered salt solutions such as Lactated Ringers may be preferable due to potential hyperchloremic kidney insult with large amounts of normal saline.

Q What is the purpose of administering a loop diuretic to a patient with AKI?

A Convert oliguric to nonoliguric renal failure

Loop diuretics may be used when attempting to convert an oliguric to a nonoliguric renal failure. Nonoliguric renal failure has a better prognosis due to control of volume and some electrolytes. Overuse or high doses of diuretics do not benefit the patient and can actually worsen renal function. Other drugs that have been used to manage AKI but are not supported in the research include low-dose dopamine and fenoldopam. Currently, there is no specific pharmacological prevention or management of AKI considered to be effective.

HINT High doses of a loop diuretic increase risk of ototoxicity and excessive diuresis with decreased renal perfusion.

Q What is the complication of poor nutrition in an AKI patient that causes an increase in release of amino acids from skeletal muscle?

A Protein catabolism

Protein catabolism occurs in AKI with the excessive release of amino acids from skeletal muscle and sustained negative nitrogen balance. Energy expenditure can increase by 30% or more if AKI is associated with sepsis and multiple organ dysfunction. It is recommended that patients with AKI should receive 25–30 kcal/kg per day with the energy intake not to exceed 30 kcal/kg/day. AKI patients will tend to develop hyperglycemia and hypertriglyceridemia.

HINT Overfeeding a critically ill patient can lead to metabolic complications such as hypertonic hydration and metabolic acidosis.

Q What is the primary treatment in patients with severe AKI?

A Renal replacement therapy (RRT)

In severe AKI, RRT is the recommended management. There are no set guidelines on when to initiate RRT, and initiation is based on individual patient risks and benefits of RRT. Recent studies indicate that early initiation of RRT may improve outcomes, but this finding requires further research (Box 7.6).

Box 7.6 Indications of Renal Replacement Therapy

Severe Metabolic acidosis	Drug overdose
Life-threatening Hyperkalemia	Volume overload
Symptomatic uremia Pericarditis Encephalopathy	Azotemia
Seizures	Intoxications

Q What is the main risk of intermittent hemodialysis (IHD)?

A Hypotension

IHD is typically delivered three to six times a week and performed over a 4- to 6-hour period. The advantage is rapid removal of toxins and life-threatening electrolytes. The disadvantage is that rapid removal or shifts of fluid can result in hemodynamic instability. Another complication of rapid removal of solutes is a sudden decrease in serum osmolality, allowing fluid to shift extravascular. This leads to cerebral edema and is called disequilibrium syndrome.

HINT Slower removal of solutes may be required in neurological patients who are more susceptible to cerebral edema.

Q What type of RRT is recommended in hemodynamically unstable patients?

A Continuous renal replacement therapy (CRRT)

CRRT is performed continuously 24 hours a day. This allows the water and solutes to be removed at a slower, more consistent rate, lowering the risk of hypotension. Hemodynamically unstable patients are candidates for CRRT, which has a lower incidence of hypotension and prevents hypervolemic occurrences between hemodialysis. CRRT is performed through a venovenous access (Box 7.7).

Box 7.7 Types of Continuous Renal Replacement Therapy

Continuous venovenous hemofiltration (CVVH)	Solutes cleared by convection No dialysate is used Rate of ultrafiltration determines convective clearance Replacement fluids may be used
Continuous venovenous hemodialysis (CVVHD)	Solutes removed by diffusion Dialysate is used Ultrafiltration used for volume control
Continuous venovenous hemodiafiltration (CVVHDF)	Combination of convective solute removal and diffusion Replacement fluids may be used

Q What is a disadvantage of CRRT for intensive care unit (ICU) patients?

A Use of anticoagulation therapy

IHD requires less anticoagulation therapy due to the rapidity of the procedure. CRRT is a slower, continuous procedure that takes place over 24 hours and is more likely to develop issues with filter clotting and requirements of more anticoagulation. Other disadvantages are the amount of nursing time, skill, and costs required to perform CRRT at the bedside.

Q Which electrolyte is most likely to become abnormally low during CRRT therapy?

A Phosphate

Hypophosphatemia (<2 mg/dL) develops frequently with CRRT. The incidence has been found to increase with longer therapy and more intense RRT. Hypophosphatemia causes muscle weakness, including weakness of the respiratory muscles, and is associated with prolonged use of mechanical ventilation.

HINT Phosphate is frequently added to the replacement fluids or dialysate solutions to prevent complication of hypophosphatemia in CCRT.

Q What is the primary complication of peritoneal dialysis (PD)?

A Peritonitis

PD can be used for CKD to allow people to manage their CKD at home but has also been used in some acute care settings, including critical care units. It can be a form of continuous RRT. One of the primary complications includes peritonitis from the indwelling PD catheter.

HINT Hemodynamically, PD is more stable than IHD.

▶ COMPLICATIONS

Q A renal dialysis patient presents with fever, chills, and chest pain. What is the most likely cause?

A Pericarditis

Uremic- or dialysis-related pericarditis is a complication of chronic renal failure and RRT. It is considered caused by accumulation of bioirritants in the pericardial sac, such as uric acid. The immune system may also play a role in development of inflammation in the pericardial space. It typically presents with chest pain (may not be as significant as other pericarditis patients), fever, chills, and pericardial friction rub. Management is typically with RRT.

HINT If large effusions or cardiac tamponade develop, it may require pericardiocentesis.

Q What electrolyte abnormality may contribute to the arrhythmias?

A Hyperkalemia

Hyperkalemia frequently results in ventricular arrhythmias and may be seen in renal failure patients. RRT is used to manage hyperkalemia but may require administration of kayexalate in between dialysis (Box 7.8).

Box 7.8 Complications of AKI and CKD

Electrolyte imbalances	Stomatitis
Pericarditis	Drowsy, lethargy to delirium
Pericardial effusions and/or tamponade	Itching, dryness (urticaria)
Pulmonary edema	Thrombocytopenia
Dysrhythmias	Anemia
Anorexia, nausea, vomiting, diarrhea	

CONTRAST-INDUCED NEPHROPATHY

Q What is a primary risk factor for development of contrast-induced nephropathy (CIN)?

A Hypovolemia

CIN is defined as an increase in baseline creatinine level by 25% or 0.5 mg/dL or greater within 24–48 hours after a procedure that requires contrast material. Almost 10% of all hospital-acquired AKI is directly related to contrast material. Hypovolemia or overall volume depletion is a primary risk for the development of CIN (Box 7.9).

HINT Recovery typically occurs 3 to 5 days after exposure unless the patient develops persistent renal failure.

Box 7.9 Risk Factors of CIN

Chronic kidney disease	Anemia
Dehydration	Cardiac disease
Diabetes mellitus	Proteinuria
Hyperglycemia	Nephrotoxic medications
Advanced age	High osmolar contrast agents
Hypertension	Greater volume of contrast agents used

Q How long before a contrast study is it recommended to discontinue nephrotoxic agents?

A 24 hours prior

It is recommended that nephrotoxic agents be discontinued 24 hours prior to performing a procedure with contrast medium. High-risk patients should be identified and preventive interventions implemented prior to the procedure.

HINT In critically ill patients, holding some of these drugs may be a risk-versus-benefit decision (Box 7.10).

Box 7.10 Nephrotoxic Agents

Nonsteroidal anti-inflammatory drugs
Angiotensin converting enzyme inhibitors/angiotensin receptor-blocking agents
Metformin
Aminoglycosides
Loop diuretics
Cyclosporine

Q What is the primary recommended intervention to prevent CIN?

A IV hydration

Precaution to prevent CIN is important in high-risk patients and creatinine levels greater than 1.8 mg/dL. Adequate IV fluid hydration before and after the procedure is beneficial and has been found to lower the incidence of CIN. The IV fluid recommended is 0.9% NaCl, with some physicians using isotonic sodium bicarbonate to alkalinize the urine in addition to fluid resuscitation. *N*-Acetylcysteine (Mucomyst) is an antioxidant of oxygen-free radicals and vasodilator in kidneys. It can be administered prior to the study and after the study in high-risk patients.

HINT   Administer fluids more cautiously in congestive heart failure (CHF) patients.

Q What is the current recommendation to prevent CIN if multiple contrast studies are required?

A 48–72 hours for repeat exposure to contrast

Another focus for prevention of CIN is on the contrast. This includes the use of non-iodinated contrast media, minimizing the volume of contrast, using iso-or hypo-osmolality and avoiding repeat exposure to contrast if possible. Recommendation is to delay repeat exposure to contrast for 48 hours in patients without risk factors and 72 hours in patients with higher risk factors such as DM.

LIFE-THREATENING ELECTROLYTE IMBALANCES

See Box 7.11.

Box 7.11 Normal Values for Electrolytes

Calcium	8.5–10.5 mg/dL (2.2–2.6 mmol/L)	Magnesium	1.5–2.3 mg/dL
Ionized calcium	4.5–5.6 mg/dL (1.1–1.4 mmol/L)	Phosphate	3.0–4.5 mg/dL
Potassium	3.5–5.0 mEq/L	Sodium	135–145 mEq/L

Values will vary based on the laboratory.

▶ PATHOPHYSIOLOGY

Q Which hormones are responsible for regulating calcium in and out of bone?

A Parathyroid hormone (PTH) and calcitonin

Calcium is primarily stored in bone. The PTH and calcitonin control movement of calcium in and out of bones using a negative feedback system based on serum calcium levels. PTH allows calcium to move intravascularly, and calcitonin increases the resorption of calcium in bone.

HINT   Calcitonin is used to manage hypercalcemia by "pushing" calcium back into the bone.

Q What is the most common cause of hypocalcemia in ICU patients when measuring total calcium?

A Hypoalbuminemia

A low albumin level is the most common reason for low total serum calcium levels in ICU patients. This may not require treatment of the low calcium levels. A low albumin lowers the total albumin but does not affect ionized calcium levels. Ionized calcium levels measure only the calcium readily available in the serum, not bound to albumin and other substances. Calcium should be corrected in the presence of normal albumin, corrected calcium or if low ionized calcium levels.

HINT Calcium is one of the electrolytes that does not want to live alone and will chelate or "marry" multiple substances. Once chelated or "married," it does not work. Only free (ionized) calcium is readily available to work (Box 7.18). Hypoalbuminemia also results in hypomagnesemia. Magnesium is also ionized or "free" and bound to proteins. Ionized levels are not frequently obtained.

Box 7.12 Causes of Hypocalcemia

Sepsis Hypoalbuminemia	Chelating agents (bind calcium) Citrate in packed red blood cells (PRBCs)
Pancreatitis	Ethylene glycol ingestion Radiographic contrast medium
Parathyroid hormone deficiency	Sodium bicarbonate
Hyperphosphatemia	Aminoglycosides
Alkalosis	Protamine sulfate
	Hypothyroidism

Box 7.13 Forms of Total Serum Calcium

Ionized	Bound to Proteins	Complexed
45% total serum calcium	40% total serum calcium	15% total serum calcium
Readily available for use	Bound to proteins	Complexed to anions such as chloride, citrate, bicarbonate, and phosphate
	Especially albumin	Ca^{++} is not available for use
	Ca^{++} is not available for use	

Box 7.14 Calculation of Corrected Total Serum Calcium

Equation: $Ca^{++} + 0.8 (4 - 2)$
Example: Patient's total Ca^{++} is 7.0 and serum albumin is 2.0
$7.0 + 0.8 (4 - 2)$
$7.0 + 1.6 = 8.6$ as the corrected Ca^{+}
$7.0 + 0.8 (2)$

Q What type of diuretic may cause hypercalcemia?

A Thiazide diuretic

Hypercalcemia is less common in ICU patients. Certain medications can cause hypercalcemia, including thiazide diuretics. Patients in the ICU require close monitoring of calcium levels and, if hypercalcemia occurs, determine the underlying cause; if it is the thiazide diuretic, the medication should be discontinued (Box 7.15).

Box 7.15 Causes of Hypercalcemia

Hyperparathyroidism	Drugs
Prolonged immobility	Thiazide diuretics
Neoplasm	Lithium
Orthopedic injuries	Sarcoidosis

Q Does insulin infusions potentially cause hypokalemia or hyperkalemia?

A Hypokalemia

The majority of potassium is intracellular and certain situations and medications can shift potassium between intracellular and intravascular spaces. Insulin "drives" potassium into the cell, lowering the serum potassium levels (Box 7.16).

Box 7.16 Causes of Potassium Shifts

Intracellular Shifts (Hypokalemia)	Intravascular Shifts (Hyperkalemia)
Insulin	Lack of insulin
Beta agonists	Beta antagonists
Alkalosis	Acidosis
Sodium bicarbonate	Tissue injury
	Cardiac arrest

Q Which electrolyte should be corrected before adequate replacement of potassium can occur?

A Magnesium

Hypomagnesemia should be corrected before correcting hypokalemia due to increased renal losses of potassium. Magnesium is needed to regulate potassium, sodium, and calcium.

HINT   Magnesium repletion is required to correct a potassium level of less than 3.0 mEq/L (Box 7.17).

Box 7.17 Causes of Hypokalemia

Low potassium intake	Diarrhea
Hyperalimentation	Diaphoresis
Diuresis	Pancreatitis and pancreatic abscesses
Hyperaldosteronism	Hypomagnesemia
Nasogastric (NG) tube to low wall suction	Delirium tremens
Vomiting	Hyperthyroidism

Q What is a cause of pseudohyperkalemia?

A Clotted blood specimen

Hemolysis of blood in the tube can falsely elevate the potassium levels. Other causes of false elevation of potassium or pseudohyperkalemia include marked leukocytosis or thrombocytosis (Box 7.18).

Box 7.18 Causes of Hyperkalemia

Dilutional	Potassium-sparing diuretics
Muscle injury Burns and trauma	Angiotensin converting enzyme inhibitors and angiotensin receptor blockers
Renal failure	Rhabdomyolysis
Adrenal insufficiency	Tumor lysis

Q What is the mechanism of hypomagnesemia during periods of diuresis?

A Decreased reabsorption

Magnesium reabsorption in kidneys has an inverse relationship to UO. High flow output results in a loss of magnesium in the urine.

HINT In renal failure, magnesium is typically normal but can be elevated due to a low-flow state. So, AKI may cause hypermagnesemia, and drugs high in magnesium should be avoided (Boxes 7.19 and 7.20).

Box 7.19 Causes of Hypomagnesemia

Malnutrition, starvation	Hyperglycemia, diabetes mellitus
NG suctioning	Acidosis
Parenteral nutrition	Hypercalcemia, hypophosphatemia
Decreased gastrointestinal absorption	Pancreatitis
Alcohol consumption	Sepsis
Diuretics	Alkalosis
Drugs binding magnesium Citrate Aminoglycosides Cyclosporine Digoxin	Insulin administration

Box 7.20 Causes of Hypermagnesemia

Renal failure
Excessive intake of magnesium-containing laxatives and antacids

Q During initial refeeding following period of starvation, which electrolyte abnormality is most common?

A Hypophosphatemia

Following starvation, an abrupt increase in carbohydrates causes a spike in the release of insulin, which drives phosphate into the cell. This is similar to the shift of potassium and phosphate following administration of exogenous insulin (Box 7.21).

Box 7.21 Causes of Hypophosphatemia

Refeeding syndrome	Vitamin D deficiency
Insulin administration	NG suction
Diuretics	Chronic diarrhea
Respiratory alkalosis	Malabsorption syndrome
Hyperparathyroidism	Extreme catabolic states
Insufficient gastrointestinal absorption	

Q What is the most common reason for hyperphosphatemia in an ICU patient?

A Acute kidney injury

AKI results in hyperphosphatemia due to inability of kidneys to excrete phosphates (Box 7.22).

Box 7.22 Causes of Hyperphosphatemia

Renal failure (acute and chronic)	Muscle injury
Excessive administration	Rhabdomyolysis
Hypoparathyroidism	Bisphosphonate therapy
Thyrotoxicosis	

Q Which of the following causes hyponatremia in the syndrome of inappropriate antidiuretic hormone (SIADH), hemodilution, or a loss of sodium?

A Hemodilution

SIADH is the result of too much antidiuretic hormone. The kidneys reabsorb water, causing dilutional sodium. There is an excess of water in relation to sodium (Box 7.23).

Box 7.23 Causes of Hyponatremia

Hypoosmolar **euvolemic** hyponatremia	SIADH Glucocorticoid insufficiency Hypothyroidism Stress Medications: Haloperidol, vasopressin
Hypoosmolar **hypovolemic** hyponatremia	Cerebral salt wasting syndrome Vomiting Diarrhea Third spacing
Hypoosmolar **hypervolemic** hyponatremia	Nephrotic syndrome Hepatic cirrhosis Cardiac failure

HINT Fluid status is the most important differentiation of the causes of hyponatremia.

Q What are the two main alterations that can result in hypernatremia?

A Free water deficit or excessive intake of sodium

Hypernatremia can be caused by an abnormal water balance or excessive intake of sodium. A free water deficit is the loss of fluid, resulting in hemoconcentration and hypernatremia. Excessive body sodium may be due to increase intake of sodium, such as administration of hypertonic (3%) NaCl (Box 7.24).

Box 7.24 Causes of Hypernatremia

Hypovolemic hypernatremia	Diuretic excess Postobstructive uropathy Intrinsic renal disease
Euvolemic hypernatremia	Diabetes insipidus Hypodopsia Insensible fluid losses
Hypervolemic hypernatremia	3% NaCl Excessive intake of sodium Primary hyperaldosteronism Cushing's syndromeHypertonic dialysis

▶ SYMPTOMS/ASSESSMENT

Q What effect does hypocalcemia have on blood pressure (BP)?

A Lowers BP

The cardiovascular effects of hypocalcemia include decrease in myocardial contractility (decreased cardiac output) and vasodilation (hypotension). The hypotension may be refractory to fluid administration and vasoconstrictive drugs. Bradycardia, which may progress to asystole or complete heart block, and prolonged QT interval are other cardiovascular effects of hypocalcemia.

HINT Calcium channel blocker's cardiovascular effects are the same as hypocalcemia; it lowers the BP and decreases myocardial contractility.

Q What is it called when the facial nerve is tapped lightly and produces involuntary twitching of facial muscles?

A Chvostek's sign

Chvostek's sign may be found in both hypocalcemia and hypomagnesemia patients. It is elicited by lightly tapping along the facial nerve. Trousseau's sign may also be present in both hypocalcemia and hypomagnesemia. This is a carpopedal spasm that occurs in response to hypoperfusion of the hand. It may be elicited with a BP cuff inflated to 20 mmHg for 3 minutes.

HINT Magnesium abnormalities are similar to calcium (Box 7.25). Mild hypercalcemia and hypermagnesemia are relatively asymptomatic (Box 7.26).

Box 7.25 Signs of Hypocalcemia and Hypomagnesemia

Circumoral and distal paresthesia or tingling
Muscle cramps progressing to muscle spasm, tremors, twitching, tetany
Seizures
Positive Chvostek's sign
Positive Trousseaus' sign
Hypotension
Bradycardia, ventricular tachycardia, and heart blocks

Box 7.26 Signs of Hypercalcemia and Hypermagnesemia

Lethargy, apathy, fatigue, depression	Nausea and vomiting
Excessive thirst	Abdominal pain
Muscle weakness, flaccidity	Hypertension
Decreased gastrointestinal motility	Shortened QT interval

Q What is the most common symptom of both hypo- and hyperkalemia?

A Ventricular arrhythmias

Both hypo- and hyperkalemia may present with cardiovascular and neuromuscular symptoms. The neuromuscular symptoms include paresthesia and weakness of the extremities, which may progress to flaccid paralysis and respiratory arrest.

Q What is the cardiovascular symptom of hypophosphatemia?

A Ventricular dysfunction

Hypophosphatemia can cause left ventricular dysfunction and may develop a dilated cardiomyopathy (Box 7.27).

Box 7.27 Symptoms of Hypophosphatemia

Weakened respiratory muscles	Acute hemolytic anemia
Confusion, lethargy	Acute left ventricular dysfunction
Gait disturbances and paresthesia	Reversible dilated cardiomyopathy

Q Hyperphosphatemia mimics what other electrolyte abnormality?

A Hypocalcemia

Hyperphosphatemia causes hypocalcemia. There is an inverse relationship between the two electrolytes. Symptoms of hypocalcemia are more prominent than signs of hyperphosphatemia.

Q What system in the body is most affected by sodium abnormalities?

A Neurological system

Both hypo- and hypernatremia can cause altered mental status. Sodium abnormalities should be suspected in a patient who develops a change in mental status and altered fluid balance (Boxes 7.28 and 7.29).

Box 7.28 Signs of Hyponatremia

Nausea	Decreased mentation
Vomiting	Seizures
Lethargy	Cerebral edema
Confusion	Coma and death

Box 7.29 Signs of Hypernatremia

Confusion	Seizures
Weakness	Decreased mentation
Lethargy	Coma and death

▶ DIAGNOSIS

Q On the cardiac monitor, the nurse recognizes that the patient has developed U waves. What electrolyte abnormality commonly causes U waves?

A Hypokalemia

As potassium progressively decreases, the ECG demonstrates characteristic changes of hypokalemia. These changes include flattened T waves, ST depression, and U waves. Characteristic ECG changes of hyperkalemia include peaked T waves and widening of QRS complex. Arrhythmias include atrioventricular (AV) conduction blocks, ventricular fibrillation, and systole.

HINT   Hypokalemia develops "U" waves, and hyperkalemia develops peaked "T" waves.

Q What type of hyponatremia presents with a urine sodium level of more than 20 mmol/L?

A Hypoosmolar hypovolemia hyponatremia

Urine sodium levels of >20 mmol/L indicate a renal loss of sodium as the cause for hyponatremia. This is not a dilutional hyponatremia and is not associated with hypervolemia. The increase in renal loss of sodium actually "pulls" water with the sodium and increases water excretion, resulting in hypovolemia.

HINT   The patient would also exhibit signs of volume depletion.

▶ MANAGEMENT

Q When should calcium be replaced in a hypocalcemic patient?

A Low-ionized calcium or symptomatic patient

Patients with low total serum calcium and normal ionized calcium levels typically do not require treatment. Patients who are symptomatic or have very low ionized calcium require treatment that includes replacing calcium.

Q Should a patient with an ionized calcium level of 0.8 mmol/L who is hypotensive receive IV calcium gluconate or calcium chloride?

A Calcium chloride

This patient has a severely low ionized calcium level and is symptomatic with hypotension. Calcium chloride contains more calcium per 10% solution than calcium gluconate and physiologically is more readily available. Calcium gluconate requires hepatic degluconation to make biologically usable calcium. Calcium chloride is the replacement calcium of choice in a symptomatic patient.

HINT   Treatment of a low electrolyte level is administration of the electrolyte.

Q What are the treatments of a severe, acute hypercalcemia?

A Hydration and diuresis

Mild hypercalcemia may not require treatment. Calcium levels between 12 and 14 mg/dL may become symptomatic and levels higher than 14 mg/dL should be treated. Hydration will dilute the calcium and encourage diuresis with furosemide. Hemodialysis may be used in extreme cases. Chronic hypercalcemia may be managed with calcitonin or drugs that inhibit resorption of bone.

HINT   Three ways to treat an elevated electrolyte: dilute, diuresis, and bind it!

Q What is used to bind potassium in a hyperkalemic patient?

A Kayexalate

Binding of potassium with kayexalate causes the excretion of potassium through the gastrointestinal route. Hyperkalemia can be treated with hydration and administration of a potassium-wasting diuretic. Another way to manage hyperkalemia is to move the potassium from the serum into the intracellular space by administering a ⊠-agonist (bronchodilator), insulin, or sodium bicarbonate. In severe cases of hyperkalemia or renal failure patients, removal of potassium is frequently with hemodialysis or continuous RRT.

HINT   Administer IV calcium chloride to patients experiencing lethal ventricular arrhythmias from hyperkalemia. This causes a direct antagonism of the hyperkalemic effect on cardiac cells.

Q What infusion may benefit patients with hemodynamic instability due to hypermagnesemia?

A IV calcium

Hydration and renal excretion with administration of furosemide are the mainstays of treatment for hypermagnesemia. Administration of IV calcium may be used if the patient is hemodynamically unstable. Acute magnesium intoxication in renal failure can be managed with hemodialysis.

> **Q** **What is the treatment of severe hyponatremia that is determined to be a true loss of sodium and not dilutional?**
>
> **A** **Hypertonic saline**

Dilutional hyponatremia is managed with fluid restrictions and diuresis. An euvolemic hyponatremia due to a renal loss of sodium should not have fluid restriction but replacement of sodium as the main treatment. Administration of a hypertonic solution too fast can cause a rapid shift in serum osmolality to a hyperosmolar state. This results in the irreversible demyelination of the neurons in the brain, particularly in the pons (Boxes 7.30 and 7.31).

Box 7.30 Treatment of Hyponatremia

Hypoosmolar **euvolemic** hyponatremia	Free water restrictions Loop diuretics Administer sodium
Hypoosmolar **hypovolemic** hyponatremia	Treat underlying cause Volume replacement
Hypoosmolar **hypervolemic** hyponatremia	Treat underlying cause Sodium restrictions Free water restrictions Loop diuretics

Box 7.31 Treatment of Hypernatremia

Hypovolemic hypernatremia	Correct volume deficits Correct free water deficits Treat underlying cause
Euvolemic hypernatremia	Correct free water deficits Treat underlying cause
Hypervolemic hypernatremia	Remove excess sodium Sodium restrictions Loop diuretics Hemodialysis (renal failure)

▶ COMPLICATIONS

> **Q** **Which neuromuscular blocking agent (NMBA) should be avoided in patients with crush injury or severe muscle trauma?**
>
> **A** **Succinylcholine**

Succinylcholine is a depolarizing NMBA. It has a rapid onset and short duration and so is frequently used for rapid sequence intubation. Depolarizing NMBA causes a rapid depolarization of all muscle, resulting in a paralysis. This can cause muscle cells to release intracellular substances such as potassium. A trauma patient with a crush injury or a patient who has sustained severe muscle trauma may already have increased release of potassium from injured muscle cells. Administering succinylcholine can cause a significant hyperkalemia and may progress rapidly to cardiac arrest.

HINT   An alternative NMBA that may be used in a patient at high risk for development of hyperkalemia is rocuronium, a short-acting, rapid-onset nondepolarizing NMBA.

> **Q** **What is the most life-threatening complication of hypocalcemia?**
>
> **A** **Prolonged QT interval**

Hypocalcemia causes a prolonged QT interval that places the patient at a greater risk for an "R on T" phenomenon and Torsades de pointes. Measure the QTc on patients with electrolyte abnormalities that place them at a risk for development of a prolonged QT interval (Box 7.32).

HINT Treat Torsades with magnesium.

Box 7.32 Electrolyte Abnormalities That Prolong QT Interval

Hypomagnesemia
Hypocalcemia
Hyperkalemia
Hyperphosphatemia

Q What is the most significant complication of hypophosphatemia in ICU patients?

A Diaphragm weakness

Hypophosphatemia contributes to acute and chronic respiratory failure and has been associated with failure of weaning from the ventilator.

Q Following the onset of AKI, which electrolyte abnormality may cause seizures?

A Hyponatremia

Hyponatremia is a result of a combination of dilutional hyponatremia and a true loss of sodium in the renal tubules. Low sodium is one of the electrolyte abnormalities that can cause seizures (Box 7.33).

HINT Think of sodium as being the neurological electrolyte.

Box 7.33 Electrolyte Abnormalities That Cause Seizures

Hypocalcemia
Hypomagnesemia
Hyponatremia
Hypernatremia
Hypoglycemia

INFECTIONS

Q What is it called when urinary tract infection (UTI) causes sepsis?

A Urosepsis

Urosepsis is an infection arising from the urinary or genital organ that results in symptomatic signs of sepsis.

▶ PATHOPHYSIOLOGY

Q What is a common cause of urosepsis in critically ill patients?

A CAUTI

Catheter-associated UTI (CAUTI) is a common cause of urosepsis in critically ill patients requiring indwelling catheters. Patients in critical care areas have an increased risk of developing multi-resistant organisms (Box 7.34)

Box 7.34 Causes of Urosepsis

Obstructive etiology
    Urethral stones
    Tumors
    Urethral strictures
    Ureterocele
	Indwelling catheters

Polycystic disease	Nephrostomy tubes
Pregnancy	Neurogenic bladder
Cystocele	Reflux

▶ SYMPTOMS

Q What is the most common pain syndrome associated with urinary tract infections?

A Flank pain

Flank pain is a common pain syndrome associated with UTI and urosepsis. This is frequently associated with nausea and vomiting (Box 7.35).

HINT   In urosepsis, the patient will also have the symptoms of sepsis.

Box 7.35 Signs and Symptoms Urinary Tract Infections

Fever	Dysuria
Nausea	Hematuria
Vomiting	Malodorous urine
Flank pain	Urinary retention
Costovertebral angle tenderness	Urinary frequency

▶ DIAGNOSIS

Q What is the initial screening lab test used to identify a potential UTI?

A Urinalysis

Urinalysis is the initial lab to send for testing. Presence of protein and elevated WBCs can indicate the presence of UTI. If the urinalysis comes back positive then a urine culture is sent to assist with the identification of the organism causing the infection.

HINT   Once the culture comes back, the antimicrobial treatment may need changes to make it more specific to the organism.

▶ MANAGEMENT

Q What is the most important intervention to prevent UTI from progressing to urosepsis?

A Antibiotic therapy

Administration of appropriate antimicrobial therapy early can prevent the progression of the infection to sepsis. Antibiotic therapy should be individualized and tailored to the initial suspected organism and then to the result of the culture and sensitivity. Fungal infections can also result in UTI and should be considered if the patient is immunosuppressed or experiencing a second infection.

HINT   The most frequent organism that causes UTI is gram-negative bacteria such as *E. Coli*.

▶ COMPLICATIONS

> **Q** What is a common neurological abnormality found in elderly patients with UTI?
>
> **A** Delirium

Delirium and altered mental status are common findings in elderly patients with UTI. It may be mistaken initially as a stroke, progressive dementia, or psychosis.

 ## ACUTE GENITOURINARY TRAUMA

▶ PATHOPHYSIOLOGY

MECHANISM OF TRAUMA

> **Q** What is the most common mechanism of injury for urethral injury?
>
> **A** Straddle injury

Blunt mechanism usually results in posterior urethral injury. An example is a straddle injury, which occurs when the bulbous urethra is compressed against symphysis pubis. Common causes are motorcycle collision, horseback riding injuries, and bicycle injuries. Penetrating mechanism is secondary to gunshot wounds, stab wounds, self-instrumentation, and perineal impalement after falls.

HINT Urethral damage is less common in women because the urethra is short, mobile, and protected by symphysis pubis. There is a greater chance of injury in males because the urethra is longer and fixed by a ligament.

> **Q** Ureteral injuries are more commonly a result of blunt or penetrating trauma?
>
> **A** Penetrating

Most common cause for ureteral injury is penetrating trauma and is rarely due to blunt mechanism of injury. Severe deceleration mechanism may cause an avulsion of ureter from the ureteropelvic junction.

HINT Colon and bowel injuries commonly occur concomitantly with ureter injuries.

> **Q** What is the most common blunt mechanism of injury that causes bladder rupture?
>
> **A** Motor vehicle crash (MVC)

MVC is the most common cause of a ruptured bladder and is associated with full bladders. Compression of a full bladder by the lap belt during a sudden deceleration impact causes the dome of the bladder to rupture into the intraperitoneal space.

HINT History of prior bladder surgery, irradiation, or malignancy may weaken the bladder and makes the bladder prone to rupture.

> **Q** What injury may be associated with posterior urethral injuries?
>
> **A** Pelvic fracture

Posterior urethral injuries may accompany pelvic fractures. Presence of a known pelvic fracture and blood at the meatus would be a significant red flag for the presence of urethral injury.

HINT Remember, blood present at the meatus would indicate the trauma nurse should not attempt to insert an indwelling bladder catheter.

> **Q** What type of genitourinary injury can occur with intercourse?
>
> **A** Penile fracture

Penile fracture can occur with forceful bending of erect penis during intercourse. Amputations of the penis or testicle can occur due to self-mutilation, assaults, and industrial trauma.

HINT   Blunt trauma to the scrotum can result in rupture of the testicles.

TRAUMATIC INJURIES

Q What traumatic injury is most commonly associated with extraperitoneal bladder rupture?

A Pelvic fracture

The majority of the extraperitoneal bladder ruptures occur with pelvic fractures. A cystography is recommended in patients with pelvic fractures due to the high association of bladder injuries.

HINT   Acetabular fractures are not commonly associated with bladder injuries.

Q Which kidney is most commonly injured in a trauma?

A Right kidney

The right kidney is the most frequently injured due to its lower position and less protection from the posterior rib cage. Increased injuries to the kidneys occur with deceleration mechanism, back and flank injuries, or rib fractures.

HINT   Kidneys are well protected from trauma by the vertebral column, surrounded by perirenal fat pads, capped by the adrenal glands, and abdominal viscera anterior.

Q What is the most commonly injured structure within the renal system?

A Kidney

The kidney is the most commonly injured organ within the renal system. Blunt mechanisms of injury account for the majority of these injuries.

HINT   Kidney damage can cause significant blood loss and a life-threatening injury.

HINT   Avulsion of the renal artery and complete loss of blood flow to the kidney is called a pedicle injury.

Q Following a straddle injury, if the Buck's fascia remains intact, the ecchymosis is confined to which structure?

A Penis

The urethra is divided into the anterior and posterior compartments. The anterior urethra is composed of the bulbar and penile urethra. The narrowest portion of the urethra is the meatus

If Buck's fascia is intact, the ecchymosis of urethral disruption is confined to the penis or perineum. The posterior urethra is composed of prostatic and membranous urethra and neurovascular erectile mechanism, which runs posterolateral and adjacent to posterior urethra

HINT   Symptoms of urethral injury depend upon if the anterior or posterior urethra is injured in the trauma.

▶ SYMPTOMS/ASSESSMENT

Q What is a common finding that would require urological imaging to be performed?

A Hematuria

Gross hematuria requires a series of urological imaging to diagnose an injury to the urological system. Microscopic hematuria in the presence of hemodynamic instability should also be an indication for an evaluation. Gross hematuria is a cardinal sign of kidney and bladder injuries.

HINT Hematuria is not always present in all urological injuries but is an indication for urological radiographic series.

> **Q** A patient presenting with hematuria and flank pain following a motor vehicle crash may have experienced injury to which urological structure?
>
> **A** Kidneys

A common presentation of kidney trauma is hematuria and flank pain. Hematuria is an important sign for injury to several of the urological structures but in combination with flank pain is a more likely injury to the kidney.

HINT Ureter injuries will not have hematuria in 20%–45% of the cases.

> **Q** The presence of vaginal bleeding following a straddle injury in a female may indicate what type of injury?
>
> **A** Urethral injury

Although women are less likely to experience urethral injuries, the presence of vaginal bleeding, external genitalia bruising, or significant incontinence in the presence of pelvic fractures should be a high suspicion of a urethral injury.

HINT Men are more likely to experience urethral injuries due to the longer, less secured urethra.

> **Q** What type of bladder injury may present with an inability to void and acute abdominal signs?
>
> **A** Intraperitoneal bladder rupture (IBR)

A complete rupture of the dome of the bladder results in extravasation of urine into the peritoneal cavity. The common presenting signs include an inability to void and acute abdominal signs such as abdominal pain/tenderness, fever, and peritoneal irritation. IBR is associated with shock symptoms of hypotension and tachycardia (Box 7.36).

HINT Extraperitoneal bladder rupture usually occurs at the lateral or base of the bladder and is associated with pelvic fractures.

Box 7.36 Symptoms Intraperitoneal and Extraperitoneal Bladder Rupture

Intraperitoneal Bladder Rupture (IBR)	Extraperitoneal Bladder Rupture (EBR)
Suprapubic tenderness	Pain with urination
Peritoneal irritation	Suprapubic tenderness
Ileus	Reddened suprapubic area
Inability to void	Necrosis of tissue suprapubic area
Hypotension	
Fever	
Abdominal pain	
Abdominal tenderness	

> **Q** What is the triad of symptoms found in urethral injuries?
>
> **A** Blood at meatus, inability to void and distended palpable bladder

The classic triad of symptoms includes blood at meatus, inability to void, and distended palpable bladder (Box 7.37).

HINT The diagnostic test to evaluate for presence of urethral injury is a retrograde urethrogram.

Box 7.37 Symptoms Anterior and Posterior Urethral Injuries

Anterior Urethral Injury	Posterior Urethral Injuries
Perineal pain	Inability to void
Blood at meatus	Blood at meatus
Penile and perineal edema	Distended bladder
Distended bladder	Butterfly perineal bruising
Inability to void (may on occasion be able to void)	High-riding prostate with rectal exam
Scrotum swelling	
Ecchymosis of scrotum	
Necrosis of scrotal tissue (late sign)	

▶ DIAGNOSIS

Q What is the gold standard diagnostic study used to identify renal injury?

A CT scan

A CT scan is the gold standard for evaluating the renal system following blunt trauma. A CT scan can be used to identify injury to the kidneys and grade the severity of the injury. A CT arteriogram may also be used to identify vascular injuries to the renal artery or renal vein. An MRI is equivalent to a CT in identifying and grading the severity of the renal injury. An MRI is more capable of differentiating an intrarenal hematoma from a perirenal hematoma. (Box 7.38)

HINT Ultrasound has not been found accurate in identifying injuries of the renal system.

Box 7.38 Renal Injury Scale

Grade I	Contusion	Microscopic or gross hematuria with normal urologic studies
Grade I	Hematoma	Subcapsula, nonexpanding without parenchymal laceration
Grade II	Hematoma	Nonexpanding perirenal hematoma confined to renal retroperitoneum
Grade II	Laceration	< 1 cm parenchymal depth of renal cortex without extravasation
Grade III	Laceration	> 1 cm parenchymal depth of renal cortex without collecting system rupture or urinary extravasation
Grade IV	Laceration	Parenchymal laceration extending through the renal cortex, medulla and collecting system.
Grade IV	Vascular	Main renal artery or vein injury with contained hemorrhage
Grade V	Laceration	Complete shattered kidney
Grade V	Vascular	Avulsion of renal hilum that devascularizes the kidney

Q What diagnostic study is most frequently used to evaluate ureteral injuries?

A Intravenous pyelogram (IVP)

Intravenous pyelogram (IVP) is a diagnostic study used to view kidneys, ureters, and bladder. Contrast dye is administered intravenous and consecutive x-rays are obtained to evaluate renal function, identify extravasation of dye from the kidneys, ureters, or bladder, devitalized segments of the kidney or abnormal ureteral deviation. IVP has a high false negative rate in penetrating injuries and is not reliable for diagnosis in that population.

HINT No single diagnostic test can be used to evaluate the renal system, and an IVP may be combined with cystogram and CT scan.

Q What diagnostic study should be performed prior to cystogram if the patient presents with blood at the meatus?

A Retrograde urethrogram

A retrograde urethrogram is used to diagnose urethral rupture by presence of extravasation of dye. It is used to evaluate the urethra. It may be performed prior to a cystogram to assure the urethra is intact without injury prior to inserting a catheter into the bladder to perform the cystography (Box 7.39).

HINT Although blood at the meatus and a high-riding prostate are commonly associated with urethral injury, the absence of such findings does not rule out the presence of urethral injury.

Box 7.39 Indications for Retrograde Urethrogram

Straddle injury
Significant deceleration mechanism
Blood at meatus
High-riding prostate
Perineal butterfly hematoma
Scrotal or perineal crepitus
Inability to pass indwelling catheter

Q What is the diagnostic study that is best used to identify a bladder rupture?

A Cystogram

CT of the abdomen is inadequate to identify a bladder rupture. A cystogram is the most accurate diagnostic study and can be used to differentiate intraperitoneal from and extraperitoneal bladder rupture. The normal bladder is teardrop in shape. It may appear distorted by the presence of a pelvic hematoma. Cystography is the most sensitive for submucosal tear of the bladder wall.

HINT CT cystography is another option to evaluate the integrity of the bladder and is about equal to a conventional cystography.

Q What is the diagnostic study of choice to identify urethral injuries?

A Retrograde urethrogram

A retrograde urethrogram is used to identify presence of both an anterior and posterior urethral injury. The presence of extravasation of dye indicates an injury.

HINT It is also important to use the retrograde urethrogram to determine if the injury is a partial or complete injury.

▶ MEDICAL MANAGEMENT

Q What is the nonoperative management of hematuria in a stable patient?

A Bedrest

Bedrest may be ordered for 24–72 hours, or until hematuria is cleared, in patients presenting with gross hematuria but are hemodynamically stable.

HINT Nonoperative management of renal trauma may include angiography and embolization to control bleeding.

> **Q** What is the most common nonoperative management of an extraperitoneal bladder rupture?
>
> **A** Suprapubic Catheter

A suprapubic catheter is placed to drain urine and allow the bladder to heal. The catheter is usually left in place for 7–10 days and then the bladder is reevaluated by cystogram for continued extravasation. If extravasation persists, the catheter may remain in place for another 7–10 days. Majority of the bladder ruptures can be managed with catheter placement and drainage alone. Intraperitoneal bladder ruptures may require surgical repair, intraperitoneal irrigation, and catheter placement.

HINT An indication for surgical management of extraperitoneal includes avulsion of the bladder neck or concomitant injury to vagina or rectum.

> **Q** What clinical finding would be a contraindication for the placement of an indwelling bladder catheter?
>
> **A** Blood at the meatus

If blood is present at the meatus, under no circumstances should a Foley be placed. Other contraindications to insertion of a bladder catheter include scrotal hematoma, perineal hematoma, or high-riding prostate.

HINT If resistance is met with insertion of a bladder catheter, stop the insertion. If the bladder catheter is inserted without a urine return, do not inflate balloon.

▶ SURGICAL MANAGEMENT

> **Q** What is an indication for surgical management of kidney injury?
>
> **A** Pedicle injury

A pedicle injury is the avulsion of the renal artery from the aorta resulting in complete loss of blood flow to the kidney. The kidney is mobile in retroperitoneum and the main renal artery connected to the aorta undergoes excessive stretch, causing arterial injury. The injury may be avulsion or the intimal layer ruptures forming a thrombus causing arterial occlusion and renal ischemia.

HINT Indications for surgical management also include ongoing hemorrhage, penetrating mechanism, and a pulsatile or expanding hematoma.

> **Q** What is the purpose of a stent being placed in ureter following surgical repair?
>
> **A** Maintain patency

A stent is placed in ureters to maintain alignment, assure patency during healing, ensure tension-free anastomosis, and prevent urinary extravasation. Surgical management of ureteral injuries typically involves debridement and anastomosis of the ureterals with the goal of water-tight closures. If large segments of the ureters are damaged, a transureteroureterostomy can be performed in which one ureter is anastomosed to the other.

HINT Extravasation of urine can cause the development of an uroma.

▶ COMPLICATIONS

> **Q** What is a complication of a delayed presentation of a ureter injury?
>
> **A** Peritonitis

Delayed presentation appears as peritonitis (Box 7.40). These symptoms include onset of fever, development of an ileus, abdominal mass, and hematuria, as well as an increase in serum creatinine levels.

HINT Delayed presentation injuries may be managed initially with endoscopic or interventional procedures followed by delayed surgical management.

Box 7.40 Complications of Ureteral Injuries

Infection
Ureteral strictures
Urinary ascites
Uroma
Fistula formation with bowel

Q **What is the most common complication of urethral injury managed with a suprapubic catheter alone?**

A **Stricture formation**

The placement of a suprapubic catheter alone without a urethral placed bladder catheter has a high incidence of stricture formation in the urethra (Box 7.41). This is typically managed with urethroplasty.

Box 7.41 Complications of Urethral Injuries

Impotency
Strictures
Incontinence
Obstruction

1. Which of the following electrolytes is most affected by aldosterone?

   A. Magnesium
   B. Potassium
   C. Calcium
   D. Phosphate

2. The cardiac monitor is showing peaked T waves. Which electrolyte abnormality can cause this electrocardiogram (ECG) change?

   A. Hypocalcemia
   B. Hypokalemia
   C. Hypomagnesemia
   D. Hyperkalemia

3. An intensive care unit (ICU) patient with sepsis has had a decrease in urine output over the last 3–4 hours. The labs show an increase in serum creatinine and blood urea nitrogen (BUN). The physician states that the urine osmolality was high and urine sodium low. What would be the most likely classification of this patient's renal failure?

   A. Prerenal failure
   B. Acute tubular necrosis (ATN)
   C. Acute interstitial nephritis
   D. Postrenal failure

4. Which of the following is the BEST treatment to prevent contrast-induced kidney injury?

   A. Sodium bicarbonate
   B. IV fluid hydration
   C. N-Acetylcysteine (Mucomyst)
   D. Furosemide (Lasix)

5. A new order is received to discontinue the nonsteroidal anti-inflammatory drug (NSAID) on your patient with a newly diagnosed acute kidney injury. Which of the following best explains the need to discontinue the NSAID?

   A. The patient will now require IV opioid pain management
   B. NSAIDs will be removed with dialysis, so they should be discontinued
   C. NSAIDs will increase the patient's gastrointestinal (GI) bleeding risk with acute kidney injury
   D. NSAIDs inhibit prostaglandins and can worsen kidney injury

1. B) Potassium
Aldosterone is a mineralocorticoid that is released in response to hypovolemia or hyperkalemia. Sodium reabsorption is linked to potassium excretion. Aldosterone does not have the same exchange system with sodium for any of the other electrolytes.

2. D) Hyperkalemia
Hyperkalemia causes peaked T waves, hypokalemia develops U waves. Hypocalcemia and hypomagnesemia prolong QT intervals.

3. A) Prerenal failure
In prerenal failure, the kidneys are hypoperfused but not injured. The kidneys can still function and are responding to aldosterone by reabsorbing sodium (low urine sodium) and concentrating urine (high urine osmolality). A septic patient could also be experiencing acute tubular necrosis (intra-renal failure), but the urine would be dilute with a high urine sodium. The risk to this patient is not as high for postrenal failure or acute interstitial nephritis.

4. B) IV fluid hydration
IV hydration is the most effective intervention to prevent injury to the kidneys from contrast used in procedures. Sodium bicarbonate and Mucomyst have also been used, but have mixed results in clinical trials and are not considered to be the first line of prevention. Lasix may actually increase injury due to nephrotoxicity.

5. D) NSAIDs inhibit prostaglandins and can worsen kidney injury
NSAIDS inhibit prostaglandins. In the kidneys, prostaglandins are needed to vasodilate the afferent arterioles during periods of renal hypoperfusion. NSAIDs can cause kidney injury or worsen renal failure with AKI. The patient may require opioids for pain management, and NSAIDs can increase GI bleeds, but neither answer is the best explanation for the order. Many drugs are dialyzed off and are timed to be administered after dialysis, not discontinued.

6. The lab calls the unit to report that a blood tube is "clotted." Which of the following labs could be falsely elevated?

   A. Potassium
   B. Creatinine
   C. AST/ALT
   D. LDH

7. A patient is diagnosed with acute kidney injury and is thought to have prerenal involvement. Which of the following would the intensive care unit (ICU) nurse expect to be the initial intervention?

   A. Initiate continuous venovenous hemodialysis (CVVHD)
   B. Start hemodialysis
   C. Start low-dose dopamine infusion
   D. Administer fluids

8. Following a subarachnoid hemorrhage, the patient's level of consciousness is decreasing. Lab work on the patient finds a sodium level of 122 mEq. The physician has ordered 3% hypertonic saline. Which of the following is a potential complication?

   A. Hypovolemia
   B. Cerebral edema
   C. Central pontine myelinolysis
   D. Vomiting

9. A trauma patient in the intensive care unit (ICU) was admitted following a tractor rollover and crush injuries. He is now demonstrating an elevated creatinine level and dark "tea"-colored urine. What is the most likely cause for his kidney injury?

   A. Contrast-induced kidney injury
   B. Acute interstitial nephritis
   C. Rhabdomyolysis
   D. Hypoperfusion

10. Which of the following interventions can result in hypokalemia by facilitating the movement of potassium into the cells?

   A. Diuretics
   B. B2 agonist bronchodilators
   C. D50 dextrose
   D. Depolarizing neuromuscular blocking agent

6. A) Potassium

Potassium is released from clot formations in blood collection tubes and can falsely elevate potassium levels. This is called "pseudohyperkalemia." The other lab values are not as affected by a "clotted" tube.

7. D) Administer fluids

Prerenal involvement indicates that this patient may be hypoperfused. The initial intervention is prompt volume replacement before hypoperfusion leads to intrarenal damage. Low-dose dopamine used to be used for renal perfusion but has not been found to improve outcomes. It is currently not recommended. Prerenal failure does not require hemodialysis.

8. C) Central pontine myelinolysis

Rapid correction of serum osmolality with the administration of hypertonic saline can produce an osmotic demyelinating syndrome called central pontine myelinolysis (CPM). Cerebral edema is a potential complication of rapidly lowering a serum osmolality. Hypovolemia and vomiting are not potential complications of hypertonic saline.

9. C) Rhabdomyolysis

Rhabdomyolysis typically occurs following crush injuries or muscle damage. It involves the release of myoglobin, causing myoglobinemia and myoglobinuria. The myoglobin is toxic to the kidneys and can produce acute kidney injury. It is characterized by tea- or cola-colored urine. This patient could have been hypoperfused or exposed to contrast studies, but the hint in the question is the color of the urine.

10. B) B2 agonist bronchodilators

Stimulation of B2 adrenergic receptors facilitates the movement of potassium (K^+) into the cells. Beta2 agonist treatments used to bronchodilate patients with asthma can cause hypokalemia. Diuretics do result in hypokalemia, but it is due to a loss of potassium in urine rather than K^+ moving into the cells. D50 dextrose and depolarizing neuromuscular blocking agents do not cause hypokalemia.

11. A 75-year-old patient presents in the emergency room with signs of septic shock. They are admitted to the ICU and being worked up for sepsis. The patient is febrile, vomiting, and complaining of low back pain. Which of the following is the most likely source of the infection?

   A. Cellulitis
   B. Urosepsis
   C. Pneumonia
   D. Meningitis

12. Which of the following is the most common mechanism of injury for urethral injury?

   A. Coup contracoup
   B. Sudden deceleration
   C. Stab wound
   D. Straddle injury

13. Which of the following diagnostic radiographs is able to view kidneys, ureter, and bladder?

   A. Intravenous pyelogram (IVP)
   B. Retrograde urethrogram
   C. Cystogram
   D. Abdominal ultrasound

14. Which of the following is the recommended management of extraperitoneal bladder rupture (EBR)?

   A. Immediate surgery
   B. Placement of stent
   C. Observation only
   D. Suprapubic catheter

15. Which of the following best describes a pedicle injury?

   A. Impalement injury genitalia
   B. Intraperitoneal rupture of bladder
   C. Avulsion renal artery from aorta
   D. Kidney rupture

11. B) Urosepsis

Urosepsis is a commonly known infection for elderly patients. Signs of urosepsis include nausea, vomiting, fever, and flank pain. The patient in the scenario does not commonly show signs of pneumonia, cellulitis, or meningitis.

12. D) Straddle injury

A straddle injury occurs when the urethra is compressed against symphysis pubis. An example of a trauma resulting in straddle injury is a motorcycle crash. Stab and gunshot wounds are also known to cause urethral injuries. It is less common with sudden deceleration but can cause avulsion of the ureter. Coup contracoup is more commonly used to describe a mechanism of traumatic brain injury.

13. A) Intravenous pyelogram (IVP)

IVP is a diagnostic study that can be used to view the kidneys, ureter, and bladder following a trauma. Retrograde urethrogram is used to evaluate the urethra. Cystogram can identify bladder injuries. Abdominal ultrasound is not really accurate in evaluating the renal system.

14. D) Suprapubic catheter

Suprapubic catheter is placed to drain the bladder and allow it to heal. An EBR may not require surgical intervention. Stents are placed for ureter injuries, not bladder.

15. C) Avulsion renal artery from aorta

A pedicle injury is the avulsion of the renal artery from aorta resulting in complete loss of blood flow to the kidney.

BIBLIOGRAPHY

Moore, P., Hsu, R. & Liu, K. (2018) Management of acute kidney injury: Core curriculum 2018. *American Journal of Kidney Disease*, 72(1), 136–148.

Hocine, A., Defrance, P., Lalmand, J., Delcour, C., Biston, P., & Piagnerelli, M. (2016). Predictive value of the RIFLE urine output criteria on contrast-induced nephropathy in critically ill patients. *BMC Nephrology*, 17(1), 36.

Goveas, B. (2017) Urosepsis: A simple infection turned toxic. *The Nurse Practitioner*, 42(7), 53–54.

Integumentary System Review

▶ LEARNING OBJECTIVES

In this chapter you will review:
- Cellulitis
- Intravenous (IV) infiltration
- Necrotizing fasciitis
- Pressure injury
- Wounds (infectious, surgical, trauma)

● CELLULITIS

▶ PATHOPHYSIOLOGY

Q **What layers of skin are affected by cellulitis?**

A **Dermis and subcutaneous**

When bacteria enter the dermis and subcutaneous tissues, it produces the superficial infection of cellulitis.

Q **What is a primary risk factor for cellulitis?**

A **Previous surgery**

Cellulitis is a skin infection that may develop as a complication in postsurgical wounds, venous ulcers, or traumatic wounds. Cellulitis is generally associated with disruption of the skin, increasing susceptibility to infections. It can be mild to life-threatening. Severity of illness correlates with the depth of skin structure.

HINT Impaired venous and lymphatic drainage can predispose to cellulitis.

Box 8.1 Cellulitis Risk Factors

▪ Previous cutaneous infection	▪ Type 2 diabetes mellitus
▪ Cirrhosis	▪ Malignancy
▪ Immunosuppression	▪ Lymphedema
▪ Venous insufficiency	

▶ SYMPTOMS/ASSESSMENT

Q **A patient presents with lower extremity wounds. Would cellulitis be more likely if symptoms were in unilateral versus bilateral extremities?**

A **Unilateral**

Cellulitis is almost always unilateral. If bilateral skin findings are present, it is more likely a result of venous stasis. Cellulitis can be nonpurulent or purulent (evidence of fluid collections or abscesses).

HINT   Postoperative wounds, typically within the first 24 hours, may appear warm, red, and tender. This is inflammation and is a normal postoperative finding.

Box 8.2 Symptoms of Cellulitis

■ Redness	■ Warmth
■ Fever	■ Swelling
■ Tenderness	■ Relatively sudden onset
■ Bullae	■ Abscess

▶ DIAGNOSIS

> **Q** What is a laboratory finding that may indicate the presence of infection and cellulitis in a wound?
>
> **A** Leukocytosis

Not all patients with cellulitis will develop leukocytosis, but it is a sign of infection and is found in approximately 50% of the patients with cellulitis. Inflammatory markers may also be elevated.

> **Q** What diagnostic study can be used to identify a fluid collection or abscess in a wound with cellulitis?
>
> **A** Ultrasound

Ultrasound of the lesion or wound is used to determine the presence and location of fluid collection or abscess.

▶ MANAGEMENT

> **Q** An uncomplicated cellulitis without an abscess can be managed with what medical therapy?
>
> **A** Antibiotics

Antibiotics are the primary management of cellulitis. IV therapy may be required initially with conversion to oral when stabilized. Abscess drainage is required in addition to antibiotics if the cellulitis has a complicated course.

HINT   Cellulitis does not usually have cultures that guide antibiotic therapy.

▶ COMPLICATIONS

> **Q** What is a complication of skin and soft tissue infections?
>
> **A** Sepsis and septic shock

Skin and soft tissue infections are common conditions and can, in severe cases, induce septic shock.

HINT   Septic shock will not resolve until all of the infected/necrotic tissue.

● IV INFILTRATION

▶ PATHOPHYSIOLOGY

> **Q** What is the difference between infiltration and extravasation of IV fluids?
>
> **A** Vesicant versus nonvesicant fluid

When the infusion is nonvesicant or nonirritating to the tissue and inadvertently delivered into the tissue, it is called infiltration. Extravasation occurs when the infusion is vesicant fluid or medication and damages the surrounding tissue. Vesicant fluids are agents capable of causing blistering, skin sloughing, or necrosis.

HINT Damage from the infiltration can extend to involve nerves, tendons, and joints.

Box 8.3 Factors Contribute to Infiltration and Severity

■ Osmolality of infusing agent (>290 mosmo/L)	■ Duration of exposure
■ Volume of infiltrating solution	■ pH of solution (outside range 5.5–8.5)
■ Chemical irritation	■ Mechanical pressure from leakage
■ Prolonged IV therapy	■ Vasoconstrictors

IV, intravenous.

Q What characteristic of the fluid infusing into the vein can increase the risk for IV infiltration or extravasation?

A Strong alkalinities or acids

Certain fluids and drugs can cause endothelial irritation leading to rupture and extravasation. Fluids that are either strong acids or alkalinities can damage cellular proteins reducing durability of the venous endothelium. High osmolality can disrupt cell function and cause cellular rupture resulting in infiltration/extravasation (Table 8.1).

HINT pH of fluids ranging from 5 to 9 is recommended for IV fluids and medications to prevent vascular injury.

Table 8.1 Drugs at Risk for Infiltration/Extravasation

Medication	pH of the Medication
Phenytoin	12
Vancomycin	2.8–4
Ampicillin/sulbactam	8–10
Etomidate	3.4
Antineoplastic drugs	
Hyperosmolar agents	

Q Which site is most commonly involved with infiltration/extravasation?

A Dorsum of hand or foot

Sites most implicated in extravasation injuries include dorsum of hand and foot IVs. Other sites of potential concern include IVs placed near joints or over bones with little soft tissue protection.

HINT Limbs with local vascular problems may have reduced venous flow, causing pooling and leakage of fluids being infused around the IV site.

▶ SYMPTOMS/ASSESSMENT

Q What is the main symptom of an irritant that is not a vesicant?

A Local pain and phlebitis

An infiltration of an irritant substance causes local inflammation, pain, burning, pruritus, swelling, or phlebitis along the vein site without tissue necrosis. Pain at the site is the first sign of infiltration.

HINT Discoloration alone does not necessarily indicate extravasation.

Box 8.4 Signs of Extravasation

■ Pain	■ Erythema
■ Swelling	■ Tenderness
■ Local blistering	■ Mottling/darkening of skin
■ Firm Induration	■ Ulceration
■ No capillary refill	

Q Are symptoms of extravasation present immediately or within days to weeks?

A Days to weeks

Initially, symptoms may appear as an irritant substance with local phlebitis, however, over several days to weeks, tissue necrosis develops. Progressive erythema, discoloration, blistering, or desquamation develops prior to tissue necrosis. This can progress to black eschar and tissue sloughing.

HINT Frequently ulcerative areas can be found underneath the necrotic eschar and are not evident until 2 weeks after injury.

Table 8.2 Grading Severity of Infiltration/Extravasation

Grade	Symptoms
Grade 1	■ Pain at infusion site ■ Difficulty flushing line ■ Minimal swelling ■ No redness
Grade 2	■ Pain at infusion site ■ Difficulty flushing line ■ Mild swelling ■ No blanching ■ Minimal redness ■ Normal capillary refill
Grade 3	■ Pain at infusion site ■ Difficulty or inability to flush line ■ Skin blanches ■ Redness at site ■ Sluggish capillary refill
Grade 4	■ Pain at infusion site ■ Marked swelling ■ Skin blanches ■ Cool to touch ■ Reduced capillary refill ■ Decreased perfusion ■ Blister

Box 8.5 At-Risk or Infiltration Injuries

■ Inability of the patient to report pain
■ Inability to visualize insertion sites
■ Peripheral IVs
■ Fragile veins, i.e., chemotherapy infusions
■ Diabetic neuropathy

IV, intravenous.

▶ DIAGNOSIS

Q What is a common sign indicating misplacement of the IV catheter?

A Increased resistance

An increased resistance to IV fluid or a reduced rate of flow can indicate the catheter is misplaced and no longer in the vein. The lack of blood return when aspirated from the catheter is not always a reliable sign of misplacement.

▶ MEDICAL MANAGEMENT

Q What is the first intervention if the nurse suspects the IV has infiltrated?

A Stop the infusion

The initial intervention for a suspected infiltration is to stop the infusion and evaluate the site. If the grade of injury is 3 to 4, then consider administering an antidote if available. Hyaluronidase is an enzyme, which can promote more rapid reabsorption of extravasated fluids. The recommended time for use is within 1 to 2 hours of extravasation.

HINT Hyaluronidase is effective with calcium chloride and total parenteral nutrition (TPN). It is not effective with vasoconstrictors.

Box 8.6 Interventions for Infiltration/Extravasation

- Removal venous access device
- Constricting bands or tapes should be removed
- Elevation of limb
- Warm or cold compresses
- Injection of antidote into damaged tissue

HINT Aspiration from the catheter prior to discontinuation may be used to remove as much of the vesicant as possible from the infiltrated site.

Table 8.3 Intervention Based Upon Grade of Injury

Grade of Injury	Interventions
Grade 1	■ Stop infusion ■ Remove IV ■ Elevate limb
Grade 2	■ Stop infusion ■ Remove IV ■ Elevate limb
Grade 3	■ Stop infusion ■ Remove any constricting tape/bandage ■ Leave IV in place for administration of an antidote ■ Photograph injury ■ Apply nonocclusive dressing ■ Elevate limb
Grade 4	■ Stop infusion ■ Remove any constricting tape/bandage ■ Leave IV in place for administration of an antidote ■ Photograph injury ■ Apply nonocclusive dressing ■ Elevate limb ■ Consult plastics

IV, intravenous.

▶ SURGICAL MANAGEMENT

> **Q** At what point would a surgical intervention be indicated following extravasation of a vesicant solution?
>
> **A** Necrotic tissue

The presence of skin necrosis and eschar may indicate the need for surgical debridement. Surgical debridement should completely remove all dead, necrotic tissue to allow only healthy tissue to remain for wound closure.

▶ COMPLICATIONS

> **Q** What is the acute severe complication of extravasation?
>
> **A** Compartment syndrome

Compartment syndrome can develop due to the infiltrated fluid and excessive swelling of the limb. The introduction of vesicant substances into tissue and nerves can result in Complex Regional Pain Syndrome.

Box 8.7 Complications of Extravasation

- Compartment syndrome
- Tissue necrosis
- Complex regional pain syndrome

⬤ NECROTIZING FASCIITIS

▶ PATHOPHYSIOLOGY

> **Q** What layer of the tissue is affected with necrotizing fasciitis?
>
> **A** Fascia

Necrotizing fasciitis is a life-threatening, rapidly progressing tissue infection.

It is an uncommon but a severe tissue infection that affects the deep fascia layer with early sparing of muscle and skin. If allowed to progress, it affects muscle and skin. The bacteria can enter through open skin from a small cut to a major trauma or surgical wound.

HINT Microthrombosis and ischemia lead to greater damage and deep tissue necrosis.

> **Q** Necrotizing fasciitis that is caused by both aerobic and anaerobic organisms is considered to be a type I or type II?
>
> **A** Type I

Type I necrotizing fasciitis is polymicrobial including both aerobic and anaerobic organisms, including gram-positive and gram-negative organisms. Type II is classically caused by Streptococcus with or without Staph infections such as *Streptococcus pyogenes* and *Staphylococcus aureus*. Type II is commonly nicknamed the "flesh-eating bacteria." Some resources include a type III that affects the skeletal muscle as gas gangrene and is a result of *Clostridium* species.

HINT Methicillin-resistant Staphylococcus aureus (MRSA) can be the cause of necrotizing fasciitis.

> **Q** What is the name of the necrotizing fasciitis that affects the perineum?
>
> **A** Fournier gangrene

Necrotizing fasciitis can be classified based upon the anatomical site of infection. Fournier gangrene is necrotizing fasciitis that affects the perineum. Anaerobic bacteria are the typical cause of this infection. Ludwig's angina involves the submandibular and sublingual spaces.

HINT   The perineum and oral cavity are frequently missed areas when looking for the cause of a systemic infection.

Q **What immune dysfunction will increase the risk of necrotizing fasciitis?**

A **Immunosuppression**

Immunosuppression of any kind, including immunosuppressive drugs, will increase the risk of infection and necrotizing fasciitis. The most common sites affected include limbs, perineum, and truncal region.

Box 8.8 Risk Factors Necrotizing Fasciitis

■ Immunosuppression:	■ Elderly
● Organ transplant	■ Previous cutaneous or soft tissue infection
● HIV	■ Previous surgery
● Immunosuppressant therapy	■ Obesity
■ Type 2 diabetes mellitus	■ Malignancy
■ HIV	■ Tracheostomy
■ Renal failure	■ Alcohol abuser
■ Malnourished	■ Peripheral vascular disease
■ Intravenous drug abuse	

▶ SYMPTOMS/ASSESSMENT

Q **What is the description of the color of the skin in area of necrotizing fasciitis?**

A **Dusky**

The initial redness of the skin turns to dusky color of necrotizing fasciitis. Quickly spreading erythema, ecchymosis with vesicles enlarging to bullae may indicate presence of necrotizing fasciitis. The bullae may be filled with fouls smelling fluid or blood and can result in significant blood loss. Once the wound advanced with necrosis and gangrene, it may no longer be painful due to destruction of the superficial nerves.

HINT   One sign of necrotizing fasciitis is the rapid progression of symptoms with pain disproportionate to clinical findings.

Box 8.9 Signs of Necrotizing Fasciitis

■ Early: Pain out of proportion to physical exam	■ Late: Loss of sensation (anesthesia)
■ Bullae (vesicles) and hemorrhagic bullae	■ Drainage from the wound
■ Tenderness beyond area of erythema	■ Crepitus
■ Cutaneous abnormal sensation	■ Cellulitis refractory to antibiotics
■ Rapid progression cellulitis	■ Dusky skin
■ Systemic toxicity	■ Fever

Q **A patient with necrotizing fasciitis frequently experiences acid–base imbalance. Which acid–base imbalance is most likely?**

A **Metabolic acidosis**

Metabolic acidosis is a common acid–base imbalance in patients with necrotizing fasciitis. Commonly associated electrolyte abnormalities include hyperkalemia and hypocalcemia. Hypoalbuminemia is common with large wounds and necrotizing fasciitis.

HINT In septic shock, coagulation abnormalities may also be experienced, and dissiminated intravascular coagulation (DIC) should be suspected.

Box 8.10 Laboratory Findings

- Leukocytosis
- Hyponatremia
- Elevated blood urea nitrogen (BUN)
- Elevated creatine phosphokinase (CPK)
- Abnormal C-reactive protein

▶ DIAGNOSIS

Q What diagnostic radiographic study is considered the best to distinguish necrotizing from nonnecrotizing infection?

A MRI

Imaging modalities such as radiographs are not effective in diagnosing necrotizing fasciitis. CT and MRI may be used to identify pockets of soft tissue gas tracking along fascial planes, fat stranding, and asymmetrical fascial thickening. Definitive diagnosis is surgical exposure with the appearance of grey fascia and tissue biopsy to identify the causative organism.

HINT Additional tests for diagnosis include needle aspiration and incision biopsy.

Box 8.11 Diagnosis Criteria for Necrotizing Fasciitis

- Extensive necrosis of the superficial fascia in the absence of macrovascular occlusion
- Systemic toxic reactions (fever, leukocytosis, positive cultures)
- Mental status changes
- Focal necrosis, microvascular thrombosis, and leukocytes in debrided tissue

▶ MEDICAL MANAGEMENT

Q What is the primary medical management of a patient with necrotizing fasciitis?

A Antibiotics

Initial management of a patient presenting with necrotizing fasciitis should be cultured and placed on a broad-spectrum antibiotic or specific to the underlying etiology if known. Once culture and sensitivity is resulted, then antibiotics are changed to more specific antibiotic for the bacteria.

HINT Delays in initiating antimicrobial therapy can increase the severity and mortality from necrotizing fasciitis.

▶ SURGICAL MANAGEMENT

Q What is the primary surgical management of a patient with necrotizing fasciitis?

A Surgical debridement

Surgical debridement or drainage is the primary treatment of necrotizing fasciitis and is usually required to manage the infection. Source control of an infection is paramount and surgical debridement is the option. Frequency of surgical debridement may vary but typically occur every 24 to 48 hours until there is no evidence of necrosis. Vascular microthrombosis and vasculitis occur even if the external skin appears healthy.

HINT Delays in surgical debridement have been found to increase mortality.

> **Q** Which dressing therapy is commonly utilized to improve closure and removal of excess drainage from the wound?
>
> **A** Negative Pressure Wound Therapy (NPWT)

NPWT can stimulate granulation tissue formation, promote angiogenesis, prepare the wound bed for repair, and facilitate wound closure. This therapy is continued until granulation tissue appears on the wound bed.

> **Q** What follow-up surgeries may be required after the necrosis is completely removed and the fascia is healed?
>
> **A** Reconstructive Surgery

Following multiple debridement surgeries, the wound may require skin grafts. Skin grafts and flap transfers can be used to close the wound. Local flap transfers are used for small wounds. Sequential stamp grafting may be more suitable for larger wounds. Free rotating grafts can be used to cover wounds with exposed bone after muscle necrosis.

HINT Stamp grafting can be used to prevent spread of infection to whole skin graft.

▶ COMPLICATIONS

> **Q** What systemic complication is commonly associated with necrotizing fasciitis?
>
> **A** Sepsis and septic shock

Sepsis and septic shock occur from the severe infection becoming systemic. This can progress to multisystem organ failure and death. Early treatment with antibiotics, fluids debridement can lower the risk and severity of sepsis.

HINT Prompt diagnosis and treatment can lower the risk of sepsis and death.

> **Q** What is the complication of a necrotizing fasciitis caused by Clostridium bacteria?
>
> **A** Gas gangrene

Clostridium species can cause infections, which produce gas gangrene. *Clostridium sordellii* infections are associated with toxic shock syndrome.

HINT Management of toxic shock syndrome caused by *Clostridium sordellii* may be treated with intravenous immunoglobulin (IVIG) therapy.

⬤ PRESSURE INJURY

▶ PATHOPHYSIOLOGY

> **Q** What is the term used to define localized tissue damage to the skin and underlying tissue usually over bony prominence that can occur in hospitalized patients?
>
> **A** Hospital-Acquired Pressure Injury (HAPI)

HAPIs are caused by prolonged or intense pressures over bony prominences or related to pressure caused by medical devices. Tissue injuries are frequently a cause of infrequent turning or repositioning. The pressure causes impaired blood flow resulting in ischemia and tissue necrosis.

HINT Patients with mobility issues are at the highest risk for development of HAPI.

Box 8.12 Common Sites Pressure Injuries

■ Buttocks	■ Hips
■ Coccyx	■ Sacrum
■ Heel	■ Patellar
■ Elbows	■ Ears
■ Occipital	■ Ankles
■ Toes	

Q What is the mechanism for tissue injury, which can occur when moving a patient up in bed?

A Shearing

The mechanism of shearing causes deep tissue injury and is commonly caused by patient movement in bed and while positioning the patient. Maceration of skin and tissue occurs with prolonged exposure to fluids, such as in patients with urine incontinence.

Box 8.13 Medical Devices Associated With Pressure Injuries

■ Orthopedic immobilizers (i.e., cervical collars, braces)	■ Nasal cannulas
■ BiPAP device	■ Catheters (Foley, central line (CL), dialysis)
■ Intermittent compression devices	
■ Tracheostomy securement devices	■ Compression stockings
■ EEG pads	■ Pulse oximeter probes

Q Which is damaged first in pressure injuries, the skin or muscle and deep tissue?

A Muscle and deep tissue

The underlying deep tissue and muscle are more susceptible to pressure and lack of oxygen than the superficial layer of skin. Often the injury is larger underneath than the appearance of the visible skin injury.

HINT This can make severity of wound classifications more difficult.

▶ SYMPTOMS/ASSESSMENT

Q What is a common pressure injury risk assessment tool used in hospitals?

A Braden Score

Skin assessment tools are used to determine the risk for skin breakdown and development of HAPI. They typically assess the moisture of the skin, presence of sharing or friction, sensory perception, and nutrition. Braden score is one example of risk assessment tool, but there is no universally accepted tool.

HINT Skin risk assessment tools commonly do not take into account risk with medical devices for pressure injury.

Box 8.14 Increased Risks HAPI

■ Impaired mobility	■ Comorbidities (vascular insufficiency, diabetes)
■ Increased skin moisture	
■ Malnutrition	■ Urinary or fecal incontinence
■ Elderly patients	■ Vasoconstrictors infusing
■ Decreased sensory	■ Nonverbal patients
■ Shear from involuntary movements or sliding in bed	■ Fever or hypothermia

HAPI, hospital-acquired pressure injury.

> **Q** What is the purpose of performing frequent skin assessments in high-risk patients?
>
> **A** Early identification of pressure injury

A pressure injury that is identified in the early stages (stage I) can be prevented from becoming a more severe or long-term complication. Identification of early injury allows for readjustments and prevention of further injury.

HINT   Identifying any areas of redness that are still blanchable allows for interventions to prevent tissue injury.

> **Q** When performing a skin assessment, an area on the sacrum is noted to be red and nonblanchable. What is the correct staging of the pressure injury?
>
> **A** Stage I

An area of intact skin that is red and found to be nonblanchable is considered a stage I pressure injury. Before this stage of injury, the reddened area is blanchable. Stage II should not be used to describe moisture-associated skin injury. Stage II heals by re-epithelization not by granulating tissue.

HINT   This staging system is not used on traumatic wounds. It is only used for pressure injuries.

Table 8.4 Staging of Pressure Injuries

Stage	Description
Stage I	▪ Intact skin ▪ Local area of redness ▪ Different color than rest of tissue ▪ Nonblanchable ▪ Painful
Stage II—Partial thickness	▪ Loss of skin with dermis exposed ▪ Wound bed is viable pink or red ▪ Moist ▪ Skin either intact or blisters
Stage III—Full thickness	▪ Adipose (fat) is visible in wound ▪ Frequently wound edges are rolled ▪ Slough or eschar may be present ▪ Undermining and tunneling may occur
Stage IV—Full thickness	▪ Exposed or directly palpable fascia, muscle, tendon, ligament, cartilage, or bone ▪ Slough or eschar visible
Unstageable pressure injury—Obscured full thickness	▪ Full-thickness tissue injury or loss in which the degree of ulcer is not confirmed because obscured by eschar. ▪ If eschar or slough is removed, a stage III or IV will be revealed
Deep pressure injury—persistent nonblanchable	▪ Intact or nonintact skin with localized area nonblanchable deep red, maroon, purple discoloration or epidermal separation revealing a dark wound bed or blood-filled blister.

HINT   If found early, skin that is still blanchable is not staged, and positioning it off the site can prevent tissue injury.

Box 8.15 Terminology of Injuries

■ Medical device-related pressure injury ■ Mucosal membrane pressure injury	■ Resultant pressure injury generally conforms to the pattern or shape of the device ■ Injury can be staged ■ Injuries that occur in the oral mucosa, GI tract, nasal passages, urinary tract, tracheal lining, and vaginal tract ■ Ulcers cannot be staged due to anatomy

GI, gastrointestinal.

▶ MEDICAL MANAGEMENT

Q What is the best prevention for HAPI?

A Frequent repositioning

Prevention is the best management for pressure injuries. If patient is immobilized or unable to turn effectively, then the best prevention is frequent repositioning. Prevention of pressure injuries caused by medical devices is appropriate selection of devices (softest tubing), placed appropriately to produce the least amount of pressure or friction.

HINT Securing devices should have sufficient padding or cushion to prevent skin injuries.

Box 8.16 Prevention of HAPI

■ Removal of medical devices as soon as possible ■ Frequent repositioning ■ Specialty beds for redistributing pressure ■ Using incontinence devices ■ Using prophylactic dressings	■ Maintaining clean, dry skin under medical devices ■ Relieving, reducing, or redistributing pressure ■ Nutrition ■ Using clean and dry sheets

HAPI, hospital-acquired pressure injury.

Q What is the major goal of wound management in patients with pressure injuries?

A Wound bed preparation

The wound bed is prepared for the optimal development of granulated tissue. The acronym TIME describes the four components of wound management. The goal is to remove the barriers to wound healing.

Box 8.17 Acronym TIME

T	Tissue management
I	Infection and inflammation control
M	Moisture balance
E	Epithelial edge advancement

Q What is the primary intervention with pressure injuries used to decrease the bacterial count in the wound?

A Wound cleansing

Wound cleansing can decrease the bacterial count in the wound. Cleansing should be gentle and not cause further damage to the tissues. Wounds noninfected may be cleansed with normal saline. Known or suspected wound infection should use antimicrobial cleansing solutions. Cleansing pressure should be adequate to clean the wound but avoid high pressures that can damage tissue or drive bacteria into the wound.

Q What type of dressing is commonly used for autolytic debridement?

A Transparent film dressing

Transparent film dressings are used when the wound requires autolytic debridement.

HINT   Do not use hydrocolloid dressing with large amounts of exudate.

Table 8.5 Dressings

Type of Dressing	Indications
Hydrocolloids	▪ Stage I–IV noninfected wounds ▪ Only small amount of drainage ▪ Do not cover enzymatic debriding agents, gels, ointments
Transparent dressings	▪ Autolytic debridement
Hydrogels	▪ Minimally draining wound and granulated tissue ▪ Painful wound
Alginate dressings	▪ Infected wounds with concurrent treatment ▪ Large draining wounds
Silver-impregnated dressing	▪ Infected or highly colonized with bacteria
Medical grade honey impregnated dressing	▪ Stage II and III
Silicone dressings	▪ Promote atraumatic dressing changes ▪ Prevents periwound tissue injury in fragile skin
Collagen matrix dressing	▪ Stage III and IV

Q Which dressing can be used in Stage III or IV with large amounts of exudate and can decrease edema in the wound bed?

A NPWT

NPWT is used in larger wounds that have excessive drainage. The negative pressure promotes healing by removing the excess fluid but maintaining a moist wound bed. It stimulates vascularization and supports the closure of the wound edges. NPWT has also been found to promote growth factor expression, angiogenesis, and growth granulated tissue.

HINT   NPWT can be used to prepare the wound bed for skin grafts.

▶ SURGICAL MANAGEMENT

Q What is the primary surgical procedure to lower the bacterial count and improve wound healing?

A Debridement

Devitalized tissue that is leathery, yellow, brown, or black should be debrided. Bacteria grow in the eschar and can further delay wound healing. There are several methods of debridement: surgical, mechanical, enzymatic, biological.

HINT   Biofilms can be present on the wound and may require debridement.

Box 8.18 Debridement Methods

Surgical	■ Scalpels
Mechanical	■ Wound irrigation
Enzymatic	■ Low-frequency sound or ultrasonic mist
Biological	■ Enzymatic debriding agents
	■ Larval therapy with sterile maggots

▶ COMPLICATIONS

Q Upon assessment of Stage III pressure injury, it is noted to have purulent drainage. What complication would be suspected?

A Infection

Infections can complicate a pressure injury and delay wound healing or cause systemic involvement.

Box 8.19 Signs of Infection

■ Erythema extending past wound edges	■ Induration of tissue
■ Increasing or change in pain or warmth	■ Purulent drainage
■ Increasing wound size	■ Systemic signs of sepsis

Q What is an infection in bone adjacent to the pressure injury?

A Osteomyelitis

Osteomyelitis is an infection in bone that is adjacent to the wound. In suspected cases, plain films, CT, and MRI scans can be used for a definitive diagnosis.

HINT MRI has the highest sensitivity and specificity for diagnosing osteomyelitis.

● WOUNDS (TRAUMA/SURGICAL)

▶ PATHOPHYSIOLOGY

Q What is a common comorbidity that can cause immunocompromised and delayed wound healing?

A Diabetes

Certain conditions increase a patient's risk for infections and complications of surgical wounds. Any condition that decreases effectiveness of host defenses is a risk factor for surgical wound infection.

Box 8.20 Conditions Increase Risk Infections Surgical Wounds

■ Immunocompromised state	■ Altered states of perfusion
■ Functional status	■ Malnutrition
■ Radiation therapy	■ Unintentional weight loss
■ Obesity	■ Longer duration of surgery
■ Emergency procedures	■ Pre-op sepsis
■ Smoking	

Q What type of surgery has the highest risk for surgical site infections (SSI)?

A Colon Surgeries

Colon surgery has the highest risk for SSI, followed by vascular surgery, cholecystectomy, and organ transplants. The greater the length of surgery will increase the risk of SSI.

Box 8.21 Increase Risk SSI

■ Longer operative procedures ■ Type of surgery (i.e., colon, vascular, transplants) ■ Emergency surgery ■ Use of blood products	■ Contaminated or dirty surgery (e.g., spillage fecal material into abdomen) ■ Hypoperfusion of organs during surgery ■ Implants

SSI, surgical site infections.

▶ SYMPTOMS/ASSESSMENT

Q What is the primary component of assessing surgical wounds for classification of wound status?

A Cleanliness and condition of wound

In surgical wounds, it is critical to clean and remove contamination from the wounds for healing and infection prevention. The CDC classification of traumatic wounds is based upon the cleanliness and condition of the wound.

HINT Colonization of a wound with pathogens is not always synonymous with infection.

Box 8.22 Classification Surgical Wounds

Class 1	■ Wounds considered clean ■ Uninfected ■ No inflammation ■ Do not enter respiratory, alimentary, genital, urinary tracts
Class 2	■ Wound clean contaminated ■ Lack unusual contamination ■ Wounds enter respiratory, alimentary, genital, urinary tracts under controlled conditions
Class 3	■ Contaminated ■ Fresh open wounds from insult sterile techniques or leakage from GI tract ■ Inflammation without purulent drainage
Class 4	■ Dirty-infected ■ De-vitalized tissue

Q A patient develops a low-grade fever 24 hours after abdominal surgery. Would this be considered a sign of SSI?

A No

Postoperative fevers are common following major surgeries. The fever is a result of the trauma and inflammation and is less likely due to SSI. If the fever develops after 96 hours, it would be a greater chance of being SSI, especially accompanied by other signs of infection.

▶ MEDICAL MANAGEMENT

Q What is the recommendation for a patient with a scheduled surgery the night before the surgery?

A Cleanse with antiseptic

Patients with planned surgical procedures are expected to shower or bathe with an antiseptic the night before the surgery. The most commonly used antiseptic is chlorhexidine. This is a preventive measure for SSI.

Box 8.23 Preoperative Interventions to Decrease SSI

- Antiseptic wash night before surgery
- Glycemic control
- Patient education regarding postoperative care
- Antibiotic prophylaxis
- Adequate nutrition

SSI, surgical site infections.

▶ SURGICAL MANAGEMENT

Q What is the recommendation for a dressing if the abdomen is left open?

A NPWT

NPWT is used following abdominal surgery when they were unable to close in the operating room. These cases may include perforation of bowel, fecal contamination, or being at risk for developing abdominal compartment syndrome.

▶ COMPLICATIONS

Q What is the complication of surgical wound that is edematous?

A Dehiscence

Wound dehiscence is typically a result of edema. It may be associated with obesity, coughing, vomiting, and straining. Wound dehiscence frequently occurs around 7th day postop. Dehiscence can lead to evisceration, SSI, and development of incisional hernia.

HINT Assessment of the incision includes approximation of edges and identifying tension.

1. Which of the following is considered an increased risk for necrotizing fasciitis?

   A. Acute respiratory distress syndrome (ARDS)
   B. Acute kidney injury (AKI)
   C. Immunosuppression
   D. Pericarditis

2. Which of the following wounds would benefit from a hydrocolloid dressing?

   A. Stage III with large amount exudate
   B. Stage II pressure injury
   C. Cover enzymatic debriding agent on Stage IV
   D. Wound requiring debridement

3. Which of the following findings would indicate the IV (intravenous) is misplaced and is no longer in vascular space?

   A. Increased resistance fluid infusion
   B. Lack of blood return
   C. Patient complaints of pain at site
   D. Presence of large-bore IV catheter

4. Which of the following dressings can stimulate granulated tissue growth and promote angiogenesis?

   A. Hydrocolloid dressing
   B. Negative pressure wound therapy (NPWT)
   C. Transparent dressing
   D. Silver impregnated dressing

5. Which area is most common for a patient to develop cellulitis?

   A. Leg
   B. Face
   C. Arm
   D. Back

(See answers next page.)

1. C) Immunosuppression
Immunosuppression, of any kind, lowers the patient's ability to fight infections. It is a risk factor for necrotizing fasciitis. ARDS, AKI, and pericarditis are disorders frequently seen in intensive care but are not an increased risk for necrotizing fasciitis.

2. B) Stage II pressure injury
Hydrocolloid dressings can be used in Stage I to IV pressure injuries but with minimal drainage. It is not recommended for large amounts of exudate. It should not be used to cover enzymatic debriding agents, gels, or ointments. Transparent film dressings are used on wounds that require autolytic debridement.

3. A) Increased resistance fluid infusion
An increased resistance to IV fluid or a reduced rate of flow can indicate the catheter is misplaced and no longer in the vein. The lack of blood return when aspirated from the catheter is not always a reliable sign of misplacement. Some medications being infused can cause pain at the site but may not indicate a misplaced IV catheter. Large-bore IV catheters would not be an indication of a misplaced catheter.

4. B) NPWT
NPWT can stimulate granulation tissue formation, promote angiogenesis, prepare the wound bed for repair, and facilitate wound closure. This therapy is continued until granulation tissue appears on the wound bed.

5. A) Leg
Although cellulitis can occur anywhere, the most common location is the lower leg. Bacteria enters disrupted areas of the skin (through a cut, wound, bite, ulcer, or dermatitis). It can occur on the face, arm, or back but the most common location is the leg.

BIBLIOGRAPHY

Centers for Disease Control and Prevention. (2016). *Surgical site infection (SSI) event: Procedure-associated module.* https://www.cdc.gov/nhsn/pdfs/pscmanual/9pscssicurrent.pdf.

Liu, Y., Guo, K., & Sun, J. (2017). Learning from clinical experience with necrotizing fasciitis: Treatment and management. *Wound Care Journal, 30*(11), 486–493. https://doi.org/10.1097/01.ASW.0000525791.33664.e0

Musculoskeletal System Review

▶ LEARNING OBJECTIVES

In this chapter, you will review:
- Compartment syndrome
- Fractures (i.e., femur, pelvis)
- Osteomyelitis
- Rhabdomyolysis
- Functional Issues

● COMPARTMENT SYNDROME

Q What are the three components within the fascia?

A Muscle, nerve, and blood vessels

Facial compartments are composed of muscle, nerve, and blood vessels. The fascial bundles are present in extremities and trunk.

Q An elevated pressure in the osteofascial compartment results in injury to which component of the bundle first?

A Muscle

An osteofascial compartment is a sheath of fascia, which binds the muscle and the neurovascular bundles. Compartment syndrome is an elevated pressure within the osteofascial compartments, which results in ischemic injury to muscle, nerve, and vascular structures (Figure 9.1). It is most commonly due to a compression or crush type injury but can also occur from an external source such as wraps, casts, or air splints (Box 9.1).

HINT The onset of compartment syndrome is usually 6–8 hours after injury.

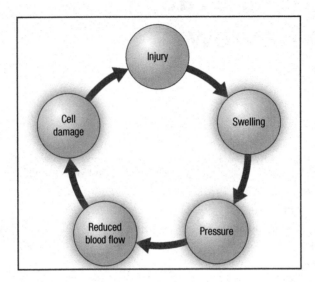

Figure 9.1 Compartment Syndrome

Box 9.1 Causes of Compartment Syndrome

Internal	External
Fractures	Compression
Swelling	Cast
Snakebite	Splint
Crush injury	Restricted positioning
IV infiltration/extravasation	

▶ SYMPTOMS/ASSESSMENT

Q What is considered to be the hallmark of compartment syndrome?

A Pain

Pain beyond pain medications is a hallmark sign of compartment syndrome, while pain on passive movement is an early sign of compartment syndrome. Pain is assessed by passively moving the distal portion of the extremity to elicit pain (i.e., calf injury can be assessed by the examiner moving the foot up and down).

HINT Compartment syndrome can produce pain beyond pain medications, paresthesia, and paralysis (or weakness of the involved extremity) early in the presentation.

Q What finding on assessment of an extremity at risk for compartment syndrome would indicate irreversible tissue injury?

A Loss of a pulse

Pulses and capillary refill will remain intact in the presence of compartment syndrome because it involves the collapse of arterioles and veins not the major arteries. Once a pulse is lost, it is too late to salvage the extremity due to irreversible tissue damage in compartment syndrome.

HINT A presentation of compartment syndrome may include a decrease in sensation of the affected extremity due to the damage of the nerves within the fascial compartment and is an earlier sign than a loss of a pulse (Box 9.2).

Box 9.2 The Ps of Assessment

Vascular	Nerve
■ Pallor ■ Pulselessness	■ Pain ■ Paresthesia ■ Paralysis

HINT   The 6th P is pressure.

> **Q** What is considered a normal compartmental pressure in an extremity?
>
> **A** 10 mmHg

Extremity compartment pressures can be measured in patients suspected of experiencing compartment syndrome. A normal compartment pressure is 10 mmHg of pressure. A compartmental pressure greater than 30 mmHg requires a surgical open fasciotomy to relieve the pressure.

HINT   The physical examination may be primarily used to recognize compartment syndrome.

> **Q** Which movements are used to assess for compartment syndrome in the forearm and wrist?
>
> **A** Flexion and extension of fingers

The Volar compartment contains flexors and pronators muscles of the forearm and wrist, median and ulnar nerve, ulnar and radial artery. Compartment syndrome occurring in the Volar compartment presents with weakness in flexors of finger and thumb. The trauma nurse can assess the Volar compartment by having the patient extend and flex their thumb and finger or perform finger abduction/adduction movements.

HINT   The patient will maintain flexion of fingers and experience pain on extension.

▶ DIAGNOSIS

> **Q** What is a commonly used laboratory finding used to assess for muscle injury following a crush mechanism of injury?
>
> **A** Creatinine Kinase (CK)

Creatinine kinase (CK) levels will elevate in patients with crush injuries due to the release of CK from the muscle when injured. Potassium can also elevate following crush injuries due to the release of intracellular components, including potassium.

HINT   Rhabdomyolysis is caused by the disruption of muscle cell membrane which release myoglobin and other components (SGOT, LDH, CK, glucose, potassium) into the bloodstream.

> **Q** Which electrolyte abnormality is most commonly associated with crush injury and acute renal failure caused by rhabdomyolysis?
>
> **A** Hyperkalemia

Potassium elevates following crush injuries due to the release of intracellular components following cellular injury. Potassium is primarily intracellular and is released with traumatic crush injuries. Hyperkalemia is most commonly found early and will typically peak within 12–36 hours after a crush injury. The hyperkalemia can be managed with kayexalate, insulin and dextrose, bicarbonate infusion, or beta agonist. Calcium gluconate can be administered as a cardioprotectant in hyperkalemic cases.

HINT   Hyperkalemia may be identified early by the presence of peaked T waves on the electrocardiogram.

> **Q** What is a sign commonly used to determine compartment syndrome in a patient unable to communicate abnormal sensation or pain affected extremity?
>
> **A** Tautness of skin

A patient unable to communicate pain or abnormal sensation in the affected extremity can contribute to a missed compartment syndrome. Patients unable to verbalize pain following an extremity injury require frequent assessment of the affected extremity for firmness, tautness of skin, and the presence of skin blisters.

HINT   The complication of an untreated compartment syndrome can be more severe than a fasciotomy.

Q What position should the nurse place the patient's extremity if compartment syndrome is suspected?

A Neutral position

An extremity suspected of having compartment syndrome should be maintained in a neutral position. Elevating the extremity may further compromise perfusion to the extremity. Allowing it to be lower than the level of the heart will increase edema and worsen compartment syndrome.

HINT   Remove any constricting dressings or casts from the extremity suspected of developing compartment syndrome.

▶ MANAGEMENT

Q What is the surgical treatment for compartment syndrome?

A Fasciotomy

Opening of the fascia will release the pressure in the muscle fascia and can prevent injury to muscle, nerves, and vessels within the compartment. Muscle necrosis can lead to contractures, loss of function, and amputations.

HINT   Each extremity has two or more compartments and varies in numbers based upon the compartment. (Table 9.1)

Table 9.1 Extremity Compartments

Extremity	Number of Compartments
Thigh	2
Calf	4
Feet	4
Forearm	2
Hand	4

Q What type of wound therapy is recommended after the open fasciotomy?

A Negative pressure wound therapy

Negative pressure wound therapy is recommended to improve healing and decrease the amount of scarring. Closure can be primary or skin grafting, typically within 7–10 days.

▶ COMPLICATIONS

Q What is a complication of a crush syndrome following a trauma to an extremity?

A Rhabdomyolysis

Crush syndrome is a condition in which prolonged muscle compression leads to muscle necrosis and the releasing of myoglobin. Rhabdomyolysis is a form of acute kidney injury in which there is a large amount of injured muscle releasing myoglobin in the blood (myoglobinemia) and is filtered through the kidneys (myoglobinuria).

HINT Rhabdomyolysis causes reddish to brownish urine, frequently described as "coke" or "tea" colored.

> **Q** What is considered a severe complication of an untreated compartment syndrome?
>
> **A** Amputation

A severe complication of an untreated compartment syndrome is an amputation due to severe muscle damage and necrosis. (Box 9.3)

HINT Performing a fasciotomy on an extremity with internal fixation can result in decreases stabilization of the fracture.

Box 9.3 Complications of Compartment Syndrome and Fasciotomy

Complications of Compartment Syndrome	Complications of Fasciotomy
■ Crush syndrome ■ Foot drop ■ Gross muscle necrosis ■ Amputation ■ Contractures (Volkman's contraction)	■ Bleeding ■ Damage neurovascular structures ■ Infection ■ Inadequate decompression

HINT Crush syndrome as a result of a compartment syndrome causes myoglobinuria, hyperkalemia, metabolic acidosis, and acute kidney injury.

● FRACTURES

▶ PATHOPHYSIOLOGY

> **Q** What type of spine fractures can occur when a person jumps from a significant height and lands on their feet?
>
> **A** Compression fractures

Compression fractures of the lumbar spine frequently occur when people fall or land on their feet from significant heights. A common triad of fractures occurs with falls that include calcaneus, thoracolumbar, and bilateral wrist fractures. The triad is due to the person landing on their feet (calcaneus fracture), the force causing compression fractures in the thoracolumbar spine, and the person falling forward on their wrists (bilateral wrist fractures).

HINT A direct impact on the top of the head can also cause compression fractures of the upper spine and is called axial loading.

> **Q** A motor pedestrian collision causes a typical pattern of injury. What is this called?
>
> **A** Waddell's triad

Motor pedestrian injury commonly presents with a pattern of injury called "Waddell's triad." The three injuries include bilateral femur fractures, blunt chest injury, and traumatic brain injury. This is classic with children that will turn to face the approaching vehicle. The impact of the vehicle bumper occurs at the level of the femur (bilateral femur fractures), the child is thrown unto the hood of the vehicle (chest trauma) and then continues off the car, landing on their head (traumatic brain injury).

HINT Adult motor pedestrians may have a slightly different pattern of injuries since they will commonly turn to avoid being hit by the vehicle.

> **Q** What is a common fracture of an elderly person following a fall?
>
> **A** Femoral neck

Fractures of the femoral neck of the hip are common in elderly patients with falls. The fracture may actually have caused their fall versus the fracture occurring due to the fall. It is typically associated with stable fractures of the pelvic ring.

HINT   The comorbidities of osteoporosis and osteoarthritis in elderly patients will increase their risk of fractures.

▶ SYMPTOMS/ASSESSMENT

Q **When assessing an extremity following a fracture, the nurse notes the patient has paresthesia. What type of injury is associated with the fracture?**

A **Nerve injury**

Both motor and sensory should be assessed following an extremity injury. The neurovascular examination of an extremity includes the 5 Ps: Pain, pallor, pulselessness, paresthesia, and paralysis. Of the 5 Ps: Pain, paresthesia, and paralysis correlate to nerve injury while pallor and pulselessness are used to assess arterial supply distal to site of injury.

HINT   A nerve that is lacerated or has sustained significant injury may cause a loss of sensation to the affected extremity distal to the site of injury.

Q **An abnormal externally rotated leg may indicate what type of fracture?**

A **Pelvic fracture**

Pelvic fractures can be a result of external rotation, lateral compression, abduction, and shearing forces. The trauma nurse should have a high suspicion for a pelvic fracture if the trauma patient has an abnormal rotation of a leg, especially an externally rotated leg.

HINT   If a patient has sustained a pelvis fracture, the trauma nurse should assess for associated injuries such as blood at the meatus (renal trauma) and hemodynamic instability (hemorrhage).

Q **When performing an extremity assessment on a trauma patient, what should the trauma nurse compare the affected extremity to?**

A **Unaffected extremity**

The trauma nurse should compare the affected extremity to the unaffected when performing assessment of the color, pulse, length of limb, sensory, and function. When assessing the trauma patient, note if the patient has a full range of motion in all extremities unless contraindicated.

HINT   Palpate pulses proximal and distal and compare the pulses to the opposite side for strength and quality.

Q **What is the bedside assessment that can be performed to assess for the stability of a pelvis?**

A **Press iliac crests together**

To assess for pelvic fractures and pelvic stability, the trauma nurse may press the iliac crests toward the midline, noting any instability of increased pain. An unstable pelvis fracture is when there is a fracture in more than one place of the pelvic ring resulting in displacements on the ring.

HINT   Never "rock" a pelvis if an injury is suspected. This may cause further damage to the internal structures.

▶ DIAGNOSIS

Q **What is the initial diagnostic study for identifying fractures?**

A **Radiographs**

Radiographs are used to identify fractures following extremity trauma. Recommended radiographs of an extremity should be of at least two views since a fracture may not be seen with just a single view. Common views obtained to identify a fracture are anterior-posterior and lateral views. CT scan of the pelvic region can also be used to confirm the radiograph findings. An arteriogram should be obtained if there is a suspected injury to the vasculature with extremity injury. A duplex doppler ultrasonography may be used as an alternative to an angiogram and can be performed in the emergency department.

HINT Crepitus noted during palpation of an extremity indicates the possibility of an underlying fracture, and a radiograph should be obtained.

▶ MANAGEMENT

Q What is the primary goal of placement of external fixators on a pelvic fracture?

A Limit blood loss

An external fixator is frequently used to stabilize pelvic fractures and limit blood loss. External fixation is accomplished with percutaneous pins connected to a rigid frame. Therapeutic embolization in interventional radiology is also used to control hemorrhage associated with pelvic fractures. Internal fixation of the pelvis is the long term management for the pelvic fracture.

HINT Damage control procedures may be required to prevent hemorrhage and death.

▶ COMPLICATIONS

Q What is a life-threatening complication of pelvic fractures?

A Hemorrhage

The pelvis contains a large vascular blood supply, including a large venous plexus, so injuries to the pelvis can result in significant blood loss and hemorrhagic shock. Posterior fractures of the pelvis have a greater incidence of hemorrhage complication than injuries to the anterior portion of the pelvis. A femur fracture may lose up to 1,500 ml of blood following an injury, and about 700–750 mL can be attributed to tibial or humeral fractures. Embolization of arterial bleeding can be used to limit the blood loss.

HINT Assess for significant blood loss that may be associated with extremity trauma and bone fractures.

Q What type of pelvic fracture has the greatest risk of complications and mortality?

A Open pelvic fracture

Complications associated with an open pelvic fracture include injury to the perineum, rectum, and genitourinary structure (bladder especially). Bladder disruption can be intraperitoneal or extraperitoneal.

Q What is a complication of a hip dislocation?

A Avascular necrosis

A complication of a hip dislocation is avascular necrosis of the femoral head. Dislocation of the knee may cause damage to the peroneal nerve and to the popliteal artery and vein. Posterior knee dislocation is associated with a higher incidence of vascular injury.

HINT Early surgical repair of hip dislocations may lower the incidence of avascular necrosis.

> **Q** What type of fracture most commonly develops the complication of an infection?
>
> **A** Open fracture

Infections following fractures occur with the greatest incidence in open fractures. Infections may involve the wounds or bone. Complication of an infection is the leading to delayed wound healing, osteomyelitis, and even sepsis (Box 9.4).

HINT Close observation of the trauma nurse for signs of sepsis is recommended following an open fracture and extremity wounds.

Box 9.4 Fracture Infection Complications

■ Avascular necrosis	■ Hemorrhage
■ Bladder rupture	■ Vascular injury
■ Nerve injury	■ Pain
■ Deformity	■ Disability
■ Muscle rupture and hernias	■ Wound infection
■ DVTs	

OSTEOMYELITIS

> **Q** What is osteomyelitis?
>
> **A** Bone infection

Osteomyelitis is bone infection, which can cause permanent disability and functional limitations if not recognized and treated early. The inflammation and infection occurs within the bone and bone marrow found in the medullary canal of bones. It may also affect adjacent soft tissue.

HINT Osteo = bone and myelo = myeloid tissue in bone marrow

▶ PATHOPHYSIOLOGY

> **Q** Which type of bones is most commonly affected with osteomyelitis?
>
> **A** Vertebral bodies

The high-risk bones for osteomyelitis in adults are the vertebral bodies of the spine. Lumbar spine is most commonly affected. Other bones affected include foot and hips. Pediatric patients are more likely to involve long bones (i.e., tibia) and especially during the growing stages.

HINT Commonly related to surgical procedures such as hip replacements or traumatic fractures.

> **Q** Which underlying disease process places the patient at a higher risk for developing osteomyelitis due to vascular insufficiency?
>
> **A** Diabetes mellitus (DM)

Diabetics are at a higher risk for vascular insufficiency and forming vascular ulcers. Ulcerative areas with infection can progress to the local bony site resulting in osteomyelitis. Other high-risk patients include patients with pressure ulcers over bony prominences, trauma, surgery, and post joint arthroplasty. (Box 9.5)

HINT The small bones of the feet are the most common site for osteomyelitis in DM patients.

Box 9.5 Factors Affect Severity of Osteomyelitis

Systemic Factors	Local Factors
■ Malnutrition	■ Vascular compromise
■ Renal failure	■ Vasculitis
■ Hepatic failure	■ Venous stasis
■ DM	■ Radiation necrosis
■ Malignancy	■ Cigarette smoking
■ Old age	■ Neuropathy
■ Immunosuppression	■ Lymphedema

Q Which microorganism is the primary cause of most osteomyelitis cases?

A *Staphyloccocus aureus*

S. aureus is a gram-positive bacteria that is found on skin. It is the most cause of osteomyelitis. Identifying the causative agent is important for antibiotic treatment to be most effective. MRSA has been increasing in frequency of bone and skin infections.

HINT Identifying the causative agent may be difficulty because the frequency of negative cultures with osteomyelitis.

Q A wound causes the spread of the infection to the bone with resulting osteomyelitis. Would this be classified as contiguous or hematogenous pathogenesis?

A Contiguous

Osteomyelitis is classified as acute or chronic. It is also classified as being caused by contiguous or hematogenous. Contiguous is spread of infection from adjacent tissue or open wounds. It is also the introduction of bacteria into bone by trauma or surgical procedures. Hematogenous osteomyelitis is the spread of infection from the bloodstream to bone. Direct inoculation occurs at the time of trauma or surgery (Figure 9.2).

HINT Most adults with hematogenous osteomyelitis have underlying chronic disease.

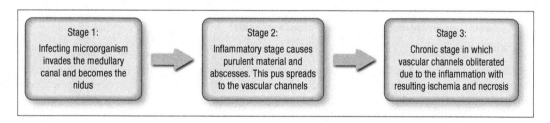

Figure 9.2 Sequence of Osteomyelitis

▶ SYMPTOMS/ASSESSMENT

Q What is the primary clinical sign of osteomyelitis?

A Pain over the affected area

Pain and tenderness over the affected bone involved is the primary clinical sign. Other symptoms can be signs of infection or sepsis (Box 9.6).

Box 9.6 Signs of Osteomyelitis

■ Fever	■ Pain-affected area
■ Loss of bone stability (surgical site)	■ Necrosis
■ Soft tissue infection	■ Swelling
■ Local redness/cellulitis	■ Decreased range of motion in joint
■ Radicular pain	■ Limited functional capability

▶ DIAGNOSIS

Q What are the primary diagnostic tests used to identify patient presents clinically with tenderness over vertebral bodies and signs of infection?

A Inflammatory serum markers

Diagnosis is typically a clinical diagnosis with supporting results of lab tests that include presence of inflammatory serum markers involving leukocytosis, elevated ESR, and C-reactive protein. Diagnostic radiographs are also utilized. Plain radiographs and CT scan are not as specific or sensitive as MRI. Radionuclide studies are also sensitive for identifying location of bone osteomyelitis.

HINT The most common findings on plain radiographs are adjacent soft tissue swelling and bone reaction. These findings are not typically found early in the disease process. X-rays become abnormal after 2–4 weeks.

Q What is the most definitive diagnosis of osteomyelitis?

A Biopsy

Obtaining a culture by biopsy should be directly from the affected bone using needle aspiration or surgical biopsy. Biopsy should be through uninfected tissue.

HINT Bone biopsy should be performed before initiation of antibiotics or 48 hours after discontinuation.

▶ MEDICAL MANAGEMENT

Q What is the primary medical treatment of osteomyelitis?

A Antibiotics

Systemic antibiotics are required as rapidly as possible to manage the infection and prevent complications of sepsis and septic shock. Antibiotic treatment consists of 4–6 week period. Hematogenous osteomyelitis is usually managed with monomicrobial treatment, while contiguous spread typically requires polymicrobial treatment.

HINT Antibiotics have poor penetration into infected fluid collections such as abscesses or necrotic bone and required surgical debridement.

▶ SURGICAL MANAGEMENT

Q A patient presents with vertebral body osteomyelitis and adjacent soft tissue involvement. What would be the probable surgical intervention for this patient?

A Drain abscess

Surgical intervention includes draining abscess in adjacent tissue, surgical debridement of necrosis, management of dead space, hardware removal, and restoration of blood supply. MRI can be used to delineate the extent of the infection. Repeat debridement may be necessary to ensure complete removal of dead bone and necrotic tissue. Revascularization of the affected limb can promote wound healing.

HINT   Hardware (i.e., screws, plates, external fixators) can be a source of secondary infection and may need to be removed.

▶ COMPLICATIONS

Q A diabetic with venous ulceration and foot necrosis continues to have chronic osteomyelitis and signs of systemic infections. What is the most likely surgical intervention?

A Amputation

The goal of treatment is to suppress the infection and maintain the limb integrity. When infections continue and bone necrosis occur, amputation of the foot may be required. (Box 9.6)

Box 9.6 Complications of Osteomyelitis

▪ Septic arthritis	▪ Systemic infection
▪ Pathological fractures	▪ Chronic osteomyelitis
▪ Squamous cell carcinoma	▪ Contiguous soft tissue infection
▪ Sinus tract formation	▪ Amputations
▪ Abscess	▪ Multiple surgeries
▪ Bone deformity	▪ Long term antibiotics
▪ Draining sinus tracts	▪ Joint instability

◉ RHABDOMYOLYSIS

Q What is the mechanism that results in rhabdomyolysis?

A Skeletal muscle injury or breakdown

Myoglobin is a protein found in skeletal and smooth muscle cells. The injury causes an alteration in the cell membrane integrity of the muscle, allowing the intracellular contents to escape into the plasma. Myoglobinuria is the presence of myoglobin in urine, which can occur if plasma levels exceed 1.5 mg/dL. Myoglobin is toxic to the kidneys, resulting in rhabdomyolysis-induced AKI.

HINT   Acidity of the urine will affect the amount of damage in the renal tubules (Box 9.7).

Box 9.7 Causes of Rhabdomyolysis

▪ Trauma	▪ Drug induced
● Crush injuries	● Cocaine
● Burns	● Heroin
▪ Muscle injury from overuse	● Barbiturates
▪ Status epilepticus generalized seizures	● Amphetamines
▪ Fever	● Diazepam
▪ Thyroid storm	● Alcohol
▪ Strenuous exercise	● Phencyclidine (PCP)
▪ Delirium tremors	● Lipid-lowering agents (statins)
▪ Ischemic injury to muscle	▪ Infections
● Prolonged immobility	● Sepsis
● Shock states	● Infectious hepatitis
● Arterial occlusion	● Viral influenza
● Postcardiac arrest	● Tetanus

Q Which two serum laboratory tests are frequently obtained to diagnose rhabdomyolysis?

A Myoglobin and creatinine kinase (CK)

Following muscle injury, myoglobin and CK levels will increase. Muscle injury causes an alteration in the cell membrane integrity of the muscle, allowing the intracellular contents to escape into the plasma. Myoglobin and CK are found in skeletal and smooth muscle cells. Other intracellular components include potassium and phosphates and can elevate following muscle injury (Box 9.8).

Box 9.8 Laboratory Values of Rhabdomyolysis

■ Elevated creatinine kinase	■ Hyperphosphatemia
■ Elevated myoglobin	■ Hypocalcemia
■ Hyperkalemia	■ Myoglobinuria

HINT Urine hematest will be positive for hemoglobin, but few or no RBCs are commonly found on urinalysis. The urine hematest is unable to differentiate hemoglobin from myoglobin.

Q What is the primary intervention used to manage rhabdomyolysis?

A Fluid resuscitation

Fluid resuscitation is the primary management used to flush the myoglobin molecules through the kidneys to decrease injury to the renal tubules. Normal saline is the fluid of choice, typically at a rate of 10–15 mL/kg/hour to achieve high urinary flow rates. Mannitol, an osmotic diuretic, can be administered if the patient becomes oliguric. It is used to increase renal perfusion, dilate renal vasculature, and "wash out" tubular debris and toxic wastes.

HINT The goal in managing rhabdomyolysis is maintaining UO greater than 100 mL/hour.

Q What urine pH is the goal when administering sodium bicarbonate to prevent injury in rhabdomyolysis?

A Higher than 6.5

Sodium bicarbonate is used to alkalinize the urine to decrease the nephrotoxicity of myoglobin. It is administered as a continuous infusion to maintain urinary pH higher than 6.5. Side effects of bicarbonates include metabolic alkalosis and hypocalcemia.

HINT Metabolic alkalosis shifts the oxyhemoglobin dissociation curve, causing hemoglobin to hold on to oxygen, resulting in hypoperfusion of tissues.

FUNCTIONAL ISSUES

Q What is considered a mobility complication of intensive care?

A ICU-acquired weakness

With the improvement of survivability in the ICU after prolonged intensive care and multisystem organ failure, there is now an increase in mobility complications post ICU. There is a high prevalence in post ICU patients that were ventilated for greater than 48 hours and even higher with multiple organ involvement. Pre-ICU comorbidities play a role in post ICU ability to function.

HINT ICU patients who have received paralytic agents and steroids are also known to be at a greater risk for ICU-acquired weakness or myelopathies.

▶ PATHOPHYSIOLOGY

Q What are two assessment tools used frequently in the ICU to limit ICU-acquired weakness after mechanical ventilation?

A Sedation and delirium tools

The level of sedation during mechanical ventilation can contribute to post ICU muscle weakness and fatigability. Sedation monitoring tools, such as RASS, can assist with the management of patient's sedation to prevent over-sedating with mechanical ventilation. Awakening the patient daily has also been found useful in preventing over-sedation. The presence of delirium has also been found to influence the length of time on a ventilator and the recovery from a critical illness. Assessment may include the use of the CAM-ICU tool to assess for delirium.

HINT   Over-sedation and development of delirium are two risk factors for prolonged mechanical ventilation contributing to the ICU-acquired weakness.

▶ SYMPTOMS/ASSESSMENT

Q What patient factor contributes the most to falls in critical care patients?

A Confused patients

Confused and agitated patients are the highest risk patients for falls in the ICU. As sedation is reduced or the patient develops delirium, the risk for falling significantly increases. RASS and CAM-ICU scores can be used to evaluate their risk for falls as well as fall risk tools. (Box 9.9)

Box 9.9 Risk Factors for Falls in ICU

■ Age-related risks (vision, gait instability)	■ Balance issues
■ Delirium	■ Alcohol withdrawal
■ Agitation	■ Illegal drugs
■ Urinary incontinence	■ Dementia
■ Polypharmacy	■ Motor weakness

▶ DIAGNOSIS

Q What is a common method for determining function in acute care patients?

A Ability to participate in ADLs

Evaluation is complex and is influenced by multiple factors (Box 9.10). One of the more common methods for evaluating a patient's function is to assess their ability to participate in activities of daily living (ADLs). There are two other frameworks used to evaluate the patient's functional abilities, including actual physical impairment of the body and performance-based measures such as sitting and walking.

Box 9.10 Evaluation of Function

■ Strength	■ Balance
■ Range of motion	■ Stability in gait
■ Proprioception	■ Cognition
■ Level of alertness	■ Psychosocial
■ Ability to follow commands	

HINT Motivation (psychosocial) plays a significant role in being able to assess as well as improve function after ICU.

▶ MANAGEMENT

> **Q** What is a nursing intervention that can be utilized to lower the risk of falls in ICU patients?
>
> **A** See Box 9.11

Majority of patient falls occur in the patient's room or bathroom.

Box 9.11 Interventions to Reduce Falls

■ Call light and personal items within reach of patient	■ Nonslip footwear
■ Bed lowest position	■ Night lights
■ Handrails in bathroom and hallways	■ Floor surface dry
■ Hospital beds and chairs locked	■ Remove clutter from the room
■ Use of bed and chair alarms	■ Pain, sedation, and delirium assessments
■ Frequent reorientation	■ Frequent rounding
■ Provide fall prevention education to patients and families	■ Side rails up for sedated patients
■ Limit use of restraints	■ Maintain all lines and tubing from tangling the patient
■ Perform fall risk assessments	■ Identify high fall risk patients in a huddle
■ Use of gait belts while ambulating	■ High-risk medication assessment
■ Toileting regimens	

▶ COMPLICATIONS

> **Q** What is a risk factor for an increased severity of injury if an ICU patient falls?
>
> **A** Anticoagulation therapy

Different severity of injuries can occur with patient falls, anywhere from a bruise to death. Certain risk factors place patients at higher risk for greater severity of injury (Box 9.12). Injury reduction is an aim in hospitals as well as fall prevention.

HINT Floor mats around the bed may not prevent a fall but can limit injury from the fall.

Box 9.12 Factors Increase Risk for Injury

■ Age (>85)
■ Pre-morbid orthopedic conditions
■ Anticoagulated state
■ Recent surgery

1. Which of the following is the most common causative microorganism of osteomyelitis?

   A. *Haemophilus influenza*
   B. *Enterococcus*
   C. *Escherichia coli*
   D. *Staphylocccus aureus*

2. Following a crush injury to your patient's lower extremity, which of the following labs would be most important?

   A. WBC count
   B. Sodium
   C. Creatinine kinase (CK)
   D. Procalcitonin

3. What is the main purpose of placing pelvic external fixators on a trauma patient?

   A. Long-term fracture management
   B. Control blood loss
   C. Decrease pain
   D. Allows early mobility

4. What is a common fracture of an elderly person following a fall?

   A. Femoral head fracture
   B. Open pelvic fracture
   C. Femur fracture
   D. Wrist fracture

5. The nurse suspects the patient has rhabdomyolysis. Which laboratory findings would support this diagnosis?

   A. Potassium 3.6 mmol/L, phosphorous 4.9 mg/dL, calcium 8 mg/dL
   B. Creatinine kinase 18,000 U/L, myoglobin 80 ng/mL, potassium 6.0 mmol/L
   C. Myoglobin 70 ng/mL, phosphorous 4.5 mg/dL, myoglobinuria
   D. Calcium 11 mg/dL, creatinine kinase 1,000 U/L, myoglobin 30 ng/mL

1. D) *S. aureus*

S. aureus often cause skin infections, which can migrate to bone from adjacent soft tissue or vascular. *H. influenza* is a gram-negative responsible for pneumonia and meningitis. *E. coli* is a gram-negative bacteria commonly found in the lower GI tract. It commonly causes urinary tract infections. Enterococcus is also commonly found in the GI tract but is a gram-positive. It can wound infections but is not as common as *S. aureus*.

2. C) Creatinine kinase (CK)

Creatinine kinase (CK) levels will elevate in patients with crush injuries due to the release of CK from the muscle when injured. Potassium can also elevate following crush injuries due to the release of intracellular components, including potassium. Sodium is not a concern with crush injuries. WBC and procalcitonin are more to evaluate for infection or inflammation.

3. B) Control blood loss

An external fixator is frequently used to stabilize pelvic fractures and limit blood loss. Therapeutic embolization in interventional radiology is also used to control hemorrhage associated with pelvic fractures. Internal fixation of the pelvis is the long term management for the pelvic fracture. Stabilizing the pelvis can decrease pain, but that is not the main purpose of placement. External fixators will not allow for early mobility.

4. A) Femoral head fracture

Fractures of the femoral neck of the hip are common in elderly patients with falls. The fracture may actually have caused their fall versus the fracture occurring due to the fall.

5. B) Creatinine kinase 18,000 U/L, myoglobin 80 ng/mL, potassium 6.0 mmol/L

Laboratory values of rhabdomyolysis include elevated creatinine kinase (normal range is 22–198 U/L), elevate myoglobin (the normal range is 25–72 ng/mL), hyperkalemia (normal range if 3.6 to 5.2 mmol/L), hyperphosphatemia (normal range is 2.5–4.5 mg/dL), myoglobinuria, and hypocalcemia (normal range is 8.6–10.3 mg/dL). The hallmark of rhabdomyolysis is an elevation in creatine kinase. Serum creatine kinase levels are usually at least five times normal and range from approximately 1,500 to over 100,000 U/L.

BIBLIOGRAPHY

Groll, M., Woods, T., & Salcido, R. (2018). Osteomyelitis: A context for wound management. *Advances in Skin & Wound Care, 31*(6), 253–262.

Parry, S., Huang, M., & Needham, D. (2017). Evaluating physical function in critical care: considerations for clinical practice and research. *Crit Care, 21,* 249.

Neurological System Review

> ▶ **LEARNING OBJECTIVES**

In this chapter, you will review:

- ▪ Stroke
    - Ischemic (embolic)
    - Hemorrhagic
    - Transient ischemic attack (TIA)
- ▪ Hemorrhage
    - Subarachnoid
    - Intracranial (ICH)
    - Intraventricular
- ▪ Seizure disorders
- ▪ Traumatic brain injury
- ▪ Acute spinal cord injury
- ▪ Brain death
- ▪ Neurological infectious diseases
- ▪ Neuromuscular disorders
- ▪ Hydrocephalus
- ▪ Delirium
- ▪ Dementia
- ▪ Encephalopathy
- ▪ Space occupying lesions
- ▪ Neurosurgery
- ▪ Testable nursing actions:
    - Intracranial pressure (ICP) monitoring and lumbar drains
    - Neurovascular interventions

● STROKE: ISCHEMIC

Q What differentiates a transient ischemic attack (TIA) from a stroke?

A Early resolution of symptoms

A stroke occurs following loss of blood flow to an area of the brain resulting in ischemic injuries and permanent cerebral infarction. TIAs are brief episodes of neurological dysfunction resulting from focal cerebral ischemia not associated with permanent cerebral infarction (Table 10.1).

HINT TIAs are considered a medical emergency and associated with a high risk for stroke.

Table 10.1 Comparison of Thrombotic and Embolic Strokes

	Thrombotic	Embolic
Pathophysiology	Atherosclerotic plaque narrows lumen of the cerebral vessel; plaque ruptures and causes thrombus from obstructing blood flow distally; common vessels include internal carotid and vertebrals	The clot originates typically in the right atrium and is thrown in to the cerebral circulation; the clot obstructs smaller vessels resulting in loss of blood flow distally; the most common location is the middle cerebral artery (MCA); other causes include patent foramen ovale, septic emboli
Presentation	Tends to have a progressive worsening of symptoms; associated more commonly with TIAs	Typically abrupt onset without progression of symptoms
Timing	May occur at rest or prior to awakening	May occur following activity or exercise

▶ PATHOPHYSIOLOGY

Q What is the term used in strokes to indicate the ischemic (reversible injury) zone?

A Penumbra

The penumbra is the reversible ischemic zone in the area of the ischemia. Injury can be reversed if perfusion is reestablished, decreasing the size of the infarction. The core is the infarction zone and is irreversible injury.

HINT   The ratio of the penumbra to the core is used in determining need for administering thrombolytic or performing thrombectomy.

Q What is hemorrhagic transformation in ischemic stroke?

A Bleeding into the core

Hemorrhagic transformation is considered to be a natural evolution of an ischemic stroke and is usually asymptomatic. Computed tomography (CT) scans following an acute ischemic stroke and especially after reperfusion can demonstrate hemorrhage in the infracted (core) area of the brain.

HINT   Because the bleeding tends to occur within the infracted zone (irreversible injury), it is usually asymptomatic.

▶ SYMPTOMS/ASSESSMENT

Q What does F.A.S.T. stand for when teaching symptoms of a stroke?

A Face, arms, speech, and time

Facial and arm weakness along with speech abnormalities are common symptoms of a stroke. Time reminds the public to call 911 immediately when symptoms occur (Box 10.1).

HINT   These are signs of an anterior circulation stroke and are more recognizable than posterior circulation stroke.

Box 10.1 Symptoms of Stroke

Ataxia	Alteration behavior
Aphasia	Visual field cuts/visual changes
Facial palsy	Agnosia
Neglect syndrome	Deviated gaze

(continued)

Box 10.1 Symptoms of Stroke (*continued*)

Cranial nerves (CN) palsies	Dysarthria
Paresis/paralysis	Dysphasia
Loss or altered sensation	Nystagmus
Changes in level of consciousness (LOC)	"Locked in" syndrome
Dizziness/vertigo	Memory loss

Q **What is a nontraditional symptom of a stroke?**

A **Shortness of breath**

Sudden pain or numbness in the face, arms, or legs, changes in mental status, generalized neurological symptoms (hiccupping, nausea, and vomiting [N&V]), sudden chest pain or palpitations, sudden tiredness, and shortness of breath are all nontraditional symptoms of a stroke. Shortness of breath is the most common.

HINT   Asymptomatic signs are more common in women, similar to cardiac.

Q **What is the neurological assessment tool used to determine the severity of the stroke?**

A **National Institute of Health Stroke Scale (NIHSS)**

NIHSS is a tool used by healthcare providers to objectively quantify the impairment caused by a stroke. On the scale, the greater number correlates to higher severity of the stroke.

HINT   NIHSS is more accurate in identifying anterior strokes and less accurate with posterior strokes.

▶ DIAGNOSIS

Q **Which radiographic study is the initial diagnostic study ordered in patients with signs of stroke?**

A **Noncontrast CT scan**

Even though the actual infarct may not be recognized on a CT scan until after 12–24 hours, the CT scan can be used to rule out hemorrhagic strokes and other causes of neurological deterioration. Some of the disorders that may mimic an ischemic stroke include: postictal state following a seizure, central nervous system (CNS) infections, intracerebral tumor, toxic–metabolic disturbances, hypoglycemia or hyperglycemia, hemorrhagic stroke, and subdural hematoma (SDH).

Q **Which studies are used to identify the ratio of penumbra to core?**

A **CT perfusion scan**

Newer imaging modalities are available incomprehensive stroke centers that use CT prefusion, MR diffusion-weighted imagery (DWI), and perfusion-weighted imagery (PWI), which will identify ischemic strokes earlier and have the ability to differentiate between reversible and irreversible injuries.

HINT   The newer magnetic resonance imaging (MRI) capability with flair may be used to determine candidates for thrombolytic therapy without a last known normal (LKN).

Q **When obtaining a recent history of symptoms, what is the single most important historical information to be obtained?**

A **Last known normal (LKN)**

The clock starts for thrombolytic therapy when the patient was at his or her previous baseline or symptom free. It is the time of onset of symptoms or when the patient was last known to be normal.

HINT   In obtaining history, it is important to determine LKN and/or onset of symptoms.

▶ MANAGEMENT

> **Q** Which of the following patient scenarios would be a candidate for thrombolytic therapy? Patient A woke up with facial drooping and upper extremity paresis. Patient B had facial drooping and upper extremity paresis 6 hours ago, which completely resolved, but he now presents in the emergency department (ED) within 30 minutes of onset of slurred speech and ataxia.
>
> **A** Patient B

The symptoms of stroke found on awakening are called "wake-up" stroke and are *not* considered to be a candidate for thrombolytics because the actual onset of the symptoms is unclear (the patient was asleep at the time) without MRI to identify flair. But if a patient reports symptoms of a stroke, which resolved completely, the time is reset (i.e., the patient is back to baseline). The onset of symptoms reoccurring is used as LKN.

HINT   This is considered to be a TIA and symptoms reoccurring would be the start of treatable stroke.

> **Q** In which situation would you allow a patient with ischemic stroke to remain hypertensive for the first 24 hours without treating for high blood pressure (BP)?
>
> **A** A patient with ischemic stroke who is *not* a candidate for thrombolytic therapy

If the patient is not a candidate for thrombolytic therapy and a hemorrhagic stroke has been ruled out, then the recommendation is to monitor BP unless systolic is greater than 220 mmHg or diastolic is greater than 120 mmHg. If the patient is a candidate for thrombolytic therapy, then the systolic BP is kept lower than 180 mmHg.

HINT   The test question may present a hypertensive stroke patient with time of onset of symptoms in the scenario and then ask how you would manage BP. First, determine whether or not the patient would be a candidate for thrombolytics.

> **Q** Within how many hours from onset of symptoms is it recommended to administer an intravenous (IV) thrombolytic in an ischemic stroke patient?
>
> **A** 3–4.5 hours

Based on the American Heart Association (AHA)/American Stroke Association (ASA) guidelines, the time can be expanded to 4.5 hours in some patients, but the goal is still within 3 hours of onset.

HINT   If it is a large vessel obstruction (LVO), mechanical thrombectomy may be performed up to 24 hours after LKN in certain circumstances.

> **Q** What is the most common time frame used for initiating mechanical thrombectomy following onset of neurological symptoms?
>
> **A** 6 hours

Endovascular therapy may also be used to recanalize and reperfuse the brain. The recommended time window following onset of symptoms for reperfusion with endovascular therapy is 6 hours. This time window can be extended if certain radiographic criteria is met.

HINT   The window expansion is based upon the volume of penumbra compared to core.

> **Q** What is always the priority of care for any stroke patient?
>
> **A** Airway and breathing

Airway and breathing is always a priority of care. Other management concerns include glucose levels, swallow evaluation, and temperature control.

HINT   Questions on the exam asking about priority of care should always consider airway and breathing as the correct answer.

PREVENTION OF ISCHEMIC STROKES

Primary stroke prevention is to prevent a stroke from occurring. Secondary stroke prevention is to prevent a stroke patient from having a recurrent stroke.

> **Q What class of medication is recommended in primary thrombotic stroke prevention?**
>
> **A Antiplatelet**

The recommended drug therapy is an aspirin (81–100 mg) a day for high-risk patients. Aspirin is not recommended for low-risk patients. An (HMG-CoA) reductase inhibitor (statin) medication is also recommended in patients with heart disease or in certain high-risk people.

HINT Clopidogrel may be used instead of aspirin if the patient has an aspirin allergy.

> **Q What class of medication is recommended in secondary thrombotic stroke prevention?**
>
> **A Antiplatelet**

Antiplatelet drugs are preferred to oral anticoagulation therapy. Other recommendations include antihypertensive medications to manage hypertensive patients and statin therapy. The recommendations include aspirin, combination aspirin/diyridamole (Aggrenox), or clopidogrel (Plavix monotherapy).

> **Q Which of the ischemic strokes is the most preventable?**
>
> **A Cardioembolic stroke**

Atrial fibrillation (AF) is the most common cause of embolic strokes and is also the most preventable type of stroke. Anticoagulation therapy is recommended for stroke prevention in this population. Warfarin (Coumadin) is the most commonly used drug. Direct thrombin inhibitors, such as dabigatran (Pradaxa) and Factor Xa inhibitors (Eliquis, Xarelto), may also be used to prevent a secondary cardioembolic stroke.

HINT Questions may include how to monitor the anticoagulation effect of these medications and recognize the complication of a hemorrhagic stroke (ICH).

▶ COMPLICATIONS

> **Q What consultation needs to be obtained to evaluate a stroke patient's risk of aspiration?**
>
> **A Speech therapy**

Swallowing difficulties and abnormal gag reflexes are common complications of a stroke. A speech therapist should perform a swallow evaluation prior to feeding a patient who has had a stroke to prevent aspiration (Box 10.2).

HINT Bedside swallow exam performed by the nurse is a screening evaluation to determine the need for more inclusive evaluation by a speech therapist.

Box 10.2 Complications of Stroke

Paresis/paralysis	Personality and mood changes
Speech problems	Depression
Swallowing difficulties	Dementia
Loss of independence	Shortened life span
Cognitive abnormalities	

⬤ STROKE: HEMORRHAGIC

Q Which type of hemorrhagic stroke is caused by an aneurysm rupture?

A Subarachnoid hemorrhage (SAH)

SAH is caused by rupture of an aneurysm or arterial venous malformation (AVM) with bleeding into the subarachnoid space. Spontaneous intracerebral hemorrhagic (ICH) stroke is caused by a ruptured cerebral blood vessel with bleeding into the brain tissue (parenchymal hemorrhage) (Table 10.2 and Box 10.3). Intraventricular hemorrhage is bleeding within the ventricles.

Table 10.2 Comparison of ICH and SAH

	ICH	SAH
Cause	Most common causes are hypertension, oral anticoagulation therapy, coagulopathies	Most common causes are rupture of aneurysm, rupture of AVM, trauma
Location of bleed	Primarily into brain tissue (parenchyma) and intraventricles (called extension)	Primarily into subarachnoid space and intraventricular space
Presentation	Headache, vomiting, hypertension, decreased level of consciousness, seizures	"Worst headache of my life," vomiting, focal neurological deficits, decreased level of consciousness (LOC)

ICH, intracerebral hemorrhage; SAH, subarachnoid hemorrhage.

Box 10.3 Common Locations for Spontaneous Intracerebral Hemorrhage (ICH)

Putamin (basal ganglia) 35%–50%	Cerebellar 5%–12%
Lobar 30%	Pontine 5%–12%
Thalamic 10%–15%	

▶ PATHOPHYSIOLOGY

Q Does a hypertensive ICH expand in size after the initial bleed?

A Yes

Rupture of the intracerebal vessel leads to accumulation of blood in the parenchyma of the brain with substantial increases in hematoma size for up to 24 hours from the initial bleed.

This increase in clot volume has been shown to be associated with clinical neurological deterioration.

HINT Lowering and managing BP early can decrease the hematoma growth and improve neurological outcomes.

Q What is commonly found surrounding an intracerebral hemorrhage?

A Cerebral edema

The bleeding causes disruption of the brain tissue. The resultant clot compresses the adjacent tissue and is followed by development of extracellular (vasogenic) cerebral edema in the periphery of the hematoma. The blood clot and the cerebral edema lead to an increase in ICP with a potential for fatal herniation syndromes. High BP can increase the volume of cerebral edema.

HINT Vasogenic cerebral edema is interstitial edema while cytotoxic cerebral edema is intracellular (Box 10.4).

Box 10.4 Pathophysiology of Cerebral Injury Following ICH

Cerebral edema
Disruption of brain tissue
Space-occupying lesion
Elevation of ICP
Fatal herniation syndromes

Q **What is the most common cause of a spontaneous ICH?**

A **Hypertension**

Hypertension is the most common cause of ICH and chronic hypertension can result in ischemic strokes, typically presenting as lacunar strokes (Box 10.5).

Box 10.5 Causes of ICH

Cerebral vasculitis
Central venous thrombosis
Vascular tumors
Coagulopathies
Anticoagulation/antiplatelet therapy
Sympathomimetic drugs
Arteriopathy
Hemorrhagic transformation ischemic strokes
Trauma
Vascular anomalies

▶ RISK FACTORS

Q **Who is at the highest risk for an ischemic stroke, an African American male or a White female?**

A **African American male**

Nonmodifiable risks include gender and race. Men have a greater risk than women for strokes. African Americans have a higher risk for stroke than Caucasians (Box 10.6).

HINT   Over the age of 85, there is a greater prevalence of strokes in women than men. This is due to the fact that women tend to live longer than men.

Box 10.6 Risk Factors for Hemorrhagic Stroke

Race (higher in African Americans)
Gender (higher in male)
Age (risk increases over the age of 55)
Hypertension
Cigarette smoking
Alcohol ingestion (dose related)
Genetics

▶ SYMPTOMS/ASSESSMENT

Case: A patient presents with sudden-onset headache and associated nausea and vomiting. Symptoms began when the patient was mowing the yard. On further assessment, it was noted that the patient was confused and had a decreasing level of consciousness (LOC).

Q Which of the above symptoms would be a red flag that this patient is experiencing an ICH?

A Sudden-onset headache associated with nausea and vomiting

The classic clinical presentation includes the onset of a sudden focal neurological deficit, commonly a headache or altered LOC, which progresses over minutes to hours. Other symptoms include nausea and vomiting, seizures, and focal neurological deficits. Onset usually occurs with activity and rarely occurs at night.

HINT Vomiting is more common with ICH than with either ischemic stroke. Symptoms rarely occur at night, whereas patients with ischemic strokes frequently awaken with symptoms.

▶ DIAGNOSIS

Q What diagnostic test would you expect the managing clinician to order on the above patient?

A Noncontrast CT scan

A noncontrast CT scan will locate the hemorrhage and determine the size and possible etiology. CT scans are considered superior to MRIs for the diagnosis of acute ICH. The volume of the hemorrhage can be estimated and is important for the prognosis.

HINT ICH score can be used to predict outcomes.

Q What associated finding on the CT scan would indicate a poor prognosis in ICH?

A Intraventricular extension

This occurs when the vessel located near the ventricles ruptures and the tissue loss occurs through the ventricular wall. Bleeding then occurs into the intraventricular system, resulting in damage to the ventricles and development of hydrocephalus.

▶ MEDICAL MANAGEMENT

Q What is the priority of care following an ICH?

A Airway and breathing

The focus of caring for a stroke patient is rapid identification, diagnosis, and management, although airway and breathing should always remain a priority. Patients with ICH have a higher risk for airway involvement due to altered mentation.

HINT Airway and breathing are always a priority of care in a patient with a decrease in LOC.

Q Following an ICH, what is the goal for BP management?

A Systolic BP less than 160 mmHg

The amount of BP control has not been established but a decrease in systolic BP to less than 160 mmHg is reasonable. Systolic BP is frequently maintained in the range of 130–150 mmHg. This range may decrease the risk of hypertensive extension of the bleed but it allows for improved cerebral perfusion.

HINT BP is frequently controlled with a titratable agent to balance the risk of hypotensive ischemia and hypertension-related rebleeding (Table 10.3).

Table 10.3 Intravenous Medications That May Be Considered for
Control of Elevated Blood Pressure in Patients With ICH

Drugs	Loading Dose	Continuous Infusion Dose
Labetalol	5–20 mg every 15 minutes	2 mg/minute (maximum 300 mg/d)
Nicardipine	NA	5–15 mg/hour
Hydralazine	5–20 mg IVP every 30 minutes	1.5–5 μ/kg/minute

Q It has been determined that the cause of an ICH is anticoagulation therapy with warfarin. What would you expect the patient to receive to reverse the bleeding?

A IV vitamin K and prothrombin complex concentrate

Management of patients presenting with ICH who are anticoagulated is to reverse or correct the coagulopathy. Prothrombin complex concentrates (e.g., KCentra) are recommended for patients on warfarin for more rapid reversal of the coagulopathy. Vitamin K is administered with the PCC due to the shorter half-life of the PCC. Other reversal agents include protamine sulfate (heparin), AndexXa (Xarelto and Eliquis), Praxbind (Dabigatran), and platelets (platelet inhibitor drugs). Management of ICH also includes treating increased ICP and protecting the brain from further injury (Box 10.7).

HINT PCC reverse the coagulopathy while the other reversal agents only reverse the specific drug itself.

Box 10.7 Other Management Therapies for ICH

Treat an increased ICP
Administer antiepileptic medications
Manage hyperglycemia (>185 mg/dL and possibly >140 mg/dL) with insulin
Treat fever with antipyretic medications

▶ SURGICAL MANAGEMENT

Q What is the location in the brain for a hemorrhage that is considered the most amenable for surgery?

A Cerebellum

Cerebellar hemorrhage more than 3 cm or a rapidly deteriorating clinical status. Surgical approaches include craniotomy with clot evacuation, stereotactic aspiration with the use of thrombolytic agents, and endoscopic evacuation. Overall, most patients with ICH will not benefit from surgery. The routine evacuation of supratentorial ICH by standard craniotomy is not recommended.

HINT Surgical options depend on the location and size of the hematoma.

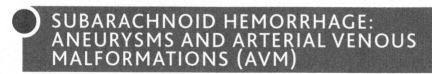

SUBARACHNOID HEMORRHAGE: ANEURYSMS AND ARTERIAL VENOUS MALFORMATIONS (AVM)

▶ PATHOPHYSIOLOGY

Q What is an aneurysm called that is round with a neck and typically located at a bifurcation?

A Sacular aneurysm

Aneurysms are classified by their shape and size. A sacular or "berry" aneurysm is round, has a neck, and is frequently found in a bifurcation or branching vessel. A fusiform aneurysm has an outpouching of the arterial wall without a neck and can occur anywhere along the vessel.

HINT   A giant aneurysm measures 2.5 cm or larger and presents with symptoms of a space lesion.

> **Q** What is the type of intracranial aneurysm caused by septic emboli commonly associated with bacterial endocarditis?
>
> **A** Mycotic aneurysm

A mycotic aneurysm is due to an infectious source. The most common source is a bacterial endocarditis.

> **Q** What is a system of dilated vessels that shunts arterial blood directly into the venous system without the capillary network?
>
> **A** AVM

AVMs are composed of the nidus, which is a fairly well-circumscribed center, as well as the feeding arteries and draining veins. Rupture of the aneurysm or AVM is frequently associated with an activity causing an increase in BP. The rupture results in bleeding, primarily into subarachnoid space, but also bleeding into the subdural or intracerebral tissue.

HINT   SAH is more commonly caused by an aneurysm rupture.

> **Q** What is the most common site of an intracerebral aneurysm?
>
> **A** Circle of Willis

This is because of all of the bifurcations and branches in the Circle of Willis. The anterior circulation accounts for 85% of the aneurysm and the posterior circulation (vertebral and basilar arteries) account for 15%.

▶ SYMPTOMS/ASSESSMENT

> **Q** What is the most common sign of an SAH?
>
> **A** Headache

Headache in SAH is frequently described as "the worst headache of my life" (Box 10.8). Warning signs are present in about 50% of the bleeds (Box 10.9). The SAH is graded on the severity of the presenting signs and symptoms.

HINT   Warning signs may present days to weeks before the rupture and is usually a headache.

Box 10.8 Other Symptoms of SAH

Loss of consciousness or change in level of consciousness	Pupillary changes Stiff and painful neck
Cranial nerve deficits (especially CN III)	Positive Kernig's and Brudzinski's signs
Visual disturbance Hemiparesis or hemiplegia	Photophobia Possible temperature elevation
Vomiting	

Box 10.9 Warning Signs of SAH

Lethargy	Cranial nerve dysfunction
Localized headache	Audible bruits
Neck pain	

Q What is the grading system most commonly used following an SAH?

A Hunt and Hess

Hunt and Hess grading is based upon clinical presentation. Grade I is minimal symptoms and grade V is the worst presentation (Box 10.10).

Box 10.10 Hunt and Hess Grading System

Grade I	Asymptomatic, mild headache, slight nuchal rigidity
Grade II	Moderate to severe headache, nuchal rigidity, no neurologic deficit other than cranial nerve palsy
Grade III	Drowsiness/confusion, mild focal neurologic deficit
Grade IV	Stupor, moderate to severe hemiparesis
Grade V	Coma, decerebrate posturing

▶ DIAGNOSIS

Q What is the initial diagnostic test for SAH?

A Noncontrast CT scan

A noncontrast CT scan is the initial diagnostic test used to screen patients presenting with headache and neurological deficits. A CT scan demonstrating a SAH indicates the need for follow-up angiography.

HINT CT angiogram may be performed, but the best diagnostic is an invasive angiogram.

Q What is the most life-threatening complication within the first 24 hours following an aneurysm rupture?

A Rebleeding

The peak incidence of a rebleed occurs within the first 24–48 hours. Securing the aneurysm with coils or clips will significantly lower the risk of rebleeding (Box 10.11).

HINT Earlier intervention is recommended to prevent rebleeding and higher mortalities.

Box 10.11 Interventions to Prevent Rebleeding (Subarachnoid Precautions)

Prevent hypertension
Avoid straining
Manage anxiety or pain
Bed rest
Quiet room
Decrease physical stimulation

▶ MEDICAL MANAGEMENT

Q Which medication is started on day one following a SAH?

A Nimodipine (Nimotop)

Nimodipine is a calcium channel blocker, which is more specific to cerebral vasculature. It is initiated the first day following the admission for SAH and is continued for 14–21 days. The primary purpose is to improve neurological outcomes following vasospasms. It increases blood flow through collateral circulation and is a neuroprotectant.

HINT Nimodipine does not prevent vasospasms but can improve neurological outcomes.

> **Q** If clinical vasospasms occur, what is the primary treatment?
>
> **A** Hypertension

Hypertension and volume expansion are used to open the cerebral vessels and improve perfusion in VS. An interventional neurologist may use angioplasty and intra-arterial antihypertensives to open the vessels in an attempt to reperfuse the brain.

HINT Triple "H" therapy is not recommended. Hypervolemia can worsen the cerebral edema and cause cardiovascular complications with volume overload.

▶ SURGICAL MANAGEMENT

> **Q** What SAH complication is managed early with an external ventriculostomy drain (EVD)?
>
> **A** Hydrocephalus

One of the main causes of early decreased mentation is the rapid development of hydrocephalus. This excessive CSF is due to the blood in subarachnoid space blocking reabsorption of the CSF through the arachnoid villi.

HINT EVDs are frequently placed early in the management of SAH.

> **Q** What is the surgical management of an intracerebral aneurysm?
>
> **A** Surgical clipping

Surgical clipping of the neck of the aneurysm has been the primary treatment of intracerebral aneurysms prior to interventional therapy. Interventional therapy is used most often to secure intracerebral aneurysms by coiling the aneurysm. Certain locations and morphology of the aneurysm is more amendable with surgical clips.

HINT Coiling or clipping of the aneurysm will secure it to prevent rebleeding.

> **Q** What is the most preferred method of managing AVM?
>
> **A** Embolization

AVM is composed of multiple arteries feeding into to one or two draining veins without capillaries in between. Embolization of the feeding arteries will decrease the size of the AVM. After multiple treatments, the AVM may be resected surgically.

HINT Surgical resection without decreasing blood supply over time can result in postoperative massive cerebral edema.

▶ COMPLICATIONS

> **Q** Your patient is 7 days post-SAH. During the day, he has a sudden decrease in LOC. Which complication is the most likely cause?
>
> **A** Vasospasms (VS)

VS is defined as the focal narrowing of the cerebral arteries. It most commonly occurs within 7–10 days following a SAH. Symptoms of VS can be any neurological deficit. Transcranial Doppler studies are performed frequently during high-risk time period. Diagnosis is confirmed with angiography but can worsen the spasm (Box 10.12).

HINT Questions frequently use the number of days after an SAH to determine the cause of a neurological change.

Box 10.12 Complications of SAH

Rebleeding
Cerebral edema
Hydrocephalus
Hyponatremia
Cerebral vasospasms

SEIZURE DISORDERS

Q What is an abnormal excessive neuronal discharge in the brain called?

A Epileptic seizure

Epileptic seizure is a transient symptom due to an abnormal excessive neuronal discharge. This definition allows for differentiation of epileptic seizures from other seizures that may not be epileptic in nature and may be accompanied by convulsions. Epilepsy is a disorder of the brain characterized by an enduring predisposition to generate epileptic seizures. Definitions of epilepsy typically include the occurrence of more than one epileptic seizure. Status epilepticus (SE) is a condition of recurrent seizures or continuous seizure activity without return to normal function (a seizure lasting > 5 minutes).

HINT   Refractory SE occurs when the seizure does not respond to two different antiepileptic medications within 20 minutes.

Q What is it called when the electroencephalogram (EEG) findings indicate seizure activity without the motor movements of a convulsive seizure?

A Nonconvulsive status epilepticus (NCSE)

NCSE is a type of status epilepticus in which the patient does not exhibit any motor movements, but the brain could be experiencing abnormal excessive neuronal activities of an epileptic seizure. It is suspected in patients with altered mental status and can be diagnosed with a continuous EEG monitor. NCSE is frequently found in patients after a generalized seizure. Any patient who is slow to awaken or remains unresponsive after a convulsive generalized seizure should have an EEG performed.

HINT   Following ICH in unresponsive patients, it is recommended an EEG is performed before considering terminal extubation.

▶ PATHOPHYSIOLOGY

Q Which lobe of the brain is most commonly involved in initiating the neuronal discharge?

A Temporal Lobe

The temporal lobe is the most common cerebral lobe involved in seizure activity. All neurological disorders can increase the risk of a seizure (Box 10.13). Other causes of epilepsy include genetic defects or metabolic disorders of the brain.

Box 10.13 List of Common Neurological Risk Factors of Seizures

Traumatic brain injury	Infectious CNS disorders
Subdural hematomas	Hypoxic or anoxic brain injuries
Brain tumors	Subarachnoid hemorrhage
Ischemic strokes	Neurodegenerative disorders
Hemorrhagic strokes	Antiepileptic medication or alcohol withdrawal

> **Q** What are three electrolyte abnormalities that can cause a seizure?
>
> **A** Hyponatremia, hypocalcemia, hypoglycemia

Electrolyte abnormalities can result in seizure activity and need to be monitored closely. Electrolyte abnormalities, hyponatremia, hypocalcemia, and hypoglycemia are the three most commonly found electrolyte abnormalities to cause seizures. Hypomagesium and hypernatremia may also cause seizures.

HINT The question may start with a scenario about a patient with an electrolyte abnormality, such as hyponatremia, and lead to questions on seizures.

> **Q** What is the name of the classification of a seizure in which the neuronal discharge is localized to an area of the brain?
>
> **A** Partial seizure

Seizures are classified as partial (focal) or generalized seizures. Generalized seizures have a neuronal discharge occurring within and rapidly engaging bilateral hemispheres. Partial seizures have a neuronal discharge that initiates in one focal site and is limited to one hemisphere. Partial seizures are further divided into simple partial or complex partial seizures. The difference between a simple and a complex partial seizure is the awareness and recall of the seizures.

HINT It is an important nursing assessment to note the patient's awareness during the seizure and whether the patient has any recall of the seizure afterward (Box 10.14).

Box 10.14 Types of Seizures

Partial Seizure	Generalized Seizure
Focal motor	Tonic–clonic (in any combination)
Jacksonian march	Absence
Somatosensory	Myoclonic
Fencer's position	Clonic
Affective	Tonic
Automatisms	Atonic
Psychic	
Postural	

> **Q** A patient may have an aura before a seizure. What seizure classification is an aura?
>
> **A** Simple partial seizure

An aura is a distinct sensory or motor event that precedes a generalized seizure. It is frequently a somatosensory simple partial seizure. Partial seizures can progress to generalized seizures.

HINT A generalized seizure preceded by an aura will typically be managed as a partial seizure.

> **Q** What is the period immediately following a seizure called?
>
> **A** Postictal

Following a seizure, the patient is usually postictal. This time usually involves prolonged sleep or rest. The patient may experience severe headache and muscle aches after muscle severe tonic-clonic contractions. The assessment of airway and breathing is important.

HINT Placing the patient in a lateral position can prevent aspiration if vomiting occurs during or after a seizure.

> **Q** After a seizure, your patient experiences a temporary blindness. What is this called?
>
> **A** Todd's paralysis

Todd's paralysis is a temporary neurological deficit, commonly a paralysis or blindness, which resolves itself spontaneously. It may last from minutes to hours after the motor seizure.

HINT   Todd's paralysis can also be a stroke mimic if the seizure is unwitnessed.

> **Q** Your patient is experiencing symptoms of seizure activity, but the EEG remains negative. What is this called?
>
> **A** Nonepileptic seizure

Nonepileptic seizures have been also been called "pseudoseizures" in the past. Seizure activity with a negative EEG can be conversion, a psychiatric disorder, or may also be fabricated seizure.

HINT   A deep cortical seizure may not demonstrate epileptic activity to surface electrodes and can be missed.

▶ SYMPTOMS/ASSESSMENT

See Box 10.15.

Box 10.15 Obtaining History of Patient's Seizures

Description of past seizures
Frequency of seizures
Seizure patterns
Precipitant of seizure
Current antiepileptic drug (AED)
Compliance status

▶ DIAGNOSIS

> **Q** What is the diagnostic test used to differentiate an epileptic seizure from nonepileptic activity?
>
> **A** EEG

An EEG is the diagnostic test of choice to recognize epileptic seizure. The most accurate result is an EEG obtained during the seizure. Accuracy decreases the farther we get from the seizure event. CT or MRI scans may be used to identify underlying pathology that would cause the seizure.

HINT   Continuous video EEG can be used to diagnose the type of seizure activity.

▶ MANAGEMENT

> **Q** What is the preferred first-line antiepileptic agent (AED) used to stop a seizure?
>
> **A** Lorazepam (Ativan)

The side effect of lorazepam is respiratory depression, but this should not deter from administering the medication to stop the seizure. It is better to secure the airway and adequately treat the seizure. This is important because the longer the seizure lasts, the greater the potential for irreversible brain damage. This is due to an increase in metabolic demands of the brain during a seizure. A second dose can be administered before adding other antiepileptic medications.

The dose and infusion rate of IV Cerebyx is expressed as phenytoin sodium equivalents (PSE) to avoid the need to perform molecular weight-based adjustments when converting between fosphenytoin and phenytoin sodium dosages (Box 10.16).

HINT   Phenytoin should not be administered faster than 50 mg/minute and fosphenytoin's maximal administration is no faster than 150 mg PSE/min because of hypotension.

Box 10.16 AEDs Used During Seizure

First line:
    Benzodiazepines (can repeat second dose)
    Ativan or Valium

Second line:
    Keppra
    Dilantin
    Cerebyx
    Vimpat

Third line:
    Versed
    Propofol
    Depacon

Fourth line: Pentobarbital

HINT   Pentobarbital is reserved as a fourth-line drug because of significant side effects of hypotension, cardiac depression, respiratory depression, and immunosuppression.

Q What is the recommended bedside monitoring for refractory status epilepticus (RSE)?

A Continuous EEG monitoring

Titration of IV infusions of AEDs is best through burst suppression on a continuous EEG. Continuous EEG is also used to recognize a nonconvulsive seizure and is recommended in cases of abnormal mental status, a comatose patient, and in survivors of cardiac arrest.

▶ COMPLICATIONS

Q Following a seizure, what complication should be closely assessed?

A Physical injury

Convulsive seizures can frequently result in physical injury from falls, repetitive impacting solid surfaces, and oral trauma.

Q What should be done with the side rails on a bed for patients with seizure precautions?

A Pad the side rails

Padding side rails can potentially help limit injuries that may occur during a seizure (Box 10.17).

Box 10.17 Seizure Precautions

Set bed in the lowest position
Bed should be locked
Side rails are in the upright position
Pad side rails
Place oral airway at bedside
Suction and oxygen equipment should be available

Q What is the most likely cause of mortality in patients with epilepsy?

A Sudden unexpected death in epilepsy (SUDEP)

Sudden death in epileptic patients is called SUDEP and is defined as a nontraumatic, non-drowning sudden death of a person with epilepsy. The greatest risk factor is frequent uncontrolled generalized seizures. SUDEP may be caused by a respiratory or cardiac event occurring during the seizure.

HINT   Continuous EKG monitoring can assist with identifying SUDEP in the hospital setting.

 # TRAUMATIC BRAIN INJURY

▶ PATHOPHYSIOLOGY

> **Q** Following a blunt mechanism of injury, what is the brain injury that occurs on the opposite side of the impact called?
>
> **A** Contracoup injury

A coup injury occurs on the side of the impact and a contracoup injury is on the opposite side of impact. The most common site for a coup–contracoup injury is an impact to the temporal area of the skull, causing a side-to-side impact of the brain in the skull.

HINT   A contracoup injury is caused by brain impacting the skull and bony protrusions.

> **Q** What is a nondisplaced fracture of the skull called?
>
> **A** Linear skull fracture

A linear skull fracture is a nondisplaced skull fracture and may be recognized on a lateral skull fracture. A basilar skull fracture cannot be identified with a lateral x-ray but is typically identified with CT scan or clinical presentation (Box 10.18).

Box 10.18 Types of Skull Fractures

Linear skull fracture	Nondisplaced fracture
Comminuted skull fracture	Fragmented disruption of skull with multiple linear fractures
Depressed skull fracture	Displaced comminuted fracture with depression
Basilar skull fracture	Fracture of the basilar skull through anterior or middle fossa

> **Q** Which two secondary injuries are the most predictive for a worsened neurological outcome following a traumatic brain injury (TBI)?
>
> **A** Hypotension and hypoxia

Brain injury is classified as primary or secondary injury. Interventions to improve outcomes are aimed at secondary injuries. Of all the secondary injuries, hypotension and hypoxia are the two most significant in worsening neurological outcomes. Immediate goals for managing TBIs are airway protection, adequate oxygenation, and improved brain perfusion. Following a TBI, there is loss of autoregulation in the area of injury resulting in focal edema and an ischemia of uninjured tissue known as a "steal" phenomenon (Box 10.19).

Box 10.19 Primary and Secondary Injuries

Primary Injuries	Secondary Injuries
Mild traumatic brain injury (TBI)	Hypoxia/anoxia
Contusions	Hypotension
Diffuse axonal injury (DAI)	Anemia

(continued)

Box 10.19 Primary and Secondary Injuries (*continued*)

Primary Injuries	Secondary Injuries
Lacerations	Hyperthermia
Subarachnoid hematoma (SAH)	Hypercapnia/hypocapnia
Subdural hematoma (SDH)	Electrolyte imbalances (e.g., hyperglycemia)
Epidural hematoma (EDH)	Cerebral edema
	Hydrocephalus

HINT   Diffuse axonal injury may be used in the scenario of a TBI patient in test questions.

> **Q What population is more likely to present with a chronic SDH?**
>
> **A Elderly**

SDH is bleeding into the subdural space. It often occurs as a result of an injury to the bridging veins and can result in rapid neurological changes (acute), delayed symptoms (subacute), and chronic presentations. Elderly people, alcoholics, and patients with dementia have brain atrophy, which allows for more room to bleed into the cranial vault before ICP increases. The populations have a higher risks of falls and head trauma.

HINT   SDH can be managed with burr holes and evacuation of the hematoma or by surgical craniotomy.

▶ SYMPTOMS/ASSESSMENT

> **Q What are the clinical signs of a basilar skull fracture?**
>
> **A Raccoon eyes and battle signs**

Clinical signs of a basilar skull fracture include bilateral periorbital ecchymosis (raccoon eyes) and/or bruising on mastoid process (battle signs). They may exhibit CSF fluid drainage from the nose (rhinorrhea) or from the ears (otorrhea). Do not use intranasal packing. Basilar skull fractures have a higher incidence of CNS infections.

HINT   All tubes (e.g., gastric tubes, endotracheal tubes, suction catheters) should be placed orally, not nasally. Nasal tubes can enter the brain through the cribriform fracture.

> **Q A rapidly expanding epidural hematoma (EDH) results in a dilated, nonreactive pupil on which side, ipsilateral or contralateral?**
>
> **A Ipsilateral pupil**

Cranial nerve III (oculomotor) is responsible for pupil size and reaction to light. Cranial nerves remain ipsilateral (except for cranial nerve IV), so injury to cranial nerve III causes a dilated, nonreactive pupil on the ipsilateral side. This is a result of uncal herniation, in which the unilateral mass pushes the temporal lobe downward through the tentorial opening.

HINT   EDH is an arterial bleed, frequently caused by injury to the middle meningeal artery following a blunt trauma. It causes rapid deterioration of neurological status, typically following a period of being lucid.

▶ DIAGNOSIS

> **Q Which primary injury is not readily visualized on noncontrast CT scans?**
>
> **A DAI**

DAI is a shearing of the axons, typically a result of mechanism of injury in which the brain rotates within the skull (e.g., rollover vehicle). DAI may not demonstrate on CT or MRI and is typically diagnosed by poor clinical neurological status with relatively normal CT scan. A sign of DAI on CT can be areas of small hyperdensitieis but is not seen in all patients.

HINT DAI in patients with low GCS have predictions of poor outcomes.

> **Q** What is the preferred method for testing fluid from the nose or ears for cerebrospinal fluid (CSF) following a trauma?
>
> **A** Halo test

The halo test involves placing the fluid from the nose or ears on gauze dressing; the blood separates from the CSF with the CSF forming a ring or halo. Glucose testing can be used to differentiate nasal drainage from CSF, but if the drainage is bloody, a halo test is not recommended because of false positives.

HINT Most questions regarding skull fractures will focus more on basilar skull fractures.

▶ SYMPTOMS/ASSESSMENT

> **Q** What are the clinical signs of a basilar skull fracture?
>
> **A** Raccoon eyes and battle signs

Clinical signs of a basilar skull fracture include bilateral periorbital ecchymosis (raccoon eyes) and/or bruising on mastoid process (battle signs). They may exhibit CSF fluid drainage from the nose (rhinorrhea) or from the ears (otorrhea). Do not use intranasal packing. Basilar skull fractures have a higher incidence of CNS infections.

HINT All tubes (e.g., gastric tubes, endotracheal tubes, suction catheters) should be placed orally, not nasally. Nasal tubes can enter the brain through the cribriform fracture.

> **Q** A rapidly expanding epidural hematoma (EDH) results in a dilated, nonreactive pupil on which side, ipsilateral or contralateral?. Which pupil is affected?
>
> **A** Ipsilateral pupil

Cranial nerve III (oculomotor) is responsible for pupil size and reaction to light. Cranial nerves remain ipsilateral (except for cranial nerve IV) so injury to cranial nerve III causes a dilated, nonreactive pupil on the ipsilateral side. This is a result of uncal herniation, in which the unilateral mass pushes the temporal lobe downward through the tentorial opening.

HINT EDH is an arterial bleed, frequently caused by injury to the middle meningeal artery following a blunt trauma. It causes rapid deterioration of neurological status, typically following a period of being lucid.

▶ MEDICAL MANAGEMENT

> **Q** What effect does CO_2 have on the cerebral vasculature?
>
> **A** Cerebral vasodilation

CO_2 is a potent vasodilator in the cerebral circulation. Hyperventilation, which reduces $PaCO_2$, has been used to lower ICP through cerebral vasoconstriction. This lowers the blood volume, thus lowering the ICP. It is not recommended to routinely hyperventilate because even though hyperventilation can lower ICP, it also decreases cerebral blood flow. Hyperventilation, with a goal of $PaCO_2$ at 32–34 mmHg, can be used in situations of increased ICP refractory to other treatments.

HINT Avoid an increase in $PaCO_2$, which elevates the ICP.

> **Q** When administering mannitol (Osmitrol), what laboratory values should be monitored closely?
>
> **A** Serum osmolality and serum sodium

Mannitol is a most commonly used osmotic diuretic in the treatment of increased ICP. It increases serum osmolality, creating a gradient between the plasma and the brain tissue. Serum osmolality and serum sodium levels can increase during repeated administration of mannitol and should be closely monitored. Mannitol should not be administered if serum osmolality becomes higher than 320 mOsm. The patient may need to be rehydrated if he or she becomes too hyperosmolar.

HINT Hypovolemia should be avoided because of the adverse effect on cerebral blood flow.

> **Q** What is the potential complication in administering hypertonic saline for increased ICP?
>
> **A** Central pontine myelinolysis

Another hyperosmolar treatment currently used to manage increased ICP caused by cerebral edema is hypertonic saline (HS) including 3%, 7.5%, and 23% saline. It does not have the diuretic effect of mannitol. HS administration can have the complication of central pontine myelinolysis (CPM) in a hyponatremic patient. (Table 10.4).

HINT Hypernatremia should be excluded before the administration of HS and held for serum sodium greater than 155 mEq/L.

Table 10.4 Treatment of TBI

Treatment	Goal	Purpose
Craniectomy	Bone flaps and hemicraniectomy	Allows room for swelling Lowers risk herniation
Fluid resuscitation	Normal saline recommended Avoid hypotonic solutions	Prevent hypovolemia and hypotension
Steroids	Not recommended for TBI May be used in other neurological disorders	Stabilizes cell membranes to decrease cerebral edema
Blood pressure management	Maintain cerebral perfusion pressure (CPP) >60 mmHg Do not aggressively attempt to keep CPP >70 mmHg	Adequate pressure to increase cerebral blood flow (CBF) Avoid complications of fluid overload (e.g., acute respiratory distress syndrome [ARDS])
Hypnotics and sedatives	Short-acting or reversible	Lowers cerebral demand Lowers intracranial pressure (ICP) May also decrease CBF
Barbiturate coma	Pentobarbital, thiopental	Lowers cerebral metabolism Lowers ICP May also decrease CBF
Temperature control	Avoid hyperthermia (fever) May or may not induce hypothermia	Lowers cerebral metabolism Neuroprotectant Decreases ICP
Glucose control	Avoid hyperglycemia Avoid hypoglycemia	Prevents furthering of cellular injury

> **Q** Which two monitoring techniques are recommended for a barbiturate coma?
>
> **A** ICP and continuous EEG with burst suppression

The induced barbiturate coma results in loss of the ability to assess a patient's neurological status, so ICP monitoring is used to determine the effectiveness of the therapy. Continuous EEG monitoring is used to guide the dosing of the barbiturate. Dosing is guided by the extent of burst suppression. Beyond the point of burst suppression, it may increase the risk of complications without offering further therapeutic benefit (Box 10.20).

HINT   Complication of barbiturates includes myocardial depression and patient's cardiovascular status should be monitored closely.

Box 10.20 Nursing Interventions to Lower ICP

Maintaining head-of-bed elevation to facilitate venous drainage
Maintaining good head alignment to facilitate venous drainage
Providing good pulmonary toiletry for oxygenation and avoiding hypercarbia
Spacing activities to limit the response of ICP

▶ SURGICAL MANAGEMENT

Q What is the procedure used if TBI patient is experiencing sustained elevation of ICP and herniating?

A Craniectomy

Craniectomy is the removal of part of the skull to prevent herniation. Bone flap is a smaller piece of skull removed, but the brain can still herniate through the bone flap. A hemi-craniectomy is the removal of half of skull, lowering risk of herniation.

HINT   Skull can be replaced later during recovery when the brain's swelling is resolved.

▶ COMPLICATIONS

Q What is cerebral edema caused by injury to the blood–brain barrier and increased interstitial fluid called?

A Vasogenic cerebral edema

Vasogenic cerebral edema is a result of injury to the brain tissue, such as trauma, brain tumors, and strokes. Cytotoxic cerebral edema is intracellular fluid in the brain caused by hypoxic or anoxic brain injuries. Both vasogenic and cytotoxic cerebral edema are commonly found in severe TBI patients.

HINT   Mannitol is most effective with vasogenic cerebral edema because it draws fluid from the interstitial space.

Q Following a depressed skull fracture, the patient develops fever and elevated WBC counts. What would be the potential complication of the depressed skull fracture?

A Meningitis

CNS infections, such as meningitis, are potential complications following a depressed and basilar skull fracture.

HINT   Signs of an infection are elevated fever and WBC count, so the infection associated with depressed skull fracture is meningitis.

Q Repetitive mild traumatic brain injuries in contact sports can result in what complication?

A Chronic traumatic encephalopathy

Chronic traumatic encephalopathy (CTE) is a complication of repetitive brain trauma frequently seen with players of contact sports. This used to be called "punch drunk" in boxing. These repetitive injuries result in deposit of tau proteins in the cortex resulting in degeneration and atrophy of the brain similar to cortical dementia (Box 10.21).

HINT CTE is similar to Alzheimer's disorder and Parkinson's disease with the pathophysiology, but this is a preventable dementia.

Box 10.21 Symptoms of CTE

Memory loss
Depression
Suicidal thoughts and suicides
Aggressive behavior
Tremors
Ataxia (gait abnormality)
Slowed movements
Speech abnormalities
Confusion

ACUTE SPINAL CORD INURY

Q A hyperflexion injury may result in rupture of which ligament?

A Posterior longitudinal

Hyperflexion injury occurs when the spine is flexed beyond the normal range of motion. An example is a front-on motor vehicle crash. The head continues forward with sufficient speed and force for the chin to touch the chest. The stretch occurs posteriorly, causing the rupture or tearing of the posterior ligaments. The anterior vertebral body may be involved as compression or wedge fracture. This injury may result in subluxation and/or disk herniation. Pediatric patient is at high risk for this mechanism of injury due to laxity of longitudinal ligaments.

HINT A "lipstick sign" is when the trauma victim has lipstick on their shirt which can indicated a hyperflexion injury.

Q A patient is diagnosed with cervical injury following a rear-end motor vehicle crash. What is the most likely mechanism for the spinal injury?

A Hyperextension

Hyperextension injuries occur when the spine is moved into an extreme hyperextension position. The stretch of the spine is now occurring anteriorly, so the anterior longitudinal ligament would be the most likely ligament to be injured (Box 10.22). The posterior vertebral body is at highest risk for fractures. Subluxation and herniated disks may also occur with this mechanism of injury. Extreme hyperextension can cause compression injury form the ligamentum flavum resulting in cord contusion and hypoxia.

HINT Whiplash is commonly caused by hyperextension mechanism of injury.

Box 10.22 Mechanism of Injury SCI

Hyperflexion	Rupture posterior longitudinal ligament Wedge fracture anterior vertebral body
Hyperextension	Rupture anterior longitudinal ligament Fracture posterior vertebral body
Rotational	Rupture posterior longitudinal ligament Dislocation of facets
Compression (axial loading)	Burst fractures

> **Q** Which of the types of odontoid fractures is considered to be a stable fracture?
> **A** Type I

Odontoid (also called the dens) is the bony structure of C2 that comes up anteriorly into the ring of C1 and allows for rotational movement of the neck. Fractures of the odontoid are classified into type I, II, III, based upon where the fracture occurred in the odontoid and I (Box 10.23). This is also used to describe stability and guides treatment of the fracture. Type I is considered the most stable of the odontoid fractures. Instability of odontoid fractures is from either cord compression or penetration of bony fragment or ligament disruption between odontoid process and the anterior aspect of C1.

HINT Type II odontoid fractures are the most common and considered most unstable of the odontoid fractures.

Box 10.23 Types of Odontoid Fractures

Type I	Tip odontoid bone above transverse ligament
Type II	Base of odontoid Between transverse ligament and body of axis
Type III	Extend into the vertebral body

▶ PATHOPHYSIOLOGY

> **Q** A patient with total loss of motor and sensory below the level of injury is called?
> **A** Complete cord injury

There is some degree of correlation between the level of function and level of radiographic injury but is not always consistent. The neurological level of injury (NLI) is the most caudal spinal cord level at which the normal motor/sensory function persists following spinal cord injury.

HINT An incomplete cord injury may initially appear functionally as a complete cord due to inflammation and edema in the cord.

> **Q** A football player presents with motor impairment greater in the upper extremities than the lower extremities following a traumatic injury. What is this incomplete injury called?
> **A** Central cord syndrome

The spinal cord injury occurs in the central portion of the cord and is characterized by greater upper extremity involvement than lower, especially involving the hands. The upper extremity axons are located in the central portion of the spinal cord, and the axons that control the lower extremity movement are located laterally in the cord. This incomplete cord syndrome is frequently caused by hyperextension injury or a fall. There is often a gradual return to function with the lower extremities first, followed by the upper extremities and finger movement last with the hand being the most common residual motor weakness. Urinary retention and sensory abnormalities vary with severity of injury.

HINT Key to recognizing this syndrome is the upper extremities weakness with lesser lower extremities weakness.

> **Q** In Brown-Sequard syndrome, there is an ipsilateral loss of what function?
> **A** Motor function

Brown-Sequard syndrome is a hemisection of the spinal cord that results in the ipsilateral loss of motor and contralateral loss of pain and temperature. It is often seen with penetrating injuries but may also be seen with epidural hematomas and traumatically herniated cervical disk (Box 10.24).

HINT This syndrome has the best prognosis with a 90% recovery of ambulation, regaining sensation and bowel/bladder function if caused by compression.

Box 10.24 Cord Injuries

Complete cord injury	Complette loss of motor and sensory below the level of injury
Anterior cord syndrome	Loss of motor Loss pain and temperature Maintain light touch and proprioception
Central cord syndrome	Greater upper than lower extremity loss
Brown-Sequard syndrome	Ipsilateral loss of motor contralateral loss of sensory

▶ SYMPTOMS/ASSESSMENT

Q The presence of sacral sparing following a traumatic spinal cord injury indicates what type of injury?

A Incomplete injury

Anal contraction with stimulation or ability to feel pinprick or touch around the anus is called "anal sparing" and indicates incomplete injury. This is a phenomenon of sensation in sacral region even though sensation is absent in thoracic and lumbar area. Sacral fibers may be protected more from compression injury thus sparing the sacral dermatomes.

HINT Assessing for sacral sparing assists with determining an incomplete from complete injury.

Q How many cervical levels is sensory assessment tested through?

A C8

There are seven cervical vertebrae and eight paired cervical nerve roots. Sensory assessment of cervical region is tested through C8. The cervical region is the only portion of the spinal column that has a greater number of paired nerve roots than vertebrae.

HINT Sensory assessment is performed using dermatome levels in spinal cord-injured patients, while motor assessment is performed using myotome levels.

Q What is the loss of motor and reflexes below the level of injury called?

A Spinal shock

Spinal shock is the loss of reflexes, and motor below the level of injury. Spinal shock occurs immediately after the injury and typically resolves within 2–16 weeks.

HINT Two of the reflexes routinely assessed in spinal cord injured patients include anocutaneous and bulbocavernosous reflex.

▶ DIAGNOSIS

Q A lateral plain radiograph can be used to diagnose what type of injury?

A Bony or vertebral fractures

A lateral x-ray is used to visualize bony abnormalities and fractures. Ligaments injuries are not identified on plain radiographs unless the spinal column is out of alignment. Flexion/extension x-rays may be obtained on an awake, cooperative patient without distracting injuries. MRI is the more definitive radiographic study used to identify ligament injuries.

HINT A patient with normal lateral cervical spine x-rays but complaints of pain in neck region should remain in cervical immobilization until flexion/extension views or magnetic resonance imaging (MRI) is obtained.

> **Q** Which radiographic study can distinguish between spinal cord hemorrhage and vasogenic edema?
>
> **A** MRI

An MRI is a gold standard for radiographic study of the spinal cord. It is able to distinguish between ischemic injury, edema, and hemorrhage within the cord.

HINT   MRI is also considered the gold standard for recognizing spinal ligament injuries.

▶ MEDICAL MANAGEMENT

> **Q** What is the primary treatment for neurogenic shock?
>
> **A** Fluid administration

The complication of neurogenic shock is systemic vasodilation with hypotension. Fluid resuscitation is the treatment of choice to correct the hypotension. If fluids do not improve the blood pressure and perfusion, vasopressors may be initiated. A goal is to maintain the mean arterial pressure between 85 and 90 mmHg to increase perfusion and improve neurological outcomes. The bradycardia associated with neurogenic shock does not typically require treatment but, if symptomatic, may place an external pacemaker.

HINT   Neurogenic shock is classified as a distributive shock.

> **Q** What respiratory parameter should be closely monitored in a spontaneously breathing acute spinal cord injured patient?
>
> **A** Forced vital capacity and/or NIF

Respiratory parameters to monitor in a patient with a spinal cord injury to determine the ability to ventilate include forced vital capacity (FVC) and negative inspiratory force (NIF). The FVC is the forced maximal breath in followed by the maximal breath out. NIF is the ability to generate enough negative pressure in the chest to allow for inspiration. The FVC and NIF are used to evaluate the respiratory muscles and ability to generate an adequate breath.

HINT   These parameters are commonly used to evaluate a person's ability to breath spontaneously effectively.

> **Q** At what level of spinal injury is the diaphragm affected and requires ventilatory support if a complete injury?
>
> **A** Fourth cervical level

The C4 level innervates the diaphragm. A patient with a cervical injury to the spinal cord at C4 level or above loses innervation to the diaphragm and usually requires intubation and mechanical ventilation. Cervical injuries at the six or seventh cervical level (C6 and C7) may still require intubation and ventilation at least in the acute period due to cord edema.

HINT   Airway and breathing is the priority of care in cervical spinal injuries.

▶ SURGICAL MANAGEMENT

> **Q** What is the primary management of a patient with burst fractures of cervical vertebrae?
>
> **A** Surgical cord decompression

Burst fractures may require surgical removal of bone to achieve cord decompression. Bony pieces may compress the spinal cord and cause neurological injury. This injury requires surgical management, and closed reduction with cervical traction is not recommended on burst fractures.

HINT   Immobilization of the spinal column is important to prevent further injury to the spinal cord from bony pieces.

▶ COMPLICATIONS

> **Q** When should a bowel regimen begin following an acute spinal cord injury?
>
> **A** Upon admission

Bowel impaction is a complication of SCI. When an acute spinal cord injured patient is admitted, the bowel regimen should be ordered and initiated. A bowel regimen includes suppository with finger stimulation timed appropriately for once-a-day bowel movement. Timing of daily suppository for once-a-day bowel training should be scheduled in acute care to facilitate rehabilitation and daily routines once the patient is discharged. A spinal cord injury above T12 may have reflex or spastic bowel while a spinal cord injury below T12 level may be hyporeflexic with a flaccid bowel.

HINT The bowel regimen should only be discontinued with severe diarrhea.

> **Q** A patient is able to void spontaneously following an acute spinal cord injury. What should the nurse assess for following the void?
>
> **A** Post-void residuals

Urinary retention is a complicatioin of SCI. If patient with a spinal cord injury is able to void spontaneously, use a bladder scan to assess for residual post voiding. If greater than 200–300 mL, straight catheterization is recommended even if spontaneously voiding. Bladder training is the removal of the indwelling bladder catheter and intermittent catheterization used in the presence of urinary retention.

HINT Bladder training is initiated as soon as patient is on maintenance fluids or oral intake.

> **Q** A patient is readmitted from rehabilitation following a cervical spinal cord injury. The patient suddenly develops hypertension with a BP of 210/120 mmHg. What would be the nurse's priority of care?
>
> **A** Find the source of stimulation and remove it

Priority of care with a hypertensive spinal cord injured patient due to autonomic hyperreflexia is to find the source of obnoxious stimulation and remove it. The critical care nurse should elevate the head of the bed to lower the pressure and assess the patient for the cause of the autonomic hyperreflexia. Once the source is identified and removed, the patient's hypertension should resolve (Box 10.25).

HINT Antihypertensive should not be the priority or first choice to manage the hypertension associated with autonomic hyperreflexia because once the source is removed, the patient would become hypotensive.

Box 10.25 Autonomic Hyperreflexia

Potential Sources of AH	Nursing Interventions
Urinary retention	Bladder scan and intermittent catheterization
Restrictive clothing	Loosen or remove clothing
Pressure sores	Reposition off of pressure scores
Fecal impaction	Remove fecal impaction

> **Q** The lack of ability for internal temperature regulation following a spinal cord injury is called?
>
> **A** Poikilothermia

Loss of thermoregulatory function occurs in cord injuries above the thoracolumbar outflow due to loss of sympathetic nervous system (SNS) stimulation. Poikilothermia is the lack of internal regulation of the body temperature found after a spinal cord injury. Spinal cord injured patients are unable to vasoconstrict and shiver to conserve heat or sweat to dissipate heat.

HINT Nursing interventions for spinal cord injured patients include controlling the body temperature through external interventions.

BRAIN DEATH

Q What type of death involves an irreversible cessation of brain function?

A Brain death

The Uniform Determination of Death Act (UDDA) defines death as follows: "An individual who has sustained either (a) irreversible cessation of circulatory and respiratory functions, or (b) irreversible cessation of all functions of the entire brainstem" (Wijdicks et al., 2010). The UDDA does not define how to determine brain death.

Most states in the United States have adopted the UDDA, but some states have added amendments stating certain criteria are needed to determine brain death. There are published practice guidelines for brain death determination, but the actual process remains variable throughout the country.

HINT   For the exam, brain death determination may be different from your hospital practice. Be familiar with the national standards.

Q What is a clinical examination performed at the bedside?

A Brainstem reflexes

There are three clinical findings required to confirm irreversible cessation of all functions of the entire brain, including the brainstem. This includes determining the coma is irreversible and has a known cause; there is an absence of brainstem reflexes; and the patient is determined to be apneic.

HINT   Brain stem reflexes include pupil reaction, Doll's eyes, and cold calorics.

Q What has to be normalized before the determination of brain death?

A Body temperature

The patient must have a body temperature above 36 °C. A drug and alcohol screen is also frequently recommended to ensure the coma is not the effect of a CNS-depressant drug. If the patient has received a neuromuscular blocking (NMB) agent, the effects must be reversed totally. This can be determined by the presence of train-of-four twitches with maximal ulnar nerve stimulation. There should be no severe electrolyte or acid–base imbalance. Achieve normal systolic pressure (>100 mmHg) to assure a reliable neurological examination.

Q How do you define a "coma"?

A Absence of all responses to any noxious stimuli

No motor response, eye opening, or eye movement with application of a noxious stimulation, other than spinal reflexes.

HINT   Some patients who are brain dead may still have nonbrain-mediated spontaneous movements and spinal reflexes.

Q What are the commonly tested brainstem reflexes?

A Pupillary response to light, ocular movements, corneal reflex, cough (tracheal reflex), and gag (pharyngeal reflex)

Bilateral pupils are frequently midsize to dilated and fixed, with no reaction to light. If the pupils are pinpoints, drug overdose should be suspected. Ocular movement is tested using the oculocephalic test (doll's eyes) and the oculovestibular test (cold calorics). Doll's eyes and cold calorics tests are done when testing for a reflex. If the reflex is there (positive), then the patient is not brain dead. If the reflex is absent (negative), it is one step toward the determination of brain death.

HINT   Doll's eyes test: The eyes should move in the opposite direction of head movement. Barbie dolls have their eyes painted on the head, so when you move their heads side to side, the eyes go in the same direction. Remember Barbie dolls are brain dead!

> **Q** Which arterial blood gas abnormality is required for an apnea test to be positive?
>
> **A** Hypercarbia

The absence of a breathing drive (apnea test) is tested with a CO_2 challenge. Documentation of an increase in $PaCO_2$ above normal levels is typical practice. Prerequisites include eucapnia and no prior evidence of CO_2 retention (e.g., chronic obstructive pulmonary disease [COPD]). Abort the test if systolic BP is less than 90 mmHg or oxygen saturation is less than 85% for longer than 30 seconds. If respiratory movements are absent and $PaCO_2$ is greater than 60 mmHg, the apnea test is positive.

HINT Other ancillary tests include EEG, cerebral angiography, nuclear scan, transcranial Doppler, CT angiography, and MRI/magnetic resonance angiography (MRA).

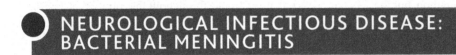

NEUROLOGICAL INFECTIOUS DISEASE: BACTERIAL MENINGITIS

▶ PATHOPHYSIOLOGY

> **Q** Where is the primary location of the infection in meningitis?
>
> **A** Meninges

Bacterial meningitis is an inflammation or an infection in the meninges, particularly involving the pia and arachnoid layer (subarachnoid space). The routes of entry for the bacteria into the meninges are listed in Box 10.26.

Box 10.26 Routes of Entry Bacterial Meningitis

Bloodstream
Middle ear infection
Sinusitis
Direct route
Mouth/nose droplets

▶ SYMPTOMS/ASSESSMENT

> **Q** What is the triad of symptoms in meningitis?
>
> **A** Nuchal rigidity, headache, and fever

Meningitis typically presents with headache, fever, and nuchal rigidity. This is considered the classic triad of symptoms (Box 10.27).

Box 10.27 Other Symptoms of Meningitis

Headache
Photophobia
Seizure
Cranial nerve palsy (e.g., CN II, III, IV, VI, VIII)
Petechiae and cutaneous hemorrhage
Brudzinski's sign
Kernig's sign

> **Q** What is it called when the hips or knees flex in response to passive neck flexion?
>
> **A** Brudzinski's sign

Brudzinski's sign and Kernig's sign are indications of meningeal irritation. Brudzinski's sign is when the examiner passively flexes the neck and the patient's hips or knees flex automatically. Kernig's sign is severe stiffness or pain in the hamstring causing an inability to straighten the leg when hip is flexed at a 90-degree angle.

▶ DIAGNOSIS

> **Q** Is the CSF glucose high or low in bacterial meningitis?
>
> **A** Low

CSF analysis is used to diagnose meningitis and determine the underlying causative microorganism. The normal glucose level in the CSF is two-thirds of the glucose in the blood. So, if the serum glucose is within normal range then the CSF glucose normal is 45 mg/dL. A ratio of CSF glucose to serum glucose less than 0.4 is a predictor of bacterial meningitis. Viral meningitis has a normal CSF glucose (Box 10.28).

HINT   Think of bacteria as being an animal; an animal has to eat. It eats glucose, whereas a virus is not an animal, and does not need to eat and will have a normal CSF glucose level.

Box 10.28 CSF Analysis of Bacterial Meningitis

Opening pressure is in the range of 200–500 mm H_2O
Elevated protein levels Elevated lactate levels
Positive Gram stain

> **Q** Which white blood cells (WBC) are expected to be elevated in bacterial meningitis?
>
> **A** Neutrophils

Neutrophils are typically elevated in a bacterial infection. Lymphocytes are typically elevated in viral infections.

HINT   Gram stains provide an accurate, rapid identification of the causative bacterium.

> **Q** What would be an indication for a head CT scan before performing a lumbar puncture?
>
> **A** Abnormal LOC, focal neurological deficit, or presence of papilledema

The presence of an abnormal neurological evaluation may indicate an increase in ICP. Performing a lumbar puncture on a patient with an increased ICP can result in brain herniation; thus, a head CT scan is needed first to identify any space-occupying lesions or presence of cerebral edema. The lumbar puncture results in a temporary decrease in CSF pressure due to removal of CSF.

▶ MANAGEMENT

> **Q** What is the priority of care in managing bacterial meningitis?
>
> **A** Administration of antibiotics

Management includes early administration of an antimicrobial agent. Any delay in treatment might be associated with an adverse outcome. Dexamethasone should be initiated with the first dose of the antimicrobial agent.

▶ COMPLICATIONS

> **Q** What is a common complication following bacterial meningitis related to a cranial nerve abnormality?
>
> **A** Hearing loss

Complications of bacterial meningitis include hearing loss, visual acuity deficits, and postmeningitis sequelae.

HINT Following meningealcoccal meningitis, a complication may include extremity amputations due to the vasculitis and thrombophlebitis.

⬤ NEUROMUSCULAR DISORDERS

MYASTHENIA GRAVIS

▶ PATHOPHYSIOLOGY

> **Q** In myasthenia gravis (MG), what do the antibodies destroy resulting in fatigable muscle weakness?
>
> **A** Acetylcholine receptors

MG is a chronic autoimmune disease that affects the neuromuscular junction causing a fatigable muscle weakness, which worsens with repetitive use of the muscles and improves with rest. Antibodies destroy the acetylcholine (ACh) receptors on the postsynaptic muscle end plate, thus decreasing the effect of acetylcholine. This reduces the number of receptor sites at the neuromuscular junction and the voltage to elicit action.

▶ SYMPTOMS/ASSESSMENT

> **Q** What is the hallmark sign of MG?
>
> **A** Muscle weakness with repetitive movement

The first time the movement is performed there are receptor sites available for acetylcholine and the contraction is strong. Further attempts of the movement become weaker until a person is unable to perform the movement. This is due to the loss of receptor sites on the muscle end plate.

HINT Examples of repetitive movements include chewing, talking, swallowing, and movement of the extremities.

> **Q** What is the primary concern when a patient with MG is admitted in a crisis?
>
> **A** Pulmonary compromise

Assessment of the patient's ventilatory capability is very important. In a crisis, a patient with MG may develop significant weakness in the diaphragm and intercostal muscles and progress rapidly to respiratory failure. Assess the quality of the voice and the ability to talk. Assess the ability to cough and suction as needed. Administer oxygen as needed and obtain arterial blood gases to monitor ventilation ($PaCO_2$).

HINT Other areas of concern include difficulty swallowing and choking caused by weakness of the laryngeal and oropharyngeal muscles. Swallow evaluations are needed.

Q Which two pulmonary function tests are used most often to evaluate ventilatory effort of patients with MG?

A Forced vital capacity (FVC) and negative inspiratory force (NIF)

Pulmonary function tests are monitored frequently, and significant changes from baseline are an indication of respiratory failure. An FVC less than 15 mL/kg or an NIF less than 20 cm H_2O are indications of the need for mechanical ventilation.

▶ MANAGEMENT

Q During crisis, what are two therapies that may be used to rapidly reverse the crisis in MG?

A Intravenous (IV) immunoglobulin (IVIG) or plasmapheresis

IVIG or plasmapheresis is indicated during an MG crisis. IVIG therapy may be preferred in patients with hemodynamic instability, in which plasmapheresis (plasma exchange) may be contraindicated. Steroids may also be initiated but can result in an exacerbation in muscle weakness within 5–10 days of initiation of the steroid and may still require the above therapies concomitantly. The cholinesterase inhibitors may actually be held initially during the crisis.

HINT Corticosteroids (prednisone) and immunomodulatory drugs (azathioprine, cyclosporine, mycophenolate) may also be used to manage MG during a crisis. Remember, this is an autoimmune disease.

▶ COMPLICATIONS

Q What is the name of the crisis induced by an overdose of cholinesterase-inhibitor drugs used to manage MG?

A Cholinergic crisis

A cholinergic crisis can also present with an increase in weakening of muscles and respiratory failure. Determining the time of the last dose is helpful in differentiating a cholinergic crisis from a myasthenia crisis. If the onset of weakness is 3–4 hours after the dose, the probable cause is an acute worsening of the disease process itself. If it is within 15–60 minutes of the last dose, it is more likely a cholinergic crisis (Box 10.29).

HINT The treatment is typically to hold the cholinesterase inhibitor medications until symptoms are resolved. Intense monitoring for signs of respiratory failure and increased weakness is necessary.

Box 10.29 Symptoms of Cholinergic Crisis

Slurred speech
Dyspnea
Increased diplopia
Increased salivation
Muscle cramping
Fasciculations
Bradycardia
Abdominal symptoms

GUILLAIN-BARRÉ

▶ PATHOPHYSIOLOGY

> **Q** What is the hallmark presentation of a patient with Guillain-Barré?
>
> **A** Ascending, bilateral paralysis

Guillain-Barré (GB) syndrome is an acute inflammatory, autoimmune polyradiculoneuropathy frequently presenting as an ascending, bilateral paralysis. The process causes demyelination of the peripheral nerves, including the cranial nerves, ventral and dorsal nerve roots, entire length of the peripheral nerves, and the autonomic nervous system (ANS). When the pathological process is completed, regeneration of the myelin sheath occurs and function is restored. Reinnervation of the muscle occurs due to new growth from the cone of the axon.

HINT   Resolution of symptoms is in the opposite direction; descending order.

▶ SYMPTOMS/ASSESSMENT

> **Q** Which of the cranial nerves are more important to assess during an acute process of GB?
>
> **A** CN IX, X, XII

Cranial nerves IX, X, and XII are responsible for the gag and swallow reflexes. As the paralysis ascends, the patient may have weakened reflexes or loss of the gag and swallow reflexes. This puts the patient at high risk for aspiration.

HINT   The other cranial nerves commonly involved are CN III, IV, and VI, which control extraocular eye movement and should be assessed on a regular basis.

> **Q** What are the signs of involvement of the autonomic nervous system (ANS)?
>
> **A** Alteration in heart rate

The autonomic nervous system (ANS) includes the sympathetic and parasympathetic nervous system. The ANS may also be affected by the demyelination of the peripheral portion of the nerves (Box 10.30).

Box 10.30 Signs of ANS Abnormalities in GB

Heart rate abnormalities (tachycardia or bradycardia)
Inverted T waves
Alteration in BP (hypo- or hypertensive)
Facial flushing
Loss of sweating ability

> **Q** Is the resolution of the paralysis ascending or descending?
>
> **A** Descending

The resolution of muscle weakness or paralysis is in the opposite direction of the onset of GB. The muscle weakness begins with gait and paralysis in the lower extremities. Muscle strength is regained in a descending fashion, with the resolution of spontaneous ventilation before the ability to ambulate.

▶ MANAGEMENT

> **Q** What is the acute medical management of GB?
>
> **A** IVIG and/or plasmapheresis

The treatment of GB is similar to that of MG. Plasmapheresis (plasma exchange) involves the removal of antibodies, which decreases the autoimmune response in the peripheral nerves (Box 10.31).

HINT   Nursing assessment and care for both MG and GB should focus on ventilatory efforts and the presence of ventilatory failure.

Box 10.31 Complications of Plasmapheresis

Clotting disorders	Hypotension
Hypocalcemia	Autonomic dysfunction
Infections	Phlebitis
Decreased serum proteins	

● HYDROCEPHALUS

▶ PATHOPHYSIOLOGY

Q What is hydrocephalus called when it occurs because of an obstruction within the ventricular system?

A Noncommunicating hydrocephalus

When there is an obstruction within the ventricular system, the flow of CSF from the ventricles to the subarachnoid space is impaired. The most common form is a mass lesion, intraventricular or extraventricular, disrupting the ventricular system. Tumors can cause blockage anywhere along the CSF flow.

Q What is the most common cause of communicating hydrocephalus in acute disease processes?

A Inabilty to reabsorb CSF

Communicating hydrocephalus occurs because of overproduction of CSF, interference with reabsorption of CSF, or venous drainage insufficiency. The ventricular system communicates with the subarachnoid space. The most common cause is damage to the arachnoid villi, which interferes with the reabsorption of CSF.

HINT   The most common cause of communicating hydrocephalus occurs in SAH and bacterial meningitis.

▶ SYMPTOMS/ASSESSMENT

Q What are two common signs of acute hydrocephalus?

A Headache and nausea/vomiting

Hydrocephalus is an increase in CSF volume and typically presents with headache and nausea and vomiting (Box 10.32).

Box 10.32 Symptoms of Hydrocephalus

Decreased LOC	Diplopia
Headache	Seizures
Nausea and vomiting	

▶ MANAGEMENT

Q What is the primary surgical treatment for the management of hydrocephalus?

A Shunt placement

A shunt provides an open communication between the ventricular system and a drainage cavity, most often the peritoneum (VP shunt). Other cavities to drain include the right atrium and pleura. The shunt can control the amount of CSF that is drained from the ventricles.

HINT   VP shunts are commonly used to treat normal pressure hydrocephalus (NPH).

▶ COMPLICATIONS

Q A patient with a VP shunt placed for chronic hydrocephalus presents with abdominal pain and fever. What would be the complication of the VP shunt?

A Peritonitis

Peritonitis is potential complication of VP shunt and can occur acutely or as a long-term complication. Peritonitis can develop due to body's response to a foreign object or bacterial infection. Symptoms include abdominal pain, erythema, fever, and leukocytosis (Box 10.33).

Box 10.33 Complications of VP Shunts

Shunt infection
Meningitis
Peritonitis
Mechanical malformation
Under drainage with development hydrocephalus
SDH/ICH

DELIRIUM

Q How is delirium best described: reversible or irreversible?

A Reversible

Delirium is a change in cognition and mentation that develops acutely and is usually reversible. It is usually a result of an underlying medical disorder, medication, or toxicity. It can be characterized as hyperactive, hypoactivitve, or mixed.

▶ PATHOPHYSIOLOGY

Q Which two neurotransmitters are attributed to physiological derangements resulting in delirium?

A Acetylcholine and dopamine

Acetylcholine and dopamine are neurotransmitters that work in opposition, increasing (acetylcholine) and decreasing (dopamine) neuronal excitability. Inflammatory and metabolic derangements are also thought to be involved in the underlying physiology of delirium.

Q What is considered a modifiable risk factor on a ventilated ICU patient?

A Narcotic and benzodiazepine administration

Respiratory failure and mechanical ventilation is a known risk factor for the development of delirium in an ICU. The need for mechanical ventilation may not be avoided, but the management of sedation can be modified. Medications are also known risk factors and commonly include narcotics and benzodiazepines. Limiting the use of these medications can decrease the risk of delirium.

HINT Risk factors for delirium can be modifiable or nonmodifiable (Box 10.34).

Box 10.34 Common Risk Factors for Delirium

Non-Modifiable	Modifiable
Baseline dementia	Sedation medication
Advanced age	Hypotenion/hypoperfusion
Disease processes	Hypoxia
Severity of illness	Respiratory failure
Predisposing comorbidities	Sepsis
	Medication induced coma
	Pain
	Isolation/disorientation
	Immobility

▶ SYMPTOMS/ASSESSMENT

Q A patient in the ICU becomes agitated and combative. How would you classify the delirium?

A Hyperactive

Hyperactive delirium is the acute onset of agitation, restlessness, and uncooperative behavior. Hypoactive is more common than hyperactive but is frequently overlooked in ICU patients and is associated with worse clinical outcomes (Box 10.35).

HINT Delirium may also present with autonomic signs such as hypertension and tachycardia.

Box 10.35 Signs of Delirium

Hyperactive Delirium	Hypoactive Delirium
Agitation	Lethargy
Anxiety	Increased sleeping during day
Restlessness	Withdrawal
Hallucinations	Poor appetite
Delusions	Depression
Combative	Somnolent
Uncooperative behaviors	

HINT Delirium can also present with a mix of alternating hyper- and hypoactivity signs.

Q Which characteristic of the criteria used to define delirium is the most common one?

A Inattention

According to the DSM-V criteria, there are four characteristics of delirium, inattention being the most common feature. The other three characteristics are acute change in mental status, disorganized thinking, and either disorganized behavior or altered level of consciousness.

HINT Delusions and hallucinations can occur but are not considered defining characteristics of delirium.

▶ DIAGNOSIS

Q **What is the primary diagnostic for recognizing delirium in critically ill patients?**

A **Clinical diagnosis**

Delirium is a clinical diagnosis. Currently no diagnostic lab, imaging, or EEG test can accurately recognize and diagnose delirium. Clinical signs of delirium and the use of delirium screening tool are the most accurate.

HINT Hypoactive delirium is commonly overlooked with the clinical assessments unless a screening tool is utilized.

Q **What is a commonly used screening tool in the ICU used to assess for the presence of delirium?**

A **Confusion Assessment Method (CAM-ICU)**

CAM-ICU is a frequently used tool to assess for presence of delirium in an ICU. It is a screening tool and a diagnostic algorithm for delirium. In addition to the CAM-ICU, a sedation assessment tool is utilized to determine level of consciousness and the ability of the patient to participate with the delirium assessment tool (Table 10.5). Another delirium tool used in the ICU is the ICDSC tool.

HINT Two most commonly used sedation tools include Richmond Agitation Sedation Scale (RASS) and Riker Sedation-Agitation Scale (SAS).

Table 10.5 Symptom Comparison: Delirium and Dementia

Delirium	Dementia
Inattention	Attention
Rapid onset cognitive changes	Cognitive changes occur over longer period of time
Greater fluctuation of symptoms	Less fluctuation of symptoms

▶ MANAGEMENT

Q **What is considered a preventive measure in mechanically ventilated patients?**

A **Early mobility**

Immobilization is a known modifiable risk factor. Early mobilization of ventilated patients in the ICU has shown to improve weaning times and incidence and severity of delirium. Another preventive goal includes improvement of sleep wake cycles.

HINT Critically ill patients require frequent reorientation to assist with preventing delirium.

Q **What is a commonly used medication to manage delirium?**

A **Haloperidol**

A commonly used medication for the management of delirium is Haloperidol. Haloperidol is an antipsychotic with minimal anticholinergic effects. Haloperidol can cause prolonged QT interval placing the patient at an increased risk of V-tach (torsades). Measuring the QT interval before initiating Haloperidol is recommended frequently throughout the therapy. Another antipsychotic used is resperidone.

HINT Haloperidol is NOT recommended for dementia psychosis.

▶ COMPLICATIONS

> **Q What effect does delirium have on weaning or liberating the patient from mechanical ventilation?**
>
> **A Increases weaning failure**

Delrium has been identified as a common cause for failing to wean from the ventilator. Delirium assessment and initiation of preventive measures is recommended in mechanically ventilated patients.

 DEMENTIA

> **Q What is the most common type of dementia?**
>
> **A Alzheimer's disease (AD)**

Alzheimer's disease (AD) is the most common type of dementia. AD is subdivided into dementia with early onset (under 65 years of age) and with late onset (over 65 years of age).

Vascular dementia is the second most common form and is the result of a stroke. There are multiple other types and causes of dementia (Box 10.36).

Box 10.36 Types and Causes of Dementia

Alzheimer's disease
Vascular dementia
Frontotemporal dementia
Parkinson's disease
Creutzfeldt-Jacob disease
Huntington's disease
Normal pressure hydrocephalus
Wernicke-Korsakoff syndrome
HIV/AIDS dementia
Alcohol-induced dementia

> **Q What are the two known risk factors for AD?**
>
> **A Age and genetics**

There is not a single risk factor but probably multiple factors that result in AD. The two known risk factors for AD are age and genetic predisposition. The risk of AD doubles every ten years after the age of 65.

▶ PATHOPHYSIOLOGY

> **Q Is AD a cortical or a subcortical dementia?**
>
> **A Cortical**

Cortical dementia is characterized by loss of neurons and synapses in cerebral cortex and certain subcortical regions resulting in gross atrophy. It typically involves degeneration of temporal and parietal lobes. AD is of the cortical dysfunction involving memory (Table 10.6).

Table 10.6 Contrasting Characteristics of Cortical and Subcortical Dementia Syndromes

	Subcortical Dementia	Cortical Dementia
Language	No aphasia	Aphasia early
Memory	Recall impaired; recognition normal or better preserved	Recall and recognition impaired
Visuospatial skills	Impaired	Impaired
Calculation	Preserved until late	Involved early
Speed of cognitive processing	Slowed early	Normal until late in disease course
Personality	Apathetic	Unconcerned
Mood	Depressed	Euthymic
Speech	Dysarthric	Normal articulation until late
Posture	Bowed	Upright
Coordination	Impaired	Normal until late
Adventitious movements	Present: chorea, tremor, tics, dystonia	Absent
Motor speed	Slowed	Normal

Q **What two areas of the brain play critical role in memory?**

A **Hippocampus and amygdala**

The hippocampus is located in the deep portion of the brain above the brainstem under the temporal lobe. It is responsible for acquiring and temporarily storing memory. Declarative memory is stored in the hippocampus. The amygdala is located under the temporal lobe and receives input from the sensory system. These structures are a part of the limbic system.

HINT   Information must be stored temporarily (short-term) for it to become a long-term memory (Table 10.7).

Q **What type of memory is doing a familiar task without actually having to think about it?**

A **Declarative memory**

There are several different types of memory. Declarative memory is being able to do a task or activity without having to think about it or think about the steps. An example is driving to and from work everyday.

Table 10.7 Type of Long-Term Memory

Type of Memory	Description	Examples
Semantic memory	Involves the conscious involvement of the learner	Example: Skill of using a telephone book
Implicit memory	Information learned without the conscious involvement of the person Memories established through early and frequent repetitions	Example: Singing the "Happy Birthday" song
Motor memory	Memory of tasks involving motor skills	Example: Riding a bike
Affective memory	Memory which is triggered by feelings or emotions	Example: Smell brings back memories

HINT   Memory and learning are not two different processes but memory is required for learning to occur.

Q **What are the two pathophysiologic changes in the brain that are characteristic of AD?**

A **Amyloid plaque and neurofibrillary tangles**

The pathological changes, which occur in AD, are caused by production of amyloid plaque and neurofibrillary tangles in the brain. Plaques are dense, insoluble deposits of amyloid-beta peptide. Neurofibrillary tangles are aggregates of microtubule-associated protein tau that are hyperphosphorylated.

HINT   Amyloid plaque and neurofibrillary tangles are characteristic findings of AD.

▶ SYMPTOMS/ASSESSMENT

Q What are the two primary symptoms of AD?

A Memory loss and cognitive decline

The symptoms seen in AD are the result of the death of many neurons in the hippocampus and cerebral cortex. This results in memory loss, impaired cognition, and behavioral changes. Memory is required for cognitive capabilities. Memory deficits are the early signs of the onset of AD and progress with the disease process. AD affects semantic memory first. Motor memory is eventually affected, with the person feeling frustrated over not being able to do even simple tasks. They may lose both fine and gross motor skills.

HINT   Affective memory may remain intact as long as the person can communicate.

Q At what stage of AD does the patient begin to pace and wander?

A Stage II

There are four stages of AD (Box 10.37). Each stage demonstrates a progressive loss including mental, physical, or emotional. The onset may be insidious and can frequently be frustrating for the person in the early stages. Stage I may not be recognized as an onset of dementia. After the diagnosis, the family may look back and identify these symptoms retrospectively.

HINT   Memory loss (recent memories) is the first symptom.

Box 10.37 Four Stages of Alzheimer's Disease

Stage I	▪ Short-term memory losses (long-term remain intact) ▪ Loss of spontaneity (less joy or enthusiasm) ▪ Sporadic loss of words (loss of words or substitution of inappropriate words) ▪ Easy to anger (may be physical as well as verbally) ▪ Less discrimination with choices (messy or unkempt, not as meticulous with clothing)
Stage II	▪ Disorientation to time and place (may be the first alarm for family members) ▪ Impaired communication (unable to express thought) ▪ Difficulty in making decisions or plans (takes longer to make minor decisions) ▪ Loss of impulse control (may act upon all thoughts regardless of consequences) ▪ Mistakes in judgment (social situations or money management) ▪ Decreased concentration (difficulty to finish a task or activity) ▪ Increased self-absorption ▪ Avoidance of new situations ▪ Delusions (may be based upon a reality in past history) ▪ Rummaging and pillaging (may hoard or stock items excessively or may pick items up that do not belong to them and put somewhere) ▪ Wandering and pacing (wander aimlessly for hours without fatigue; pacing is accompanied by signs of anxiety, tension and strain)

(continued)

Box 10.37 Four Stages of Alzheimer's Disease (*continued*)

Stage III	■ Sundowning (sleep disrupted with wandering in the middle of the night) ■ Catastrophic reactions (to various events and can result in verbalization, pacing and physical reaction) ■ Failure to recognize family and friends ■ Hyperorality (unexplained movements of mouth and tongue) ■ Preservation (continual activity after the stimulus is removed; i.e., continue to chew even though the food is ready to swallow) ■ Latency (inability to begin an activity) ■ Agnosia (inability to recognize commonly used tools, i.e.; toothbrush) ■ Apraxia (inability to perform a task with an item; i.e., unable to brush teeth with toothbrush)
Stage IV	Unable to communicate in meaningful way No recognition of self or others Total dependence

▶ DIAGNOSIS

Q What is the primary test used to diagnose memory losses and dementia?

A Mini-Mental State Examination (MMSE)

MMSE is a neurophysiologic test used to determine onset or presence of dementia. It involves copying drawings, remembering words, reading, and subtracting serial numbers.

Q What is the definitive diagnosis of AD?

A Autopsy

Definitive diagnosis is on autopsy only. Autopsy reveals plaque formation and neurofibrillary tangles to confirm the diagnosis. A probable diagnosis is made based upon history and physical, diagnostic tests, cognitive testing, and mental status evaluation.

▶ MANAGEMENT

Q What is the primary pharmacological management for AD?

A Cholinesterase inhibitors

Cholinesterase is an enzyme that breaks down acetylcholine (ACh) after it crosses the synapse. The drug suppresses this enzyme so that acetylcholine is not broken down as rapidly, thereby increasing concentration of ACh. This may temporarily slow the rate of decline in memory and thinking ability in early stages (mild to moderate). Examples include donepezil hydrochloride (Aricept), galantamine (Razadyne), rivastigmine (Exelon) and Exelon patch. The other drug approved to treat AD is an NMDA receptor antagonist. NMDA receptors are for glutamate, which is an excitatory neurotransmitter. Excessive amounts of glutamate can lead to cell death (excitotoxicity). An example includes memantine (Akatinol).

HINT A common side effect of cholinesterase inhibitors is nausea and vomiting (cholinergic excess).

▶ COMPLICATIONS

Q What is a common complication of dementia patient that occurs in the evening and can increase the likelihood of falls in hospital?

A Sundowning

Sundowning is a type of agitation that occurs with older patients and patients with dementia. In the evenings or during the night they become more disoriented and agitated. This agitation can frequently contribute to patient falls in the hospital.

HINT   Turning on lights well before sunset and closing the curtains at dusk will minimize shadows and may help diminish confusion that occurs with sundowning.

⬤ ENCEPHALOPATHY

Q How is encephalopathy defined?

A Generalized cortical dysfunction

There are multiple underlying etiologies that cause this generalized cortical dysfunction. Encephalopathy can be as a result of systemic metabolic and toxic involvement brain injury (Box 10.38).

Box 10.38 Characteristics of Encephalopathy

Fluctuations of level of consciousness (LOC)
Poor attention span (inattention)
Hallucinations and delusions
Changes in psychomotor activity

▶ PATHOPHYSIOLOGY

Q What is the underlying cause of posterior reversible encephalopathy syndrome (PRES)?

A Hypertension

Hypertensive crisis can cause altered mentation (encephalopathy), confusion, visual disturbances, and headaches. This is a reversible syndrome when managed early by controlling the patient's BP. PRES is a result of hyperperfusion causing a disruption of the blood brain barrier and vasogenic edema in the occipital parietal lobes.

HINT   PRES is the encephalopathy that involves progressive headaches and visual disturbances.

Q Which type of encephalopathy is caused by vitamin B-1 deficiency?

A Wernicke's encephalopathy

Wernicke's encephalopathy is often seen in alcoholics because of the effect alcohol has on vitamin B-1 uptake and utilization. Other causes include malnutrition, hemodialysis, and HIV/AIDS patients.

HINT   Complication of bariatric surgeries includes reduced thiamine absorption resulting in vitamin B-1 deficiency and Wernicke's encephalopathy.

Q What is the underlying physiology thought to result in Hashimoto's encephalopathy?

A Autoimmune

The physiology of Hashimoto's encephalopathy is not completely understood but is associated with autoimmune or inflammatory abnormalities. There is a relationship between Hashimoto's and thyroiditis (Box 10.39).

Box 10.39 Underlying Causes of Encephalopathy

Alcohol-induced encephalopathy
Hypertensive encephalopathy
Anoxic/hypoxic encephalopathy
Wernicke's encephalopathy
Hepatic encephalopthy

(*continued*)

Box 10.39 Underlying Causes of Encephalopathy (*continued*)

AIDS encephalopathy
Toxic/metabolic encephalopathy
Hashimoto's encephalopathy
Infectious encephalopathy
Uremic encephalopthy

▶ SYMPTOMS/ASSESSMENT

Q A patient with hepatic failure presents with asterixis and definitive personality changes. What grade of severity is the hepatic encephalopathy?

A Grade II

Hepatic failure can be graded in severity, ranging from I to IV (Box 10.40). Grade II involves personality changes, inappropriate behavior, and asterixis or commonly called "liver flap."

HINT   Uremic encephalopathy can also present with asterixis.

Box 10.40 Grading Hepatic Encephalopathy

Minimal	Psychometric or neuropsychological alterations of tests exploring psychomotor speed/ executive functions or neurophysiological alterations without clinical evidence of mental change
Grade I	Trivial lack of awareness Euphoria or anxiety Short attention span Impairment of addition/subtraction Altered sleep patterns
Grade II	Lethargy or apathy Disorientation of time Obvious personality change Inappropriate behavior Asterixis
Grade III	Somnolence or near stupor Responsive to stimuli Confused Gross disorientation Bizarre behavior
Grade IV	Coma

Q A patient with history of hypertension presents with altered mentation and visual disturbances. Which type of encephalopathy is most likely the cause?

A PRES

Posterior reversible eencephalopathy syndrome (PRES) is a hypertensive crisis resulting in symptoms of progressive headache, visual disturbances, nausea, and papilledema (Box 10.41).

HINT   PRES is hypertensive encephalopathy.

Box 10.41 Specific Symptoms of Certain Encephalopathies

PRES	Visual disturbances Progressive headaches Papilledema Nausea
Wernicke's	Ataxia Ophthalmoplegia Peripheral neuropathy
Hypoxic/anoxic	Myoclonus activity Seizures
Hepatic	Personality changes Asterixis Bizarre behavior Coma
Hashimato	Myoclonus Seizures Visual hallucinations Psychosis
Uremic	Myoclonus Nystagmus Hyperreflexia Papilledema

▶ DIAGNOSIS

Q Which diagnostic study is the best for identifying PRES when a patient presents with hypertension and altered mentation?

A MRI

Cerebral changes in PRES include bilateral occipital cerebral edema, which is best identified with MRI.

Q Which diagnostic test is typically used to differentiate encephalopathy from other neurological disorders, including seizures?

A EEG

Encephalopathy demonstrates bilateral slowing on EEG without epileptic spikes. Patients with altered mentation from postictal state will typically demonstrate findings of epileptic activity.

HINT Following anoxic brain injury, myoclonic and seizure activity can occur. An EEG can be used to differentiate between the two.

Q In hepatic failure, what lab is utilized to assist with the diagnosis of hepatic encephalopathy?

A Ammonia level

Elevated ammonia levels is the underlying cause of the encephalopathy associated with hepatic failure. Ammonia levels assist with the recognition of hepatic encephalopathy, but the level is not a strong prediction of severity. The clinical signs of encephalopathy is used to stage or determine the severity of the encephalopathy.

▶ MANAGEMENT

Q What is the most common medical management of Wernicke's encephalopathy?

A Thiamine replacement

Parental thiamine replacement is the medical management for Wernicke's encephalopathy.

HINT Do not administer glucose to thiamine-deficient patients because it causes acute worsening of the deficiency and rapid neurological deterioration.

Q What is the primary management of a patient post cardiac arrest with an anoxic brain injury?

A Target temperature management (TTM)

Controlled hypothermia with TTM following an anoxic brain injury is used to improve neurological outcomes after cardiac arrest. TTM is the only neuroprotectant found to improve neurological outcomes in cardiac arrest (Box 10.42).

Box 10.42 Common Interventions for Certain Encephalopathies

PRES	Antihypertensive therapy to lower the BP
Wernicke's	Parental replacement of thiamine
Hypoxic/anoxic	Targeted temperature management (TTM)
Hepatic	Cathartics (Lactulose) Antibiotics (Neomycin, Rifaximin)
Hashimoto	Corticosteroids Immunosuppression
Uremic	Hemodialysis

▶ COMPLICATIONS

Q What is the complication if Wernicke's encephalopathy is not treated with thiamine replacement?

A Korskoff's syndrome

Wernicke-Korsaff syndrome is progressive, irreversible cognitive state due to lack of thiamine replacement. It is an amnesic state, involving both antegrade and retrograde amnesia. The term refers to two different syndromes representing different stages of the Wenicke's encephalopathy.

HINT Wernicke's syndrome is acute and reversible while Korskoff's is chronic and irreversible brain injury.

⬤ ICP MONITORING AND LUMBAR DRAINS

▶ ICP MONITORING

Q Where is an intraventricular catheter placed for CSF drainage and ICP monitoring?

A Anterior horn of lateral ventricle

ICP monitoring is commonly used when managing a patient with a neurological disorder resulting in an increase in ICP. In combination with BP, it is currently the best way to continuously monitor cerebral perfusion. ICP monitors can be placed in several areas of the brain, including the epidural space, subarachnoid space, intraparenchymal, and intraventricular. Intraventricular catheters are considered the gold standard because they are placed directly into the ventricles, for more accurate pressure readings and ability to drain CSF.

HINT The intraventricular catheters can also be used to manage increased ICP by draining CSF.

Q What is the most common reason for placement of an ICP monitor?

A Decrease in LOC

There are many different neurological scenarios that warrant the placement of an ICP monitor. The most common indications include a TBI with a Glasgow Coma Scale (GCS) score of 8 or less and a significantly abnormal CT scan (Box 10.43).

Box 10.43 General Indications for ICP Monitoring

Hydrocephalus: communicating and noncommunicating	Infections: meningitis, encephalitis
Subarachnoid hemorrhage (SAH): acute hydrocephalus or Hunt and Hess Grade ≥ III	Brain relaxation in the operating room (OR)
Cerebral edema	Space-occupying lesions
Mass lesions	

HINT   ICP monitoring not only provides information regarding pressure and perfusion but also shows compliance of the brain. ICP waveform analysis is used to determine compliance.

Q What ICP waveform abnormality would indicate a decrease in brain compliance?

A P2 component greater than the P1 component

The normal ICP waveform is a three-peaked wave, similar in shape to the arterial waveform. The peaks are labeled P1, P2, and P3. The P1 component is the highest in amplitude, followed by P2 and P3 in a descending manner. As the ICP increases, the amplitude of all the peaks also increases. When the P2 component becomes greater than P1, it is an indication of noncompliance in the cranium and may require intervention at this time.

Q What is the external landmark used to level the transducer of the ICP monitor?

A Tragus of the ear

It is recommended that the same external landmark be used consistently for leveling an external transducer. Tragus of the ear is most commonly used. The external landmarks approximate the transducer level to the foramen of Monro, which is the zero reference level.

Q How do you control the amount of CSF drainage from an external ventricular drain (EVD)?

A Raise or lower the drainage system

Drainage of CSF is based on hydrostatic pressure. Leveling the fluid-filled EVD at or above the zero reference level controls the amount of drainage.

HINT   It is based upon gravity drainage, the lower the EVD the greater the amount of CSF drainage.

Q How do you calculate CPP?

A CPP = MAP – ICP

MAP is the driving force and ICP is the opposing force. The difference between the two is the pressure needed to perfuse the brain. A decrease in MAP or an increase in ICP can result in hypoperfusion. A normal CPP is greater than 60 mmHg. A CPP between 40 and 60 mmHg is hypoperfusion and a CPP less than 40 mmHg indicates anoxic brain injury. The goal is typically to maintain CPP greater than 60 or 70 mmHg, depending on the neurological disorder.

Q What is a complication of overdrainage of CSF?

A Hemispheric shift

If the CSF is drained too rapidly or an overdrainage occurs, it can cause a shift of the brain laterally and an uncal herniation (Table 10.8).

HINT   A shift from overdrainage can also cause vascular tearing and subdural hematoma.

Table 10.8 EVD Complications and Management

Complication	Prevention	Management
Infection	Antibiotic-impregnated ventricular catheters Aseptic technique of placement of catheter Aseptic technique of flushing the EVD tubing with initial setup Strict sterile dressing change	Cerebrospinal fluid (CSF) analysis if infection is suspected Antimicrobial therapy Remove infected catheters, if possible
CSF leak	Assess catheter site and dressing for CSF drainage	Inform physician immediately if ventriculostomy dressing is wet May place a suture or remove the catheter
Aneurysm rebleed	Monitor ICP and ICP drainage carefully Prevent CSF overdrainage	Rapid recognition and notification of the physician Control blood pressure
Hemispheric shifts	Monitor ICP and ICP drainage carefully Prevent CSF overdrainage	Rapid recognition and notification of the physician Clamp the EVD

CSF overdrainage
Subdural
  hematoma
  formation
Herniation
	Maintain the EVD drip chamber at the prescribed level
	Inform patient/family not to change level of bed without assistance
	Ensure zero reference is maintained
	Clamp EVD any time there is a procedure that may cause CSF overdrainage
		Rapid recognition and notification of the physician
		Clamp the EVD

Hemorrhage	Assure international normalized ratio (INR) is within normal range prior to catheter placement	May require surgical management
Misplacement of catheter	Ensure postprocedural CT scan, if ordered, is performed in a timely manner Perform ICP waveform assessment Assure catheter drainage is CSF by performing a halo test	Removal and replacement of catheter

▶ LUMBAR DRAINS

Lumbar drainage devices (LDDs) are systems that are placed in the subarachnoid space at the lumbar level (L_2–L_3 level or below) and are used to obtain CSF samples or drain CSF. LDDs are commonly used in the treatment of dural fistulae, shunt infections, and in the diagnostic evaluation of idiopathic normal-pressure hydrocephalus (NPH) (Box 10.44).

Box 10.44 Relative and Absolute Contraindications for LDDs

Relative Contraindications	Absolute Contraindications
Coagulopathy	Increased intracranial pressure (ICP)
Brain abscess	Unequal pressures between supratentorial and infratentorial compartments
History prior to lumbar spine surgery	Infected skin over needle-entry site
History of prior lumbar vertebral fracture	Spinal epidural abscess
	Intracranial mass
	Obstructive noncommunicating hydrocephalus
	Spinal arteriovenous malformation

Q What is a common complication following placement of a lumbar drain?

A Postprocedural puncture headache

A common complication of a lumbar puncture or drain is a headache following the procedure. This may be managed by keeping the head of the bed flat and administering analgesics. If this does not alleviate headache, a blood patch may be performed (Box 10.45).

HINT A patient with an epidural catheter for pain management could have similar potential complications to those needing lumbar drains.

Box 10.45 Complications of Lumbar Drain

Radicular nerve pain
CSF leak
CNS infection (e.g., meningitis)
EDH
Catheter fracture
Herniation
Cerebral venous thrombosis
Overdrainage of CSF
Occlusion of tubing

Q What should you do with the LDD when making changes in the patient's position?

A Clamp the drainage system

A position change can affect the amount of drainage. Clamping the catheter's drainage system while making changes in the patient's position will prevent over drainage from occurring. Over drainage can result in SDH and tension pneumocranium. After repositioning, the LDD should be leveled and the drainage assessed.

1. Which of the following is the cause of an embolic stroke in which the thrombi originate in the leg veins?

   A. Endocarditis
   B. Atrial fibrillation
   C. Patent foramen ovale (PFO)
   D. Left ventricular wall myocardial infarction (MI)

2. Your patient has been having tonic-clonic seizure for 5 minutes. Which of the following treatments would be the best initial intervention?

   A. Propofol
   B. Phenobarbital
   C. Ativan
   D. Dilantin

3. Which of the following is the most common peripheral neuropathy in the intensive care unit (ICU) patient?

   A. Guillain-Barré syndrome
   B. Critical illness polyneuropathy (CIP)
   C. Myasthenia gravis
   D. Multiple sclerosis

4. A patient recovering from bacterial meningitis has developed a cranial nerve deficit and long-term complications from the injury. Which of the following cranial nerve is the most commonly involved with meningitis, and what is the long-term complication?

   A. CN VII, facial drooping
   B. CN II, difficulty swallowing
   C. CN I, smelling losses
   D. CN VIII, hearing losses

5. Which of the following secondary injuries in traumatic brain injury (TBI) will result in the most significant worsening of neurological outcomes?

   A. Hyperglycemia
   B. Hypercapnia
   C. Hyponatremia
   D. Hypoxia

6. Following an ischemic stroke, the intensive care unit (ICU) nurse performs a neurological assessment and notes that the patient is unable to form words. The patient follows commands, is oriented to person and place, and the pupils are equal bilaterally. Which of the following best describes this patient's neurological deficit?

   A. Agnosia
   B. Expressive aphasia
   C. Global aphasia
   D. Receptive aphasia

1. C) Patent foramen ovale (PFO)
All of the conditions referenced in these answers can cause an embolic stroke, but the patent foramen ovale (PFO) is the one in which the thrombi typically originate in the leg veins (venous thrombi). PFO is an opening between the left and right atrium. As a venous clot travels from the legs, it may cross through the opening into the left atrium to become a systemic embolus.

2. C) Ativan
Ativan, a benzodiazepine, is the most commonly used first-line drug to stop a seizure. The most effective drugs for rapid termination of generalized seizures are benzodiazepines, as they typically terminate the seizure within 2–3 minutes.

3. B) Critical illness polyneuropathy (CIP)
CIP is a secondary condition that occurs in critically ill patients. It is both motor and sensory, and is thought to be caused by inflammation. High-risk factors include mechanical ventilation, use of paralytic agents and sedatives, and steroids. Guillain-Barré is a peripheral neuropathy but is less commonly cared for in the ICU than CIP. Myasthenia gravis and multiple sclerosis are not peripheral neuropathies.

4. D) CN VIII, hearing losses
CN VIII (acoustic) is the cranial nerve most commonly injured by meningitis. It frequently results in long-term hearing losses. CN II (optic) may also be commonly involved, but injury to this nerve results in visual disturbances rather than difficulty swallowing. CN VII (facial) and CN I (smell) are not commonly involved with meningitis. Other CNs that may be affected with meningitis are CN III, IV, and VI, which are involved with extraocular eye movement.

5. D) Hypoxia
Hypoxia and hypertension have been found to be the two most powerful determinants of neurological outcome following a traumatic brain injury. Hyperglycemia, hypercapnia, and hyponatremia may also worsen outcomes, but hypoxia has a more significant effect on neurological outcomes.

6. B) Expressive aphasia
In expressive aphasia the patient has difficulty forming speech and putting together sentences. The patient is able to understand conversation and can follow commands. In receptive aphasia, the patient is unable to understand language and cannot follow verbal commands. The patient may be able to express words, but they do not make sense. Global aphasia is an inability to understand language and an inability to express speech. Agnosia is the inability to process sensory information.

7. Which of the following is best described as being an antibody-mediated destruction of acetylcholine receptors on the muscle end plates?

   A. Guillain-Barré syndrome
   B. Myasthenia gravis (MG)
   C. Multiple sclerosis
   D. Amyotrophic lateral sclerosis (ALS)

8. Which of the following symptoms can be a sign of diffuse anoxic brain injury?

   A. Confusion and agitation
   B. Myoclonus activity
   C. Asymmetrical pupils
   D. Nausea and vomiting

9. While administering mannitol to lower intracranial pressure (ICP), which of the following should the intensive care unit (ICU) nurse monitor closely to prevent serious complications?

   A. Potassium levels
   B. Osmolality levels
   C. Computed tomography (CT) scan results
   D. ICP readings

10. While caring for a patient in the intensive care unit (ICU) following a severe traumatic brain injury, the patient is noted to have bilateral periorbital ecchymosis and cerebrospinal fluid (CSF) leak. Which of the following is the most likely diagnosis?

    A. Depressed skull fracture
    B. Basilar skull fracture
    C. Mandibular fracture
    D. Diffuse axonal injury

11. A new orientee in the intensive care unit (ICU) asks the nurse how fast can she administer phenytoin (Dilantin) intravenous. What is the best response?

    A. Administer IV push as rapidly as possible during a seizure
    B. Administer by intravenous route no faster than 50 mg/minute
    C. Do not administer IV, only oral route indicated
    D. Administer IV piggyback mixed with D5W over 1 hour

12. When performing an apnea test to assist with the determination of brain death, which of the following has to occur to determine the absence of spontaneous breathing efforts?

    A. Hypotension
    B. Hypercapnia
    C. Hypoxia
    D. Absence of reflexes

13. Which of the following intracranial pressure (ICP) waveform changes indicates a noncompliant brain and may be found prior to an increase in ICP?

    A. Increase in X descent
    B. Development of A waves
    C. Dampened waveform
    D. The P2 wave is greater than the P1 wave

(See answers next page.)   383

7. B) Myasthenia gravis (MG)

MG is a neuromuscular disorder that affects the acetylcholine receptors, resulting in fluctuating muscle weakness and fatigue. Guillain-Barré syndrome and multiple sclerosis involve the myelin sheath along neurons; ALS involves upper and lower motor neurons.

8. B) Myoclonus activity

Myoclonus activity (irregular, jerking movements) can be a sign of diffuse anoxic brain injury. Anoxic brain injuries typically result in unresponsiveness (coma) rather than confusion and agitation, and bilateral midposition unreactive pupils. Asymmetrical pupils are typically caused by unilateral injuries or masses.

9. B) Osmolality levels

Osmolality levels should be monitored closely while administering mannitol. A current osmolality level should be known before the next dose of mannitol is administered. Severe hyperosmolar states can worsen neurological outcomes. Potassium is important because of the diuresis, but the osmolar state is monitored closely to prevent potential complications. CT scan results and ICP readings can be assessed to determine the effectiveness of the mannitol treatment.

10. B) Basilar skull fracture

Patients with basilar skull fractures frequently develop bilateral periorbital ecchymosis (raccoon eyes) or mastoid process bruising (Battle sign) and a CSF leak. Depressed skull fractures typically are associated with hematomas. Facial fractures can frequently involve the basilar skull and present with similar bruising and CSF leak, but this is not typical for a mandible fracture. Diffuse axonal injury is trauma to the brain tissue.

11. B) Administer by intravenous route no faster than 50 mg/minute

Phenytoin can be administered intravenous (IV push or piggyback), but the rate of administration should not exceed 50 mg/minute, even during a seizure. Too-rapid administration can result in cardiac depression and hypotension.

12. B) Hypercapnia

The apnea test is used to assist with the determination of brain death and assess for any spontaneous breathing. Hypercapnia, also known as hypercarbia (or an increase in $PaCO_2$ by >20 mm Hg), is required to assure adequate triggering of a spontaneous breath. Hypotension and hypoxia can occur and may cause the apnea test to be stopped due to instability but do not need to occur to trigger a breath. Absence of reflexes is also used in brain death determination, but this is not a part of the apnea test.

13. D) The P2 wave is greater than the P1 wave

The ICP waveform has three waves: P1, P2, and P3. In a normal ICP waveform, the P1 component is the highest, followed in descending order by the P2 and the P3 components. If the P2 wave is greater than the P1 wave, brain noncompliance is present and may be seen before the ICP elevates. A dampened waveform may indicate problems within the system, or a low ICP. A waves are high ICPs that occur over a prolonged period of time. Y descents are found on pulmonary artery (PA) waveforms, not ICP waveforms.

14. Which reflex is commonly assessed when determining brain death?

    A. Anocutaneous reflex
    B. Babinski reflex
    C. Bulbocavernosus reflex
    D. Oculovestibular reflex

15. A subarachnoid hemorrhage (SAH) patient is being managed in the intensive care unit (ICU) following an aneurysm clipping. The family is asking why the patient has to remain in the ICU for 14 days. What is the best explanation the ICU nurse can provide to the family for the length of stay?

    A. Cerebral edema is still a concern following a bleed and the doctor is being cautious by having the patient stay in ICU for 14 days
    B. Vasospasms are a potential complication and may occur up to 14 days after the bleed
    C. There is no reason for this extra stay, because the patient is doing really well
    D. I will ask the physician and maybe she can explain the rationale for the length of stay

16. During neurogenic shock, which of the following dysrhythmias would be most expected?

    A. Sinus tachycardia
    B. Supraventricular tachycardia
    C. Complete heart block
    D. Sinus bradycardia

17. A patient was admitted to the ICU following a MVC and TBI with basilar skull fracture. They develop leukocytosis and fever. Which of the following would be the most likely cause?

    A. Meningitis
    B. Pneumonia
    C. CAUTI
    D. CLABSI

18. A patient presents with a "lipstick sign" in the emergency room following a motor vehicle front-end collision. Which of the following injuries is most commonly associated with hyperflexion injury?

    A. Burst fracture
    B. Rupture posterior ligament with subluxation
    C. Whiplash injury
    D. Spinal cord compression

19. Which of the following vertebral fractures would be considered stable and managed without surgical intervention?

    A. Atlantoccipital dislocation
    B. Hangman's fracture
    C. Type I Odontoid
    D. Burst fracture

20. During your assessment of a patient with a spinal cord injury, you note the patient has no motor movement of their legs and do not respond to painful stimulus but are able to feel light touch bilateral. Which of the following conditions best identifies this patient's injury?

    A. Anterior cord syndrome
    B. Complete cord injury
    C. Central cord syndrome
    D. Brown sequard cord syndrome

(See answers next page.)

14. D) Oculovestibular reflex

The oculovestibular (cold calorics) reflex and oculocephalic (doll's eyes) reflex are two reflexes used in the determination of brain death. Anocutaneous and bulbocavernosus reflexes are assessed in patients with spinal cord injury to determine the return of reflexes. A Babinski reflex is abnormal in comatose patients.

15. B) Vasospasms are a potential complication and may occur up to 14 days after the bleed

Typically, following an aneurysm rupture, SAH patients are kept in close observation for at least 14 days after the hemorrhage. This is because vasospasms can occur as late as 14–21 days post hemorrhage.

16. D) Sinus bradycardia

Neurogenic shock symptoms of vasodilation, hypotension, and bradycardia occur in SCI due to the damage to the sympathetic nervous system. At the cervical level, complete injury interrupts sympathetic outflow to the heart while the parasympathetic outflow remains intact via vagus nerve causing bradycardia in neurogenic shock. Sinus tachycardia is found in all other shock states. SVT and complete heart block are not common dysrythmias with neurogenic shock.

17. A) Meningitis

Following a basilar or depressed skull fracture, the patient is at an increased risk for meningitis. Presentation includes leukocytosis and fever. Aspiration pneumonia is common with TBI patients, but there is not any indication of pneumonia in the scenario. CAUTI and CLABSI are not the likely answers because there is no reference to presence of catheters.

18. B) Rupture posterior ligament with subluxation

Hyperflexion injuries occurring from front-end collisions can result in rupture of the posterior longitudinal ligament due to the stretch posterior. Without the posterior longitudinal ligament, instability occurs with anterior subluxation. Whiplash most frequently occurs with rear end collision. Burst fractures of the vertebra occur with a loading mechanism or compression. Spinal cord compression occurs with a narrowing of the spinal canal.

19. C) Type I Odontoid

Type I Odontoid fracture is the very tip of the odontoid bone and is not at risk for cord compression. It is considered a stable fracture. Atlantoccipital dislocation is an unstable subluxation between the occiput and C1. Hangman's fracture is the bilateral fracture of the ring of C2. It can result in anterior subluxation. Burst fractures can cause cord compression and are unstable fractures.

20. A) Anterior cord syndrome

Anterior cord syndrome results in the loss of motor, pain, and temperature but maintaining light touch and proprioception. Complete injury would be a loss of motor and all sensory. Central cord syndrome involves the upper extremities great than the lower. Brown-Sequard cord syndrome is the ipsilateral loss of motor and contralateral loss of sensory.

21. A patient is admitted to the ICU following MVC with a SCI. The nurse notes the patient is hypotensive and bradycardic. Which of the following is the cause of the patient's hemodynamic instability?

   A. Spinal shock
   B. Autonomic hyperreflexia
   C. Neurogenic shock
   D. PRES

22. A hemipalegic patient with a history of SCI is in the unit for a small bowel obstruction. The patient's BP is 225/110 mmHg. Which of the following is the hypertensive crisis that is associated with SCI?

   A. PRES
   B. Neurogenic claudication
   C. Spinal shock syndrome
   D. Autonomic hyperreflexia

23. Which type of encephalopathy is associated with vitamin B-1 deficiency?

   A. Wernicke's
   B. Hashimoto's
   C. PRES
   D. Uremic

24. Following bariatric surgery, what is the physiology for the potential development of Wernicke's syndrome?

   A. Alcohol intoxication
   B. Anemia
   C. Vitamin D deficiency
   D. Thiamine deficiency

25. Which of the following is the most accurate statement regarding the difference between dementia and delirium?

   A. Delirium results in hyperactivity and dementia hypoactivity
   B. Delirium affects mainly attention and dementia affects mainly memory
   C. Delirium symptoms fluctuate and dementia progressively worsens
   D. Delirium affects all ages and dementia affects the elderly only

21. C) Neurogenic shock
Neurogenic shock occurs in SCI due to injury of the sympathetic nervous system. The parasympathetic remains intact causing vasodilatin, hypotension, and bradycardia. Spinal shock is the loss of motor, reflexes, and sensory at or below the level of injury even if the injury is an incomplete. It is due to the trauma of cord with edema and swelling. Autonomic hyperreflexia causes hypertension and occurs after spinal shock resolves. PRES is a brain injury due to hypertensive crisis.

22. D) Autonomic hyperreflexia
Autonomic hyperreflexia is a long-term complication of SCI. Painful stimulus below the level of injury causes an autonomic response with hypertension. This can be a life-threatening hypertensive crisis. PRES is a complication of hypertension, not a cause. Neurogenic claudication is pain in legs while walking due to spinal nerve involvement. Spinal shock results in hypotension, not hypertenison.

23. A) Wernicke's
Wernicke's encephalopathy is commonly associated with alcoholics and is caused by alteration in uptake and utilization of vitamin B-1. PRES is an encephalopathy associated with hypertensive crisis. Hashimoto's is associated with thyroiditis. Uremic encephalopathy is associated with renal failure and uremia.

24. D) Thiamine deficiency
A common complication of bariatric surgeries is reduced absorption of thiamine resulting in vitamin B-1 deficiency and increased risk of Wernicke's encephalopathy. Alcohol intoxication can also cause Wernicke's encephalopathy but is not associated with bariatric surgery. Vitamin D deficiency and anemia does not cause Wernicke's encephalopathy.

25. B) Delirium affects mainly attention and dementia affects mainly memory
Delirium is partially defined as inattention. It mainly affects attention (inattention) while dementia affects memory initially followed by more cognitive involvement. Delirium can present with either hypoactivity or hyperactivity. Both delirium and dementia symptoms can fluctuate. Delirium can affect all ages but is more common in elderly. Dementia though can occur as early onset and not only affect the elderly.

BIBLIOGRAPHY

Connolly, E. S. Jr, Rabinstein, A. A., Carhuapoma, J. R., Derdeyn, C. P., Dion, J., Higashida, R. T., ... & Vespa, P. (2012). Guidelines for the management of aneurysmal subarachnoid hemorrhage: A guideline for healthcare professionals from the American Heart Association/American Stroke Association. *Stroke, 43*(6), 1711–1737.

del Zoppo, G. J., Saver, J. L., Jauch, E. C., & Adams, H. P. Jr. (2009). Expansion of the time window for treatment of acute ischemic stroke with intravenous tissue plasminogen activator. *Stroke, 40,* 2945–2948.

Fisher, R. S., Van Emde Boas, W., Blume, W., Elger, C., Genton, P., Lee, P., & Engel, J. Jr. (2005). Epileptic seizures and epilepsy definitions proposed by the International League Against Epilepsy (ILAE) and the International Bureau for Epilepsy (IBE). *Epilepsia, 46,* 470–472.

Goldstein, L. B., Bushnell, C. D., Adams, R. J., Appel, L. J., Braun, L. T., Chaturvedi, S., ... & Pearson, T. A. (2011). Guidelines for the primary prevention of stroke: A guideline for healthcare professionals from the American Heart Association/American Stroke Association. *Stroke, 42*(2), 517–584.

Hemphill, J. C. III, Greenberg, S. M., Anderson, C. S., Becker, K., Bendok, B. R., Cushman, M., ... & Woo, D. (2015). Guidelines for the management of spontaneous intracerebral hemorrhage: A guideline for healthcare professionals from the American Heart Association/American Stroke Association. *Stroke, 46*(7), 2032–2060.

Kanner, A., Ashman, E., Gloss, D., Harden, C., Bourgeois, B., Bautista, J., Abou-Khalil, Burakgazi-Dalkilic, E., Park, E., Stern, J., Hirtz, D., Nespeca, M., Gidal, B., Faught, E., & French, J. (2018) Practice guideline update summary: Efficacy and tolerability of the new antiepileptic drugs II: Treatment resistant epilepsy. *Neurology, 91*(2)

Powers, W., Rabinstein, A., Ackerson, T. Adeove, O., Bambakidis, N., Becker, K., Biller, J., Brown, M., Demaerschalk, B., & Hoh, B. (2019) Guidelines for the early management of patients with acute ischemic stroke: 2019 update to 2018 guidelines for the early management of acute ischemic stroke. *Stroke, 50*(12), e344–e418.

Tunkel, A., Hasbun, R., Bhimraj, A., Kaplan, S., Scheld, M., van de Beek, D., Bleck, T., Garton, H., & Zunt, J. (2017). 2017 Infectious Diseases Society of America's Clinical Practice Guidelines for Healthcare-Associated Ventriculitis and Meningitis. *Clinical Infectious Diseases, 64*(6), e34–e64.

Wijdicks, E., Varelas, P. N., Gronseth, G. S., & Greer, D. M. (2010). Evidence-based guideline update: Determining brain death in adults. *Neurology, 74,* 1911–1918.

Behavioral and Psychosocial Review

▶ **LEARNING OBJECTIVES**

In this chapter, you will review:
- ▪ Substance use disorders
- ▪ Agitation
- ▪ Anxiety
- ▪ Moderate sedation
- ▪ Pain
- ▪ Suicidal ideation and/or behaviors
- ▪ Depression
- ▪ Aggression
- ▪ Abuse/neglect
- ▪ PTSD
- ▪ Medical nonadherence
- ▪ Restraint use in the ICU
- ▪ Testable Nursing Actions: Restraints

⬤ SUBSTANCE USE DISORDERS

Q What is the major difference between an addiction and a dependence on a drug?

A Compulsive cravings

An addiction is an acquired chronic disorder characterized by compulsive use of drugs with a craving resulting in physical, psychological, and social harm. This craving and abuse continue despite the evidence of harm. It is a loss of control and denial of potential for harm and is characterized by the persistent use of dysfunctional drugs. The definition for addiction includes a compulsion or an overpowering drive to take the drug in order to experience the psychological effects.

HINT Chronic use of an opioid does not mean the patient is addicted.

Q What is the adaption to drugs at the cellular level such that when the drug is removed abruptly, withdrawal symptoms occur?

A Dependence

Dependence on a substance is the result of chronic drug administration and has a characteristic set of signs and symptoms called withdrawal syndrome. Dependence can occur with and without addiction. The incidence of physical dependence on substances (including alcohol) is greater than most healthcare workers realize and needs to be monitored closely to prevent complications of withdrawal.

HINT Abuse can coexist independently from both dependence and addiction.

> **Q** What is the illicit use of a substance outside the legitimate medical practice called?
>
> **A** Abuse

Abuse is when a substance is used, either prescribed or illicit, outside of normal practice or without medical justification.

> **Q** When a person has multiple prescriptions for pain and anxiety prescribed by several different physicians, what is this typically called?
>
> **A** Drug seeking

There are three main reasons for people seeking drugs. One is because they have a drug addiction and are seeking substances for their cravings and a "high." Other drug seekers may be obtaining drugs to sell but are not actually taking the substances themselves. There are also a large number of drug seekers who are people truly in pain but are not being managed appropriately for their pain. They are commonly seen as addicts but actually have a pseudoaddiction on the drug because of unrelieved pain or fear of reemergence of the pain.

HINT People in pain may do extraordinary things to obtain pain medications to adequately control their pain.

> **Q** What are the most commonly prescribed addictive drugs in the world?
>
> **A** Hypnotics and sedatives

Hypnotics and sedatives are the most commonly prescribed drugs in the world with addicting properties. Alcohol is the most widely used substance.

HINT Alcohol is a sedative/hypnotic, so there is cross-tolerance and cross-dependence between alcohol and other sedatives.

> **Q** What is the major characteristic of alcohol abuse (not just use)?
>
> **A** Dangerous behaviors

Alcohol abuse is defined as a pattern of recurrent alcohol use associated with dangerous behaviors (e.g., driving while intoxicated, fighting, or being sexually promiscuous) or a failure to meet one's obligations at home or work.

HINT Abuse is not determined by a set amount or frequency of alcohol consumption.

▶ PATHOPHYSIOLOGY

> **Q** What part of the brain is responsible for "addictions" to substances?
>
> **A** Subcortical area

Addiction affects the subcortical area including the hypothalamus. The subcortical areas of the brain are not involved in higher cognitive processing, but these are areas of the brain that motivate and mediate instinctual drive-based and emotionally charged behaviors. Despite the different types of drugs that are addicting, the common characteristic of all of the potentially addictive drugs is a specific neuronal pathway called the mesolimbic dopamine pathway. It is located in the "reward center" of the brain. Drugs that affect this pathway cause a release of dopamine, which then stimulates the release of endogenous opioids, the result of which is profound euphoria and elevated moods associated with drug intoxication and drug-seeking behavior.

> **Q** When does physical dependence on a substance become apparent?
>
> **A** Sudden cessation

Physical dependence occurs over time as the body adapts to the repeated dosing of the drug. Physical dependence becomes apparent with withdrawal or sudden reversing and rapid fall in drug levels. Suddenly, unopposed by the drug's effects, the adaptive changes become nonadaptive and physical symptoms appear.

HINT   Some drugs have minimal to no physical dependence or withdrawal symptoms, even in addicted people.

> **Q** What is the excitatory neurotransmitter receptor that alcohol inhibits?
>
> **A** *N*-Methyl-D-asparate (NMDA)

Acute alcohol ingestion inhibits NMDA receptors, reducing excitatory glutamate transmission, and has an agonist (enhancing) effect on gamma-aminobutyric acid (GABA), the inhibitory neurotransmitter. Initially, alcohol produces euphoria, exaggerated feelings of well-being, and reduced self-control, and then produces sedation. Long-term use of alcohol causes chronic suppression of excitatory receptors (NMDA), so the brain increases the synthesis of excitatory neurotransmitters. Abrupt cessation of alcohol use causes a rebound stimulatory effect and accounts for the symptoms of withdrawal (Box 11.1).

HINT   Alcohol withdrawal syndrome (AWS) is a result of unopposed hyperexcitable neurons. This contributes to delirium tremens (DT) and withdrawal seizures.

Box 11.1 Neurotransmitters in the Brain

Gamma-aminobutyric acid (GABA)	Inhibitory neurotransmitter
Glutamate	Excitatory neurotransmitter
N-methyl-D-aspartate (NMDA)	Excitatory receptors
Serotonin	Excitatory transmission
Dopamine	Excitatory transmission
Norepinephrine	Excitatory transmission

▶ SYMPTOMS/ASSESSMENT

> **Q** What is an important component of the initial assessment of all patients admitted into the intensive care unit (ICU)?
>
> **A** Obtain accurate history

Prevention of AWS is the first step to decreasing mortality. An accurate drinking history to determine potential dependence on alcohol assists with prevention and early recognition of the symptoms of AWS. Ask the patient about his alcohol use, including the frequency and number of drinks daily (Box 11.2).

HINT   Consider obtaining further information regarding the amount of alcohol intake from a family member.

Box 11.2 Questions to Ask Regarding Alcohol Consumption

What alcoholic beverages are consumed?	How many years have you been drinking?
How many per occasion are consumed?	Any history of alcohol withdrawal?
How often do you drink?	History of other substance abuse?
When was the time of your last drink?	History of major psychological conditions?

> **Q** What is a commonly used assessment/screening tool for alcohol use/abuse?
>
> **A** CAGE questionnaire

The CAGE questionnaire is short and easy-to-use screening tool to be incorporated into a routine admission history of alcohol use. One "yes" answer to these questions suggests that the patient needs to be observed more closely, two "yes" answers are highly correlated with alcohol abuse or dependence, and three "yes" answers indicate alcohol abuse with an increase in sensitivity to 100%.

HINT   One of the problems with the CAGE assessment is that it does not distinguish between past and present alcohol use (Box 11.3).

Box 11.3 CAGE Questionnaire

C	Have you felt you can **cut** down on your drinking?
A	Have people **annoyed** you by criticizing your drinking?
G	Have you ever felt bad or **guilty** about your drinking?
E	Have you ever had a drink first thing in the morning to steady your nerves or to get rid of a hangover? **(eye-opener)**

Q **What do most people do when asked about how many drinks they have had per day or when asked about taking illicit substances?**

A **Deny or minimize**

Most people want to either deny or minimize the amount they drink when discussing their alcohol intake or use of illicit substances. Ask questions in a nonjudgmental and matter-of-fact way with other general questions. For example, ask about the alcohol intake following questions on caffeine consumption (Box 11.4).

HINT   Ensure the patient knows that everyone is being asked these questions.

Box 11.4 Definition of "One" Drink

12 ounces of beer	2½ ounces cordial or liqueur
8½ ounces of malt liquor or fortified beer, ale (40-ounce bottle)	2½ ounces cordial or liqueur
5 ounces of wine	1½ ounces of spirits, 80-proof vodka, gin, whiskey, or brandy
3½ ounces fortified wine (sherry or port)	

▶ DIAGNOSIS

Q **What laboratory test will elevate within 4–8 weeks with alcohol ingestion?**

A **Mean corpuscular volume (MCV)**

Elevated MCV may indicate alcohol abuse. Index of red blood cell (RBC) size (macrocytosis) increases with alcohol intake within 4–8 weeks. This occurs in 90% of all alcoholics. The mechanism is unknown, but it may be caused by poor nutrition.

Q **What pattern of elevated liver enzymes indicates alcohol-induced liver failure?**

A **Aspartate aminotransferase (AST) is two times higher than alanine aminotransferase (ALT)**

Alcohol-induced liver dysfunction will elevate both AST and ALT. The pattern specific for liver failure is an AST two times greater than ALT. This pattern is generally not seen in other causes of liver failure. Homocysteine levels are elevated in nonabstinent alcoholics, and the levels may be associated with withdrawal seizures.

HINT   Homocysteine levels may be a useful biomarker of risk of alcohol withdrawal seizures.

> **Q When do symptoms of AWS peak following the last drink?**
>
> **A 24–48 hours**

Autonomic hyperactivity appears within hours of the last drink and usually peaks within 24–48 hours. Withdrawal signs typically start between 5 and 10 hours after the last drink. Symptoms of AWS can range from mild, self-limiting to severe and life threatening (Box 11.5). Chronic alcoholics typically experience progressively shorter intervals between their last drink and progressive worsening symptoms of AWS during each subsequent episode. This phenomenon is called a "kindling effect" (Figure 11.1)

Box 11.5 Symptoms of AWS

Mild	Major
Autonomic hyperactivity	Hallucinations
Tachycardia	Tactile
Mild anxiety	Visual
Hypertension	Auditory
Gastrointestinal (GI) disturbances	Seizures
Diaphoresis	Tonic–clonic
Insomnia	Delirium tremens (DTs)
Vivid dreams	Confusion
Headaches	Disorientation
Anorexia, nausea, and vomiting	Impaired attention
Hyper-reflexia	Severe autonomic activity
Hyperventilation	Hallucinations
Low-grade fever	Respiratory or cardiovascular collapse

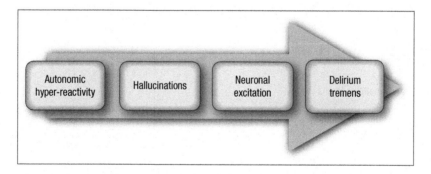

Figure 11.1 Progression of AWS.

> **Q What tool is used clinically to determine the severity of AWS?**
>
> **A Clinical Institute Withdrawal Assessment for Alcohol Scale, Revised (CIWA-Ar)**

CIWA-Ar is a tool used to determine the severity of AWS and to guide therapeutic intervention. A score of less than nine indicates that the patient must be observed. If the score is greater than nine, a benzodiazepine should be administered. Determination of the score is then repeated each hour until less than 10 and dosing of benzodiazepine is continued until less than nine. At this point, scoring can be every 8 hours, then discontinued when score is less than six on four consecutive assessments.

HINT Use of a symptom-triggered dosing protocol with the use of CIWA-Ar may reduce treatment time and amount of drug used versus administering a fixed dose (Box 11.6).

Box 11.6 CIWA-Ar

Patient: _____ Date: _____ Time: _____
(24-hour clock, midnight = 00:00)
Pulse or heart rate, taken for 1 minute: _____ Blood pressure: _____
NAUSEA AND VOMITING: Ask: "Do you feel sick to your stomach? Have you vomited?" Observation.
0 no nausea and no vomiting
1 mild nausea with no vomiting
4 intermittent nausea with dry heaves
7 constant nausea, frequent dry heaves and vomiting
TACTILE DISTURBANCES: Ask: "Have you any itching, pins-and-needles sensations, any burning, any numbness, or
do you feel bugs crawling on or under your skin?" Observation.
0 none
1 very mild itching, pins and needles, burning or numbness
2 mild itching, pins and needles, burning or numbness
3 moderate itching, pins and needles, burning or numbness
4 moderately severe hallucinations
5 severe hallucinations
6 extremely severe hallucinations
7 continuous hallucinations
AUDITORY DISTURBANCES: Ask: "Are you more aware of sounds around you? Are they harsh? Do they frighten
you? Are you hearing anything that is disturbing to you? Are you hearing things you know are not there?"
Observation.
0 not present
1 very mild harshness or ability to frighten
2 mild harshness or ability to frighten
3 moderate harshness or ability to frighten
4 moderately severe hallucinations
5 severe hallucinations
6 extremely severe hallucinations
7 continuous hallucinations
VISUAL DISTURBANCES: Ask: "Does the light appear to be too bright? Is its color different? Does it hurt your
eyes? Are you seeing anything that is disturbing to you? Are you seeing things you know are not there?"
Observation.
0 not present
1 very mild sensitivity
2 mild sensitivity
3 moderate sensitivity
4 moderately severe hallucinations
5 severe hallucinations
6 extremely severe hallucinations
7 continuous hallucinations
HEADACHE, FULLNESS IN HEAD: Ask: "Does your head feel different? Does it feel like there is a band around your
head?" Do not rate for dizziness or lightheadedness. Otherwise, rate severity.
0 not present
1 very mild
2 mild
3 moderate
4 moderately severe
5 severe
6 very severe
7 extremely severe
TREMOR: Arms extended and fingers spread apart. Observation.
0 no tremor
1 not visible, but can be felt fingertip to fingertip
4 moderate, with patient's arms extended
7 severe, even with arms not extended

(continued)

Box 11.6 CIWA-Ar (*continued*)

PAROXYSMAL SWEATS: Observation.
0 no sweat visible
1 barely perceptible sweating, palms moist
4 beads of sweat obvious on forehead
7 drenching sweats
ANXIETY: Ask: "Do you feel nervous?" Observation.
0 no anxiety, at ease
1 mildly anxious
4 moderately anxious, or guarded, so anxiety is inferred
7 equivalent to acute panic states as seen in severe delirium or acute schizophrenic reactions
AGITATION: Observation.
0 normal activity
1 somewhat more than normal activity
4 moderately fidgety and restless
7 paces back and forth during most of the interview or constantly thrashes about
ORIENTATION AND CLOUDING OF SENSORIUM: Ask: "What day is this? Where are you? Who am I?"
0 oriented and can do serial additions
1 cannot do serial additions or is uncertain about date
2 disoriented for date by no more than 2 calendar days
3 disoriented for date by more than 2 calendar days
4 disoriented for place/or person
Total **CIWA-Ar** Score _____ Rater's initials _____ Maximum possible score 67
The **CIWA-Ar** is *not* copyrighted and may be reproduced freely. This assessment for monitoring withdrawal
   symptoms requires approximately 5 minutes to administer. The maximum score is 67 (see instrument). Patients
   scoring less than 10 do not usually need additional medication for withdrawal.

▶ MANAGEMENT

Q What is the drug of choice for preventing and/or treating AWS?

A Benzodiazepines

The mechanism of action for benzodiazepines is to enhance depression of neurotransmitter GABA, which replaces the effect of alcohol. Lorazepam or diazepam may be used to reduce the risk of AWS. Neuroleptics have also been used to manage AWS but may not be as effective as benzodiazepines. They do not treat the autonomic effects of AWS. Pregabalin or tiapride are nonbenzodiazepine drugs that may be used in AWS. They prevent the hypersecretion of excitatory neurotransmitters found in AWS.

HINT   Lorazepam has a shorter half-life than diazepam, which may help prevent oversedation.

Q Administration of thiamine to patients with a history of alcohol use is done to prevent which syndrome?

A Wernicke–Korsakoff's syndrome

Wernicke's encephalopathy (WE) and Korsakoff's syndrome are a result of thiamine deficiency. Administration of intravenous (IV) thiamine is used routinely to prevent Wernicke–Korsakoff's syndrome. Multivitamins are frequently added in the management of patients with a history of alcohol use (Box 11.7).

Box 11.7 Causes of Thiamine Deficiency in Alcohol Use

Dietary deficiency	Increased excretion
Reduced absorption	Interrupts metabolism of thiamine

Q Patient with AWS develops tetany and positive Chvostek's sign. What common electrolyte abnormality seen with alcohol use may present with these symptoms?

A Hypomagnesemia

Hypomagnesemia is a common electrolyte abnormality of patients with alcohol use and AWS. Symptoms of low magnesium include tetany and positive Chvostek's sign. Other electrolyte abnormalities that need to be monitored and corrected include hyponatremia, hypokalemia, and hypophosphatemia.

> **Q** What are the two problems that occur with managing pain in a substance abuse patient?
>
> **A** Give too little or too much

There are *two major errors* that occur in the hospital when managing pain in patients with a history of drug and/or alcohol addiction. The errors can be at both extremes of the spectrum. The patient's reported pain is not believed by the healthcare providers, and the request for pain medication is denied. Or the patient is treated as a nonaddictive patient and opioid intake is allowed to escalate beyond reasonable estimates to control the pain (Box 11.8).

Box 11.8 Hints for Managing Pain in Substance Abusers

Avoid excessive negotiation but allow some decisions to be made by the patient
Be prepared to administer higher doses (development tolerance)
Give nonopioids in combination with opioids
Accept patient's reported pain and treat following appropriate assessments
Do not try to treat the addiction while the patient is in pain
Substance abusers may have a low tolerance for pain
Do not administer an agonist antagonist opioid (sudden reversal of opioids)
Monitor for symptoms of withdrawal
Avoid detoxification during treatment of acute pain

HINT When opioids are no longer required, taper slowly to minimize the emergence of withdrawal symptoms.

▶ COMPLICATIONS

> **Q** What is the primary symptom of the complication of Korsakoff's syndrome?
>
> **A** Amnesia

Without treatment of thiamine, 75% of WE patients develop permanent severe amnestic syndrome (Korsakoff's syndrome; Boxes 11.9 and 11.10).

Box 11.9 Symptoms of Korsakoff's Syndrome

Retrograde amnesia
Anterograde amnesia (inability to assimilate new information)
Decreased spontaneity
Decreased initiative
Confabulation (filling in memory gaps with distorted facts)

Box 11.10 Symptoms of Wernicke's Encephalopathy

Delirium	Ophthalmoplegia (paralysis of eye muscles)
Nystagmus	Memory abnormalities
Ataxia	

> **Q** What is a common high-risk complication of AWS?
>
> **A** Seizures

Patients who are at high risk for AWS-induced seizures include those with a prior history of withdrawal seizures, high alcohol consumption, and multiple previous detoxifications. Many alcohol-dependent patients have causes other than alcohol withdrawal that contribute to or cause seizures. An electroencephalogram (EEG) can differentiate between AWS seizures and epilepsy. The EEG of AWS patients demonstrates normal low-amplitude waves, whereas EEGs of patients with epilepsy shows generalized spike and wave points.

> **Q** What is the complication of AWS that has exacerbation of autonomic symptoms?
>
> **A** DTs

DTs is one of the most serious manifestations of AWS. It is characterized by fluctuating disturbances of consciousness and change in cognition occurring over a short period of time. Symptoms are due to exacerbation of autonomic system and can result in death (Box 11.11).

Box 11.11 Symptoms of DTs

Sweating	Hypertension
Nausea	Tachycardia
Palpitations	Hyperthermia
Tremor	Tachypnea

AGITATION

▶ PATHOPHYSIOLOGY

> **Q** What is the primary goal in managing agitation and delirium?
>
> **A** Control at the lightest level of sedation

Maintaining light levels of sedation is associated with improvements in clinical outcomes of ICU patients. These improvements include shorter ICU stays, shorter overall hospital days, lower ventilator days, and fewer complications from mechanical ventilation. Sedation is titrated with the goal of light sedation instead of deep, unless clinically contraindicated.

HINT   Lighter levels of sedation (as well as unrelieved pain) may increase signs of stress response (i.e., tachycardia and hypertension) and should be monitored closely.

> **Q** What is an acute change in neurological function with alterations of mental status with disorganized thinking?
>
> **A** Delirium

Delirium is a syndrome characterized by an acute onset of cerebral dysfunction with a change of fluctuation in baseline mental status, inattention, and either disorganized thinking or an altered level of consciousness (LOC). The cardinal signs of delirium are a disturbed LOC and a change in cognition. Presence of delirium is an independent predictor of poor outcome (Box 11.12).

Box 11.12 Cardinal Signs of Delirium

Disturbed level of consciousness (LOC)	Decreased awareness of environment Reduced ability to sustain focus or attention
Change in cognition	Memory deficit Disorientation Language disturbances Hallucinations or delusions

HINT   A misconception of delirium is that it requires hallucinations or delusions. Delirium can be present without these symptoms. Hyperactive delirium is more often associated with hallucinations and delusions.

> **Q Which medications are commonly associated with delirium?**
>
> **A Sedatives**

Administration of sedatives and opioids to ICU patients contributes to the development of delirium. Disease states such as sepsis may induce delirium (Box 11.13).

Box 11.13 Factors Contributing to Delirium

Sedatives	Immobilization
Opioids	Sensory overload
Physical restraints	Certain medications
Sleep deprivation	Drug or alcohol withdrawal
Disease states (i.e., sepsis, multiple organ dysfunction syndrome)	Mechanical ventilation

> **Q What medical history may increase the risk of developing delirium in the ICU?**
>
> **A Dementia**

There are four known risk factors and many other suspected risks for the development of delirium in the ICU (Box 11.14). Pre-existing dementia is the medical history known to be a significant risk factor for the development of delirium.

HINT   Delirium that occurs in a dementia patient is frequently called "sundowner's syndrome." Age (older patients) is a known risk factor in non-ICU patients and probably is a contributing risk in ICU delirium.

Box 11.14 Known Risk Factors for Delirium

Dementia	History of alcoholism
History of hypertension	High severity of illness on admission to the ICU

▶ SYMPTOMS/ASSESSMENT

> **Q A patient who is restless and agitated in the ICU may have what complication?**
>
> **A Delirium**

Delirium is defined as a temporary state of mental confusion, whereas psychosis is a severe mental disorder characterized by loss of contact with reality. Delirium is characterized by restlessness and agitation (Box 11.15).

Box 11.15 Symptoms of Delirium

Short attention span	Sleep disturbances
Restlessness and agitation	Abnormal psychomotor activity
Persecutory delusions	Emotional disturbances (fear, anxiety, anger, depression, apathy)
Vivid hallucinations	

HINT Patients with delirium may be agitated, calm, or lethargic (Box 11.16).

Box 11.16 Signs of Agitation

Exhibits continual movement	Pulling out lines and tubes
Fidgeting	Disorientation
Moving from side to side	Does not follow simple commands

▶ DIAGNOSIS

Q What is the Ramsey Scale used for in the ICU?

A Determine sedation levels

There are several tools used in the ICU to determine sedation levels. Sedation scales can be used to titrate the level of sedation, maintaining a lighter sedation except in certain situations that require deeper sedation. The Ramsey Scale is one of the sedation assessment tools used in the ICU (Box 11.17).

HINT These sedation scales are not accurate in comatose patients or patients receiving neuromuscular blocking agents. The Richmond Agitation Sedation Scale (RASS) and Sedation Agitation Scale (SAS) are two of the more valid and reliable assessment tools with high inter-rater reliability (Tables 11.1 and 11.2).

Box 11.17 Sedation Scales

Ramsey Scale	New Sheffield Sedation Score
Motor Activity Assessment Scale (MASS)	Adaption to the Intensive Care Environment (ATICE)
SAS	Minnesota Sedation Assessment Tool
RASS	Vancouver Interaction and Calmness Scale (VICS)
Sedation Intensive Care Score (SEDICS)	

Table 11.1 Richmond Agitation Sedation Scale (RASS)

Score	Term	Description
+4	Combative	Overtly combative, violent, immediate danger to staff
+3	Agitated	Pulls or removes tube(s) or catheter(s); aggressive
+2	Very agitated	Frequent nonpurposeful movement, fights ventilator
+1	Restless	Anxious, but movements not aggressive or vigorous
0	Alert and calm	
−1	Drowsy	Not fully alert but has sustained awakening (eye-opening/ eye contact) to voice (>10 sec)
−2	Light sedation	Briefly awakens with eye contact to voice (< 10 sec)
−3	Moderate sedation	Movement or eye-opening to voice (but no eye contact)
−4	Deep sedation	No response to voice, but movement or eye-opening to physical stimulation
−5	Unarousable	No response to voice or physical stimulation

Table 11.2 Sedation Agitation Scale (SAS)

Score	Term	Descriptor
7	Dangerous agitation	Pulling at endotracheal tube (ETT), trying to remove catheters, climbing over bedrail, striking at staff, thrashing side to side
6	Very agitated	Requiring restraint and frequent verbal reminding of limits, biting ETT
5	Agitated	Anxious or physically agitated, calms to verbal instructions
4	Calm and cooperative	Calm, easily arousable, follows commands
3	Sedated	Difficult to arouse but awakens to verbal stimuli or gentle shaking, follows simple commands but drifts off again
2	Very sedated	Arouses to physical stimuli but does not communicate or follow commands, may move spontaneously
1	Unarousable	Minimal or no response to noxious stimuli, does not communicate or follow commands

Q What objective measurement of brain function is used to measure depth of sedation in patients receiving neuromuscular blocking agents?

A Bispectral Index (BIS) monitor

The BIS monitor is available for monitoring brain function and can be used as an objective measurement of sedation levels. It is more commonly used on mechanically ventilated patients on neuromuscular blocking agents. Once paralyzed for therapeutic purposes, the nurse is unable to use assessment scales for sedation. Other objective measures of brain function include auditory evoked potentials or Narcotrend Index.

HINT The subjective sedation scores are recommended in patients not receiving a neuromuscular blocking agent.

Q What tool is available for monitoring delirium in the ICU?

A Confusion Assessment Method for ICU (CAM-ICU)

CAM-ICU is a valid and reliable tool used in the ICU to monitor for delirium. It is recommended that all patients in the ICU be monitored routinely for delirium.

▶ MANAGEMENT

Q What is the purpose of daily "wake up" on patients receiving sedation?

A Maintain lighter level of sedation

Daily "wake up" ensures the patient is at a lighter level of sedation. Protocols are used in most hospitals to interrupt sedation daily until the patient awakens, and then resedate. The interruption has not been found to cause significant physiological stress and may decrease length of stay (LOS) in the ICU and mechanical ventilator days. Deep sedation is one reason for delayed emergence from sedation. Other causes include prolonged infusion, older age, hepatic dysfunction, or renal failure.

HINT This technique is frequently called "sedation vacation."

Q Which of the sedatives frequently used in the ICU is recommended in patients requiring intermittent awakenings?

A Propofol

Propofol is a nonbenzodiazepine frequently used to provide sedation in mechanically ventilated patients. It has a very quick onset and short half-life so patients will wake up faster once the propofol infusion has been stopped. Benzodiazepines may also be used for sedation in the ICU but may have a longer half-life (Table 11.3).

HINT Propofol is commonly used in neurological patients requiring frequent neurological assessments due to its shorter emergence. However, propofol's duration of clinical effect is much shorter because propofol is rapidly distributed into the peripheral tissues.

Table 11.3 Agents Used for Sedation in the ICU

Agent	Onset (IV Route; min)	Half-Life (hour)
Lorazepam	15–20	8–15
Diazepam	2–5	20–120
Midazolam	2–5	3–11
Propofol	1–2	2–24
Dexmedetomidine	5–10	2–3

Q Which sedative does not have respiratory depression and can be used on a nonintubated patient?

A Dexmedetomidine

Dexmedetomidine is a selective α-receptor agonist. It is different from other sedatives because it has been found to have analgesic effects and may lower the dose of the opioid. It does not affect the respiratory system and so may be given to nonventilated patients. It is the only sedative approved by the Food and Drug Administration (FDA) in nonintubated ICU patients. Propofol is not recommended for nonventilated patients. Benzodiazepines and propofol have sedating, hypnotic, amnesic, and anxiolytic effects without analgesic effects. Their primary side effects include hypotension and respiratory depression. Dexmedetomidine's side effects include hypotension and bradycardia.

HINT Patients sedated with dexmedetomidine wake up with minimal stimulation and are more interactive.

Q What nonpharmacological intervention may lower the number of ICU days and decrease the incidence of delirium?

A Early mobilization

Early and aggressive mobilization of ICU patients reduces the depth of sedation, decreases length of hospital stay and ICU days. Mobilization and ambulation of patients on mechanical ventilation have been found to lower the number of mechanical ventilation days. Pharmacological management has included haloperidol, but there is no study confirming that haloperidol reduces delirium in ICU patients. Use of dexmedetomidine for sedation in mechanically ventilated patients may lower the incidence of delirium when compared to benzodiazepines (Box 11.18).

HINT A complication of haloperidol is prolonged QT interval with increased incidence of Torsades de pointes.

Box 11.18 Interventions to Promote Sleep in the ICU

Control lighting at night
Cluster patient activities (allow periods of undisturbed sleep)
Decrease stimuli at night

▶ COMPLICATIONS

> **Q** Which patient population is more likely to be sensitive to benzodiazepines?
>
> **A** Elderly

Elderly patients are more sensitive to the sedating effects of benzodiazepines and can have adverse reactions, including agitation and delirium. The patient may have a different reaction to a different benzodiazepine.

> **Q** What food allergies would indicate that a patient is at risk for an allergic reaction to propofol?
>
> **A** Egg or soybean

Propofol is dissolved in a 10% lipid emulsion that contains egg lecithin and soybean oil. This can precipitate allergic reactions if a person has an allergy to either eggs or soybeans. Other potential complications of propofol that are due to the lipid emulsion are hypertriglyceridemia and acute pancreatitis.

HINT   Propofol infusion syndrome (PRIS) is a rare but life-threatening condition (Box 11.19). Complications of PRIS include acute kidney injury, rhabdomyolysis, and liver dysfunction.

Box 11.19 Symptoms of PRIS

Worsening metabolic acidosis	Arrhythmias
Hypotension despite vasopressors	Hyperkalemia
Hypertriglyceridemia	

> **Q** What is a potential complication of agitation in an intubated patient?
>
> **A** Self-extubation

Agitation can cause harmful effects on the patient and, potentially, healthcare providers (Box 11.20).

Box 11.20 Complications of Agitation

Self-extubation	Injury to self
Increased oxygen consumption	Injury to healthcare providers
Hemodynamic instability	Unable to participate in care

⬤ MODERATE SEDATION

> **Q** What is the level of arousal when a patient is given a moderate sedation?
>
> **A** Respond purposefully to verbal commands

Moderate sedation is used for diagnostic and therapeutic procedures. There are different levels of sedation, ranging from minimal sedation to anesthesia. A patient's response to stimulation determines the level of sedation. The ability to maintain an airway and ventilate is also included in the definitions of the levels of sedation (Table 11.4).

Table 11.4 Levels of Sedation

Level of Sedation	Arousal	Airway/Ventilation
Minimal	Responds normally to verbal commands Impaired cognitive function and coordination	Unaffected

Moderate	Responds purposefully to verbal commands or
	   light tactile stimulation
	Amnesia may be present
		No intervention required
		Protected reflexes are present
		   (cough, gag)

Deep	Cannot be easily aroused or responds purposefully
	   to stimulation
	Amnesia may be present
		May require assistance to maintain
		   airway
		Spontaneous ventilation may be
		   inadequate

Anesthesia	Drug-induced loss of consciousness Unarousable even with painful stimulation	Often requires intubation and ventilation

HINT   Anesthesia is not considered moderate sedation.

Q What are the two major goals of moderate sedation?

A Provide relief of anxiety and pain control

The major goals of moderate sedation, at all levels, include providing relief from anxiety (sedation) and pain control. Deep sedation may be used also to minimize or prevent patient movement during the procedure.

Q What is the greatest concern when providing moderate sedation?

A Respiratory depression

Maintaining the ability to have effective spontaneous ventilation is an important aspect of moderate sedation. Medications administered to obtain moderate sedation have side effects of respiratory depression, and multiple drug administration may have a synergistic effect. The ability to maintain an airway and effective ventilation are goals during moderate sedation and both should be monitored closely (Box 11.21).

Box 11.21 Risk Factors for Moderate Sedation

Morbidly obese
Elderly
History of severe cardiovascular or pulmonary disease
Obstructive sleep apnea
Substance abuse
Smoking history

Q Prior to initiation of moderate sedation, what must be obtained from the patient or family?

A A signed consent form

An informed consent form must be obtained that explain the benefits and risks of administration of moderate or deep sedation (Box 11.22).

Box 11.22 Preprocedure Assessment

Relevant history
Assessment of systems (emphasis on pulmonary and cardiovascular systems)
Airway assessment
Ensuring nothing by mouth (NPO) status
Pain assessment
Determine level of anxiety

HINT An airway assessment is recommended prior to a procedure in case complications of moderate sedation occur, and the patient requires emergency intubation.

Q During the procedure, how frequently should vital signs be assessed and documented when using moderate sedation?

A Every 5 minutes

The assessment and documentation of vital signs, oxygen saturation, $EtCO_2$ (if in use), and level of sedation should be done every 5 minutes during the procedure or more frequently if significant changes or events occur.

HINT Alarms should be on at all times and documented.

Q What are the two most commonly used classes of medications used to obtain moderate sedation?

A Opioids and benzodiazepines

Opioids provide not only analgesia but also sedation. They may be used alone or in combination with a benzodiazepine. Benzodiazepine is an anxiolytic used to control anxiety and provide amnesia and hypnotic effects for the procedure. Commonly used opioids are morphine and fentanyl. Diazepam and lorazepam are frequently used benzodiazepines. Other sedatives that may be used include ketamine, methohexital, and propofol. Naloxone is used to reverse complications of opioids, and flumazenil is used for the reversal of benzodiazepines.

HINT Administer reversal agents slowly in small increments to reverse the side effect (respiratory depression) without reversing the sedation or analgesic effect of the medication.

Q In addition to respiratory depression, what other complication can commonly occur with the administration of moderate sedation?

A Hypotension

Airway and ventilation complications are the most common, but hypotension can also occur. This is commonly a result of histamine release causing vasodilation and hypotension (Box 11.23).

Box 11.23 Complications of Moderate Sedation

Respiratory depression
Loss of airway
Hypotension
Drug overdose
Anaphylaxis
Nausea and vomiting
Aspiration

PAIN

▶ PATHOPHYSIOLOGY

> **Q What type of pain is typically undertreated in critically ill patients?**
>
> **A Procedural pain**

Procedures are frequently performed in the ICU and result in periods of intense pain. Frequently analgesia is present for maintenance in ICU following a trauma, surgery, or burns, but treatment of intermittent pain due to procedures is not consistent and is ineffective. Removal of chest tubes is an example of a painful procedure commonly not adequately managed.

HINT   Preemptive analgesia should be administered before the procedure to alleviate pain.

▶ SYMPTOMS/ASSESSMENT

> **Q When should pain assessment be performed on an ICU patient?**
>
> **A Routinely, on all ICU patients**

Pain assessment should be routinely performed on a regular basis. It is considered to be the fifth vital sign and should be performed as frequently as obtaining vital signs (as frequently as hourly in an ICU patient). Good management of pain is dependent on the assessment for pain on a frequent basis. Patients in the ICU can experience pain even at rest. Pain levels increase with movement, coughing, and procedures. Pain is frequently remembered after discharge from the ICU and contributes to posttraumatic stress disorder (PTSD).

HINT   Women have greater pain following a cardiac surgery as compared to men.

▶ DIAGNOSIS

> **Q What are two pain assessment tools used in the ICU to determine pain in nonverbal patients?**
>
> **A Behavioral Pain Scale (BPS) and Critical Care Pain Observation Tool (CPOT)**

BPS and CPOT are two tools commonly used in the ICU to assess for the presence of pain in nonverbal patients who are unable to self-report pain but who are capable of motor activity. BPS and CPOT have been found to be the most valid behavioral assessment scales (Table 11.5 and Box 11.24). Reliable assessment of pain is the basis of pain management. Although self-report is preferred over observation, patients on mechanical ventilation, those with decreased LOC, and/or sedation may not have the ability to self-report pain. The least reliable assessment of pain is change in vital signs and should not be used to determine pain levels. Vital sign changes can be a red flag to perform a pain assessment.

HINT   Behavioral assessment tools may not be as reliable in brain-injured patients.

Box 11.24 Behavioral Pain Scale (BPS)

BPS Includes:
  Facial expression
  Upper limb movement
  Compliance with ventilation

Table 11.5 Critical Care Pain Observation Tool (CPOT)

Indicator	Description	Score	
Facial expression	No muscular tension observed	Relaxed, neutral	0
	Presence of frowning, brow lowering, orbit tightening, and levator contraction	Tense	1
	All of the above facial movements plus eyelids tightly closed	Grimacing	2
Body movements	Does not move at all (does not necessarily mean absence of pain)	Absence of movement	0
	Slow, cautious movement, touching or rubbing the pain site, seeking attention though movements	Protection	1
	Pulling tubes, attempting to sit up, moving limbs/thrashing, not following commands, striking at staff, trying to climb out of bed	Restlessness	2
Muscle tension (evaluation by passive flexion and extension of upper extremities)	No resistance to passive movement	Relaxed	0
	Resistance to passive movements	Tense, rigid	1
	Strong resistance to passive movement, inability to complete them	Very tense or rigid	2
Compliance with ventilator (intubated patients) *or* vocalization (extubated patients)	Alarms not activated, easy ventilation	Tolerating ventilator or movement	0
	Alarms stop spontaneously	Coughing but tolerating ventilator	1
	Asynchrony, blocking ventilation, alarms frequently activated	Fighting with ventilator	2
	Talking in normal tone or no sound	Talking in normal tone or no sound	0
	Sighing, moaning	Sighing, moaning	1
	Crying out, sobbing	Crying out, sobbing	2
Total range		0–8	

▶ MANAGEMENT

Q Which opioid analgesic has a complication of neurotoxicity?

A Meperidine

Meperidine administration can result in the accumulation of the neurotoxic metabolite normeperidine. Neurotoxic findings include tremors, shakiness, myoclonus, and seizures. Meperidine is not frequently used for pain management in the ICU because of neurotoxicity. IV opioids are recommended as first-line drugs to manage pain in the ICU. Nonopioids can be used to supplement and lower the dose of the opioid (Box 11.25).

HINT Combining a nonopioid with an opioid can decrease the side effects of the opioid. When treating neuropathic pain, administer either an anticonvulsant (gabapentin) or an antidepressant (carbamazepine).

Box 11.25 Common Analgesics Used in the ICU

Morphine	Remifentanil
Fentanyl	Ketorolac
Hydromorphone	Intravenous (IV) acetaminophen
Methadone	Local and regional anesthetics

> **Q What is the recommended mode of delivery for analgesics following abdominal aortic aneurysm repair?**
>
> **A Thoracic epidural**

Abdominal aortic surgeries have shown excellent pain management, with a thoracic epidural catheter being placed prior to surgery. This route is superior to IV opioids with fewer complications in certain patient populations. Thoracic epidural pain management may also benefit patients with multiple rib fracture. This allows the patient to breathe deeply and cough without pain, which lowers the incidence of developing pneumonia.

▶ COMPLICATIONS

> **Q What physiological occurrence leads to the majority of the complications of unrelieved pain?**
>
> **A Stress response**

Unrelieved pain results in the activation of the stress response and the sympathetic nervous system. This produces tachycardia, vasoconstriction, and reduced arterial and tissue oxygenation (Box 11.26).

Box 11.26 Complications of Unrelieved Pain in the ICU

Stress response	Immunosuppression
Hypermetabolic catabolism	Chronic neuropathy pain
Impaired wound healing	Posttraumatic stress disorder
Increased risk of wound infections	Myocardial ischemia

⬤ SUICIDAL BEHAVIOR

> **Q Which patient population should receive a screening for depression or suicidal thoughts?**
>
> **A All patients**

The Joint Commission (TJC) has urged hospital and healthcare providers to watch for attempted suicides in patients with no history of psychiatric problems or history of previous attempts. The alert stresses that it is not just psychiatric patients who kill themselves, citing as an example someone recently diagnosed with cancer going into the emergency room (ER) because the cancer-related pain has become unbearable and commits suicide in the ER. Almost 25% of suicides within the hospital occur in nonpsychiatric settings, such as ERs, oncology units, ICU, and long-term care hospitals. Screen all patients for depression and suicidal thoughts when they are admitted to a hospital or into the ICU.

HINT The methods most often used in hospitals are hanging, suffocation, intentional drug overdose, and strangulation.

▶ PATHOPHYSIOLOGY

> **Q** What is the most common underlying belief of a person who attempts or commits suicide?
>
> **A** Hopelessness

Suicide occurs in response to feelings of hopelessness. Feelings of hopelessness result from the belief that suffering will never stop and, as a result, nothing positive will ever come of the future. Death is viewed as an option to end the suffering and prevent a future without hope.

> **Q** What increases the likelihood of suicidal thoughts in patients with medical illnesses?
>
> **A** Pain

Patients diagnosed with cancer or those who are in intense, intractable pain may feel worn out and hopeless. There is a need for routine evaluation and monitoring of suicidal behavior in both severe acute and chronic pain. Medical illness raises the risk for suicide because the presence of an illness or injury, especially associated with persistent pain, strains coping abilities. It increases the likelihood the patient will attribute the failures to cope with as personal inadequacy. There is an uncertainty about the future and worry that the medical condition will cause further loss and deterioration of the self.

HINT The presence of an illness, injury, or pain often leads to feelings of depression, especially in individuals sensitive to loss of control (Box 11.27). Thirty to forty percent of people who commit suicide have made a previous attempt.

Box 11.27 Increased Risks for Suicidal Behavior

Family history of suicide	Substance abuser
Previous suicide attempt	History of psychiatric problems
Prescription of potentially lethal medications	Suicidal ideation
Diagnosis of cancer or chronic illness	Suicidal behavior
Physical health problems	PTSD
Traumatic brain injury	Delirium or dementia
Severe pain (chronic or acute)	Social stressors: financial strain, unemployment
Poor prognosis or prospect of certain death	Disability

▶ SYMPTOMS/ASSESSMENT

> **Q** A patient in the ICU is recovering from surgery. The patient states his family would "be better off without him." What is this statement?
>
> **A** Verbal suicide threat

Verbal suicide threats need to be recognized. When performing suicide risk assessment, start with questions that assess the person's feelings about life. Then ask specific questions about death, self-harm, and suicide. Examples of verbal suicide threats include: "Life is not worth living," "I wish I would go to sleep and not wake up."

HINT The nurse should take seriously all statements made by a patient that indicate, either directly or indirectly, the desire to die.

> **Q** A patient in an acute care hospital may have different warning signs than a patient in a psychiatric hospital. What is an important assessment that should be ongoing with all ICU patients?
>
> **A** Watch for warning signs

Frequently, patients who commit suicide or self-harm in an acute care environment, like an ICU, may not have significant risk factors but typically will have demonstrated warning signs. In critically ill or injured patients, coping skills that normally have been functional may not be effective. The threat is perceived as being overwhelming and feelings of hopelessness and depression become more common. Most in-hospital suicides are impulsive, without apparent planning. At least once a shift, ask about suicidal intent in patients with warning signs (Box 11.28).

HINT Suicide assessment by the ICU nurses should become a part of the daily assessment (Boxes 11.29 and 11.30).

Box 11.28 Warning Signs

Irritability	Anxiety
Verbal suicide threat	Impulsiveness
Agitation	Global insomnia
Complaints of unrelenting pain	Lack of interest in future plans or current treatment
Refusing visitors or medications	
Refusing to eat	Excessive fear and worries
Acute signs of depression	Delusions or hallucinations
Expressing feelings of hopelessness and helplessness	Requesting early discharge

Box 11.29 Questions Regarding Suicidal Thoughts

In the past 2 weeks, have you had thoughts you would be better off dead?
In the past 2 weeks, have you had thoughts of hurting yourself in any way?
Have you made a suicide attempt in the past?
Do you have a current plan?
When you have thought of hurting yourself, what would you do?
How often have those thoughts occurred?

Box 11.30 Use of Mnemonic "In Sad Cases" in Depression Signs

IN	Interest (life not worth living)	C	Concentration
S	Sleep	A	Agitation/slowed
A	Appetite	S	Stricken with guilt
D	Depressed	E	Energy
		S	Suicide (thinks, plans, has means)

▶ MANAGEMENT

Q If a patient mentions feeling hopeless, what would be the best response?

A Talk openly

Talk openly about depression, death, and suicide with patients. Communication needs to include listening to the patient. Ask direct questions without being judgmental. Determine whether the patient has a plan to carry out the suicide. Do not counsel the patient yourself but get professional help (Box 11.31).

HINT The more detailed the plan, the greater the risk. Do not leave a person who is talking about suicide alone.

Box 11.31 Interventions to Prevent Suicide

Remove items that could be used for suicide (Sharp objects, cleaning solvents)	Referral to mental health professional for further assessment
Place patient on 1:1 observation	Follow up appropriately at the time of discharge
Initiate elopement precautions	

Q What is a common method for attempting suicide in an acute care hospital environment?

A Hanging

Hanging has been a common method for suicide or self-harm in the acute hospital setting. The availability of means to perform self-harm by hanging is present in ICU and other areas of the hospital. This includes cords, call button cords, sheets, bandages, and IV tubing. Staff training should include knowledge of potential means of suicide in the ICU and how to prevent access to these means (Box 11.32).

HINT Perform close observation, at least every 15 minutes, in high-risk patients and document the observations. Remove potentially hazardous items from the patient's room and secure patient's belongings.

Box 11.32 Methods of Suicide in the Hospital

Hanging	Drug overdose
Jumping out of windows	Strangulation
Cutting with a sharp object	

DEPRESSION

Q What are periods of profound depression and/or mania that interfere with living called?

A Mood disorders

Mood disorders include bipolar disease and depression. These are considered pervasive alterations in temperament characterized by profound periods of depression or exaggerated mania or both. These extreme variations of mood interfere with the daily lives of those afflicted with these mood disorders, potentially causing problems with interpersonal relationships and livelihood of those involved.

HINT Mood disorders are the most commonly diagnosed psychiatric disorder in which those affected attempt or commit suicide.

Q How is a major depressive disorder different from feeling "down" for several days?

A More severe

Major depressive disorders are more severe than feeling "down" for several days, which commonly occurs in most people. It is a severe state of despair and gloom that is a debilitating condition. In major depressive disorder, there is a significant change from the person's normal behavior and functioning for several weeks or more. They typically experience feelings of hopelessness and joylessness with thoughts that life is not worth living. Without treatment, symptoms may recede over time but can reoccur in time.

HINT Major depressive disorder is different from chronic, long-term depression, which is called dysthymia.

Q What are two coexisting disorders that are associated with a high increased risk of depression?

A Medical disorders and psychiatric disorders

Medical disorders may include any medical diagnosis or severe life-threatening disorders. People with medical disorders are more likely to develop depression than they would if they were in a healthy state. There is a high rate of depression in patients with chronic illnesses, pain, diagnosis with poor prognosis, and end of life. Some degree of depression is actually normal in bereavement, but severe feelings of "darkness" and ideation of suicide are considered a major depressive disorder. Psychiatric disorders are also commonly associated with major depression. Depression can lead to an increase in mortality from other diseases such as coronary artery disease and cancer.

HINT   Elderly living in nursing homes have a high rate of major depression due to loneliness, loss, illness, pain, and facing death as a reality.

▶ PATHOPHYSIOLOGY

Q What is the theory called in which a person is depressed because this person believes her problems are her own fault, and there is nothing she can do to change them?

A Learned helplessness

Learned helplessness is a theory that considers the reason that people experience depression. The theory proposes that anxiety about situations or problems leads to depression. The patients believe they are at fault for their problems (guilt). According to the theory, they also believe that there is nothing they can do to change their own situation or problems. Other theories that consider major depressive disorders include cognitive and psychoanalytic theories.

HINT   Genetic factors may play a role in the development of depressive disorders but are not completely responsible without other factors involved.

Q Are serotonin levels found to be low or high in major depressive disorders?

A Low

Serotonin is a neurotransmitter that has many roles in behavior, mood, cognition, and aggressiveness. Major depressive disorders are found to have a deficiency of serotonin and its precursor, tryptophan. Serotonin, norepinephrine, and dopamine are destroyed by an enzyme called monoamine oxidase (MAO) (Table 11.6). MAO inhibitors are antidepressants that increase serotonin levels by inhibiting the enzyme MAO. Neuroendocrine function has been found to play a role in depressive disorders. Adrenal cortisol secretion is increased during periods of depression.

HINT   Selective serotonin reuptake inhibitors (SSRIs) are antidepressants that increase serotonin levels by inhibiting presynaptic reuptake.

Table 11.6 Neurochemical Involvement in Depression

Neurochemical	Role	Level of Depression
Serotonin	Affects mood, behavior, and cognition	Low
Norepinephrine	Energizes body in stress	Low
Dopamine	Motivation and pleasure center of brain	Low
Acetylcholine	Alters mood, sleep, and neuroendocrine function	High

▶ SYMPTOMS/ASSESSMENT

Q What are three key elements that should be included in a brief assessment for depression?

A Mood, energy, and pleasure

Mood is an individual's overall current outlook on life. A low mood is gloomy, down-hearted, and sad. Findings of low energy levels include listlessness, and patients frequently state they are tired for no reason. The element of pleasure is assessed by determining the patient's feelings of self-worth and hope. Low pleasure (anhedonia) is found if the patient is feeling hopeless, joyless, helpless, and worthless. Low findings in all three of these key elements indicate a current state of depression, and a more comprehensive assessment is recommended (Box 11.33).

HINT When obtaining an assessment history, listen to what and how the patient provides the information as well as his body language. Many patients with low self-esteem and depression have poor hygiene on admission to hospital and show signs of self-neglect.

Box 11.33 Components of Comprehensive Assessment of Depression

Personal history of depression, suicide attempts, psychiatric disorders
Family history of depression, suicide, and psychiatric disorders
Obtain more details of current episode of depression
General appearance
Motor activity during interview
Determine affect
Ability to process information
Decision making and problem solving
Self-concept

Q Psychotic features of a major depressive condition may include false perceptions and false ideas. What are these two conditions called?

A Hallucinations and delusions

Psychotic features may sometimes occur with major depression. These include experiencing hallucinations, which are false perceptions of reality, and delusions, which are false ideas. Other symptoms that may occur during profound depression include catatonic and melancholic features (Box 11.34).

Box 11.34 Symptoms of Major Depressive Disorder

Catatonic features	Peculiar movements
	Stupor
	Meaningless repetition of words
	Repetition of movements
Melancholic features	Lack of pleasure in anything
	Excessive or inappropriate guilt
	Marked slowness
Common symptoms	Extreme negativism
	Appetite changes
	Weight loss
	Insomnia
	Lack of energy
	Slow mental processing
	Withdrawn and inactive
	Fixed facial expression
	Limited movement

(continued)

Box 11.34 Symptoms of Major Depressive Disorder (*continued*)

Common symptoms	Minimal eye contact
	Flat affect
	Apathy
	No verbal responses at times
	Poor judgment
	Diminished ability to concentrate
Atypical symptoms	Agitation
	Anxiety
	Easily provoked to anger
	Restlessness
	Hypersomnia
	Leaden feelings in legs

HINT Depression may be greatest in the morning or on awakening (diurnal).

▶ DIAGNOSIS

Q **What is a common rating scale used to assess depression?**

A **Beck's Depression Inventory II**

Beck's depression scale is frequently used in the acute care setting to rate the degree of depression. It is a 21-item assessment tool that takes approximately 5 minutes to administer. The Geriatric Depression Scale and the Patient Health Questionnaire are also depression screening tools used in acute care settings.

HINT In 2008 the American Heart Association (AHA) recommended screening for depression in all patients with acute coronary syndrome and strokes.

▶ MANAGEMENT

Q **A patient on a tricyclic antidepressant (TCA) presents with dry mouth, sweating, and blurred vision. What is the most likely cause of these symptoms?**

A **Anticholinergic syndrome**

TCAs produce anticholinergic syndrome as a side effect. TCAs cause a higher incidence than SSRIs. Anticholinergic syndrome includes dry mouth, sweating, blurred vision, weight gain, and sexual dysfunction. TCAs inhibit reuptake norepinephrine and serotonin, allowing for more time at postsynaptic receptor.

HINT TCA takes up to 2–6 weeks to begin being effective as an antidepressant. (Box 11.35).

Box 11.35 Common Side Effects of Tricyclic Antidepressants (TCAs)

Orthostatic hypotension	Weight gain
Sedation	Dry mouth
Tachycardia	Constipation
Headache	Urinary hesitancy
Blurred vision	Sweating
Tremor	

Q What class of drug is considered to be a first-line agent to treat major depression and has less cardiovascular effects than TCAs?

A SSRIs

SSRI is recommended to treat major depressive disorders. They have lower cardiotoxicity than TCA and are safer for older patients. SSRIs have a lower rate of anticholinergic symptoms (Box 11.36).

Box 11.36 Common Side Effects of SSRIs

Anxiety	Tremor	Sexual dysfunction
Sedation	Nausea and vomiting	Constipation or diarrhea
Headaches		

Q Which antidepressant has a potential significant side effect of hypertension?

A MAO inhibitors (MAOIs)

MAOIs are responsible for inhibiting the enzyme MAO, allowing an increase in serotonin levels. Drugs and foods high in tyramine can interact with the MAOI, causing hypertension and strokes. Foods high in tyramine include smoked or fermented products such as bacon, ham, and most cheeses.

HINT Therapeutic drug levels may take up to 4 weeks after initiation of MAOI therapy.

Q What is the major goal of the nurse when speaking to a depressed patient?

A Affirm patient's worth

When speaking with a patient experiencing depression, establish a trusting relationship and affirm the patient's worth (Box 11.37).

Box 11.37 Interpersonal Skills With a Depressed Patient

Establish a trusting relationship
Convey message of "being" there for the patient
Affirm the patient is valuable
Allow patient time to talk about his or her feelings
Display unconditional positive regard for patient
Empathy

▶ COMPLICATIONS

Q What is the major complication of severe major depressive disorder?

A Suicide

Recurrence rates of depression and suicides are high in people with severe major depressive disorder. Suicide precautions should be initiated, and the patient must be monitored closely (Box 11.38).

Box 11.38 Other Complications of Major Depression

Compulsive behaviors (eating disorders, gambling, substance abuse)	Malnutrition
Substance abuse	Social isolation

AGGRESSION

Q What acts constitute violence in the workplace?

A Verbal to physical assault

Violence in the hospital can range from verbal to physical assault. Workplace violence is an act in which a person is abused, intimidated, threatened, or assaulted while working at his or her place of employment. The healthcare setting leads all other industries in the percentage of nonfatal assaults against workers (Box 11.39).

Box 11.39 Examples of Aggressive Behaviors/Violence in the Workplace

Verbal threats	Sarcastic comments
Shouting or yelling	Belittling gestures
Pushing, hitting, kicking, or physical harm	Aggressive body postures
Cursing and offensive language	Spitting or biting
Slamming doors, throwing objects, or punching walls	

Q What is an example of a patient who would be considered "inherently" violent?

A Prison inmate

A prison inmate being cared for in the ICU may have what is called an inherent risk for violence. Other cases may include known psychotic patients. Continual observation for aggression or violence may be indicated in these cases. Other cases of patient or family violence are situational. Something in the situation causes the nonviolent person to become aggressive and even violent. This occurs more frequently in hospital settings (Box 11.40).

HINT   Provoking situations include issues that cause frustration, such as delays in patient care.

Box 11.40 Types of Violence in the Workplace

Violence by stranger	Violence by coworker
Violence by patient or family member	Violence by someone in a personal relationship

Q What is a common reason in the ICU that can result in anger and aggressive behaviors?

A Stress

The ER and ICU are high-dependency areas prone to being very stressful and causing stress to patients and family members. Stress can lead to anxiety, anger, and aggression. Anxiety can result in frustration and feelings of helplessness. In the ICU, family members often are anxious and exhibit frustration regarding visitation rules, wanting to talk to the doctors, and fear for their loved ones. They often feel powerless about the situation and about loss of their own autonomy. Anger often follows these feelings and may even bring some perceived "power" back to the person.

HINT   Healthcare providers may experience aggression from clients influenced by drugs, alcohol, stress, or physical trauma.

▶ SYMPTOMS/ASSESSMENT

Q A family member begins to raise his voice and pound on the table. What are these signs?

A Signs of anger

There are five warning signs of escalating behaviors leading to violence. These include confusion, frustration, blame, anger, and hostility. Anger is characterized by visible changes in body posture and is very risky behaviors that lead to violence (Boxes 11.41 and 11.42).

Box 11.41 Signs of Anger

Argumentative	Cursing
Difficult to please	High-pitched voice
Sarcasm	Acting-out behavior
Pacing and motor agitation	

Box 11.42 Warning Signs of Escalating Behaviors

Confusion	Bewilderment
	Distracted
Frustration	Impatience
	Feelings of sense of defeat
Blame	Placing responsibilities on other people
	Find fault in others' actions
	Place blame directly on healthcare providers
Anger	Visible changes in body posture
	Threatening behaviors
Hostility	Threats of physical action
	Actual acts of physical harm

▶ MANAGEMENT

Q What is the best management for aggressive behaviors?

A Prevention

One of the most important aspects of managing aggressive behaviors is to recognize signs that signal distress and intervene before these aggressive behaviors occur. Most situations of aggressive behavior and violence have warning signs of escalating emotions (such as anger) and may be diffused with appropriate interventions.

HINT Learn how to recognize, avoid, or diffuse potentially violent situations (Box 11.43). When dealing with angry or hostile patients/family members, always be prepared to evacuate or isolate. Do not get cornered in the room; remain near the door for faster exit.

Box 11.43 Interventions for Warning Signs

Confusion	Listen to concerns
	Provide honest answers and accurate information
Frustration	Clarify questions
	Reassure them

(continued)

Box 11.43 Interventions for Warning Signs (*continued*)

Blame	Obtain consultations of experts
	Use other healthcare providers
	Arrange family conferences
	Refocus on facts
Anger	Allow venting or expressing feelings
	Do not argue
	Do not offer solutions
Hostility	Evacuate to safety
	Call security

Q What is a commonly taught technique used as an early intervention in potentially aggressive incidents?

A De-escalating

Certain behaviors and responses can help de-escalate situations that can escalate to violence. These responses should be routinely practiced in dealing with patients and family members. If at any time the situation appears to escalate beyond the comfort zone, disengage and walk away. Hospital security should be called for assistance in those situations (Box 11.44).

Box 11.44 De-escalating Techniques

Remain calm, speak slowly and clearly
Be confident
Focus on what the person is saying
Listen with empathy
Encourage the person to talk
Acknowledge the person's feelings
Establish ground rules and calmly describe consequences of violent behavior
Break down the problem into smaller, more manageable issues
Ask for his or her recommendations to correct the situation
Do not allow the person to block your exit
Acknowledge concerns and accept criticism
Avoid physical contact and long periods of fixed gazes
Avoid sudden movements that might be interpreted as being threatening
Acknowledge the seriousness of the situation
Maintain space between yourself and the person
Do not bargain with the person
Maintain an open posture
Be vigilant throughout the encounter

Q If a patient becomes angry at the nurse for having to attempt to start an IV a second time, what is the best reaction of the nurse?

A Validate the patient's anger

Anger is a human emotion, and a rational expression of anger can be appropriate in some situations. Discouraging angry feelings may cause the person discomfort and escalate his or her feelings. Acknowledge the person's angry feelings. Responding with anger back at the patient will only escalate the situation. Understanding anxiety and addressing the underlying cause of anger will decrease the chance of escalating anger (Boxes 11.45 and 11.46).

HINT Nurses need to avoid personalizing the anger, even if directed at them.

Box 11.45 Interventions for Angry Behaviors

Listen to the patient or family member	Attempt mutual problem solving
Do not dismiss the person's concerns	Assist with identifying the source of anger
Recognize anxiety and intervene early	Call in a second staff member when there are signs of patient getting agitated
Allow the person to express anger	May use the call button to call for assistance
Encourage patients to have more control	Avoid being defensive

Box 11.46 Actions to Minimize Security Risks

Be aware of your surroundings
Trust your instincts
Remove yourself from uncomfortable situations
Remain close to the door during incidents

▶ COMPLICATIONS

Q What potential negative effects on the workplace environment occur over time with repeated incidences of dealing with violence?

A Low morale

Frequent experience with anger and violence in the hospital can lead to low morale among nursing staff, increased stress, and burnout in nurses. Working in a hostile environment leads to staff turnover (Box 11.47).

Box 11.47 Effects of Violence in Hospitals

Minor or major physical injuries	Low morale of nurses
Physical disability	Increased job stress
Psychological trauma	Increased nursing turnover

● ABUSE/NEGLECT

Q Who is frequently the first person to report elder abuse in home situations?

A Healthcare providers

Older people are less likely to self-report abuse. It is typically the healthcare providers who recognize the signs of elder abuse and report the situation to adult protective services. They may be the only people outside of the family to interact with the person (Box 11.48). Suspected as well as confirmed cases should be referred. Identifying, reporting, and treating elder abuse is a responsibility of all healthcare providers. If it is severe enough, call the police and assure that the perpetrator does not have access to the patient.

HINT Mandatory reporting laws for confirmed elder abuse exist in all 50 states and 44 states have mandatory laws to report suspected cases.

Box 11.48 Reasons for Lack of Self-Report of Abuse

Fear of retaliation	Protecting their family
Fear of being placed in a nursing home	Being ashamed or feelings of guilt
Feelings of being powerless	Lack of knowledge on how to report

Q What constitutes elder mistreatment or abuse?

A Physical, emotional, or sexual abuse

Persons 60 years of age or older may experience physical, emotional, and/or sexual mistreatment or abuse. According to the World Health Organization (WHO), elder abuse is "a single, or repeated act, or lack of appropriate action, occurring within any relationship where there is an expectation of trust which causes harm or distress to an older person." Neglect and financial exploitation are both considered elder abuse. Neglect is not meeting the patient's needs and failure to protect the person from harm. Emotional abuse may include threats, humiliation, and verbal abuse.

HINT   Remember, these patients frequently rely on the perpetrator to provide them with shelter, food, money, and clothing.

Q What is the most common reason for lack of reporting abuse in the critical care areas?

A High acuity or unconsciousness

Critical care nurses usually have only brief periods of time with the patient, and due to the criticality of the patient's status, they may not have explored the potential for abuse. Patients may be unconscious and unable to report to the nurse. Screening for abuse routinely will assist with identifying abuse cases. Abuse can occur in domestic or institutionalized settings.

HINT   Families may know of the situation or are the ones actually abusing the patient, so they may deny the abuse.

▶ PATHOPHYSIOLOGY

Q What underlying illness of the patient has been found to increase risk of abuse?

A Dementia

Patients with dementia are at a greater risk of being physically and emotionally abused. Short-term memory losses, agitation, and aggression associated with dementia place high stress on the primary caregivers and increase the risk of abuse.

HINT   Keep the risk factors in mind as a "red flag" for potential elder-abuse situations (Box 11.49). A greater workload and responsibility of the primary caregiver increases the risk of abuse.

Box 11.49 Risk Factors for Elder Abuse

Presence of dementia	History of mental illness of primary care provider
Shared living conditions	Alcohol misuse/abuse of primary care provider
Social isolation	Physical impairment
Financial difficulties	Lack of support for the primary caregiver
Greater dependence on primary care provider	Older

▶ SYMPTOMS/ASSESSMENT

Q When would be the ideal time to talk with an alert and oriented patient about potential abuse?

A When alone

Establishing a good rapport and a trusting relationship with patients will allow them to feel safer about disclosing mistreatment and abuse. Most of the time, they will not talk about the abuse while the family is present. Once the family leaves, opening the conversation about abuse may help the patients discuss their situation.

HINT Encourage patients to talk and empower them to prevent further abuse. Document everything pertinent from the interview. It may be used later in a court of law for criminal or guardianship proceedings. In elderly patients, use similar rules that are used when assessing pediatric abuse. Always think, do the injuries match the story?

▶ MANAGEMENT

Q What should the critical care nurse do if she suspects a patient was in an abusive situation at home?

A Report the suspected abuse

The report of the suspected abuse can be directly to the adult protective services or to the ICU manager or social worker. Nurses should know hospital policy and whether there is a protocol in place for reporting suspected or confirmed cases of abuse. Legally and ethically, nurses have a responsibility to protect the patients from further harm or injury.

HINT Nurses need to continually be aware of their suspicions and intuitions regarding potential abuse.

▶ COMPLICATIONS

Q What psychological disorder can be caused by an abusive situation?

A Depression

Abuse diminishes self-respect, pride, and dignity leading to depression, social isolation, and higher rates of dementia in the elderly. It may contribute to failure to thrive syndrome and higher mortality from illnesses or injuries.

HINT Abuse places the person at a higher risk of suicide.

 PTSD

Q What is the underlying issue that can lead to a post-traumatic stress disorder in the ICU?

A Experience traumatic event

Critical illness is a traumatic event and can lead to PTSD. Critical illness and the critical care environment can lead survivors to experience the symptoms of PTSD after hospital discharge. PTSD is a mental health disorder. It can be defined as the development of characteristic symptoms following exposure to extreme traumatic stressor and the person's response to the event involves intense fear, helplessness, or terror (Box 11.50).

HINT Cognitive processing at the time of the critical illness is important for the development of PTSD.

Box 11.50 Critical Care Stressors for PTSD

Isolation	Sedation
Painful procedures	Sleep deprivation
Feelings of helplessness	Fear of dying/imminent threat of death
Loss of control	

▶ PATHOPHYSIOLOGY

> **Q** What is an identified risk factor for the critically ill patient to develop PTSD after hospital discharge?
>
> **A** Delusional memories

The patients' recall of delusional events and less of the factual events have been found to be linked to greater incidence of PTSD later after hospitalization (Box 11.51). Amnesia for the period of critical care is related to the severity of the PTSD. Some studies have found, patients more awake while on mechanical ventilation had less incidence and severity of PTSD. Fractions of memory and memory of events that did not occur increase the difficulty for patients to understand what happened to them during that time period,

Box 11.51 Risks for Development of PTSD in Critically Ill Patients

Delusional memories	Fractional memory
Hallucinations	Delirium
History of depression and mental health issues	Minimizing sedation
Coping skills	ICU length of stay
Sepsis and MSOD	Lack of social support
Intubation and mechanical ventilation	Physical restraints
Sleep deprivation	Intraoperative recall of events

▶ SYMPTOMS/ASSESSMENT

> **Q** Which sleep disorder is most commonly found in post ICU patients with PTSD?
>
> **A** Nightmares

Nightmares are a common sleep abnormality that is a sign of PTSD. These nightmares can lead to the fear of sleeping and eventually sleep deprivation.

Box 11.52 Signs of PTSD

Nightmares	Flashbacks/Intrusive recollections
Mentally and emotionally relive the event	Avoid reminders of the event (people, places, etc.)
Avoidance of feelings/emotional withdrawal	Hyperarousable
Easily startled, "jumpy"	Severe anxiety
Emotional (difficulty controlling anger and irritability)	Difficulty concentrating

▶ DIAGNOSIS

> **Q** What is the primary diagnosis of PTSD?
>
> **A** Clinical Signs

PTSD diagnosis is based upon clinical signs and symptoms. The presence of symptoms of PTSD after experiencing a traumatic event is the diagnosis of PTSD. Based upon the Diagnosis and Statistical Manual of Mental Disorders, PTSD is the development of characteristic symptoms following exposure to extreme traumatic stressor…the person's response to the event must involve intense fear, helplessness or horror.

▶ MANAGEMENT

Q What nursing intervention can potentially improve and lower the PTSD after critical illness?

A Improve patient's understanding of events

One area that can potentially lower the incidence and severity of PTSD is implementing interventions that improve the patient's understanding and recollection of true events (Box 11.53). ICU diaries are being used more for hospital staff and family to write down events that happened for the patient to read after improvement. This provides factual information about their stay in the ICU, which allows the patient to reconstruct their memory on more factual memories.

HINT Even patients that are sedated or unresponsive can develop delusional memory and should be managed the same as those lightly sedated and awake.

Box 11.53 Interventions to Improve Memory of Critically Ill Patients

Explain all procedures to the patient	Reorient the patient frequently
Allow open family visitation	Maintain ICU diaries
Counseling sessions after discharge	Allow patient to talk about their memories

▶ COMPLICATIONS

Q What is a potential sequela of depression and PTSD after a critical illness?

A Suicide

Suicide is associated with PTSD and depression (Box 11.54)

Box 11.54 Complications of PTSD

Suicide	Drug and alcohol abuse
Loss of self-identity	Decreased quality of life

⬤ MEDICAL NONADHERENCE

Q A patient is admitted with hypertensive crisis due to nonadherence with their medications. What is a common reason for nonadherence to medical management of a chronic illness?

A Side effects of the medication

Nonadherence to treatments and management of chronic illness is common and can be associated with many different reasons. Medication nonadherence is a lack of taking the medication, not taking according to instructions or mixing the medications without a physician's knowledge. Patients may not always be forthcoming or honest when asked about adherence to the medical regimen (Box 11.55).

HINT Multiple medications or medications that are required to be taken more frequently are more likely to contribute to nonadherence of medication.

Box 11.55 Reasons for Medical Nonadherence

Lack of motivation	Side effects of medications
Denial	Cognitive impairment
Drug or alcohol abuse	Cultural issues
Treatments complex	Cost of medications

(continued)

Box 11.55 Reasons for Medical Nonadherence (*continued*)

Lack of understanding of directions	More than one medication
Highly anxious patients	Fear of becoming dependent
Failed to refill medication	Take lower dose than prescribed

Q How is the difference between noncompliance and nonadherence?

A Intentional versus non-intentional

Noncompliance is the intentional or deliberate refusal of the patient. This can include denial, disagreement with the healthcare provider, or ignore the recommendations. Nonadherence is a term used which includes unintentional refusal by the patient. This may be due to confusion, helplessness, or dementia.

Q What is a method for improving medical compliance in chronic illness?

A Education

Patients are more likely to adhere to medications if they understand the purpose and significance of the medications. Quality interactions, ongoing communication, and education are key to improving medical adherence. Medical terminology is a foreign language to most patients. Education needs to be at a level the patient can understand.

Box 11.56 Methods to Improve adherence

Provide clear and understandable instructions	Simplify instructions in layman terms
Medication adherence contract	Link medication schedule with daily activities
Automated phone call/text reminders	Once a day medication if possible
90-day prescriptions	Automatic refill programs

Q What is a major complication of medical noncompliance or nonadherence?

A Death

Nonadherence and noncompliance can lead to poor health outcomes, increased hospitalizations, and death.

● RESTRAINT USE IN THE ICU

Q What restraining therapy should be used in ICU?

A Least restrictive but effective

Restraints can cause issues with patient comfort and dignity as well as complications of falls, limb injuries, and skin breakdown. The recommended restraint is the one that is least restrictive but still effective. Alternatives to restraints should be considered when appropriate and underlying problems treated that may decrease the need for restraints. Bed alarms may be used to alert the nurse of the patient getting out of bed and may lower the need for restraints (Box 11.57).

HINT Restraints should not be routinely used on all ICU patients. The need should be determined on a case-by-case basis.

Box 11.57 Interventions to Lower the Need for Restraints

Adequate pain management	Involvement in activities
Treat delirium or agitation	Adequate lighting in room
Assess for fever or hypoxia	Frequent toileting offered
Ambulate (if possible)	Allow family to sit with patient
Alternative therapy (pet therapy, aromatherapy, massage)	

Q How often should restraint for medical purposes renewal be reordered?

A Every 24 hours

Restraining orders are limited to 24 hours and require daily orders for renewal. The rationale for the need for restraints should also be documented daily. An order should be obtained within 1 hour of initiating restraints.

Q What type of restraint is an analgesic when administered for sedation purposes?

A Chemical restraint

Analgesics, sedatives, hypnotics, and neuroleptic drugs may assist with decreasing the need for restraints, but these are still considered chemical restraints. These drugs are not purely chemical restraints but are a part of therapeutic treatment that may lower the need for physical restraints.

Q What is the primary purpose of restraints in the ICU?

A Patient safety

Restraint use in the ICU is primarily for patient safety to prevent inadvertent discontinuation of endotracheal tubes or other invasive lines or tubes. Restraints may also be used to prevent falls and injuries in patients with delirium or dementia. Restrained patients require frequent observation to prevent complications. Families and patients need to receive information about the purpose of the restraints.

HINT The nurse must balance responsibility to protect the patient's rights and the obligation to prevent injury to the patient.

1. A patient who has a history of progressive dementia is becoming agitated. Which of the following is the LEAST appropriate intervention?

   A. Restrain the patient to prevent self-injury
   B. Use gentle touch and a reassuring voice when talking with the patient
   C. Allow such patients to do as much for themselves as possible
   D. Ask the family to remain with the patient at all times, if possible

2. What is considered to be the primary addiction center of the brain?

   A. Frontal lobe
   B. Hypothalamus
   C. Pituitary gland
   D. Temporal lobe

3. A patient in the intensive care unit (ICU) for pancreatitis has a history of dementia. She is confused but cooperative. Which of the following recommendations is most appropriate for assessing pain in this patient?

   A. Use behavioral signs only to assess for pain
   B. Ask the patient directly about her pain
   C. Have the family tell you if the patient is in pain or needs pain medications
   D. Use vital sign changes to assess for pain

4. Haloperidol is ordered on a patient with agitation and acute psychosis. Which test should obtain as a baseline prior to initiating the medication?

   A. Doppler flow study
   B. 12-lead ECG
   C. Echocardiogram
   D. EEG

5. Which of the following is considered a "stressor" that would contribute to development of PTSD in ICU patients?

   A. Fear of dying or imminent threat of death
   B. Hospitalization
   C. Surgical procedures
   D. Vasoactive medications

6. Amnesia for the period of time of critical illness correlates with severity of PTSD after critical illness. Which of the following is highest risk for critical care PTSD?

   A. Use of sedation
   B. Delusional memories
   C. Recall of actual events
   D. Ability to communicate

1. A) Restrain the patient to prevent self-injury

Gentle touch, soothing music, reading, and walks (if possible) can decrease agitation. Allowing patients to do as much for themselves as possible supports independence and the patient's ability to care for himself or herself. Using family as sitters can help with an agitated patient and prevent the need for restraints. If possible, try not to restrain the person during a period of agitation.

2. B) Hypothalamus

Addiction affects the hypothalamus. It is in the subcortical region of the brain and is responsible for sleep, hunger, moods, sex drive, and circadian rhythms.

3. B) Ask the patient directly about her pain

Objective report of pain by the patient, even a patient with dementia, is the best method of pain assessment. In this case, the patient is cooperative even though confused, and should be able to tell the nurse if she is in pain. Behavioral signs and family input can also be used, but should not be the only pain assessment. Vital signs are the least reliable means of assessing pain.

4. B) 12-lead ECG

A 12-lead ECG can be used to measure the QT interval. A complication of Haloperidol is prolonged QT interval and increased risk of V-tach (torsades). Prior to initiating Haloperidol, a baseline QT should be obtained. An EEG is not required prior to administering Haloperidol. Doppler flow study and echocardiograms are not used to monitor the side effects or complications of Haloperidol.

5. A) Fear of dying or imminent threat of death

Symptoms of PTSD occur after exposure to extreme traumatic stressors, and the person's response to the event involves intense fear, helplessness, or terror. Hospitalization and surgical procedures, by themselves, are not traumatic stressors. Vasoactive medications are not considered a stressor that will cause PTSD.

6. B) Delusional memories

The patients' recall of delusional events and less of the factual events have been found to be linked to greater incidence of PTSD later after hospitalization. Administration of sedatives and PTSD depends upon the level of sedation and accurate recall of the events. Ability to communicate during critical illness will lower risks of post-critical care PTSD.

7. Which is the nurse's priority when evaluating a severely depressed patient?

    A. Affirm the patient's worth
    B. Show empathy for the patient
    C. Allow the patient to talk about their feelings
    D. Best to stay positive while talking to the patient

8. The nurse is assessing the patient for alcohol dependence and is asking the patient multiple questions as part of an assessment. The patient stops the nurse to ask, "what do you mean by one drink?" Which explanation by the nurse is correct?

    A. "8 ounces of beer"
    B. "6 ounces of wine"
    C. "2.5 ounces cordial"
    D. "5 ounces of malt liquor"

9. The nurse is explaining to a nursing student what is happening in their depressed patient's brain. Which statement would be correct to use in education?

    A. Serotonin energizes the body in stress and is low in patients with depression
    B. Dopamine affects mood, behavior, and cognition, and it is low in patients with depression
    C. Norepinephrine provides motivation and pleasure in the brain, and it is low in patients with depression
    D. Acetylcholine alters mood, sleep, and neuroendocrine function and is high in patients with depression

10. The patient received a dose of midazolam 2 min ago and asked the nurse how long it will be before they feel relief. Which response from the nurse is correct?

    A. "Just wait about 15 more minutes"
    B. "It will take about five more minutes"
    C. "You should already feel a difference"
    D. "You should start to have relief any minute now"

7. A) Affirm the patient's worth

The major goal of the nurse when speaking with a depressed patient is to affirm the patient's worth. This can be accomplished by establishing a trusting relationship, allowing the patient to talk about their feelings, displaying positivity regarding the patient and showing empathy. Each of these actions plays an important role in affirming the patient's value and worth, but alone will not accomplish the priority goal.

8. C) "2.5 ounces cordial"

A liqueur, or cordial, is a sweetened distilled spirit. It fits into the definition of one drink as 2.5 ounces of cordial. 12 ounces of beer, 5 ounces of wine and 8.5 ounces of malt liquor also counts as one drink.

9. D) Acetylcholine alters mood, sleep, and neuroendocrine function and is high in patients with depression

Acetylcholine alters mood, sleep, and neuroendocrine function and is high in patients with depression. Serotonin affects mood, behavior, and cognition and is low in patients with depression. Norepinephrine energizes the body in stress and is low in depressed patients. Dopamine provides motivation and is the pleasure center of the brain. Levels are low in patients with depression.

10. D) "You should start to have relief any minute now"

The onset of midazolam is 2–5 min. Since it has already been 2 min, the patient would start to feel relief any minute. The onset of Lorazepam is 15–20 min, so responding with about 15 more minutes would be if the patient had received this medication. Responding with five more minutes would be more in line with a Dexmedetomidine administration as the onset is 5–10 min. "You should already feel a difference" is slightly derogatory and does not give the patient the best answer.

● BIBLIOGRAPHY

Barr, J., Fraser, G. L., Puntillo, K., Ely, E. W., Gélinas, C., Dasta, J. F., … & Jaeschke, R. (2013). Clinical practice guidelines for the management of pain, agitation, and delirium in adult patients in the intensive care unit. *Critical care medicine, 41*(1), 263–306.

Garrouste-Orgeas, M., Flahault, C., Vinatier, I. (2019). Effect of an ICU diary on Posttraumatic Stress Disorder Symptoms among patients receiving mechanical ventilation. *Jama, 322*(3), 229–239.

Gélinas, C., Fillion, L., Puntillo, K. A., Viens, C., & Fortier, M. (2006). Validation of the critical-care pain observation tool in adult patients. *American Journal of Critical Care, 15*(4), 420–427.

Hartsell, Z., Drost, J., Wilkens, J., & Budavari, I. (2007). Managing alcohol withdrawal in hospital patients. *Journal of the American Academy of Physician Assistants, 20*(9), 20–25.

Kross, E. K., Pollak, K. I., & Curtis, J. R. (2019). Addressing the psychological symptoms of critical illness: the importance of "Negative" trials in guiding next steps. *Jama, 321*(7), 649–650. https://doi.org/10.1001/jama.2019.0072

Marra, A., Pandharipande, P., & Patel, M. (2017). ICU delirium and ICU related PTSD. *Surgical Clinics of North America, 97*(6), 1215–1235.

Rittenmeyer, L. (2012). Aggression in high dependency care environment. *Critical Care Nursing Clinics of North America, 24*, 41–51.

Wade, D. M., Mouncey, P. R., Richards-Belle, A., Wulff, J., Harrison, D. A., Sadique, M. Z., … & Rowan, K. M. (2019). Effect of a nurse-led preventive psychological intervention on symptoms of posttraumatic stress disorder among critically ill patients: A randomized clinical trial. *Jama, 321*(7), 665–675. https://doi.org/10.1001/jama.2019.0073

Warlan, H & Howland, L. (2015). Posttraumatic stress syndrome associated with stays in the intensive care unit: Importance of nurse's involvement. *Critical Care Nurse, 35*(3), 44–52.

World Health Organization. (n.d.). *Ageing and life course: Elder abuse.* Retrieved from http://www.who.int/ageing/projects/elder_abuse/en/index.html

Multisystem Review

● SEPSIS AND SEPTIC SHOCK

Q What is the presence of bacteria in the bloodstream called?

A Bacteremia

A bacteremia is the viable presence of bacteria in the bloodstream. Blood cultures are positive for bacteria. A fungemia is the presence of fungus in the bloodstream. A positive culture is one of the signs of an infection. An infection initiates the inflammatory response and onset of sepsis (Box 12.1).

Box 12.1 Signs of an Infection

- Presence of white cells in normal sterile body fluid
- Positive culture (urine, blood, sputum)
- Perforated viscous
- Radiographic evidence of pneumonia in association with purulent sputum

Q What is the white blood cell (WBC) criteria used to define sepsis?

A WBC greater than 12,000 or less than 4,000 or greater than 10% bands

Sepsis is the inflammatory response to a known infection. Sepsis occurs if two or more of the defined criteria are present. Systemic inflammatory response syndrome (SIRS) is the systemic inflammatory response to a variety of severe clinical insults. SIRS is defined by the same criteria used to define sepsis but without signs of infection and a negative blood culture (Box 12.2).

HINT Sepsis is a disease process managed in all areas of the hospital and is not exclusive to critical care.

Box 12.2 Criteria for Sepsis

- Temperature > 38.3 °C (101 °F) or < 36 °C
- Heart rate > 90 beats/min
- Respiratory rate > 20 breaths/min or $PaCO_2$ < 32 mmHg
- WBC > 12,000 cells/mm³ or < 4,000 mm³ > 10% immature granulocytes (bands)

Q What is septic shock?

A Sepsis with hypotension and/or hypoperfusion

Severe sepsis is sepsis accompanied by hypotension and/or hypoperfusion. Severe sepsis is also called sepsis-induced tissue hypoperfusion or organ dysfunction. Hypotension is systolic blood pressure (BP) less than 90 mmHg, mean arterial pressure (MAP) less than 65 mmHg, or a decrease in BP by greater than 40 mmHg from baseline. Hypoperfusion may include but is not limited to oliguria, increased lactate levels higher than 4 mmol/L, or acute alteration in mental status. The sepsis bundles use a lactate level greater than 4 mmol/L to recognize hypoperfusion (Box 12.3).

Box 12.3 Signs of Hypoperfusion

- Acute altered mental status
- Blood glucose >140 mg/dL in patients without diabetes
- Arterial hypoxemia (PaO_2/FiO_2 ratio <300)
- Acute oliguria (<0.5 mL/kg/hr for at least 2 hrs)
- Creatinine increase >0.5 mg/dL above baseline
- Coagulation abnormalities (international normalized ratio [INR] >1.5 or activated partial thromboplastin time (aPTT) >60 sec)
- Ileus
- Thrombocytopenia (platelet count <100,000)
- Hyperbilirubinemia (total bilirubin >2 mg/dL)

HINT Septic shock is defined by hypotension and hypoperfusion despite adequate resuscitation.

Q What causes multiple organ dysfunction in sepsis?

A Hypoperfusion

Multiple organ dysfunction syndrome (MODS) is the presence of altered organ function, involving two or more organs, in an acutely ill patient such that homeostasis cannot be maintained without intervention. It is progressive but potentially reversible and is a result of hypoperfusion and injury to the organs.

HINT The incidence of mortality is related to the number of organs involved in MODS and the severity of organ dysfunction (Table 12.1).

Table 12.1 Signs of Organ Dysfunction

System	Major Sign
Pulmonary	PaO_2/FiO_2 ratio < 300
Renal	Increased serum creatinine > 2.0 or creatinine increase > 0.5 mg/dL or 44.2 µmmol/L
Hepatic	Increased bilirubin levels > 4 mg/dL
Hematology	Decreased platelet counts < 100,000/µL INR > 1.5 aPTT > 60 sec
Central nervous system	Altered Glasgow Coma Scale (GCS)

▶ PATHOPHYSIOLOGY

Q What is the most common microorganism that causes sepsis?

A Gram-positive bacteria

Gram-positive bacteremia has surpassed the gram-negative bacteria. A common gram-positive bacteria found in hospitals is methicillin-resistant *Staphylococcus aureus* (MRSA; Box 12.4).

Box 12.4 Gram-Negative Bacteria

Escherichia coli	Enterobacter
Klebsiella pneumoniae	Serratia
Pseudomonas aeruginosa	Proteus

HINT   Gram-negative bacteria colonize the gastrointestinal (GI) tract and oral secretions (Box 12.5). Central-line sepsis is commonly a result of gram-positive bacteremia.

Box 12.5 Gram-Positive Bacteria

- Staphylococcus
- Streptococcus

Q Which microorganism is the most common cause of a secondary infection?

A Fungus (Candida)

Fungal infections frequently present as a second episode of an infection. This is due to the use of antibiotics to treat the first infection, which alters the normal flora and allows opportunistic infections to develop. Another high-risk patient is an immunosuppressed patient. Fungal sepsis (fungemia) has a higher mortality than bacteremia and is harder to diagnose. The presence of a fungemia may not result in a positive blood culture. Management is frequently based on presumptive therapy, which is to "presume" there is a fungemia and treat with antifungal medication. New tests may be used to assist with the diagnosis of Candida (1,3 β-d-glucan assay [Grade 2B], mannan, and antimannan antibody assays).

HINT   Sepsis with a negative blood culture is frequently caused by fungal infections

SYMPTOMS/ASSESSMENT

> **Q** An increase in bands greater than what percentage indicates severe sepsis?
>
> **A** Greater than 10%

Bands are immature WBCs. If more than 10% of the circulating WBCs are bands, this indicates an overwhelming infection and sepsis. Other WBC changes potentially indicating sepsis include WBC count greater than 12,000 or less than 4,000.

HINT For example, if the complete blood count (CBC) differential finds 45% bands it indicates that 45% of the circulating WBCs are immature and not functional.

> **Q** In severe septic shock, does the left ventricular (LV) ejection fraction (EF) increase or decrease?
>
> **A** Decrease

Proinflammatory cytokine, tumor necrosis factor (TNF), is released following the presence of a microorganism and initiates the inflammatory response. TNF has a negative contractility effect on the myocardium and results in a decrease in EF. The cardiac output (CO) is usually high in sepsis because of systemic vasodilation lowering the resistance (Box 12.6).

HINT Use of a right ejection fraction–oximetry (REF-ox) pulmonary artery catheter in sepsis patients has shown a decrease in EF even during periods of high COs. Right ventricular EF commonly ranges from 30% to 40% during early sepsis.

Box 12.6 Symptoms of Sepsis/Sepsis Shock

■ Tachycardia ■ Tachypnea ■ Leukocytosis or leukopenia or increased bands ■ Fever ■ Decreased systemic vascular resistance (SVR) ■ Hypotension (vasodilation) ■ Increased CO ■ Decreased EF	■ Metabolic acidosis ■ Respiratory alkalosis ■ Pulmonary artery hypertension ■ Altered mental status ■ Edema or positive fluid balance ■ Hyperglycemia (> 140 mg/dL or 7.7 mmol/L) in a nondiabetic patient ■ Signs of organ dysfunction ■ LV dilation

▶ DIAGNOSIS

> **Q** What diagnostic determines the microorganism(s) involved in causing an infection and the best antibiotics needed to treat the infection?
>
> **A** Culture and sensitivity

Diagnosis of sepsis is the presence of two or more of the defining criteria for sepsis. Once sepsis is recognized, cultures determine the causative microorganisms and their susceptibility to certain antibiotics. Recommendation is at least two sets of blood cultures (both anaerobic and aerobic bottles) with at least one drawn percutaneously and one drawn from a vascular access device that is more than 48 hrs old. Both sets of blood cultures can be obtained at the same time as long as they are from two different sites. Cultures from other potential sites of infection (urine, sputum, cerebrospinal fluid [CSF], wounds) are obtained and are sent with the blood cultures for testing.

HINT If the same organism is recovered from both the samples, there is a better likelihood that the organism is responsible for the sepsis.

> **Q** What other lab tests beside the CBC can be used to determine the presence of an infection?
>
> **A** Plasma C-reactive protein and prolactin

Plasma C-reactive protein and prolactin are biomarkers for diagnosis of infection. They may be used as additional information but are not, at this time, shown to distinguish from infection and other causes of inflammation.

HINT   Procalcitonin levels may be beneficial in determining when to discontinue the antibiotics.

▶ MEDICAL MANAGEMENT

Q   What is the overall best management goal for sepsis?

A   Prevention

Prevention of an infection or sepsis is still the best management. Hand washing is the main area of prevention found to lower the incidence of infections across the continuum of patient types and ages (Box 12.7).

Box 12.7 Sources of Hospital-Associated Infections

▪ Catheter-associated urinary tract infection ▪ Central line-associated bloodstream infections ▪ Ventilator-associated pneumonia	▪ Hospital-acquired pneumonia ▪ Intra-abdominal source

Q   What is the current recommendation to prevent a catheter-associated urinary tract infection (CAUTI)?

A   Minimize the use and duration of the urinary catheter

Urinary tract infections are the most common type of health care-associated infections. Current practice is to mostly avoid an indwelling urinary catheter insertion, if possible. If a urinary catheter is required in surgery, the goal is to discontinue it within 24 hours. Removing the indwelling catheter as soon as possible will lower the incidence of urinary tract infections. The most common causative microorganisms are *Escherichia coli* and *Candida*. It is not recommended to change bags or indwelling catheters on a routine basis. The catheter can be changed if clinical indications are present, including infection or contamination of the system (Box 12.8).

HINT   Remember all lines and tubes in the patient are a source of infection and should be removed as soon as possible. (Box 12.9).

Box 12.8 Appropriate Reasons for Urinary Catheter Use

▪ Accurate input and output in critically ill patients ▪ Need to monitor urine output ▪ Unable to use bedpan or urinal Coma ▪ Sedation and paralytics	▪ Large volume of fluid infusions or diuretics ▪ Urological surgical patients ▪ Urinary retention or obstruction

Box 12.9 Prevention of Urinary Tract Infections

▪ Aseptic insertion technique and use of sterile equipment ▪ Keep bag off the floor ▪ Keep bag lower than the bladder ▪ Properly secure to prevent movement of bladder	▪ Maintain a closed drainage system ▪ May use antiseptic/antimicrobial impregnated catheters ▪ Empty collecting bag regularly

> **Q** What nursing intervention has been found to lower the incidence of ventilator-associated pneumonia (VAP)?
>
> **A** Oral care with chlorhexidine

Oropharyngeal decontamination with chlorhexidine is recommended to lower the incidence of VAP. Selective digestive decontamination has also been proposed to lower the risk of VAP (Box 12.10).

Box 12.10 Methods of Prevention of VAP

■ Proper hand washing	■ Subglottic suctioning
■ Oral decontamination	■ Prevent unplanned extubations/reintubations
■ Digestive decontamination	■ Avoid saline lavages
■ Head of the bed (HOB) elevated	

> **Q** How quickly should antibiotics be started following a diagnosis of sepsis?
>
> **A** Within 1 hour

Antibiotics are the main treatment of sepsis and may halt its progression and improve outcomes if administered early in the course of sepsis. Cultures should be obtained prior to the administration of antibiotics unless doing so would cause significant delay in the administration of antibiotics. Antibiotics can result in sterilization of the cultures within a few hours, making identification of the causative organisms more difficult. They should be obtained sooner than 45 minutes after the diagnosis of sepsis. Emperic Broad-spectrum antibiotics should be used to be effective against all likely organisms. Once culture results are obtained, antibiotics should be changed to a more specific antibiotic for the organism's susceptibility, with the goal being within 3–5 days.

HINT Recommendation is to maintain a 5- to 7-day course of antibiotic therapy. May increase the number of days in case of slow clinical response or continued presence of the infected source.

> **Q** In early goal-directed therapy of severe sepsis, what is the central venous pressure (CVP) goal of the initial fluid resuscitation in a spontaneous breathing patient?
>
> **A** CVP 8–12 mmHg

Severe sepsis is persistent hypotension or hypoperfusion after the initial bolus of fluid. Early goal-directed strategy includes monitoring CVP and $ScvO_2$ to determine the adequacy of resuscitation. A CVP of 8–12 mmHg is recommended for spontaneous breathing patients and slightly higher on ventilated patients (12–15 mmHg) because of positive pressure effects in the chest. $ScvO_2$ can be monitored intermittently or continuously. The goals should be obtained within 6 hrs on recognition of sepsis. Goals can be obtained with fluid administration, blood products, dobutamine infusion, and/or lower oxygen demands with sedation or paralysis. Another parameter used to monitor hemodynamics is stroke volume variance (SVV), which will determine fluid responsiveness.

HINT Lactate levels may also be monitored with a goal to normalize serum lactate (Box 12.11). A decrease in heart rate is also a good indication of successful resuscitation.

Box 12.11 Goals of Resuscitation in Severe Sepsis

■ CVP 8–12 mmHg in spontaneous breathing
■ CVP 12–15 mmHg ventilated
■ MAP ≥ 65 mmHg
■ Urine output ≥ 0.5 mL/kg/hr
■ $ScvO_2$ 70% or SvO_2 65%

> **Q What fluids are recommended for initial resuscitation in sepsis?**
>
> **A Crystalloids**

Current recommendation for fluid resuscitation in severe sepsis or sepsis-induced hypoperfusion is crystalloids given within first 3 hours. This is recommended because of lack of benefit for albumin used initially, which is more expensive than a crystalloid. If the patient requires substantial amounts of fluid to meet the goals of volume resuscitation, then albumin administration can be used with crystalloids. Initially, the fluid challenge should be a minimum of 30 mL/kg bolus with more fluids, if needed, to meet the predetermined goals of volume resuscitation.

HINT Hydroxy ethyl starches (Hetastarch) are not recommended in resuscitation of sepsis patients because of their worsening effect on kidneys.

> **Q What vasopressor is considered to be the first choice in maintaining MAP greater than 65 mmHg?**
>
> **A Norepinephrine (Levophed)**

Vasopressor therapy is recommended to maintain MAP greater than or equal to 65 mmHg. Below this perfusion pressure, autoregulation in the critical vascular beds is lost. The vasopressor recommended as a first-line treatment is norepinephrine. If an additional vasopressor is required, epinephrine or vasopressin may be added to maintain pressure or to lower the dose of norepinephrine. Vasopressin is not recommended as a single first-line vasopressor in sepsis. Dopamine may be an alternative vasopressor to norepinephrine but only in certain patients who are at very low risk for tachyarrhythmias. Low-dose dopamine should not be used for renal protection. A patient with absolute or refractory bradycardia may receive dopamine as the first-line vasopressor. Phenylephrine is not recommended in the treatment of septic shock unless associated with serious arrhythmias or CO is known to be high or when other vasopressor agents have failed to achieve the target MAP.

HINT An arterial line is recommended for continuous and more accurate BP readings. Central venous access is required for the administration of vasopressors.

> **Q When should corticosteroid therapy be considered in a patient with sepsis?**
>
> **A Refractory to vasopressors**

A patient who responds to fluids and/or vasopressor therapy by improving hemodynamic parameters (BP) and lactate levels does not require corticosteroid treatment. If hemodynamic stability cannot be achieved, even after resuscitation and vasopressors, 200 mg/day of hydrocortisone as a continuous infusion is recommended. Continuous infusions may control blood glucose more effectively than intermittent boluses with less significant hyperglycemia. Once vasopressors are not required, hydrocortisone may be tapered down and discontinued. The adrenocorticotropin hormone (ACTH) test is not recommended to determine indication for corticosteroid therapy.

HINT Side effects of hydrocortisone are hypernatremia and hyperglycemia.

> **Q According to the Sepsis Campaign guidelines, when should the insulin protocol be initiated in a sepsis patient?**
>
> **A Glucose greater than 180 mg/dL**

Current recommendations for glucose control are to treat with sliding-scale insulin if blood glucose levels are greater than 180 mg/dL at two consecutive times. Maintain glucose less than 180 mg/dL while avoiding hypoglycemia. Blood glucose levels may be checked every 4 hours when stable and every 1–2 hours while elevated. Maintaining strict glucose levels of less than 110 mg/dL is not recommended because of the incidence of hypoglycemia.

HINT Point-of-care glucose tests may not be as accurate as plasma glucose levels from the laboratory and should be interpreted cautiously, especially in patients with low hematocritis.

> **Q** At what serum pH would sodium bicarbonate therapy be administered in septic shock patients with lactic acidosis?
>
> **A** Less than 7.15

There is no benefit to treating pH with sodium bicarbonate until pH decreases less than 7.15. The side effects of sodium bicarbonate cause the risks of administration to be greater than the benefit (Box 12.12).

Box 12.12 Complications of Sodium Bicarbonate

▪ Fluid overload	▪ Hypercarbia
▪ Hypernatremia	▪ Decrease serum ionized calcium
▪ Increased lactate levels	▪ Greater affinity of hgb to red blood cells (RBCs)

▶ SURGICAL MANAGEMENT

> **Q** In the case of a known source of infection, what is the best management?
>
> **A** Remove the source of infection

Radiographics are frequently used to find the location of the infection. If the infectious source is amendable, then drainage, percutaneous drainage, or surgical excision may be required. Source control as rapidly as possible can lower the incidence of mortality (Box 12.13).

HINT   If the source is determined to be an intravenous (IV) access source, the catheter must be removed promptly after obtaining other access.

Box 12.13 Foci Infections That Are Surgically Amendable

▪ Abscesses (including intra-abdominal)	▪ Intestinal ischemia
▪ Gastrointestinal perforation	▪ Necrotizing soft tissue
▪ Cholangitis	▪ Empyema
▪ Pyelonephritis	▪ Septic arthritis

▶ COMPLICATIONS

> **Q** What is the primary physiology for a hypoperfused state in sepsis?
>
> **A** Inability of the cells to use oxygen

Initial hypoperfusion is a result of distributive shock (vasodilation) and hypovolemia (increased vascular permeability). Even after fluid resuscitation and BP are restored, hypoperfusion may persist. It is largely attributed to an inability of the cells to use the oxygen delivered to the tissues. Another major contributing factor is maldistribution of blood flow, which occurs at the regional level (splanchnic, renal, and mesenteric) as well as at the microvascular level.

HINT   Remember the aphorism, "You can lead a horse to water but you cannot make it drink." In sepsis, you can optimize the delivery of oxygen to the tissues/cells, but you cannot make them take in the oxygen (Box 12.14).

Box 12.14 Causes of Inadequate Tissue Oxygenation

▪ Decreased oxygen delivery (DO_2)	▪ Inability to offload O_2 from hgb
▪ Inability to extract oxygen	▪ Arteriovenous shunt
▪ Blockage of normal cellular metabolism	▪ Endothelial injury
▪ Greater distance between capillary and tissue (edema)	▪ Loss of vascular tone

> **Q** What is the GI complication due to use of multiple antibiotics in treating sepsis?
>
> **A** *Clostridium difficile*

C. difficile is a superinfection that may occur as a result of using multiple antibiotics, broad-spectrum antibiotics, and lengthy duration of treatment. Narrowing the spectrum and shortening the time of antibiotics therapy may lower the risk of opportunistic infections such as Candida or superinfections such as *C. difficile* and resistant bacteria (vancomycin-resistant enterococcus faecium).

HINT   Antibiotics can change the normal GI flora. Probiotics may be used to limit some of this altered flora.

> **Q** What is the most common cause of death in septic shock?
>
> **A** Multiple organ dysfunction syndrome

MODS is a complication of tissue and organ hypoperfusion that occurs in severe sepsis and septic shock. MODS is defined as the presence of altered organ functions in acutely ill patients such that homeostasis cannot be obtained without intervention. The number of organs affected predicts mortality. Any organ can be affected by sepsis-induced hypoperfusion (Box 12.15).

HINT   This is also commonly called multisystem organ failure (MSOF).

Box 12.15 Common Organs Involved in MODS

■ Acute respiratory distress syndrome	■ Septic encephalopathy
■ Acute kidney injury	■ Systolic and diastolic dysfunction of myocardium
■ Hepatic failure	■ Disseminated intravascular coagulation
■ Gastrointestinal tract	■ Metabolic dysfunction with hyperglycemia

> **Q** What plays a central role in microvascular dysfunction that occurs in MODS?
>
> **A** Endothelium

The endothelium regulates vasomotor tone, coagulation, vascular permeability, and balance between pro- and anti-inflammatory cytokines. Biomarkers that measure endothelial activity (plasminogen activator inhibitor-1) demonstrate increased levels following activation of the inflammatory system and correlate the severity of MODS.

> **Q** What tool can be used to determine the rate and extent of organ failure?
>
> **A** Sequential organ failure assessment (SOFA)

The SOFA scoring system is used to determine the extent of organ function or rate of failure.

HINT   When scoring, if none match the patient, the score is set at 0 for that section. If more than one match, then the highest score is used (Table 12.2).

Table 12.2 SOFA

Respiratory System	
PaO_2/FiO_2	SOFA Score
< 400	1
< 300	2
< 200 **and** mechanically ventilated	3
< 100 **and** mechanically ventilated	4

(*continued*)

Table 12.2 SOFA (*continued*)

Nervous System	
Glasgow Coma Scale	**SOFA Score**
13–14	1
10–12	2
6–9	3
<6	4
Cardiovascular System	
MAP or Vasopressor Requirement	**SOFA Score**
MAP < 70 mmHg	1
Dopamine < 5 *or* dobutamine (any dose)	2
Dopamine > 5 *or* epinephrine ≤ 0.1 *or* norepinephrine ≤ 0.1	3
Dopamine > 15 *or* epinephrine > 0.1 *or* norepinephrine > 0.1	4
Liver	
Bilirubin	**SOFA Score**
1.2–1.9	1
2.0–5.9	2
6.0–11.9	3
> 12	4
Coagulation	
Platelets × 10³	**SOFA Score**
< 150	1
< 100	2
< 50	3
< 20	4
Renal System	
Creatinine or Urine Output	**SOFA Score**
1.2–1.9	1
2.0–3.4	2
3.5–4.9	3
> 5	4

DISTRIBUTIVE SHOCK: ANAPHYLAXIS

Q How is anaphylaxis different from an anaphylactoid reaction?

A Immunoglobulin E (IgE) mediated

Anaphylaxis and anaphylactoid reactions are both acute, life-threatening hypersensitivity reactions, but anaphylaxis is immune-related, whereas an anaphylactoid reaction is not. Anaphylaxis involves IgE binding to an antigen that the person was previously exposed to. Anaphylactoid does not have the immune component but is similar in assessment, diagnosis, and treatment.

HINT   Both are called life-threatening hypersensitivity reactions.

> **Q** How quickly can the symptoms of hypersensitivity reactions occur following exposure to the provoking agent?
>
> **A** Within minutes

The onset of symptoms can occur within minutes to hours. Typically, symptoms will peak in severity within 5–30 min. The episode frequently lasts fewer than 24 hours but can be protracted or reoccur after initial resolution.

▶ PATHOPHYSIOLOGY

> **Q** In both hypersensitivity reactions, what is triggered causing the release of chemical mediators?
>
> **A** Mast cells

Mast cells are activated in both anaphylaxis and anaphylactoid reactions, releasing several chemical mediators. Overall, the mediators increase capillary permeability and cause peripheral vasodilation. Increased capillary permeability can cause airway swelling and angioedema. Peripheral vasodilation results in hypotension, which is labeled as distributive shock (Box 12.16).

HINT   The most life-threatening component of a hypersensitivity reaction is angioedema.

Box 12.16 Chemical Mediators Released in Anaphylaxis

- Bradykinin
- Platelet-activating factor
- Prostaglandins
- Leukotrienes

> **Q** What are the two most common causes of anaphylaxis?
>
> **A** Food and insect stings

Food sensitivities, insect stings, and antibiotics are the most common causes of an IgE-mediated anaphylaxis reaction. These occur after previous exposure to a provoking agent. Stinging insects such as bees, wasps, and fire ants contain a substance in their venom that initiates the IgE antibody response. Penicillin is the most common antibiotic to cause an anaphylaxis reaction. Other common antibiotics include cephalosporin and sulfonamides (Box 12.17).

Box 12.17 Common Food Allergies That Cause Anaphylaxis

■ Peanuts	■ Milk
■ Shellfish	■ Eggs
■ Fish	■ Seeds
■ Tree nuts	

HINT   Some food allergens are so severe that just touching or inhaling the odor of those foods can cause a hypersensitivity reaction (Boxes 12.18 and 12.19).

Box 12.18 Causes of IgE-Mediated Hypersensitivity Reactions

■ Food allergies	■ Muscle relaxants
■ Insect stings	■ Latex
■ Pollen	■ Snake bites
■ Antibiotics	

Box 12.19 Causes of Nonimmunological Hypersensitivity

- Contrast media
- Opioids
- Aspirin and nonsteroidal anti-inflammatory drugs (NSAIDs)

▶ SYMPTOMS/ASSESSMENT

> **Q What is the most life-threatening symptom of anaphylaxis reactions?**
>
> **A Angioedema**

Angioedema can cause the loss of the airway from edema and is the most life-threatening symptom of anaphylaxis. Symptoms include wheezing and dyspnea. Urticaria is a common associated symptom. Sudden loss of consciousness can also be an initial sign, and patients may report a feeling of "impending doom" (Box 12.20).

Box 12.20 Symptoms of Anaphylaxis

■ Airway swelling	■ Abdominal pain
■ Hoarseness	■ Hypotension
■ Urticaria and pruritus	■ Dizziness and syncope
■ Dyspnea	■ Chest tightness and pain
■ Wheezing	■ Headache
■ Nausea and vomiting	■ Seizure
■ Diarrhea	■ Flushing

▶ MANAGEMENT

> **Q What is the initial drug used to treat an anaphylaxis reaction?**
>
> **A Epinephrine**

Epinephrine 1:1,000 dilution 0.2–0.5 mg dose can be administered subcutaneously or intramuscularly. If there is severe hypotension, epinephrine can be administered as a continuous infusion. It is an α- and β-agonist, but it will also decrease release of mast cells. Hypotension is treated with fluid resuscitation and vasopressors, and supplemental oxygen is administered. Steroids and antihistamines (Benadryl) sometimes provide even greater relief of symptoms.

HINT Antihistamines block the H_1 receptor, so adding an H_2 receptor blocker (Ranitidine) can enhance effectiveness.

> **Q What drug can limit the effectiveness of epinephrine?**
>
> **A β-blockers**

Patients taking β-blockers may be resistant to epinephrine demonstrating continued hypotension and bradycardia. The bradycardia may require atropine to manage. Other drugs that may interfere include angiotensin-converting enzyme (ACE) inhibitors and monoamine oxidase (MAO) inhibitors.

> **Q A patient states he has an allergy to contrast dye but requires a diagnostic procedure. What can be given prior to administration of contrast to decrease the allergic reaction?**
>
> **A Steroids and antihistamines**

Pretreatment can be performed with steroids and antihistamines prior to giving contrast dye to a sensitive patient who requires a diagnostic procedure.

▶ COMPLICATIONS

> **Q** What is a potential cardiovascular complication caused by hypotension and hypoxia?
>
> **A** Myocardial infarction

Airway obstruction is the most common complication of anaphylaxis. Other complications are not common. Severe hypotension and hypoxia from airway edema can cause acute myocardial infarction (AMI).

TOXIC INGESTIONS/DRUG OVERDOSE/ TOXIN EXPOSURE

> **Q** What mixed-drug combination is the most common overdose?
>
> **A** Opioids, alcohol, and sedatives

Opioids, sedatives, and alcohol include a mixed combination of drugs and are the most common overdose in the emergency department (ED). The hallmark symptom is a depressed level of consciousness (LOC). Acetaminophen is the most common single-drug overdose. Overdoses may be intentional and unintentional.

HINT   Most overdoses involve more than one class of drugs and may have a mixed presentation.

▶ PATHOPHYSIOLOGY

> **Q** What is the physiology for the development of metabolic acidosis with cyanide poisoning?
>
> **A** Inhibits cytochrome oxidate

Inhibition of cytochrome oxidate results in interference in oxidative phosphorylation and cellular energy production. The anaerobic metabolic pathway produces lactic acid with the development of lactic acidosis. Cyanide also interferes with oxygen consumption with the development of tissue hypoperfusion.

HINT   Nipride infusions can induce methemoglobinemia and elevated thiocyanate levels.

▶ SYMPTOMS/ASSESSMENT

> **Q** What are the two most important assessments in the initial evaluation of drug or toxin overdoses?
>
> **A** Vital signs and neurological assessment

Vital signs are important in assisting with the determination of the causative substance, severity of the overdose, and in guiding initial management. Tachypnea is a nonspecific finding, but a respiratory depression guides the need for immediate intubation. Neurological assessment, including LOC, pupils, ocular movement, and motor skills, is useful in determining the substance and acuity of the patient. Frequent neurological assessments are recommended to follow changes over time (Table 12.3).

HINT   Bowel sounds may also be used.
　　　　Hypoactive = opioids or anticholinergics
　　　　Hyperactive = organophosphates

> **Q** Which two alcohol ingestions have the greatest morbidity and mortality?
>
> **A** Ethylene glycol and methanol

Table 12.3 Symptoms of Common Toxins

Drug	Blood Pressure (BP)	Heart Rate (HR)	Respiratory Rate (RR)	Temp.	Pupils	Nystagmus	Seizures
Anticholinergics	I	I	I	I	I	U	I
Sympathomimetics cocaine, amphetamines	I	I	I	I	I	U	I
Cyclic antidepressants	D	I		I			I
Salicylates			I	I			I
Opioids	D		I	D	D (except meperidine)		
Carbon monoxide		I	I	D		I	
Organophosphates	D	D	I		D		I
Alcohol			D		I	I	I
Sedatives, hypnotics	D	D	D	D		I	

I, increase; D, decrease; U, unchanged.

Ethylene glycol and methanol ingestion can result in significant metabolic abnormalities, seizures, and coma. Visual disturbances are "red flags" for methanol ingestion and the presence of calcium oxalate crystals in urine are "red flags" for ethylene glycol (Box 12.21).

HINT Ethylene glycol = antifreeze
Methanol = solvent, antifreeze, fuel
Acetone = paint thinners, nail polish remover
Isopropyl alcohol = disinfectant
Ethanol = drinking alcohol, fuel

Box 12.21 Symptoms of Ethylene Glycol and Methanol Ingestion

■ Pulmonary edema ■ Hypotension ■ Ataxia ■ Seizures ■ Coma ■ Abdominal pain	■ Nausea and vomiting ■ Visual disturbances (methanol) Photophobia, blindness, blurred vision ■ Calcium oxalate crystals in urine (ethylene glycol) ■ Anion gap metabolic acidosis ■ Osmolal gap

HINT Anion gap metabolic acidosis may not be present initially.

Q Which of the overdoses presents with "wet" symptoms?

A Cholinergic overdose

A cholinergic overdose presents with "wet" symptoms of increased lacrimation, salivation, urination, emesis, and diarrhea (Box 12.22).

Box 12.22 Symptoms of Cholinergic Overdose

■ "Wet" symptoms ■ GI upset ■ Bronchorrhea ■ Bradycardia	■ Fasciculations ■ Confusion ■ Miosis

HINT   SLUDGE: salivation, lacrimation, urination, defecation, GI upset, emesis.

> **Q A sympathomimetic overdose causes what BP changes?**
>
> **A Hypertension**

Sympathomimetic drugs (such as cocaine, amphetamines, methamphetamines) cause a sympathetic response. Extreme hypertension and tachycardia are common cardiovascular symptoms of overdose. Presentation of new-onset seizure should warrant a toxicology screen for a sympathomimetic drug.

HINT   In a sympathomimetic drug overdose, everything "speeds up," including mentation (Box 12.23).

Box 12.23 Symptoms of Sympathomimetic Overdose

■ Hypertension	■ Hallucinations (visual and tactile)
■ Tachycardia	■ Acute psychosis
■ Arrhythmias	■ Mydriasis
■ Seizures	■ Diaphoresis
■ Central nervous system (CNS) excitation	■ Hyperthermia

> **Q A patient presents with decreased LOC and depressed respirations. What is the most likely overdose?**
>
> **A Sedatives or hypnotics**

Sedatives and hypnotics are the most widely prescribed drugs. An overdose presents with decreased LOC and respiratory depression. Hypotension may also be present. These patients frequently require emergency intubation to protect an airway.

HINT   Opioid overdose presents very similarly to sedative overdose. Opioids also frequently present with miosis (constricted pupils).

> **Q A patient overdoses with Benadryl. Would the pupils be constricted or dilated?**
>
> **A Dilated (mydriasis)**

Benadryl is an anticholinergic drug. Anticholinergic overdose presents with mydriasis, hyperthermia, and tachycardia. Anticholinergic drugs block the neurotransmitter acetylcholine and inhibit the parasympathetic nervous system. This results in greater sympathetic stimulation, causing papillary dilation (Box 12.24).

HINT   Miosis = small pupils
Mydriasis = dilated pupils

Box 12.24 Symptoms of Anticholinergic Overdose

■ Dry skin	■ Tachycardia
■ Hyperthermia	■ Delirium
■ Mydriasis	■ Thirst
■ Diaphoresis	■ Urinary retention

> **Q A patient presents to the ED with nausea and vomiting, headache, and decreased LOC. A pulse oximetry shows 100% saturation, but the arterial blood gas (ABG) comes back only 88% saturated. What is the most likely cause of this presentation?**
>
> **A Carbon monoxide poisoning**

Carbon monoxide is a colorless and odorless gas that can cause headache, dizziness, nausea, seizures, and coma. Carbon monoxide binds with hemoglobin to form carboxyhemoglobin. It has a 240 times greater affinity for hemoglobin than oxygen, so it reduces the amount of hemoglobin available to carry oxygen. Pulse oximetry cannot distinguish between oxygen and carboxyhemoglobin, so it will typically demonstrate 100% saturation. Laboratory blood gases can determine what is bound to hemoglobin and provide an accurate oxygen saturation level. The discrepancy is indicative of carbon monoxide poisoning. Confirmation of the diagnosis is increased arterial or venous carboxyhemoglobin levels.

HINT History of possible exposure to carbon monoxide is also important for determining the diagnosis.

▶ DIAGNOSIS

> **Q** What is the initial diagnosis typically based on?
>
> **A** Clinical presentation

The clinical presentation is typically used to make an initial diagnosis of drug overdose or toxin exposure. The exact substance may not be known initially, and determining the substance is not a priority over resuscitation and treatment. Blood and urine will be sent for drug and toxin screens to assist with a more specific diagnosis. Qualitative toxicology screens are performed on urine samples and indicate only the presence or absence of the substance. A quantitative study provides the substance as well as the serum levels and can direct treatment in some cases. Blood alcohol levels are also obtained.

HINT Treatment is not delayed awaiting toxicology screens to come back. Qualitative toxicology screens do not change the initial management (Box 12.25). Cyclic antidepressants can be measured but do not correlate with the severity of toxicity.

Box 12.25 Quantitative Studies Assist in the Management of the Following Overdoses

■ Acetaminophen	■ Phenytoin
■ Carbamazepine	■ Lithium
■ Carboxyhemoglobin	■ Digoxin
■ Ethanol	■ Valproic acid
■ Methanol	■ Antidepressants
■ Ethylene glycol	

> **Q** If information about an overdose can be obtained, what is the most important information for determining the significance of toxin levels?
>
> **A** Time of ingestion

History should include the substance ingested or exposed to, amount ingested, and the time of ingestion. The time of ingestion is important to determine how significant the presenting clinical symptoms are and to interpret the drug or toxin levels. Note any unusual odors on the patient's breath, clothing, emesis, and nasogastric aspiration.

HINT Also determine whether the drug is regular or of sustained-release form. Sustained-release drugs will need to be monitored and treated longer until the drug is out of the system.

> **Q** What two lab results are important to determine the presence of anion gap metabolic acidosis?
>
> **A** ABG and electrolytes

ABG provides information on oxygenation and ventilatory ability. Hypoxemia, hypercarbia, and metabolic acidosis are common findings that may need correcting. If there is metabolic acidosis, calculate the anion gap.

HINT Obtain a 12-lead electrocardiogram (ECG) if cardiotoxic drug ingestion is suspected.

> **Q** What is an osmolal gap?
>
> **A** Comparison of serum osmolality to calculated serum osmolality

Calculate an osmolality and compare it to the serum osmolality obtained from the laboratory. A positive osmolal gap is greater than 10 mOsm/kg (Boxes 12.26 and 12.27).

Box 12.26 Osmolal Gap Calculation

(2 × Na⁺ + Glucose/18) + (blood urea nitrogen [BUN]/2.8)

Box 12.27 Example of Positive Osmolal Gap Toxins

- Methanol
- Ethanol
- Ethylene glycol
- Acetone
- Isopropyl alcohol

▶ MANAGEMENT

Q What is the priority of care in drug overdoses?

A Airway

Initial priorities in managing drug overdoses follow the ABCs: airway, breathing, and circulation. Emergency management may include intubation and mechanical ventilation to protect the airway. The most common reason for hypotension in toxic ingestions is venous pooling, so treatment is fluid resuscitation.

HINT Exceptions include skin contamination with organophosphates, which can incapacitate health care providers, and cyanide poisoning, which requires a cyanide antidote kit.

Q What three interventions are commonly recommended in a patient with decreased LOC?

A Glucose, thiamine, and naloxone

Following ABCs, a patient presenting with a decreased LOC may receive glucose, thiamine, and naloxone as initial treatment. To treat potential hypoglycemia, 50% glucose (25–50 g IV) is administered because hypoglycemia can cause unresponsiveness. Thiamine (100 mg IV) and naloxone (0.4–2 mg IV) are given to reverse potential opioid overdose. Flumazenil can reverse benzodiazepines but is not typically given routinely for an overdose or decreased LOC. Rapid reversal of benzodiazepine overdose can cause seizures from withdrawal.

HINT Naloxone is indicated in the classic presentation of opioid overdose: miosis, respiratory depression, and decreased LOC.

Q What is the recommended primary GI decontamination method following oral ingestion of a drug overdose or toxin?

A Activated charcoal (AC)

AC absorbs the substances and allows greater elimination through the GI tract. The best results occur when administered within 1 hour of ingestion of the substance. The dose is 1 g/kg, and it is most commonly administered through gastric tubes. Cathartics, such as sorbitol, may be given in conjunction with AC to shorten transit time in the GI tract and to lower the amount of drug absorbed. Induced vomiting with ipecac is not recommended in most patients due to risk of aspiration or protracted vomiting. Caustic agents should never be managed with induced vomiting. Gastric lavage is not recommended for all patients and should only be done within 1 hour of ingestion. Whole-bowel irrigation can be performed with large volumes of polyethylene glycol electrolyte solutions.

HINT A contraindication for AC is a perforated bowel. Contraindications for lavage are acid or alkali ingestions.

Q What is the procedure for accelerating renal excretion of drugs?

A Diuresis and alteration of urine pH

Diuresis with IV fluids and diuretics can accelerate elimination through the kidneys. Certain drugs will increase excretion if the urine is alkaline. Sodium bicarbonate infusions are used to alkalinize the urine. Hemodialysis may be considered in life-threatening ingestions involving substances excreted by kidneys.

Q What is the antidote for acetaminophen?

A N-Acetylcysteine (NAC)

Glutathione normally metabolizes toxic metabolites of acetaminophen. NAC is a substitute for glutathione causing a greater metabolism of toxic byproducts. NAC can be administered by oral or IV route within 24 hours of ingestion (most effective within 8 hours). The oral route has a strong sulfur smell and is not well tolerated without episodes of vomiting. IV route is a bolus followed by an infusion for 21 hours. It has a higher incidence of an anaphylactoid reaction. Acetaminophen levels can be obtained and are used to determine the need for administration of NAC. Levels greater than 10 µmmol/L are considered high, and in combination with elevated liver enzymes, they indicate the need for NAC.

HINT Rumack–Matthew nomogram is used to plot the levels to determine the need for NAC.

Q What are the drugs that inhibit metabolism of ethylene glycol or methanol to toxic metabolites?

A Ethanol or fomepizole

Alcohol dehydrogenase metabolizes ethanol alcohol over other alcohols. Administration of ethanol will prevent metabolism of ethylene glycol or methanol to toxic metabolites. Ethanol infusion will worsen decreased LOC. Fomepizole is a competitive inhibitor of alcohol dehydrogenase and allows elimination through renal excretion or hemodialysis without a decrease in LOC. Methanol ingestion may also receive folic acid to eliminate formic acid.

HINT AC does not bind alcohols but may be administered if suspected drug overdose is combined with alcohol consumption. Hemodialysis is more effective in managing metabolic acidosis than sodium bicarbonate (Box 12.28).

Box 12.28 Indications for Hemodialysis

- Visual impairment
- Renal failure
- Pulmonary edema
- Severe or refractory metabolic acidosis
- Alcohol level > 25 mg/dL

Q What drug may be given to reverse the cardiovascular effects of a β-blocker overdose?

A Glucagon

Beta-adrenergic blockers produce bradycardia and hypotension in an overdose. Glucagon is considered the first-line treatment because of its positive chronotropic and inotropic effects. It can be administered by IV bolus or as a continuous infusion until the symptoms are corrected. Calcium gluconate may be used to reverse the hypotension. The management of a calcium channel blocker overdose is similar and requires frequent monitoring of ionized calcium levels.

HINT Consider placing a transcutaneous pacemaker during initial treatment.

Q What is the primary treatment for carbon monoxide poisoning?

A Administration of 100% oxygen

Administration of 100% oxygen should be initiated as soon as a possible diagnosis of carbon monoxide poisoning is made. The patient may need to be intubated if he shows a decreased LOC. The use of hyperbaric oxygen may be used in certain situations if the patient is unresponsive to the initial treatment of 100% oxygen.

HINT   Hyperbaric oxygen may decrease the incidence of cognitive deficits associated with carbon monoxide exposures.

Q What class of drugs may be avoided in managing hypertension of acute cocaine intoxication?

A β-1 selective β-blocker

Hypertension of cocaine intoxication is caused by pure α stimulation. Administering a β-1 selective β-blocker results in unopposed α-adrenergic activity and complications of coronary artery vasoconstriction and possibly worsening of hypertension. Labetalol may be the drug of choice due to its combination of an α-blocker and a β-blocker. The first-line treatment for anginal chest pain is nitroglycerin followed by either phentolamine or calcium channel blockers.

HINT   Treat complications of cocaine toxicity with, for example, IV hydration to prevent rhabdomyolysis.

Q What is the treatment for wide QRS complexes in cyclic antidepressant overdoses?

A Sodium bicarbonate

Cyclic antidepressant overdose can cause wide QRS complexes (>0.10 sec) and can result in ventricular tachycardia (Torsades de pointes). The intraventricular delays are caused by the cyclic antidepressant slowing the influx of sodium into myocardial cells. Sodium bicarbonate uncouples the cyclic antidepressant from myocardial cells. Sodium bicarbonate also treats myocardial depression. Recent studies have found success with hypertonic saline in treating the wide QRS complex and hypotension. An overdose of selective serotonin reuptake inhibitors (SSRI) is usually not as severe as the cyclic antidepressants and is managed similarly.

HINT   Magnesium is used to manage Torsades de pointes.

▶ COMPLICATIONS

Q What is the major complication of an acetaminophen overdose, both intentional and unintentional?

A Liver failure

Liver failure is caused by an accumulation of the toxic metabolite N-acetyl-p-benzoquinone imine (NAPQI) in excess of the substance glutathione that is required to conjugate NAPQI for easier removal. Conjugation of the metabolite into a water-soluble state allows for renal excretion. The excess unconjugated substance binds to the hepatocytes causing inflammation, necrosis, and cell death. This can occur with an acute overdose of acetaminophen or with chronic abuse with accumulation over time.

HINT   Nonintentional overdose usually occurs because of lack of education regarding the dose limit of acetaminophen in a 24-hour period coupled with all the medications that contain acetaminophen.

Q What is an acute cardiovascular complication of a sympathomimetic overdose?

A AMI

Sympathomimetic drug overdose causes stimulation of the sympathetic nervous system with extreme hypertension and tachycardia. This significantly increases the workload of the heart and myocardial resistance. Tachycardia decreases diastolic time and coronary artery perfusion. The increase in demand and decrease in supply results in myocardial ischemia. Other life-threatening complications are intracerebral hemorrhage, stroke, rhabdomyolysis, necrotizing vasculitis, and death. Dilated cardiomyopathy is a long-term cardiovascular complication.

HINT   AMI can occur even in young people without coronary artery disease who have had a sympathomimetic overdose.

Q What syndrome can occur with an overdose of SSRI?

A Serotonin syndrome

Serotonin syndrome can be life-threatening and may be caused by other drugs as well as SSRIs (MAO inhibitors, lithium, meperidine). The syndrome can present with hyperthermia, hypertension, tachycardia, tremors, and seizures (Box 12.29). It is best prevented by administering AC soon after an initial overdose. If it does occur, manage the life-threatening symptoms, which includes intensive cooling, antihypertensives, anticonvulsants, sedation, and intubation with mechanical ventilation. Cyproheptadine is a serotonin antagonist that may be given to treat serotonin syndrome, but efficacy has not been proven at this time.

HINT   Serotonin syndrome does not require administration of dantrolene or bromocriptine.

Box 12.29 Symptoms of Serotonin Syndrome

■ Agitation	■ Diarrhea
■ Decreased LOC	■ Tremor
■ Hypertension	■ Muscle rigidity
■ Tachycardia	■ Myoclonus
■ Diaphoresis	■ Seizures
■ Hyperthermia	

⬤ ASPHYXIA/ANOXIC BRAIN INJURY

Q What is different about hypoxic–ischemic brain injury (HI–BI) when compared to an ischemic stroke?

A Global ischemia

An ischemic stroke results in a more regional ischemia based on the vascular territory. HI–BIs affect blood flow to the entire brain, so HI–BI has a more global effect on the ischemia.

HINT   HI–BI has also been called anoxic injury or anoxic encephalopathy.

Q What is the most predominant outcome following survival of HI–BI?

A Coma or vegetative state

Generalized brain hypoxia or anoxia results in greater injury to the cortical structures such as the lobes of the cerebral cortex and the memory center of the hippocampal area, then to the brainstem structures. Patients may have a decreased LOC but still have reflexes and spontaneous respirations due to the intact brainstem.

HINT   These patients are not brain dead because of the continued brainstem function.

▶ PATHOPHYSIOLOGY

Q What is the excitatory neurotransmitter that increases following an anoxic brain injury?

A Glutamate

Following an anoxic injury, the inhibition of adenosine triphosphate (ATP) occurs, resulting in anaerobic metabolism leading to efflux of glutamate. Glutamate is a neuroexcitatory substance that causes further damage to the neurons, influx of calcium, apoptosis, and cellular death.

HINT Calcium channel blockers have been used during periods of hypoxia as a neuroprotectant by blocking the influx of calcium (Figure 12.1).

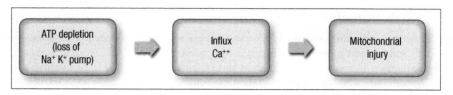

Figure 12.1 Physiology of ischemia.

Q What is released following reperfusion resulting in further cellular death?

A Free radicals

A reperfusion injury occurs once blood flow is reestablished to an organ or tissue. Affected mitochondria produce oxygen free radicals during periods of ischemia. Following reperfusion, free radicals and inflammatory mediators are released and exacerbate tissue necrosis by lipid peroxidation (Box 12.30).

Box 12.30 Causes of Anoxic Brain Injuries

▪ Postcardiopulmonary resuscitation (CPR)	▪ Attempted suicide by hanging
▪ Respiratory arrest	▪ Loss of airway in significant amount of time
▪ Cardiac arrest	▪ Airway obstruction
▪ Near drowning	▪ Carbon monoxide poisoning
▪ Strangulation	▪ Profound hypotension

Q What type of cerebral edema occurs with a HI–BI?

A Cytotoxic cerebral edema

Cytotoxic cerebral edema indicates the extra water is intracellular. This is typically caused by a hypoxic–ischemic injury. The lack of ATP (energy source at the cellular level) interferes with the $Na^+ K^+$ pump, allowing a greater amount of sodium to influx into the cell. Water follows sodium and results in intracellular swelling and edema.

▶ SYMPTOMS/ASSESSMENT

Q What are tested to evaluate brainstem function?

A Cranial nerves

Neurological evaluation of the cerebral cortex includes assessment of the level of arousal and mentation. Brainstem assessment includes cranial nerves and reflexes.

HINT It is important to exclude factors that may affect the neurological examination (Box 12.31).

Box 12.31 Factors That Obscure the Neurological Examination

▪ Hypothermia	▪ Ongoing nonconvulsant seizure
▪ Illicit drugs prior to hospitalization	▪ Postictal
▪ Ongoing cerebral hypoperfusion	▪ Electrolyte abnormalities
▪ Sedatives and analgesics	▪ Metabolic derangements
▪ Neuromuscular blocking agents	

▶ DIAGNOSIS

> **Q** What diagnostic test has been most widely used to assess LOC and guide prognosis after a HI–BI?
>
> **A** Electroencephalogram (EEG)

An EEG has been used most frequently in conjunction with clinical neurological examinations to determine LOC and to assist with determining the prognosis after an HI–BI. The reactivity of EEG waves to external stimulation is more important than the baseline reading in HI–BI evaluations. Sedation, metabolic derangements, and sepsis can alter the EEG findings, making them less prognostic.

HINT The presence of reactivity on EEG with an external stimulus indicates a better prognosis.

> **Q** What diagnostic test may be used to assess the integrity of afferent pathways?
>
> **A** Somatosensory evoked potentials (SSEPs)

SSEPs assess the integrity of afferent pathways from the brain stem and thalamocortical pathways to the primary somatosensory cortex. Injury in the subcortical area of the brain may cause a slowing of the pathway, whereas injury in the cortical portion causes an absence of impulses within the pathway. This is not influenced by sedation or metabolic derangements like EEG.

> **Q** How long after an insult will a computed tomography (CT) scan demonstrate diffuse cerebral edema?
>
> **A** Within 48 hours

CT scans may find diffuse cerebral edema due to cytotoxicity. Generally, cerebral edema is found within 48 hours following the insult. MRI, with diffusion-weighted imagery (DWI) and FLAIR capabilities, may be used to determine the extent of injury within 24 hours.

▶ MANAGEMENT

> **Q** What is the primary medical management of an anoxic brain injury?
>
> **A** Therapeutic hypothermia (TH)

TH has been found in postcardiac arrest resuscitation to improve outcomes if initiated early and maintained for 12–24 hrs. This technique is also frequently used on HI–BI patients as adjunctive treatment in addition to maintaining an airway, treating cerebral edema, administering anticonvulsants, and preventing complications. Hyperbaric oxygen may be tried as an adjunctive therapy following stabilization of the patient.

▶ COMPLICATIONS

> **Q** What is a common complication of a HI–BI that typically occurs soon after an insult?
>
> **A** Seizure

There is a relatively high incidence of seizures within 24 hours following a global ischemic injury to the brain. They may also occur within several weeks of the insult. This is because of an increase in excitatory neurotransmitters (glutamate) following an injury, which has been found to lower the seizure threshold (Box 12.32).

HINT The seizure is typically a complex partial seizure or a myoclonic seizure.

Box 12.32 Complications of HI–BI

- Seizure
- Movement disorders
    - Parkinsonism
    - Dystonia
    - Tremor
    - Athetosis
- Motor weakness, paresis, or paralysis
- Cognitive impairment
    - Impaired attention
    - Memory impairment
    - Language difficulties
- Posthypoxic leukoencephalopathy (demyelination)
- Neuropsychiatric problems (delirium, psychosis, akinetic mutism)

THERMOREGULATION

Q What is the primary indication for Targeted Temperature Management (TTM)?

A After cardiac arrest

Targeted temperature modulation (TTM) is aimed to minimize post-anoxic injury and improve neurological outcomes. It encompasses mild hypothermia and maintenance of normothermia. Out-of-hospital cardiac arrest with ventricular fibrillation is the primary indication for TTM (mild). The American Heart Association also includes in-house postcardiac arrest with any arrhythmia for comatose patients with return spontaneous circulation and out-of-hospital cardiac arrest with pulseless electrical activity and asystole.

HINT TTM should be initiated as soon as possible after ROSC to minimize reperfusion injuries.

Q What is the primary mechanism of TTM in preventing brain injury during reperfusion?

A Decreases metabolism

The reduction in metabolism in the brain results in a decrease in oxygen demand. Immediately following resuscitation, during the reperfusion stage, this decrease in oxygen demand improves brain oxygenation. Other benefits of TTM may include stabilization of cell membranes and the blood–brain barrier, inhibition of oxygen free radicals during reperfusion, and reducing brain inflammation.

HINT Hypothermia reduces cerebral oxygen consumption by a rate of 6% per 1°C change in temperature.

Q What is the temperature goal for TTM following a cardiac arrest and return of ROSC?

A 33°C to 36°C

Cooling a patient's core temperature from 33 °C to 36 °C has shown an increase in survival rates and improved neurological outcomes. Early initiation following successful resuscitation improves success of therapy. TTM is maintained for at least 24 hrs and up to 48 hrs. It is recommended that at least two sites be used for monitoring body temperature.

HINT Cooling below 33 °C is difficult due to shivering and increase risk of arrhythmias.

Q What method of temperature monitoring is recommended with TTM to assure accuracy of the temperature?

A Core temperature

Core temperature provides the closest approximation to brain temperature. Temperatures should be obtained from the bladder, esophagus, or endovascular. Other methods such as axillary, oral, or infared ear or forehead should be avoided. Some delay in body temperature adjustment with the rectal probe makes it less accurate.

HINT Continuous temperature monitoring is recommended during TTM.

> **Q** What are the three phases of TTM?
>
> **A** Induction, maintenance, and rewarming

Induction is the rapid reduction of body temperature with internal and/or external cooling methods. The maintenance-phase goal is to maintain hypothermic temperature for minimum of 24 hours. Maintaining the goal temperature steadily is important in this phase for improved outcomes. The rewarming phase is controlled and is purposeful rewarming of the patient. Avoid too rapid of rewarming due to potential neural axonal injury. Careful control of the temperature for at least 48 hours following the end of rewarming to prevent fever. Fever, post TTM, is associated with poorer neurological outcomes.

HINT Rewarming is recommended to occur at a rate of 0.15° to 0.25°C/hour (Table 12.4).

Table 12.4 Three Phases of TTM

Induction	Maintenance	Rewarming
■ Obtain baseline Hemodynamics Electrolytes	■ Maintain body temperature within goal range	■ Controlled and purposeful Goal is to rewarm after 24–48 hours. Prevent overshooting of temperature
■ Rapid reduction in body temperature Surface cooling Internal cooling	■ Manage electrolyte abnormalities. Avoid overshooting electrolyte correction	■ Monitor: Hemodynamics Electrolytes
■ Prevent shivering	■ Frequent vital signs ■ Monitor electrolytes and coagulation studies ■ Provide sedation and analgesia ■ Prevent or manage shivering	■ Administer fluids if hypotensive ■ Monitor temperature for rebound hypothermia

> **Q** Which cooling method, surface or intravascular, has been shown to cool faster during the induction phase?
>
> **A** Intravascular cooling

Intravascular cooling can use the technique of either metal or circulating cold water-filled balloon conductors or infusion of cold saline. The advantage of intravascular cooling is more rapid cooling, which is more effective in the induction phase than surface cooling. The disadvantages are it is invasive and more expensive. Surface cooling may use air, volatile liquids, or cold water and/or ice. It is less invasive but may cause greater fluctuations in body temperature. Selective brain-cooling devices are now available, such as intranasal cooling and devices that specifically cool the head.

HINT Some studies have shown that a more rapid induction has a greater success with improving neurological outcomes.

> **Q** What is the most common complication of TTM?
>
> **A** Shivering

Shivering is a natural response to hypothermia but can impede induction and maintenance of goal body temperature. Shivering generates heat and increases consumption two to five times greater than normal. Lowering body temperature produces vasoconstriction, which is a compensatory mechanism to prevent heat loss. Vasoconstriction keeps core organs 2–4 °C higher than the peripheral tissues. Once vasoconstriction is no longer working to maintain heat, then shivering begins as a compensatory mechanism to increase body temperature (Box 12.33).

HINT A higher rate of shivering is found in males and patients with low magnesium levels.

Box 12.33 Adverse Effects of Shivering

■ Increase body temperature ■ Patient discomfort ■ Increase metabolism ■ Increase oxygen demand and consumption ■ Increased production of CO_2	■ Tachycardia ■ Hypertension ■ Tachypnea ■ Increased intracranial pressure (ICP)

Q What is the purpose of counter surface warming?

A To prevent shivering

Counter surface warming can be used to prevent shivering. Skin temperature influences at least 20% of the shivering threshold, so blowing warm air on skin (across the face or body) at 40–43 °C will increase the shivering threshold (Box 12.34).

Box 12.34 Prevention of Shivering

■ Counter surface warming
■ Rapid cooling past the threshold of 35 °C
■ Keep hands and feet covered with gloves and socks
■ Adequate sedation

Q What assessment tool may be used to determine the presence and degree of shivering?

A Bedside Shivering Assessment Tool (BSAT)

BSAT is a validated four-point scale that has been found to accurately predict energy expenditure. It quantifies the assessment of shivering and can be used to determine the efficacy of current management. It is easy to use (palpate neck and chest region) and can be performed hourly and more often during the induction and rewarming phases.

HINT Shivering begins in the trunk and spreads to the extremities (Table 12.5).

Q Which drug classification is used most frequently to manage shivering?

A Analgesics and sedatives

Meperidine has been found to decrease shivering and vasoconstriction thresholds. It has the adverse effects of neurotoxicity and lowering of the seizure threshold. Meperidine may be used in combination

Table 12.5 Bedside Shivering Assessment Tool (BSAT)

Score	Severity	Description
0	None	No shivering noted on masseter, neck, or chest wall
1	Mild	Localized to neck and/or thorax only
2	Moderate	In addition, involves gross motor movements of upper extremities
3	Severe	Gross motor movements of trunk, upper, and lower extremities
P	Paralyzed	Pharmacologically paralyzed

with other drugs, including buspirone (Buspar) and/or propofol (Diprivan), to work synergistically to lower the threshold. Buspar is a 5-HT 1a agonist and has been found to be effective in reducing shivering. Other drugs that may be used include tramadol (Ultram), ondansetron (Zofran), α2 agonist, and magnesium infusions. Neuromuscular blocking agents may be used to stop shivering but are typically used only if other methods are ineffective. Medications used to prevent shivering should continue until normothermia is achieved.

HINT The goal is to decrease the shivering threshold, that is, lower the point at which shivering begins.

Q What happens to potassium levels during the induction of hypothermia?

A Decrease

Potassium shifts intracellularly during the induction of hypothermia. This lowers serum potassium levels. Other electrolyte abnormalities include hypophosphatemia and hypomagnesemia (Box 12.35).

HINT Avoid overreplacing electrolytes because during rewarming the electrolytes will shift back into the serum, causing hyperkalemia, hypermagnesemia, and hyperphosphatemia.

Box 12.35 Complications of Hypothermia

■ Shivering	■ Cardiac arrhythmias
■ Electrolyte disturbances	■ Lowers drug metabolism rates in liver
■ Coagulopathy	■ Pneumonia
■ Bradycardia	■ Hyperglycemia
■ Decreased myocardial contractility	■ Sepsis

Q What is the severe complication of hypothermia that can worsen outcomes?

A Coagulopathy and bleeding

Hypothermia can affect the coagulation cascade and cause coagulopathy and bleeding. The temperature goal for TTM may be individualized, and risk of bleeding is used to determine the maintenance temperature.

HINT The lower the body temperature is maintained, the greater the risk of coagulopathy and bleeding.

Q What are two ECG changes that may occur with hypothermia?

A Elevated J point and Osborne wave

There is elevation of the J point (backside of the QRS complex) 1–2 mm from baseline. An Osborne wave is a positive deflection occurring immediately behind the QRS complex. Either of these ECG changes may be found with hypothermia.

HINT An elevated J point should not be mistaken as an elevated ST segment.

LIFE-THREATENING MATERNAL/ FETAL EMERGENCIES

▶ PATHOPHYSIOLOGY

Q What is a common cardiomyopathy that can be experienced in a normal pregnancy?

A Hypertrophy

The uterus increases in volume with increasing gestation. The increased volume pushes up on the diaphragm and results in the heart rotating along its long axis, and the cardiac apex is displaced laterally.

Myocardial volume and afterload increase causing cardiac hypertrophy. Cardiac output (CO) and heart rate increase during normal pregnancy around 5–8 weeks gestation. CO will peak during labor due to increased venous return with each contraction.

HINT Mitral and tricuspid regurgitation is a common valvular abnormality found in normal pregnancy due to the changes.

Q What does the functional residual capacity (FRC) do during late pregnancy?

A Decreases

The FRC is the volume remaining in the lungs at end expiration. This is partially due to the elevated diaphragm. FRC correlates to the work of breathing.

HINT Elevated progesterone levels during pregnancy lead to a state of chronic hyperventilation and hypocarbia.

Q What causes a "physiologic anemia of pregnancy"?

A Dilutional Anemia

Plasma volume increases more than RBC mass leading to a decrease in maternal hematocrit. This is a dilutional anemia and is a normal physiological occurrence in pregnancy. WBC counts increases slightly at term and platelets decrease.

HINT Gestational thrombocytopenia may be found in some third-trimester pregnancies with platelet counts of 70,000–150,000.

Q What is the physiological change that increases a pregnant woman's risk for thromboembolic events?

A Hypecoagulable state

The greater risk of thromboembolic events is caused by several vascular and coagulation factor changes leading to the hypercoagulability.

HINT Pregnant ICU patients should be screened for presence of deep vein thrombosis (DVT) and have aggressive VTE prophylaxis.

Q What does the acronym HELLP stand for indicating a complication in pregnancy?

A <u>H</u>emolysis, <u>E</u>levated <u>L</u>iver enzymes, <u>L</u>ow <u>P</u>latelets

HELLP syndrome includes microangiopathic hemolytic anemia, elevated liver enzymes, and low platelets. HELLP usually occurs before 37 weeks of gestation and can overlap pre-eclampsia. HELLP can result from generalized endothelial and microvascular injury from complement and coagulation cascade activation. This results in increased vascular tone and platelet aggregation leading to liver hemorrhage and necrosis.

HINT Acute Fatty Liver of Pregnancy (AFLP) is considered an extension of HELLP.

Q What is the leading cause of maternal death worldwide?

A Obstetric Hemorrhage

Obstetric hemorrhage is the leading cause of mortality. It is defined as >500 mL blood loss in vaginal delivery and >1000 mL blood loss with a cesarean delivery (Box 12.36).

HINT Most obstetric ICU admissions are due to hemorrhage.

Q What is a placenta previa?

A Placenta previa is when the placenta is overlying the internal cervical os. A placenta accreta is when the placenta invades the myometrium and fails to separate following delivery. These are two more common causes of obstetrical hemorrhage.

Box 12.36 Causes of Obstetric Hemorrhage

■ Uterine atony	■ Placenta abruption
■ Abnormal placentation (previa/accreta)	■ Uterine rupture
■ Genital tract lacerations	■ Uterine inversion
■ Coagulopathy	

HINT The greatest risk factor for either abnormal placentation is serial cesarean births.

> **Q** Severe sepsis and septic shock can occur peripartum and can increase maternal mortality. What is a common prenatal infection?
>
> **A** Chorioamnionitis (CA)

CA is an infection of the amniotic fluid, membranes, and/or placenta. It results from ascending polymicrobial infection in the setting of rupture of membranes or advanced cervical dilatation (Box 12.37).

Box 12.37 Causes of Peripartum Infections

■ Prenatal Infections	■ Postpartum Infections
■ Chorioamnionitis (CA)	■ Endometritis
■ Septic abortion	■ Wound infection
■ Pyelonephritis	■ Necrotizing fasciitis
■ Pneumonia	■ Pelvic abscess
■ Septic pelvic thrombophlebitis	■ Pyogenic sacroiliitis

▶ SYMPTOMS/ASSESSMENT

> **Q** What is the primary sign of amniotic fluid embolism?
>
> **A** Hypoxic respiratory failure

Amniotic fluid embolism syndrome results in maternal severe hypoxic respiratory failure, acute lung injury, hypoxic pulmonary vasoconstriction, and acute right heart failure. It is associated with shock, disseminative intravascular coagulopathy (DIC) and seizures (Box 12.38).

HINT Symptoms usually present within 24 hrs of delivery.

Box 12.38 Risk Factors Amniotic Fluid Embolism

■ Maternal age	■ Uterine overdistension
■ Cesarean delivery	■ Uterine rupture
■ Placental abruption	■ Severe cervical lacerations

> **Q** What is required to be present for the diagnosis of preeclampsia?
>
> **A** Hypertension

Preeclampsia is defined as a new onset of hypertension and either proteinuria or end-organ dysfunction at more than 20 weeks gestation in previously normotensive women. It can also be defined as severe hypertension in women with a history of chronic hypertension with either of the other two symptoms. Early recognition and diagnosis will improve maternal outcomes (Box 12.39).

HINT May use urine protein/creatinine ratio of more than or equal to 0.3 to diagnose proteinuria.

Box 12.39 Symptoms of Severe Pre-Eclampsia

- SBP > 160 mmHg and/or DBP > 110 mmHg
- Proteinuria > 5 g per 24 hr
- Oliguria < 400 mL per 24 hr and elevated creatinine
- Cerebral irritability or visual changes
- Hepatic abnormality (Epigastric or RUQ pain, elevated LFT)
- Pulmonary edema
- Thrombocytopenia (< 100K)

Q What symptom is used to define eclampsia?

A Seizures

Eclampsia is the presence of generalized tonic clonic seizure in women with preeclampsia without a seizure disorder. Onset of seizures is often preceded by severe, unrelenting headache, nausea, or vomiting.

HINT Seizures are usually self-limiting in patients with eclampsia.

Q What is recommended to monitor the fetus in maternal critical illness?

A Fetal heart tones (FHT)

Continuous monitoring of a fetus is recommended when of viable gestational age. Maternal hypoxia, hypotension, or acid-base imbalances can affect the oxygenation of the fetus. The fetus is dependent upon uterine bloodflow for oxygenation. Uterine blood flow is not autoregulated, so it is dependent upon maternal systolic BP. Fetal heart patterns should be monitored by an experienced obstetrical nurse or physician.

HINT Vasopressors can decrease uterine blood flow even while increasing maternal BP due to the vasoconstriction.

Q What is the most common presentation of a patient with acute fatty liver of pregnancy (AFLP)?

A History 1-2 weeks of nausea and vomiting

ALFP occurs in late pregnancy or immediately postpartum. It may be associated with coagulopathy and encephalopathy (Box 12.40).

HINT Risk factors include autosomal deficiency of LCHAD, multiple pregnancies, and coexisting HELLP.

Box 12.40 Symptoms of AFLP

Nausea and vomiting	Anorexia
Malaise	Jaundice
Ascites	Progressive hepatic encephalopathy
Transient diabetes insipidus	Proteinuria
Hypertension	Hypoglycemia
Metabolic acidosis	Renal failure

Q Which obstetrical emergency presents with a boggy, soft uterus after delivery?

A Uterine atony

Signs of uterine atony after delivery includes a boggy, soft uterus often with the lower uterine segment filled with blood clot (Box 12.41).

Box 12.41 Risk Factors Uterine Atony

- Precipitous or prolonged labor
- Labor augmentation
- Overdistended uterus
- Grand multiparity
- Prior history uterus atony

> **Q** An obstetrical patient presents with severe, persistent abdominal pain and vaginal bleeding. What would be the most likely cause?
>
> **A** Placental abruption

Placental abruption presents with severe, persistent abdominal pain which differs from the classic crescendo-decrescendo labor pain. It may be associated with vaginal bleeding. Ultrasound may be able to locate a retroplacental clot. At the time of cesarean delivery, the uterus will appear bluish discoloration.

HINT Fetal heart rate tracings will be associated with placental abruption.

▶ DIAGNOSIS

> **Q** What is considered the diagnosis for preeclampsia?
>
> **A** Clinical diagnosis

The diagnosis of preeclampsia is primarily based upon clinical findings. Laboratory work to confirm proteinuria or end-organ dysfunction is used.

> **Q** What laboratory tests are being monitored for the diagnosis of HELLP?
>
> **A** Platelets and liver enzymes

HELLP is an acronym for hemolysis, elevated liver enzymes, and low platelets (Box 12.42).

Box 12.42 Laboratory Evidence of HELLP

- Abnormal peripheral smears (burr cells, shistocytes, echinocytes)
- Hemolysis (elevated indirect bilirubin, LDH > 600, low haptoglobin)
- Elevated liver transaminase
- Thrombocytopenia

> **Q** What peripartum complication is diagnosed with echocardiogram?
>
> **A** Peripartum cardiomyopathy

Peripartum cardiomyopathy with heart failure can occur in the last month of pregnancy or within 5 months of delivery in the absence of know cardiac disease. Echocardiogram shows decreased contractility and left ventricular wall enlargement without hypertrophy. LV ejection fraction is less than 45%. Chest x-rays will show an enlarged cardiac silhouette.

HINT BNP levels are elevated but can elevate in a healthy pregnancy.

> **Q** What diagnostic exam is used to determine the presence of chorioamnionitis (CA)?
>
> **A** Amniocentesis

Amniocentesis is used to obtain a sample of amniotic fluid for culture and gram stain. This is performed if the obstetric patient presents with systemic signs of infection, uterine tenderness, and foul smelling vaginal drainage.

HINT Management is with antibiotics.

▶ MEDICAL MANAGEMENT

> **Q What is the definitive treatment of preeclampsia?**
>
> **A Delivery of the fetus**

The definitive treatment of severe eclampsia is the delivery of the fetus, even if premature. Seizure prophylaxis is recommended in severe preeclampsia and is continued for up to 24 hrs post delivery. The hypertension should be controlled with antihypertensives while avoiding hypotension.

HINT   Magnesium sulfate infusions prior to cesarean delivery may be used for seizure prophylaxis and prevention of additional seizures.

> **Q What therapy is indicated in peripartum cardiomyopathy is the LV ejection fraction is less than 35%**
>
> **A Anticoagulation therapy**

Pregnancy typically results in hypercoagulable state. With the increased incidence of clotting and a decrease in ejection fraction, LV thrombus can occur. Other management is the same as treating cardiomyopathy in a nonpregnant person. It can include diuretics, digoxin, beta blockers and vasodilators.

> **Q What is a nursing intervention for uterine atony?**
>
> **A Fundal massage**

A boggy, soft uterus is noted with assessment and management includes fundal massage and evacuation of the fundus as first-line treatment. Uterotonic medications can be administered during fundal massage. Obstetric balloon devices can also be used to temporarily tamponade uterine bleeding.

HINT   Retained products of conception can prolong hemorrhage.

▶ SURGICAL MANAGEMENT

> **Q What is typically required, following onset of amniotic embolus syndrome, in regards to the fetus?**
>
> **A Emergency C-section**

Emergency delivery of the fetus by caesarean is recommended with amniotic fluid embolus syndrome. It may possibly require ligation of uterine/internal iliac arteries and even hysterectomy.

HINT   Sudden cardiac arrest in a healthy woman post delivery is likely caused by an amniotic embolus.

> **Q What surgical treatment can be performed if medical management has failed to control the hemorrhage in a patient with uterine atony?**
>
> **A Uterine artery ligation**

Patients with hemorrhage due to uterine atony may require surgical treatment. This can include uterine compression sutures or uterine artery ligation before considering hysterectomy to control the blood loss.

HINT   Some hospitals have the capability to perform angiographic embolization of the uterine artery to control bleeding.

▶ COMPLICATIONS

> **Q What is the severe complication of pre-eclampsia?**
>
> **A Eclampsia**

Eclampsia is the severe complication of pre-eclampsia and is characterized by seizures in the absence of other neurological disorders. Eclampsia can progress to hepatic failure, hemorrhage, and infection.

> **Q** In maternal cardiac arrest that is not immediately responsive to BLS and ACLS, what is considered to improve maternal survivability?
>
> **A** Emergency cesarean delivery

Prompt consideration of emergency cesarean delivery during maternal cardiac arrest is recommended. The initiation of cesarean delivery is recommended to begin within 4 minutes with the goal of delivering a viable fetus within 5 minutes of the maternal cardiac arrest.

HINT   Removal of the fetus can improve maternal hemodynamics and resuscitation.

> **Q** What is the severe complication of HELLP?
>
> **A** Liver rupture

Liver rupture is the severe complication of HELLP that requires immediate surgery. Emergency surgery is not delayed for diagnostic imaging studies.

SLEEP DISRUPTION

▶ PATHOPHYSIOLOGY

> **Q** What effect does frequent sleep interruptions have on rapid eye movement (REM) sleep?
>
> **A** Decreases REM sleep

Sleep consists of two phases: rapid eye movement (REM) and nonrapid eye movement (NREM) REM sleep is required for restoration of mental and physical well-being. Little to no REM sleep occurs in ICU patients because of frequent stimulation and awakenings. They experience shorter amounts of sleep than reported at home and frequently perceive quality of sleep as poor.

HINT   Poor sleep patterns may already be experienced by elderly patients who are exacerbated being in the ICU.

> **Q** What are two predominant environmental factors in the ICU that contributes to sleep interruptions and sleep deprivation?
>
> **A** Lights and Noise

Lighting in the ICU can disturb ICU patient's sleep patterns. The noise in the ICU includes conversations, alarms, phones, pagers, television, and equipment (i.e., mechanical ventilators) (Box 12.43).

HINT   Benzodiazepine has been found to alter sleep quality and decrease REM time.

Box 12.43 Factors Contribute to Sleep Deprivation

▪ Lights	▪ Noise
▪ Delirium	▪ Sundowning
▪ Pain	▪ Sleep apnea
▪ Patient care activities	▪ Mechanical ventilation
▪ Diagnostic procedures	▪ Psychosis/Delirium
▪ Analgesics and sedatives	▪ Critical Illness
▪ Limb restraints	

▶ SYMPTOMS/ASSESSMENT

> **Q** What is considered the best assessment of sleep quality in an awake, oriented and communicative patient in the ICU?
>
> **A** Self-report

Self-report of sleep quality is the best assessment if the patient is able to communicate. Using the patient's own appraisal of their sleep is beneficial because they are able to compare usual sleep quantity and quality to usual sleep. If patient is able to communicate, note any complaints of difficulty falling asleep, interrupted sleep, or not feeling rested.

HINT Assessment of past sleep habits is helpful to determine differences between patient's home and hospital sleep quality.

> **Q** What is a monitor used in the critical care units that can be used to measure the level of consciousness?
>
> **A** BIS monitor

Bispectral index (BIS) monitor is a measure of level of Consciousness (LOC) by algorithmic analysis of patient's EEG on a scale of 0–100 that represents cortical electrical activity. BIS scores correlate with different stages of sleep.

HINT Richmond Agitation and Sedation Score (RASS) may be used to evaluate sleep on an ICU patient.

▶ MANAGEMENT

> **Q** What is the endogenous hormone released by the pineal gland in response to dim lighting in early evening?
>
> **A** Melatonin

Melatonin is released by the pineal gland in response to evening time when the light is dimming prior to nighttime. It is considered the hormone for sleep. Melatonin has been used to manage insomnia and circadian rhythm disorders (Table 12.6).

HINT Higher doses of melatonin have cause irritability and anxiety.

Table 12.6 Medications Used to Manage Sleep Disturbances

Drug Class	Comments
Benzodiazipine	▪ Cautious use in elderly ▪ May develop tolerance, dependency, cognitive impairment ▪ Decreases REM sleep time
Nonbenzodiazepine receptor aonist	▪ Lower risk of tolerance, sleep alteration ▪ Most indicated acute insomnia ▪ Reduce dose for elderly
Antidepressants	▪ Not approved by FDA for insomnia ▪ Suppress REM sleep
Antihistamines	▪ Not recommended for insomnia ▪ Anticholinergic effects ▪ Associate with residual daytime sleepiness

Box 12.44 Interventions to Promote Sleep in ICU Patients

■ Avoid unnecessary baths between hours 2:00 and 5:00 a.m. ■ Back massage ■ Sleep promotion protocols ■ Observed quiet time or blocked sleep time ■ Obtain a routine chest x-ray and labs either at 10:00 pm or 5:00 a.m. (avoid hours between 2:00 and 4:00 a.m.) ■ Provide large clocks easily visible by patient ■ Provide ear plugs and eye masks for patients at night ■ Music therapy or background of comforting sounds (i.e., ocean sounds) ■ Aromatherapy	■ Position patient for comfort ■ Manage pain and anxiety ■ Turn down lights during sleep time ■ Turn televisions off or down ■ Turn alarms down during quiet or sleep time ■ Perform basic p.m. tasks similar to routine at home ■ Allow family member to stay with the patient ■ Post sign on door "Sleeping, please be quiet" ■ Close doors during sleep time ■ Use relaxation or imagery techniques

Q What is a sleep-promoting nursing intervention that can reduce nighttime sleep disruption?

A Organize patient care activities

Organizing the patient care activities at night to limit the amount of time the patient is disturbed for lab draws, medications, procedures, etc. This can decrease the number of sleep interruptions, improving the quality of sleep,

▶ COMPLICATIONS

Q What is the most common psychological complication of sleep deprivation in the ICU?

A Delirium

Sleep deprivation and disruption commonly cause delirium in ICU patients. Delirium can delay ventilator weaning, increase LOS in ICU and negatively affect outcomes (Box 12.45).

Box 12.45 Adverse Effects of Sleep Deprivation

■ Altered or reduced cognition ■ Lowered seizure threshold ■ Decreased ability to wean from ventilator ■ Mood instability ■ Lower pain thresholds	■ Muscle weakness or fatigue ■ Delayed wound healing ■ Suppressed immune system ■ Emotional distress ■ Delirium

● POST INTENSIVE CARE SYNDROME (PICS)

Q What three areas does Post Intensive Care Syndrome (PICS) affect in a person following discharge from the intensive care unit?

A Physical, Cognitive, and Mental

PICS is a physical, cognitive, and mental disorder that occurs during ICU stay or after ICU or hospital discharge. Advances in technology and the ability to keep critically ill patients alive longer have increased the recognition and incidence of PICS. PICS can affect long-term prognosis.

HINT PICS may also be experienced by family members of critically ill patients.

▶ PATHOPHYSIOLOGY

Q What is the primary physical result of PICS?

A Prolonged muscle weakness

ICU-acquired muscle weakness is the acute muscle weakness of all extremities in a symmetrical pattern that is caused by critical illness. It is also called critical illness myopathy. This has also been shown to be a predictor of failure to wean from the ventilator. The muscle weakness is caused by injury both to muscle and nerve. The injury ranges from ischemia, microthrombosis, endoneural edema, inflammation, and mitrochondrial dysfunction (Box 12.46).

HINT   PICS can last from months to years post discharge.

Box 12.46 PICS

Physical	Cognitive	Mental
■ Critical care myopathy ■ Critical care polyneuropathy ■ Muscle deconditioning	■ Impaired memory ■ Impaired executive functioning ■ Verbal fluency ■ Attention deficits ■ Visual-spatial disabilities	■ Depression ■ Anxiety ■ Post-traumatic stress disorder

Q What is a common cognitive abnormality in the ICU that is known to contribute to the development of PICS?

A Delirium

There is strong evidence of delirium increasing risk for long-term cognitive dysfunctions following an ICU stay (Box 12.47). Elderly are prone to cognitive impairment during and following intensive care.

HINT   There is an association between altered cognition in the ICU (delirium) and the development of dementia soon after discharge.

Box 12.47 Contributors to Critical Care Weakness

■ Chronic disease
■ Neuromuscular pathology
■ Pain
■ Hyperglycemia
■ Psychological disturbances
■ Advanced age
■ Severity of illness
■ Corticosteroids
■ Neuromuscular blockers

▶ SYMPTOMS/ASSESSMENT

Q What physical examination could be found in patients in the ICU that have developed PICS with a myopathy?

A Distal weakness of extremities

Physical examination may include distal muscle weakness on the extremities, sensory deficits, and depressed or absent deep tendon reflexes (DTRs).

▶ DIAGNOSIS

> **Q** What diagnostic study would be useful in determining the presence of muscle weakness or nerve involvement in suspected PICS?
>
> **A** Electromyography-Nerve Conduction Velocities (EMG-NCV) studies

Patients with PICS and neuromuscular involvement will have EMG-NCV studies that demonstrate decreased amplitudes of sensory and motor nerve action potentials.

HINT The 6 min walk test is used to assess degree of weakness and is useful test of global physical recovery in former ICU patients.

> **Q** What is a potential predictor of cognitive impairment in PICS patients?
>
> **A** EEG

Low-frequency activity is often found on patients with poor cognitive outcomes following critical illness. EEG may be able to provide prognostic information regarding cognition.

▶ MANAGEMENT

> **Q** What is a recommended intervention in ventilated patients to lower the episode of delirium and PICS?
>
> **A** ABCDE Bundle

The ABCDE bundle is recommended with mechanically ventilated patients to decrease the number of ventilated days. It includes delirium screening and early mobilization. Other interventions which may decrease PICS include family involvement with the patient and ICU diaries.

HINT Early physical and cognitive rehabilitation may improve muscle strength, prevent muscle deconditioning and improve executive functioning.

> **Q** What does the initials FGH stand for when added to the ABCDE bundle mneumonic in ventilated patients in the ICU?
>
> **A** F= Family and transitions of care
> G= Good handoff communication
> H= Handout educational material on PICS

The ABCDE mneumonic has been used in critical care for improving liberation from mechanical ventilation. The addition of FGH to the mneumonic is in relation to PICS is to address issues with family and transitions of care, good handoff communication, and handouts of educational material for PICS.

> **Q** How does an ICU diary written by family and staff decrease PTSD?
>
> **A** Provides factual information

Patients often report memory or recollections of events that were not factual and often delusional. The lack of memory for actual events may mean the patient processes these delusions and unreal experiences (frequently persecutory in nature) as being factual. This can lead to long-term psychological issues including PTSD. ICU diaries can help provide the patient with the factual events, limiting some of the delusions.

▶ COMPLICATIONS

> **Q** What is the primary consequence of the PICS after discharge?
>
> **A** Poor quality of life

Poor quality of life is considered the greatest adverse effect of the PICS following hospital discharge. Quality of life encompasses both physical and psychological aspects of one's overall well-being.

HINT   Primary caregivers may often experience psychological issues that negatively affect quality of life as well as the patient.

● PAIN (ACUTE/CHRONIC)

▶ PATHOPHYSIOLOGY

Q What are the three different types of pain?

A Sensory, cognitive, emotional

Sensory pain is the neurophysical aspect of pain. Emotional pain is the response of the person to pain. It includes anxiety, fear, depression, anger, guilt, frustration, panic, and suffering as some of the emotional responses to pain. Cognitive pain involves thinking, judging, interpreting, and deciding on the meaning of the pain.

Q What are the cutaneous pain receptors called?

A Nociceptors

Nociceptors are specialized nerve endings that detect noxious stimuli (and perceived stimuli) and transform into pain-producing impulses which travel through sensory neurons to the spinal cord. Pain receptors are present throughout the body including: Skin, periosteum, joint surfaces, arterial walls, veins, subcutaneous tissues, muscle, fascia, and viscera (Box 12.48).

HINT   Damaged tissues release sensitizing substances.

Box 12.48 Sources of Pain

Cutaneous	▪ Superficial parts of the body such as skin and subcutaneous tissue ▪ Well supplied by nerves and has well-defined localized pain
Deep	▪ Include nerve receptors originating in bone, vessels, nerves, muscles, and other supporting tissue ▪ Poor nerve supply results in dull pain
Visceral	▪ Pain that occurs from the body organs ▪ Sensitive to stretching, inflammation, and ischemia. ▪ Causes referred pain.
Neuropathic	▪ Pain caused by injury or damage to the nerve fibers in the periphery ▪ or by damage to the CNS resulting in the interruption of the ability for the nerve fibers to conduct sensory information

Q Which part of the brain is the main pain center in the brain?

A Thalamus

Thalamus is the main pain center in the brain. Awareness of pain occurs in the lower centers of the brain. Cortical areas in the brain are the sites of the final pain information processing and are responsible for one's awareness of the reality of pain.

Q What is the excitatory neurotransmitter that results in painful impulses?

A Substance P

Substance P excites, resulting in the painful impulses. Endorphins and enkephalins (endogenous opioids) inhibit the release of substance P. Produced in the brain and are morphine-like peptide substances.

HINT   Prostaglandins appear to sensitize the pain receptors.

▶ SYMPTOMS/ASSESSMENT

Q What is the most reliable way to determine presence and severity of pain?

A Self Report

Self-report is the most reliable indicator of the presence of pain and intensity of pain. The patient is expert regarding his own pain. Nurses are _not_ the best judge of pain and can cause inadequate pain relief with their own personal judgment.

HINT   Vital sign changes are not a reliable assessment of pain.

Q Using the PQRST approach for pain assessment, what does R stand for in the acronym?

A Region and Radiation

The R in the acronym PQRST stands for region (where is the pain located) and radiation (where does the pain radiate) (Box 12.49).

Box 12.49 PQRST Approach

P	Provocative and Palliative
Q	Quality
R	Region and Radiation
S	Severity
T	Timing

Q What is a common assessment tool used on a patient in the ICU that is unable to communicate due to intubation?

A Behavioral Pain Scale

A behavioral pain scale can be used in the ICU if a patient is unable to communicate. Facial expressions, limb movement, vocalization (nonintubated), and compliance with the ventilator are frequently used signs when monitoring for pain in noncommunicative patients. The inability to communicate pain does not mean pain is not being experienced by the patient.

HINT   If the intubated patient can follow commands the pain assessment tool "FACES" can be used for assessing severity of pain.

▶ MEDICAL MANAGEMENT

Q At what level do the nonsteroidals (NSAIDs) affect for pain management?

A Peripheral

NSAIDs primarily work at the site of injury or peripheral. They inhibit prostaglandin production and decrease pain receptors. Prostaglandin, when released, will sensitize nerves carrying pain impulses and worsen pain. Morphine-like drugs (Mu agonists) bind to the mu opioid receptors and block the release of substance P. They primarily work at the CNS level (brain and spinal cord).

HINT   Inflammation can cause the release of prostaglandins.

Q What is the life-threatening complication with the use of opioid analgesics?

A Respiratory depression

Respiratory depression and respiratory arrest are life-threatening complications of opioids when used as analgesics. Clinically significant respiratory depression is accompanied by other signs of altered mentation such as sedation and mental clouding (Box 12.50).

Box 12.50 Complications of Opioids

- Respiratory depression
- Decreased intestinal depression
- Nausea and vomiting
- Hypotension
- Sedation
- Delayed gastric emptying
- Confusion and delirium

Q What is the class of medication used in first-line management of neuropathic pain?

A Antiepileptic drugs (AED)

AED, such as gabapentin, is considered the first-line treatment for neuropathic pain. Neuropathic pain is not well managed with opioids and often contributes to opioid dependency and addiction.

HINT   Second-line drugs for neuropathic pain are tricyclic antidepressants.

SURGICAL MANAGEMENT

Q Which invasive route for pain medication is commonly recommended in patients with open abdominal aortic aneurysm surgery?

A Thoracic epidural analgesia

Thoracic epidural analgesia is recommended for abdominal aortic aneurysm and traumatic rib fractures to manage pain. It has been shown to decrease respiratory complications and improved clinical outcomes.

HINT   Elderly patients with traumatic rib fractures have been found to benefit from epidural analgesics.

Q What is the primary property of propofol when used in the critical care setting?

A Sedation

Propofol is an anesthetic that is used as a short acting sedative in critical care unit. Propofol results in sedation, hypnosis, and amnesia. It is also an anticonvulsant and antiemetic.

HINT   Propofol does not have any analgesic properties.

Q What is the advantage of dexmedetomidine (Precedex) in liberating patients from the ventilator?

A No respiratory depression

Precedex is a potent alpha-adrenergic reeceptor agonist, which has sedation and analgesic properties. Precedex has no respiratory depression and can be used during liberation of the patient from the ventilator. It is a sympatholytic drug, so bradycardia and hypotension are potential effects.

▶ COMPLICATIONS

> **Q** Undertreated pain can have negative consequences. What is the effect of the release of catecholamines with pain?
>
> **A** Vasoconstriction

Pain causes increase plasma catecholamines levels causing vasoconstriction, impaired tissue oxygenation, and increased myocardial oxygen demand.

HINT Pain can also result in a catabolic state with breakdown of muscle.

⬤ ACID–BASE IMBALANCES

> **Q** On an arterial blood gas (ABG), what are the three components that are used to determine the acid-base balance?
>
> **A** pH, CO_2, HCO_3

The three components of the ABG used to determine the acid-base balance is the pH, CO_2 and HCO_3 (bicarbonate). There are four cardinal acid-base disorders: metabolic acidosis, metabolic alkalosis, respiratory acidosis, and respiratory alkalosis (Table 12.7).

Table 12.7 Physiology Acid-Base Abnormalities

Acid-base disorder	Physiology
Metabolic acidosis	Remove base OR Add acid
Metabolic alkalosis	Add base OR Remove acid
Respiratory acidosis	Hypoventilation
Respiratory alkalosis	Hyperventilation

> **Q** What is an example of a metabolic acidosis that results in an anion gap?
>
> **A** Diabetic ketoacidosis

Diabetic ketoacidosis and lactic acidosis are two common causes of an anion gap in metabolic acidosis. A classic technique to determine the cause of the metabolic acidosis is to determine if anion gap exists. Two common acids resulting in an anion gap are lactate and β-hydroxybutyrate. Cations are positive (base), and anions are negative (acid) (Boxes 12.51 and 12.52).

HINT Elevated chloride levels result in metabolic acidosis but do not affect the anion gap.

> **Q** Your patient is determined to have metabolic alkalosis; what would you expect in the respiratory compensation?
>
> **A** Hypoventilation

Box 12.51 Calculation Anion Gap

Traditional Calculation	Common Calculation
$(Na^+ - K^+) - (Cl^- + CO_2)$	$Na^+ - (Cl^- + CO_2)$

Box 12.52 Etiology of Metabolic Acidosis

Anion Gap	Non-Anion Gap

Lactic acidosis	Gastrointestional
	    Diarrhea
	    Pancreatic drainage
	    Ileostomy drainage

Ketoacidosis
    Diabetic
    Starvation
    Alcohol
	Kidney related
	    Acute kidney injury
	    Renal tubular acidosis

Intoxications
    Methanol or ethylene glycol poisoning
    Salicylate overdose
	Endocrine related
	    Adrenal insufficiency
	    Hypoaldosteronism

	Pharmacotherapy Excessive volumes of hypertonic saline

Hypoventilation results in the retaining of CO_2 to compensate for metabolic alkalosis. This is a reflexive change in minute ventilation. It does not reflect respiratory dysfunction but is an expected physiological response to metabolic alkalosis.

Q What is a common cause of metabolic alkalosis in critically ill patients with mechanical ventilation, gastric tubes to suction and abdominal drains?

A Gastric tube to suction

Gastric fluid loss is a common cause of metabolic alkalosis in patients with gastric tubes connected to suction. Another common cause is active diuretic therapy or corticosteroid therapy. Typically, metabolic alkalosis is a result of loss of an acid with the gain of a base being less common (Box 12.53).

HINT   Administration of exogenous alkali can lead to metabolic alkalosis in patients with impaired renal function.

Box 12.53 Causes of Metabolic Alkalosis

- Diuretic use
- Chronic diarrhea or laxative use
- Severe potassium or magnesium depletion
- Cushing syndrome or primary aldosteronism
- Vomiting or NG suction

Q What respiratory abnormality results in respiratory acidosis?

A Hypoventilation

A decrease in ventilatory rate or depth will result in respiratory acidosis due to the accumulation of CO_2. Following the rise in CO_2, bicarbonate will increase to compensate. The kidneys will normally retain bicarbonate at the glomerulus by secreting hydrogen ions into the renal tubular lumen.

HINT   The renal effect on plasma bicarbonate takes several days to completely adjust the pH in respiratory alkalosis.

Q The patient presents with the diagnosis of myasthenia gravis. An arterial blood gas is ordered and an elevated CO_2 is identified. What is the underlying cause of the respiratory acidosis?

A Neuromuscular abnormalities

There are three underlying etiologies, which result in respiratory acidosis. This includes primary pulmonary derangements, primary neurological abnormalities (commonly neuromuscular disorders), and metabolically mediated causes (Box 12.54).

Box 12.54 Causes of Respiratory Acidosis

Pulmonary Disorders	Neurological Abnormalities	Metabolic Disorders
■ COPD ■ Status asthamticus ■ Severe pneumonia ■ Severe cardiogenic pulmonary edema ■ Smoke inhalation ■ Pneumothorax or hemothorax	■ Traumatic brain injury ■ Spinal cord injury ■ Myasthenia gravis ■ Guillain-Barré syndrome ■ Amyotrophic lateral sclerosis ■ Muscular dystrophy	■ Myxedema coma ■ Thyrotoxic crisis ■ Severe hypokalemia or hyperkalemia

Q What effect does hyperventilation have on bicarbonate levels?

A Decreases Bicarbonate levels

Hyperventilation lowers the CO_2 levels resulting in a respiratory alkalosis (Box 12.55). The kidneys regulate bicarbonate reabsorption by regulating adjusting hydrogen ion secretion into the renal tubular lumen. Persistent hypocapnia enhances bicarbonate excretion thus lowering the bicarbonate levels.

HINT Low CO_2 levels (hypocapnia) and low bicarbonate levels indicate simple chronic respiratory alkalosis.

Box 12.55 Causes of Respiratory Alkalosis

Pulmonary Causes	Neurological Causes	Metabolic Causes	Drug Related
Asthma	Traumatic brain injury	Severe sepsis	Salicylate acidosis
Pulmonary edema	Brain tumors	Hepatic failure	Caffeine overdose
Pulmonary embolism	CNS infections		

1. Which of the following is a result of an exaggerated immunoglobulin E (IgE) response to an external trigger?

   A. Immune hemolytic anemia
   B. Anaphylactoid reactions
   C. Anaphylaxis
   D. Transplant rejection

2. Which of the following medications is considered to be the most effective treatment for anaphylaxis?

   A. Glucagon (GlucaGen)
   B. Epinephrine
   C. Diphenhydramine (Benadryl)
   D. Albuterol (Proventil)

3. Which of the following is used to treat the cardiac depression that occurs with overdoses of beta antagonist drugs?

   A. Atropine
   B. Glucagon
   C. Epinephrine
   D. Racemic epinephrine

4. Which of the following statements best describes severe sepsis/septic shock?

   A. Hypotension in severe sepsis is due to vasodilation and low systemic resistance
   B. High cardiac output in severe sepsis is a result of increased myocardial contractility
   C. The decrease in cardiac output is the major factor contributing to tissue hypoperfusion in sepsis
   D. Sepsis causes a metabolic acidosis with a normal anion gap

5. Which of the following drugs is an antidote for acetaminophen?

   A. Lactulose
   B. Methadone
   C. Disulfiram (Antabuse)
   D. N-Acetylcysteine (NAC)

1. C) Anaphylaxis

Anaphylaxis is an acute syndrome produced by the release of inflammatory mediators from basophils and mast cells. It is an exaggerated IgE response to an antigen. Anaphylactoid reactions have similar clinical presentations but do not involve the elevation of IgE. Immune hemolytic anemia is a result of elevated IgG levels. Transplant rejection is a delayed immunological response and involves cell-mediated immunology.

2. B) Epinephrine

Epinephrine blocks the release of inflammatory mediators from sensitized basophils and mast cells. It is the most effective drug for anaphylaxis. Glucagon is used when anaphylactic reactions are refractory to epinephrine. Antihistamines, such as Benadryl, are often used for cutaneous anaphylactic reactions and should be given in combination with other medications. Albuterol may be given to alleviate bronchospasm but is not the primary drug for anaphylaxis.

3. B) Glucagon

Glucagon antagonizes the cardiac depression caused by beta blockers. Glucagon produces a positive inotropic and chronotropic effect that is equivalent to a beta agonist, but it does not use the beta receptors to do so. Atropine would actually worsen the bradycardia and hypotension. Epinephrine and racemic epinephrine are not effective, because the beta receptors that they stimulate are blocked from the beta antagonist.

4. A) Hypotension in severe sepsis is due to vasodilation and low systemic resistance

In severe sepsis/septic shock, the patients become hypotensive due to vasodilation and capillary permeability. The low systemic resistance causes a high cardiac output, but there is actually a decrease in myocardial contractility. Ejection fractions are low due to the release of a myocardial depressant factor. The tissue hypoxia is a result of inability of the tissues to utilize the oxygen. Anaerobic metabolism with elevated lactate levels is a result of the tissue hypoxia and does produce an anion gap.

5. D) *N*-Acetylcysteine (NAC)

NAC is the antidote for acetaminophen overdoses or toxicity. It is most effective when started within 8 hrs of acetaminophen ingestion. Disulfiram is used to treat alcoholism. Methadone has been used to treat heroin abusers. Lactulose is used to lower ammonia levels in patients with liver failure.

6. Following an anoxic brain injury, which of the following is the most common complication?

   A. Seizure
   B. Hemorrhagic stroke
   C. Hypotension
   D. Acute respiratory distress syndrome (ARDS)

7. Serotonin syndrome can be caused by an overdose of which of the following drug classifications?

   A. Selective serotonin reuptake inhibitors (SSRIs)
   B. Calcium channel blockers
   C. Beta blockers
   D. Angiotensin-converting enzyme (ACE) inhibitors

8. HELLP is a complication that can occur during pregnancy. What does the H indicate in HELLP?

   A. Hypertension
   B. Hemolysis
   C. Heterotrophic
   D. Hypoxia

9. What is the definitive treatment for severe eclampsia?

   A. Continuous antihypertensive
   B. Fluid boluses
   C. Administration PRBC
   D. Delivery fetus

10. Which of the following causes of obstetrical life-threatening hemorrhage is least common?

    A. Uturus atony
    B. Genital tract laceration
    C. Placental abruption
    D. Placenta previa

6. A) Seizure

Seizure is the most common complication of anoxic brain injury from any cause. Hypotension can occur following resuscitation, but it is not the most common complication. Hemorrhagic stroke and ARDS are not considered complications of anoxic brain injuries.

7. A) Selective serotonin reuptake inhibitors (SSRIs)

SSRIs are a class of antidepressants. Serotonin syndrome is a potentially life-threatening complication of SSRI use. It presents with hyperthermia, hypertension, tachycardia, tremors, and seizures. Calcium channel blockers, beta blockers, and ACE inhibitors do not affect serotonin levels.

8. B) Hemolysis

HELLP acronym is used to describe a syndrome that can occur during pregnancy. HELLP stands for "Hemolysis" "Elevated Liver Enzymes" "low Platelet."

9. D) Delivery of the fetus

The definitive treatment of severe eclampsia is the delivery of the fetus, even if premature. Antihypertensives are used to manage the symptoms but are not a definitive treatment. Fluid boluses and administration of PRBC are not treatments of severe eclampsia.

10. B) Genital tract laceration

Most obstetrical admissions to the ICU are hemorrhage related. The most common causes of obstetrical hemorrhage include uterine atony, placental abruption, and abnormal placentation (previa). Genital tract lacerations are a cause of hemorrhage but are less common.

11. Which of the following is the most reliable assessment of pain?

    A. Observation of pain behaviors
    B. Family stating the patient has pain
    C. Presence of tachycardia
    D. Self-report

12. Which of the following is the mechanism of action for NSAIDs to manage pain?

    A. Work on the dorsal horn
    B. Block Mu receptors
    C. Inihibit prostaglandins
    D. Suppress the thalamus

13. Which of the following side effects does not occur with the use of dexmedetomidine (Precedex)?

    A. Sedation
    B. Respiratory depression
    C. Bradycardia
    D. Hypotension

14. Which of the following has been found to contribute to the cognitive component of Post Intensive care syndrome (PICS)?

    A. Steroids
    B. Neuromuscular blocking agents
    C. Delirium
    D. Beta blockers

15. Frequent sleep interruptions in the ICU can result in which of the following?

    A. Decreased REM sleep
    B. Improved cognition
    C. Dementia
    D. Results in sleep apnea

(See answers next page.)

11. D) Self-report

Self-report is the most reliable indicator of the presence of pain and intensity of pain. Observation of painful behaviors is a component of the assessment but is not the most reliable. Vital sign changes are the least reliable.

12. C) Inhiibit prostaglandins

Prostaglandin, when released, will sensitize nerves carrying pain impulses and worsen pain. NSAIDs inhibit prostaglandins. Opioids work on the MU receptors and affect the dorsal horn in the spinal cord. The thalamus is the primary pain center but affected by opioids.

13. B) Respiratory depression

Precedex is a potent alpha-adrenergic receptor agonist which has sedation and analgesic properties. It is a sympatholytic drug, so bradycardia and hypotension are potential effects. Precedex has no respiratory depression and can be used during liberation of the patient from the ventilator.

14. C) Delirium

There is strong evidence of delirium increasing risk for long-term cognitive dysfunctions following an ICU stay or PICS. Steroids and neuromuscular agents can contribute to PICS but contributes to the muscular weakness, not cognitive function. Beta blockers do not affect PPICS.

15. A) Decreased REM sleep

Little to no REM sleep occurs in ICU patients because of frequent stimulation and awakenings. They experience shorter amounts of sleep than reported at home and frequently perceive quality of sleep as poor. Dementia is a long-term cognitive issue versus delirium. Loss of REM sleep can decrease cognition not improve it. It does not contribute to sleep apnea.

BIBLIOGRAPHY

Dellinger, R. P., Levy, M. M., Rhodes, A., Annane, D., Gerlach, H., Opal, S. M., ... & Moreno, R. (2012) Surviving sepsis campaign: International guidelines for management of severe sepsis and septic shock. *Critical Care Medicine, 41*(2), 486–552.

Pisani, M., Freise, R., Gehlback, B., Schwab, R., Weinhouse, G., & Jones, S. (2015). Sleep in the Intensive Care Unit. *American Journal of Respiratory and Critical Care Medicine,* 191, 7.

Presciutti, M., Bader, M., & Hepburn, M. (2012). Shivering management during therapeutic temperature modulation: Nurse's perspective. *Critical Care Nurse,* 32(1), 33–42.

Taccone, S., Picetti, E., & Vincent, J. (2020). High quality targeted temperature management (TTM) after cardiac arrest. *Critical Care,* 24(6).

Telias, I. & Wilcox, M. (2019) Sleep and circadian rhythm in critical illness. *Critical Care,* 23(82).

Professional Caring and Ethical Practice

▶ LEARNING OBJECTIVES

In this chapter, you will review:

- Synergy model
- Advocacy and moral agency
- Caring practice
- Collaboration
- Systems thinking
- Response to diversity
- Facilitation of learning
- Clinical inquiry

● SYNERGY MODEL

> **Q** According to the synergy model, what drives the characteristics or competencies of the nurses?
>
> **A** Patient and family needs

The needs of patients and families drive the competencies of the nurses. Synergy occurs when the nurse's competencies match the characteristics and needs of the patient. Optimal outcomes occur when the nurse and the patient are in synergy. Patient and nurse work together, synergistically, toward a common goal.

HINT The emphasis of the synergy model for clinical practice is that the patient's needs always come first.

> **Q** Following onset of sepsis, an intensive care unit (ICU) patient develops acute kidney injury (AKI) and acute respiratory distress syndrome (ARDS). Which patient characteristic is the greatest concern at this time?
>
> **A** Complexity

Patients and families all have similar needs, but each person brings unique characteristics to the current situation. Individualization of care focused on the patient's needs or characteristics depends on where the patient is on the continuum of health and illness. Patient characteristics can evolve or change over time and are based on a continuum. Complexity is the intricate entanglement of two or more systems. A patient with sepsis and multiple organ dysfunction (MOD) is a high-complexity patient because of the influence of each system's failure on the other (see http://ajcc.aacnjournals.org).

HINT The higher acuity patients will tend to have greater complexity. All patient characteristics are intertwined and cannot be viewed alone.

> **Q** What level of expertise does a nurse have who has been practicing for 25 years in the ICU and is able to look at the whole picture and make decisions based on her experience and knowledge?
>
> **A** Expert (Level 5)

The level of competency of a nurse depends on her experience, knowledge, desire to learn, and to meet the patient's needs. Competencies may range from novice to expert in each of the nurse characteristics. The goal of nurses should be to practice at the highest level of competency.

HINT   Level 5 is the highest level or level of an expert and should be the goal for ICU nurses (see http://ajcc. aacnjournals.org). The professional and caring practice questions are based on the patient and nurse characteristics.

⬤ ADVOCACY AND MORAL AGENCY

Q What occurs when two or more unattractive courses of action are possible and either course opposes the other?

A Ethical or moral dilemma

Ethics encompasses all aspects of life, including our conduct, behavior toward ourselves, toward others, and toward the environment. Ethical dilemmas exist when two or more unattractive courses of action are possible, but neither have an overwhelming rationale choice. Equally compelling alternatives and a moral argument can be made for and against each alternative.

HINT   Ethical dilemmas in hospitals have been increasing in frequency and intensity (Box 13.1).

Box 13.1 Common Ethical Dilemmas in the ICU

Contradictory beliefs (patient, family, healthcare providers)	Removal of life-sustaining therapies
Lack of clear clinical or legal guidelines	Assisted suicides
Futility issues	Scarce resources for allocation
Do-not-resuscitate (DNR) and do-not-intubate (DNI) issues	Increased costs for new technology and patient care

Q What occurs when the nurse believes that she knows the ethically correct action in a situation but a different action is occurring?

A Moral distress

Moral distress is common in the healthcare environment with the complexity of ethical dilemmas that occur. Moral distress occurs when the nurse believes that she knows the ethically correct action to take in the situation, but a conflicting action is being pursued due to other members of the healthcare team or family members. ICU nurses need to be aware of their own personnel beliefs and to be aware of the differences in professional and personal values. The optimal is allowing the nurse to practice in a manner that maintains her own sense of self-respect while maintaining the dignity of the patients.

HINT   The American Association of Critical Care Nurse (AACN) views moral distress as a key issue for critical care nurses (Box 13.2).

Box 13.2 AACN's Four "A"s in Moral Distress

Ask
Affirm
Assess
Act

Source: AACN (www.aacn.org).

> **Q** What are frequently used to determine the "right" actions in an ethical dilemma?
>
> **A** Ethical principles

Ethical principles, professional guidelines, and ethical processes are used to determine the "right" action. Moral principles are approaches used in ethics to determine what is right and wrong. There are certain ethical principles more commonly used in healthcare ethical dilemmas.

HINT   Remember, ethical decisions are not absolute in what is right and wrong, and reasonable people can still disagree with the action. That is why it is called a dilemma.

> **Q** What is the ethical principle of an obligation to maximize benefits and minimize harm?
>
> **A** Beneficence

Beneficence is the obligation to promote the welfare of others by maximizing benefits and minimizing harm. Beneficence is frequently used in ethical dilemmas in the hospital and refers to the healthcare practitioner's responsibility to benefit the patient, usually through acts of kindness, compassion, and mercy.

HINT   This is the principle often used to analyze futile care and withdrawal of life support (Box 13.3).

Box 13.3 Ethical Principles

Utilitarianism	It is based on the following two principles:
	1. The greatest good for the greatest number
	2. The end justifies the mean
	The situation determines whether the act is right or wrong
Deontology (formalistic)	This principle is based on moral rules and unchanging principles
	Morality is defined by the act, not the outcome.
	The principles are:
	1. People should be treated as ends and never as a means
	2. Human life has value
	3. One is to always tell the truth
	4. Above all, do no harm
	5. All people are of equal value
Justice	This principle is that every person is to be treated similarly, avoiding discrimination on the basis of age, sex, perceived social worth, financial ability, or cultural/ethnic background
	Incorporates ideas of fairness and equality
Beneficence	Refers to the healthcare provider's responsibility to benefit the patient, usually through acts of kindness, compassion, and mercy
	Action maximizes the benefit and minimizes the harm
Nonmaleficience	This principle requires that actions do not inflict harm
	The definition of harm becomes crucial when applying this principle
Autonomy	The belief is that the competent patient has the right to determine his or her own care
	The right to refuse therapy
	It recognizes that each person has worth as an individual and the capacity to choose
	The patient's values and wishes should be upheld unless they impose unfair burden on healthcare providers or institutions

(continued)

Box 13.3 Ethical Principles (*continued*)

Paternalism	Based on the belief that healthcare professionals have a duty to benefit the patient, outweighing the right of independent choice
	The principles include:
	1. Benefits provided outweigh autonomy
	2. Patient's condition severely limits ability to choose autonomously
	3. Intended action may be universally justified in relevantly similar circumstances
Fidelity	Duty to be faithful to others by keeping promises and fulfilling contracts and commitments.
	Moral obligation of the nurse to have a duty to his or her patients
Veracity	Duty to tell the truth and not to lie or deceive others

Q What ethical principle is being used when the healthcare team obtains informed consent for a procedure?

A Autonomy

Decision-making in the ICU has been divided into paternalism and autonomy. The goal has been toward autonomy, encouraging patients and families to make their own decisions regarding healthcare. During times of crisis, using a pure autonomy model for decision-making may put undue stress on family. The family may require more assistance from healthcare providers in making critical decisions. A newer model of shared decision-making may help patients and families in critical situations to make a more informed decision with less anxiety and more appropriate input from physicians in some cases. This has been found to improve collaboration between healthcare providers and families.

HINT Family members may be required to take sole responsibility for decision-making regarding end of life with limited information or understanding. Nurses play an important role in assessing the family's level of knowledge and in providing an education for the family.

Q When an ethical dilemma occurs in the ICU, what is the first step in resolving the dilemma?

A Data collection

Many decisions made in the ICU have an ethical component. Decisions need to be made based on a learned skill, not just an emotional response. Making such decisions should involve using a systematic process and ethical principles to provide direction. Without guidance, the decisions are made on emotions, intuitions, or fixed policies. Data collection is the first step in resolving a moral or ethical dilemma. It involves gathering medical facts, including the prognosis, alternatives, and assessment of patient/family knowledge. Social facts are also collected, including the living environment, family and significant others, economic concerns, and current or previously stated wishes.

HINT Steps of resolving an ethical dilemma are similar to the nursing process (Box 13.4).

Box 13.4 Steps in Determining Ethical Dilemma

Step 1: Data collection	Gather medical facts, including the prognosis, alternatives, and assessment of patient/family knowledge Gather social facts, including the living environment, family and significant others, economic concerns, current or previously stated wishes
Step 2: Identify the conflict	Weigh the values and determine where they conflict or complement, determine who and what are involved in the conflict State the family's, patient's, and healthcare provider's ethical position
Step 3: Define the goals	Are goals patient-centered, realistic, achievable, and collaborative? Examples are the goal of prolongation of life, relief of pain, maximum recovery

(*continued*)

Box 13.4 Steps in Determining Ethical Dilemma (*continued*)

Step 4: Identify ethical principles	List the principles and rank order them to identify the primary principle. There may be conflicting principles.
Step 5: Review alternative courses of action	Compare the alternatives to the goals, predict possible consequences of the alternatives, and prioritize acceptable alternatives.
Step 6: Choose the course of action	This is the alternative that breaks the fewest ethical principles.
Step 7: Develop and implement a plan of action	Following determination of action, a plan is developed to determine how to carry out the action and is performed.
Step 8: Evaluate the plan	Follow up after the action is implemented to determine if pre-set goals were reached. If not, determine what could have improved the action to meet the goals.

Q When a patient is in an irreversible coma, and the physicians have declared that treatment can not cure or improve quality of life that would be satisfactory to the patient, what is it called?

A Futile care

Futile care is any clinical circumstance in which the physician and his or her consultants, consistent with the available medical literature, conclude that further treatment cannot, within a reasonable probability, cure, ameliorate, improve, or restore quality of life that would be satisfactory to the patient (Box 13.5).

HINT Examples of futile-care situations include an irreversible coma or persistent vegetative state or terminal illness, where application of life-sustaining procedures would serve only to delay the inevitable.

Box 13.5 Criteria Used to Determine Futility of Care

Severity of illness	Expected long-term outcomes
Comorbidities	Duration of therapy
Life expectancy	Cost of treatment
Predicted quality of life	

Q What is a legal document that identifies someone who will have the power to make medical treatment decisions in the event the patient is unable?

A Durable power of attorney for medical purposes

The Patient Self-Determination Act (PSDA) went into effect in 1991, requiring all healthcare facilities receiving Medicare or Medicaid funds to provide written information to the adult patient about his or her rights according to the state law to make treatment decisions and execute advanced directives. A durable power of attorney for medical purpose is a legal document, which identifies someone who will have the power to make medical treatment decisions in the event the patient is unable. This is initiated at a time when the patient loses the capacity to participate in the decision-making process (Box 13.6).

HINT Advanced directives were developed to ensure a patient's right for autonomy and to provide high-quality care at the end of life.

Box 13.6 Common Reasons for Not Having a Power of Attorney

Reluctance to talk about death
Patient waiting for physician to initiate the conversation
Difficulty in completing the required forms
Unaware of power of attorney
Nurses unaware or do not initiate conversation

CARING PRACTICE

Q What do patients experience in the ICU because of constant noise, alarms, and hearing unfamiliar voices?

A Sensory overload

Patients in the ICU experience sensory overload due to constant noise and alarms. Sensory overload contributes to sleep deprivation, anxiety, agitation, and delirium in ICU patients. Other negative experiences reported by patients in the ICU include fear, anxiety, sleep deprivation, lack of privacy, pain, and discomfort (Box 13.7).

HINT Patients experience a more positive outcome in ICUs that incorporate natural lighting, soothing sounds, meaningful stimuli, and pleasant views.

Box 13.7 Causes of Sensory Overload

Frequent alarms	Constant stimulation
Blinking lights	Bright lights
Unfamiliar sounds	Unpleasant smells
Machinery sounds	Multiple lines and tubes
Unfamiliar voices	Restraints
Clinicians talking at the bedside	Hurried pace in crowded space

Q What are two of the most disruptive noises patients report hearing in the ICU?

A Talking and alarms

Noise is an environmental hazard that causes patient discomfort. Loud conversation by healthcare providers is one of the most frequently reported noises the patient recalls after being in an ICU. Nurses do not realize sometimes how loud they are when talking to each other in the unit and at the patient's bedside. This is reported to be disruptive to patients. Alarms are also frequently reported as being disruptive (Box 13.8).

HINT Nurses are not always aware of their loudness in conversation and should take an objective assessment of the ICU environment. Noisy environments can lead to sleep deprivation, psychosis, and delirium (Box 13.9).

Box 13.8 Causes of Loud Noises

Staff conversations	Telephones ringing
Alarms going off all the time	Televisions on all of the time
Banging doors	Noisy machines and equipment (i.e., intra-aortic balloon pump, ventilators)

Box 13.9 Adverse Effects of Noisy Environment

Sleep disruption	Vasoconstriction
Activation of sympathetic nervous system	Hyperarousal
Impaired wound healing	Delirium

Q What do patients in the ICU commonly perceive as a loss that creates anxiety?

A Loss of control

Patients in the ICU commonly experience a loss of control that creates anxiety. Providing order and predictability can create an illusion of some control by the patient. This is called anticipatory guidance that keeps the patient from being surprised at a routine. Once the patient is able to make simple decisions, allow the patient to make small choices. Give some control back to the patient in areas in which he or she can make decisions. Other common causes of anxiety in the ICU include a loss of function or self-esteem, sense of isolation, and a fear of dying.

HINT   Allowing small choices can assist the patient's coping with larger procedures in which little choice is present (Box 13.10). Patients should also have the right to make decisions about visitors, who can visit, and for how long.

Box 13.10 Examples of Patient Choices

Do you want a bath now or in 20 minutes?
At what angle do you want your head of bed?
Do you want to turn to your right or left side?
Do you want your pain medication now or in 20 minutes?

Q **What do families typically express in regard to their feelings while their loved ones are in the ICU?**

A **Helplessness**

The suddenness of injury or illness may cause family members to have uncertainty about the situation. They may approach the ICU nurse with multiple questions and concerns. The family is thrown into a whirlwind of activity and commonly experience feelings of helplessness. They are often unprepared for the whole impact of the injury or illness. Frequently, families experience a "roller coaster" of emotions during the ICU stay. They may be happy that their loved one is alive but upset about the injury or losses; there are good days and bad days with many ups and downs.

HINT   Family members may ask "unanswerable" questions and usually do not expect an answer. It shows their deep and inner fears (Box 13.11).

Box 13.11 Family Member Reactions to Illness

Shock	Distrust
Anxiety	Guilt
Denial	Remorse
Hostility/anger	Depression

Q **What is a common coping mechanism that family members have following a critical illness or injury in order to regain some control?**

A **Vigilance**

The initial emotional reaction of fear, shock, or panic is sometimes followed by irrational acts and demanding behaviors. Vigilance becomes a coping mechanism by family members in an attempt to regain some control of the situation. Family members commonly want to be at the bedside or in the ICU waiting room 24 hours a day. They may express concern about being gone because of what can happen, they may miss meeting the physician, or their loved ones may wake up while they are gone.

Vigilance includes constantly seeking information to ensure that tasks are being carried out (i.e., "I thought they were going to CT this morning?" "Has she had dinner yet?").

HINT   Establishing a trusting relationship immediately relieves some of the anxiety, then family members are more likely to feel comfortable enough to leave the hospital (Box 13.12). Explain to the family that this is more a "marathon" than a "short sprint," and they need to save energy for when the patient leaves the ICU or hospital.

Box 13.12 Interventions for Families

Obtain correct phone numbers and keep at bedside	Show interest in how the family is doing
Take initiative and call family frequently with updates	Be courteous
Teach about what to expect while in ICU	Allow family members to express negative feelings
Set up physician and family visits or conferences	Ask what the family needs
Establish a trusting relationship	Do not give false reassurances
Follow through with tasks	Allow family members to assist in providing basic aspects of care (brush teeth, comb hair, assist with bath, help with meals)
Provide honest information about the condition of the patient	
Explain why things are done the way they are	Provide consistent information to family

Q What intervention can an ICU nurse do to decrease the number of calls about the status of a patient?

A Establish a contact person

A common issue ICU nurses encounter is constant calls from family and friends seeking updates. Setting up a contact person from the family for the healthcare providers to provide updates will decrease the number of calls into the ICU. Remember, frequent calls to the immediate family can increase their stress and time spent updating other relatives and friends (Box 13.13).

HINT Encourage immediate family members to have downtime; "allow" them to screen their calls.

Box 13.13 Recommendations for Frequent Calls With Family

Establish chain of calls to deliver information to larger number of people
One person will make outgoing calls when an update is given
Develop an updated outgoing message on phone daily
Develop a website for updates, information, and progress
Establish a guest page
E-mail updates as a group e-mail

Q What should families be told about bedside conversations in the patient's room?

A Avoid talking about the patient's medical condition

Family members and healthcare providers should avoid talking beside the patient's bed about the patient's medical condition. Patients may be able to hear even if they are not responding or appear to be disoriented. Families frequently do not know what to say to the patient or what to talk about at the bedside. Some families just stand at bedside and are afraid to touch their loved ones because of all of the lines and tubes. ICU nurses can encourage them to talk to the patient directly and touch their loved ones (Box 13.14).

HINT Patients report increased anxiety and fear when overhearing conversations about procedures at the bedside.

Box 13.14 Interventions to Encourage Conversations With Patients

Encourage family and friends to normalize conversations
Talk about daily happenings at work and home
Encourage families to keep a diary at home and then talk to the patient from the diary
Avoid talking only about the illness, injury, or treatments
If patient is unresponsive, talk about her hobbies, likes, or favorite activities
Avoid talking beside the patient's bed about the patient's medical condition

> **Q** **What is the most common need or priority of family members in the ICU?**
>
> **A** **Need for information**

The number one identified need of the family members is the need for information. Family members frequently ask for lab results, vital signs, or watch monitors. They may fixate or focus on certain things such as blood pressure, heart rate, or temperature. Families experience increased frustration when they get different information from different healthcare providers. Continuity of nursing assignments provides consistency for patients and families. The nurse is more aware of family needs and better able to reinforce teaching already provided to family. Nurses need to create an atmosphere of understanding, concern, and empathy with the family (Box 13.15).

HINT   Most families do not want "sugar-coated" answers; they want to be told the truth. Honesty and full disclosure of prognosis are recommended.

Box 13.15 Common Needs of Families

Need to feel hope	Need for honesty
Need to receive information about the patient	Need to see the patient frequently
on a daily basis	Need to know the patient is comfortable and without pain
Need to feel the nurses and physicians care about the patient	Need for support from the healthcare personnel
Need to know the prognosis	Consistency in nurses and physicians

> **Q** **What visitation policy can offer a more healing environment and family-focused care?**
>
> **A** **Flexible (open) visitation policy**

The ICU environment should be a family-focused care culture. Allowing a more open visitation policy provides families with a greater feeling of being welcome to be with their loved ones. Increasing the visitation times can strengthen the relationship between the family and the nurse. Research has also shown benefits of allowing families to remain at the bedside based on the patient's physiological responses (decrease anxiety, intracranial pressure). There is a need for less restrictive and individualized visitation in ICUs (Box 13.16).

HINT   Advocate the adjustment of visitation hours to meet the needs of family members. Novel visitation policies include allowing young children to be accompanied by adults and pet-assisted therapy in the ICU.

Box 13.16 Advantages of Open Visitation

Families feel more assured about the care that their loved ones are receiving	Allows ability to regain sense of control
More aware of any changes that occur with their loved one	Improves family coping skills
Not knowing what is happening on the "other side" of the doors produces anxiety	Strengthens relationships with the nurses
Provides a sense of direction	

> **Q** **Family presence during resuscitation may benefit the family member. What is an important aspect to success of family presence during resuscitation?**
>
> **A** **Support person remains with family member**

In family presence during resuscitation programs, usually one family member is allowed to remain in the room during resuscitation. Success of the program depends on the ability to keep a support person with the family member to explain what is happening, provide emotional support, and evaluate the person's response. This program originally started in trauma resuscitation and has expanded to resuscitation in cardiopulmonary arrests in the hospital (Box 13.17).

Box 13.17 Benefits of Family Presence During Resuscitation

Family members observe the efforts of the healthcare providers	The mystery of activities behind "closed doors" is reduced
Family members can provide comfort and words of encouragement to the patient	Assist with decision-making about code versus DNR (family may halt code)
Ability of the family to have closure Acceptance of the outcome is facilitated	Facilitation of bonding between patients' family members and healthcare providers
Families perceive that they are actively involved in the resuscitation of their loved one	Holistic approach is fostered Lowered legal malpractice suits

HINT   Families allowed to remain in the room during resuscitation typically express feelings that they know the healthcare staff did everything possible to save their loved one. Most concerns have been unfounded in research involving family presence during resuscitations (Box 13.18).

Box 13.18 Identified Fears of Staff in Family Presence

Fear of increased stress of healthcare personnel involved	Fear of litigation
Uncertainty of helpfulness of family member during the procedure or resuscitation	Long-term effects on family's emotional status; posttraumatic stress disorder Violation of patient's privacy
Fear that the family member will interrupt/disrupt the resuscitation	Lack of the family member's understanding of tasks and procedures being performed
Family members may be offended and potentially engage in negative behaviors	Increased required number of staff involved in the code
Staff might feel inhibited from performing necessary tasks	

COLLABORATION

Q **What negative effect on patient outcomes has been found when nurses practice in an unhealthy work environment?**

A **Medication errors**

An unhealthy work environment can lead to increased medication errors and poor patient-care delivery. Errors in delivering patient care will negatively affect outcomes for patients. There is a link between healthy work environments, excellent nursing care, and patient outcomes. A healthy work environment should be focused on safety, caring, and respect for each other, including all healthcare providers, patients, and families (Box 13.19).

Box 13.19 Negative Effects of an Unhealthy Work Environment

Medication errors
Poor delivery of care
Patient-care errors
Stress to healthcare professionals
Higher nurse turnover

> **Q What is the biggest underlying issue found in an unhealthy work environment?**
>
> **A Poor communication**

Each bad situation relates back to poor communication and ineffective relationships among healthcare providers. Healthcare providers need to improve working relationships and communicate on a more professional level. Outbursts and disruptive behavior may prevent a nurse from calling a physician to report patient changes or question an order. This may lead to medication or patient-care errors. According to the AACN, a healthy work environment, has six standards that must all be instituted to establish a healthy work environment and improve patient outcomes (Box 13.20).

Box 13.20 Six Standards for a Healthy Environment by the AACN

Skilled communication	Appropriate staffing
True collaboration	Meaningful recognition
Effective decision-making	Authentic leadership

> **Q When engaged in skilled communication, what is an important aspect the nurse must have to ensure the mutual respect of their colleagues?**
>
> **A Listen to the other individual's perspectives**

It is important to treat others with respect and to develop a mutually respectful relationship. Listening to other healthcare professionals' perspectives during the discussion will improve the skilled communication and assist with the development of mutual respect.

HINT   The focus is not to "win" but to find an agreeable solution with a desirable outcome (Box 13.21).

Box 13.21 Aspects of Skilled Communication

Healthcare organization should provide education on skilled communication	Use mutual respect
Focus is to find solutions and desirable outcomes	Congruence between word and action
Protect and advance professional relationships	Zero tolerance for abuse and disrespectful behavior
Listen to all relevant perspectives	

> **Q What is a common time for breakdown of communication between nurses to occur?**
>
> **A Shift change**

Shift change is a common time for breakdown of communication to occur. This was quoted to be the "single largest source of medical error" with errors ranging from administering wrong medication to resuscitating a DNR patient. A significant amount of information is passed along among nurses during period of report and change of patient care from one nurse to another. Ensuring important information regarding the previous shift events and future care is important to ensure continuity and to avoid missing important changes in the patient's status.

HINT   Communication during shift report may be inadequate if nurses are tired and stressed (Box 13.22). Distraction is a significant cause of medication errors. Assuring a "quiet zone" while obtaining and administering medications is important to prevent medication errors.

Box 13.22 Use of Mnemonic "I PASS the BATON"

Introduction	Introduce self (if needed)
Patient	Name, identifiers, age, sex, location, physicians involved in care
Assessment	Presenting chief complaint, vital signs, current system review, symptoms, and diagnosis

(continued)

Box 13.22 Use of Mnemonic "I PASS the BATON" (*continued*)

Situation	Current status, circumstances, including code status, recent changes, responses to treatment
Safety	Critical lab values, reports, allergies, fall risk, isolation
Background	Comorbidities, previous episodes, current medications, family history
Actions	What actions were taken or required?
Timing	Level of urgency and explicit timing, prioritizing of actions
Ownership	Who is responsible?
Next	What will happen next? Anticipated changes, what is the plan?

Q What is the standardized framework for members of the healthcare team to communicate about a patient's condition?

A Situation, Background, Assessment, Recommendation (SBAR)

SBAR is a standardized framework for members of the healthcare team to communicate about a patient's condition. SBAR was originally used by nuclear submariners during exchange of command. It frames a conversation and facilitates communication with physicians. It has been found to lower adverse events (Box 13.23).

Box 13.23 Barriers of Communication Among Healthcare Providers

Language barriers (accents differ even in English-speaking people)	Conflict with personalities
Varying communication styles	Workload
Distraction	Stress

Q What needs to be considered in planning family conferences in regard to health information privacy regulations?

A Determining those approved for medical information

When planning a healthcare conference to discuss the patient's clinical status and treatment plans, ensure that the family members involved have the patient's approval to obtain healthcare information regarding the patient. During family meetings, open-ended questions are used to determine what the family understands about their loved one's condition. Repeating or reflecting on what the family said will allow a chance for them to correct any misunderstandings. Hearing all the family members' thoughts and opinions before making a decision can facilitate a consensus even if the final decision may be against their own beliefs.

HINT Reflection is a good technique when determining patients' or family members' understanding about the illness or treatments.

Q When making decisions regarding end of life and withdrawal of life support, whose perspective or opinion should be considered?

A The patient's

In situations when the patient is unable to make decisions regarding life support, the family will make those decisions. The decision should still be made based on the wishes of the patient. A living will may indicate the extent of life support the patient would want. Without a living will, sometimes asking the family, "What do you think your loved one would want in this situation?" will encourage them to make decisions based on what they think their loved one would want.

⬤ SYSTEMS THINKING

Q Holistic nursing care is healing oriented and is centered on which relationship?

A Relationship with patient

Holistic nursing is patient-centered care directed toward healing, not diseases. It protects, promotes, and optimizes healing while attempting to alleviate suffering. It is comprehensive and recognizes the totality of the patient by interconnecting the body, mind, spirituality, energy, culture, relationships, and environment. It promotes comfort, empowerment, healing, and the well-being of the patient.

HINT Holistic nursing emphasizes self-care and autonomy. A role of a holistic nurse is to ensure that the patient is aware of alternatives and the implication of treatment options.

Q What is a complementary intervention used to manage anxiety?

A Deep-breathing exercises

Managing anxiety in ICU patients includes instructing them in deep-breathing exercises. Other exercises may include relaxation or imagery techniques. Holistic nurses incorporate both conventional and complementary/alternative/integrative modalities (CAM) into practice (Boxes 13.24 and 13.25).

Box 13.24 Complementary Techniques to Manage Anxiety/Pain

Deep-breathing exercises	Aromatherapy
Relaxation techniques	Massage
Guided imagery	Pet therapy
Deep-muscle relaxation	Humor
Music therapy	

Box 13.25 Examples of CAM

Natural products	Practice of traditional healers
Mind–body medicine	Energy therapies (i.e., magnet therapy, light therapy)
Spinal manipulation	Homeopathy
Movement therapies and massage	Acupuncture and acupressure

Q What is the quest to discover the ultimate meaning and purpose of one's life called?

A Spirituality

Spirituality is the culmination of a person's quest to discover the ultimate meaning and purpose of his or her life. Spirituality reflects the essence and substance of that person. Religion is the belief in and worship of a superhuman controlling power, especially a personal God. Religion can impact the development of spirituality and provides some answers to spiritual questions. ICU nurses should assess spiritual issues while reassuring patients there is no pressure on them to discuss issues they do not want to discuss. Active listening is sometimes the best intervention to help a patient clarify his or her wishes, hopes, and beliefs (Boxes 13.26 and 13.27). Religion may provide support to patients and their families and can be a significant part of their coping mechanism. Healthcare providers will want to explore the patient's contact with formal religious institutions, as well as informal spiritual beliefs. Knowledge of a patient and his or her family's religious beliefs are particularly important for healthcare professionals whose patients are struggling with serious illnesses.

HINT Spirituality is a part of the holistic care. The ICU nurse can provide support, solace, spiritual strength, and presence. Prayer has been found to be a powerful tool to help patients cope with critical illness and impending death.

Box 13.26 Common Spiritual Issues

Desire for forgiveness	Need for affirmation of a person's value/meaning
Need to forgive	Hope for a peaceful and painless death
Desire for closure	Concern for loved one's left behind

Box 13.27 Spiritual Questions Commonly Encountered in ICU

Why me?	What will the last hours be like?
Is my illness a punishment?	Is there a God?
Why was I placed on Earth?	What happens after death?
Is there hope?	Will I be punished for my sins?
How can I be forgiven?	Will I be alone?
How can I forgive?	Will I be remembered?

Q What is a common issue in caring for an awake and alert patient on a mechanical ventilator?

A Communication

Effective communication is known to assist with establishing a trusting relationship. Effective communication with intubated patients on mechanical ventilation is a challenge to critical care nurses. Slowing down, demonstrating patience, and allowing time for the intubated patient to communicate is a large step in improving effective communication (Box 13.28).

Box 13.28 Communication Adjuncts for Intubated Patients

Nonverbal signals
Writing tablets
Communication boards

RESPONSE TO DIVERSITY

Q During the admission assessment, the family states that the patient is from a tribe in Africa. What is the nurse's initial priority in providing care that is compatible with the patient's cultural beliefs?

A Perform a cultural assessment

Cultural sensitivity often begins with a cultural assessment that includes finding information on the patient's cultural beliefs, views, and cultural norms. Individuals can vary within a particular culture with regards to beliefs or norms, so the patient should be recognized as an individual within a cultural context. Identifying how the patient has responded to an illness in the past and exploring what effect the critical injury or illness will have on the patient is essential to determine the patient's perceptions. Healthcare beliefs regarding chronic illness, seeking medical attention, and death and dying may vary among cultures and ethnic backgrounds (Box 13.29).

HINT   Determine whether there is anything the nurses should or should not do when providing care that is sensitive to the individual's values and beliefs. Awareness and acceptance are at the heart of cultural sensitivity.

Box 13.29 Components of Cultural Assessment

Place of birth	Health beliefs and practice
Number of years in the United States	Who is the primary decision-maker?
Primary and secondary language	View on death and dying
Religious practices	Role in the family

> **Q What is it called when one practices patient-centered care while understanding the patient's needs from the patient's perspective?**
>
> **A Cultural competence**

Cultural competence is not knowing or having a complete understanding of all ethnic and cultural beliefs and world viewpoints but the ability to assess and determine the individual patient's beliefs and needs. Open-ended questions may assist with determining the person's beliefs that influence his or her understanding of their illness and healthcare. Chaplains and social workers may also be resources to collaborate with to understand particular ethnic or cultural belief systems (Box 13.30).

HINT   The custom in several cultures is for the family to be informed of the poor prognosis and allow the family to decide whether the patient should be told, whereas American healthcare providers put strong emphasis on patient's rights (Table 13.1).

Box 13.30 Challenges in the ICU

Cultural or religious diets Religious belief against use of blood transfusions	Self-inflicting injuries (i.e., rubbing coins on body to create welts)
Stoicism or vocal responses to pain	Sacred threads or jewelry
Particular practices involving end of life and death	Herbal or complementary treatments
Safety risks	Interpretation of eye contact
Patriarchal cultures and the Health Insurance Portability and Accountability Act (HIPAA) laws	Interpretation of touch or hands-on care
	Male nurses caring for female patients

Table 13.1 Examples of Potential Compromises With Cultural Beliefs

Challenges	Potential Remedies
Lighting candles under bed	Use of flashlights instead of candles
Belief that one should die facing east	Physically move bed to accommodate belief
Sacred threads on wrist	Tape to avoid need to remove before surgery

> **Q What is it called when one believes that all Hispanic women are vocal when in pain?**
>
> **A Stereotyping**

Stereotyping is making the assumption that everyone within a certain ethnic background or culture will have the same beliefs and reactions to certain situations. There is a difference between stereotyping and generalization. Generalization is the recognition of a cultural pattern (i.e., Hispanic women are vocal when in pain) that requires follow-up to assess whether this individual follows that pattern. Generalization is a starting point and can benefit the care provided to the patient and family. Stereotyping, on the other hand, can lead to undue stress, decreased quality of care for patients and their families, and should be avoided. Stereotyping could lead to undertreating pain in Hispanic women. Individual assessment of a typical pain response will avoid overgeneralization based on culture.

HINT   Be aware of beliefs and differences in cultures but ensure individualized assessment and care.

> **Q** What is frequently a significant barrier between different ethnic backgrounds?
>
> **A** Language

Frequently, language is a significant barrier between healthcare providers and patients of a different ethnic background. Patients may be relatively new to America and speak very little English. Using medical interpreters will facilitate communication and improve a trusting relationship. Children of the patient may be more fluent in English but should not be used as an interpreter in the healthcare setting. Exposure of the child to sensitive healthcare information and role reversal can cause undue stress and adverse effects. Other concerns are the accuracy of the interpretation, especially the medical terminology, competency, and potential conflict of interest that may exist. Competent translators require knowledge of two different languages, medical terminology, and maintain ethical and professional practice standards.

HINT Provide written patient education materials in other languages in addition to English.

> **Q** A Spanish-speaking patient is scheduled for surgery in the morning. What would be an important step in obtaining a signed consent for surgery?
>
> **A** Use hospital translator

It is recommended that an interpreter be used when obtaining signed consent forms from a patient or family member with limited or no English-language abilities. Consent forms can be translated into multiple languages, but an interpreter should still be used to assist with obtaining a signed consent, assess the patient's understanding, and assist in translating questions that the patient may have regarding the procedure. Cultural beliefs may impact their understanding of the procedure and the use of a translator allows for facilitation of dialogue between the patient and healthcare providers, and allows for patient/family to ask questions and express concerns about the scheduled surgery or procedure (Box 13.31). Nurses need to know how to access language services in their hospital. This may be an in-house person or via telephone or video.

HINT Remember, deaf and hearing-impaired patients or family members may require sign-language interpreters.

Box 13.31 Strategies When Using Translator

Provide background information to translator before session	Avoid medical jargon
Explain purpose of session to translator	Look directly at the patient/family and not at the interpreter
If possible, have interpreter talk to patient/family before session begins	Observe patient's/family's facial expressions and body language (nonverbal language) in response to the discussion
Develops a trusting relationship Able to determine individual beliefs, not stereotyping	Be patient
Speak in shorter sentences and avoid long explanations	Have family repeat back to the interpreter to verify understanding

> **Q** In addition to language interpretation, what else may translators be able to assist with?
>
> **A** Understanding cultural beliefs

Different cultures have different rules of behavior. Interpreters fluent in the language are frequently from the same cultural background and can function as a cultural broker as well as perform interpretation. Cultural brokers are a resource when patient's cultural beliefs affect patient care. Hospitals are increasingly being staffed by people from different countries with diverse cultural backgrounds. These healthcare providers can also function in the role of a cultural broker.

HINT These cultural differences in healthcare providers, however, can also create conflict and misunderstanding, which can result in tension among the staff and affect patient care.

> **Q** A septic patient is of the belief that he is ill because his soul was stolen, and he wants a shaman to come in to find the soul. Should he receive antibiotics, the shaman, or both?
>
> **A** Both

The mind is very powerful and can help heal the body. If the patient's belief is that the soul is stolen and he will not get better until it is recovered, he may not get better with medical management alone. The treatment of allowing the shaman to find the patient's soul will benefit the patient along with the antibiotics. Treatment should be appropriate to etiology and benefit the patient by treating his beliefs. The nurse needs to increase the effort of understanding how the patient views the illness, allowing interventions to be tailored to those beliefs.

HINT Do not allow ethnocentrism to interfere with caring for a patient. Who knows which belief is either right or wrong?

FACILITATION OF LEARNING

> **Q** When teaching a patient or family member, what should be avoided or used sparingly?
>
> **A** Medical terminology

Avoid or limit the use of medical terminology. Healthcare providers are perceived as "speaking a different language." Physicians tend to either use short answers or answers full of medical terminology, and nurses frequently adopt the role of "interpreter." Nurses should regularly attend patient/physician conferences or rounds to assist with interpretation and clarification. Plain language should be used in both verbal and written information provided for the patient and family.

HINT Families are more likely to ask questions of the nurses than the physicians.

> **Q** When assessing learning needs of a patient in the ICU, what is an important factor to determine?
>
> **A** Readiness or ability to learn

In critically ill patients, a significant component of the learning assessment is to determine whether the patient is ready and able to learn. If sedated and ventilated or unable to respond, they may not be ready for learning. Families, however, may become the focus of the education in the ICU (Box 13.32).

Box 13.32 Assessment Components of Patient/Family Education

Who needs to be taught?	Health literacy
What needs to be taught?	Identify factors that may impede learning
How does it need to be taught?	Identify interventions to address these factors
Readiness to learn	

HINT Health literacy is a common issue that impedes learning. Written material is more effective if written at sixth- to eighth-grade levels.

> **Q** When teaching, should basic information be provided first, or should the more pertinent complex information be provided at once?
>
> **A** Basic information

Knowledge expands on basic understanding and previous knowledge. Teaching or development of learning materials should be organized from basic to complex information. The simple ideas and understandings are introduced first, followed by more complex or harder concepts. Teaching a complex motor skill is facilitated by taking the total skill and breaking it down into simple steps.

HINT It takes practice to become proficient at performing skills.

> **Q** What is the primary principle of an adult learner that needs to be considered when teaching patients or family in the ICU?
>
> **A** Need to know

Adults need to know why it is important to learn something new. If the knowledge is perceived as important, greater effort will be committed to learning it. The learner needs to be aware of his or her deficiencies in knowledge. Adults are also self-directed learners and are responsible for their own decisions regarding learning (Box 13.33).

Box 13.33 Principles of the Adult Learner

Need to know	Orientation to learning
Self-directed	Internal motivation to learn
Influence of learner's life experience	Use active participation in learning
Progress from known to unknown	Require reinforcement of behavior
Readiness to learn	

HINT Life experiences shape values, beliefs, and attitudes that influence learning.

> **Q** What are the two important aspects of providing education to patient and families?
>
> **A** Simplicity and reinforcement

Keeping instruction and education simple with minimal medical jargon facilitates understanding and learning. A good technique is to begin teaching sessions with open-ended questions used to evaluate current level of understanding. Medical topics can be complex and intimidating to teach. Keeping it simple can assist the teacher and learner with difficult topics. Choose three or four essential concepts of a given topic to teach. Reinforcement is the concept of repeating the information multiple times during the session. Provide written material to reinforce learning sessions.

HINT Frequently, informal teaching at the bedside is the best opportunity to provide education ("teachable moments"). Patient care and patient education are inseparable.

> **Q** What frequently interferes with the ability of a patient and family to concentrate and learn?
>
> **A** Anxiety and stress

Anxiety can markedly decrease the ability of the patient or family to concentrate and learn. Frequently, family members repeat questions even after answers and explanations are provided due to stress and anxiety. This affects their readiness to learn (Box 13.34).

Box 13.34 Barriers to Learning

Stress or anxiety	Presence of pain
Lack of support systems	Literacy and health literacy
Lack of time	Language barriers
Lack of confidence by nurse	Cultural differences
Lack of motivation by patient/family	

> **Q** What can the ICU nurse do to facilitate the transfer of the patient from the ICU to a lower acuity area?
>
> **A** Education

Critical care nurses need to prepare the patient and family for the eventual transfer from the ICU to a lower acuity area. This is a milestone in recovery but may be viewed by the patient or family as being stressful. They may experience relief and joy about the transfer if they believe the patient has improved, but if they believe the patient still requires close monitoring, the transfer may trigger fear of an inadequate level of monitoring. This may produce resistance to the transfer by family. The patient and family will experience less stress if the ICU nurse has spent time educating them about the step-down or floor routines, staffing patterns, and visiting hours. Reassure the patient and family of the competency of the nurses even if the level of monitoring has changed.

HINT   Acknowledge the anxiety of the transfer and emphasize the transition is a positive sign of recovery.

Q What should occur after the patient or family is taught a new concept or medication?

A Evaluation of learning

Evaluation of learning is important in determining the effectiveness of the education. Evaluating learning can indicate need for further reinforcement of key concepts. Questions to the learner regarding the information reviewed provides immediate feedback as to the effectiveness of the instruction.

HINT   When evaluating the learning of a motor task, use return demonstration.

 ## CLINICAL INQUIRY

Q What is it called when practice is based on the best available research data from well-designed studies?

A Evidence-based practice (EBP)

EBP is the use of the best available research data to guide practice and develop guidelines. EBP uses one's expert level of knowledge and experience to apply the data to clinical situations. Patient's and family's preferences are combined with this knowledge to individualize the plan of care. EBP optimizes patient's outcomes and assists nurses with keeping up with frequent changes in healthcare. EBP demonstrates a change from the historical practice based on authoritative opinions to emphasize findings from research and studies (Boxes 13.35 and 13.36).

HINT   Use of protocols, clinical pathways, and algorithms facilitate incorporating EBP to the bedside. Review the "Practice Alerts" posted on the AACN website for EBP recommendations by the AACN.

Box 13.35 Barriers to Implementation of EBP

Lack of knowledge	Changing behavior met with resistance
Inability to understand statistical analysis	Change is a slow process
Lack of time	Lack of management commitment
Heavy patient assignments	Lack of organizational support
Lack of skills/resources	Large amounts of research and data available

Box 13.36 Research Terminologies

Qualitative	Research that seeks to provide understanding of human experience, perceptions, motivations, intentions, and behaviors based on description and observation
Quantitative	Traditional scientific methods, which generate numerical data and usually seek to establish causal relationships between two or more variables, using statistical methods to test the strength and significance of the relationships
Randomized controlled trials (RCTs)	Prospective, randomized, experimental studies using control groups
Meta-analysis RCT	Summary of relevant RCT

HINT Randomized controlled trials (RCTs) are considered the most reliable form of evidence. RCTs and meta-analysis of RCTs are considered level I evidence (the highest).

Q What is the first step to using EBP in the hospital?

A Identify knowledge gaps

Knowing that there is a knowledge gap between research and actual practice is the first step in initiating change based on EBP. Critical and continuous evaluation of practice is the best opportunity to identify gaps or needed changes in practice (Box 13.37).

HINT EBP training can benefit nurse's competency in initiating EBP and increase participation in EBP activities.

Box 13.37 Steps to Evidence-Based Practice

Identify knowledge gap	Determine validity of research study
Formulate questions	Apply research findings to patient care
Conduct literature searches	Appropriately involve patient in decision-making

Q What framework can be used when a nurse performs a clinical inquiry on a clinical practice issue?

A Patient, intervention, comparison, outcome (PICO)

The PICO framework assists the nurse in formulating the question regarding the clinical practice issue. Some clinical questions may be simple, whereas others are more complex. Once the question is formulated, then the next step is to review the literature (Table 13.2).

Table 13.2 PICO

PICO	Example
P = Patient/Population/Disease	Patients ready to be weaned from ventilator
I = Intervention	Pressure support
O = Outcome	Safety, effectiveness, and number of ventilator days

HINT PICO may be used as a first step to assist with literature review (Box 13.38).

Box 13.38 Steps of Clinical Inquiry

Identify the knowledge gap	Determine how findings relate to practice
Formulate the question	Apply the findings in practice
Review literature	Evaluate the change in practice (i.e., outcomes, compliance)

Q What are patient-centered, multidisciplinary plans of care that use EBP?

A Clinical practice guidelines (CPG)

CPGs are patient-centered, multidisciplinary, multidimensional plans of care that help the healthcare team to move toward EBP and improve the process of how care is delivered. It involves collaborative practice groups working with developing CPG (Box 13.39).

HINT Clinical interventions must be based on strong evidence demonstrating improved outcomes or benefits to the patient.

Box 13.39 Benefits of CPG

Improves practitioner accountability	More cost effective
Increases coordination of care	Greater ability to evaluate care is provided
Decreases unnecessary variations in practice	Improves transition through healthcare settings
Improves quality of care	

> **Q What is the tool used in the clinical setting that guides care in a specific clinical problem?**
>
> **A Clinical pathway**

Clinical pathways (also called critical pathways or clinical maps) are document-based tools that provide a link between evidence and practice. They are structured, multidisciplinary plans of care that detail essential steps and provide a timeline. They detail the steps in the course of treatment (algorithms, protocols) and evaluate variances from the pathway. A variance is an omission of an action, an inappropriate action, or an action that did not occur according to the timeline (usually late). Clinical pathways may be better suited for patients who are more predictable. Reviewing the variance record can be used to improve the quality of care, make changes in practice to improve outcomes, and provide a means of continuous quality improvement.

HINT   Critical areas of the clinical pathway can be highlighted to guide nurses in the important steps found to improve outcomes (Box 13.40).

Box 13.40 Components of Clinical Pathway

Timeline
Steps of care or interventions
Intermediate and long-term goals
Variance record

> **Q What is a common goal when using EBP medicine?**
>
> **A Quality improvement**

EBP, CPG, and clinical pathways all strive to improve patient outcomes and maximize clinical efficiency. They also help to reduce variance in care by promoting standardization and provide care according to accepted standards of care.

HINT   Remember, guidelines are guidelines and should not be viewed as "prescriptive" but can be overridden by good clinical judgment.

1. Which of the following is the best method to assess a patient's level of anxiety?

   A. Observe for signs of agitation
   B. Ask the patient to rate their anxiety level
   C. Use the Richmond Agitation Sedation Scale (RASS) tool
   D. Ask a family member if the patient is experiencing anxiety

2. Which of the following is considered a limitation to the ethical principle of autonomy, and is an indication to use a different principle in decision-making?

   A. When a person is likely to injure self or others
   B. When the decision is not in the patient's best interest
   C. When the physician has a different plan of care and is in agreement with other consultants
   D. When the family has strong beliefs that are contradictory to the patient's beliefs

3. Which of the following is the primary goal of implementing evidence-based practice (EBP) in the clinical setting?

   A. Decrease nursing time required at the bedside
   B. Facilitate communication between physicians
   C. Improve patient care and outcomes
   D. Provide patients with a plan of care

4. A family arrives in the intensive care unit (ICU) to see their loved one for the first time. They are asking questions and becoming more agitated. Which of the following best explains the behavior of this family?

   A. Feelings of helplessness
   B. Guilt feelings
   C. Poor coping skills
   D. Denial

5. A patient is admitted to the intensive care unit (ICU) following a motor vehicle crash (MVC). The patient is unresponsive and on a mechanical ventilator. The family has expressed a need to stay with the patient or remain in the waiting room 24 hrs a day so that they can be available for their loved one at all times. Which of the following would be the best response by the intensive care unit (ICU) nurse?

   A. Reassure the family that the physician is the best and their loved one will be okay
   B. Tell the family there is nothing they can do to help and that they should not remain in the waiting room all day
   C. Explain to the family that they also need to get rest so that they can be more prepared when their loved one may require more of their care
   D. Encourage the family members to stay with the patient 24 hours a day

1. B) Ask the patient to rate their anxiety level

Anxiety is subjective. The best method of assessment is to ask the patient if they are anxious, and to rate the anxiety on a scale of 1–10. Agitation does not always accompany anxiety. The RASS tool is used to assess sedation, not anxiety. Family members may not be aware of the patient's anxiety and are not as reliable as the patient.

2. A) When a person is likely to injure self or others

Autonomy is the right of self-determination, independence, and freedom. Actions are determined based upon the patient's beliefs and desires. Autonomy is overridden in healthcare only when the patient is likely to injure self or others. As an example, a patient who has attempted suicide may be admitted and treated, even if treatment is against the patient's wishes. The patient's decision is prioritized over the physician's and family's desires, even if that decision is not considered to be in the patient's best interest by others.

3. C) Improve patient care and outcomes

EBP refers to use of the best available research data to guide practice and develop guidelines. Evidence-based practice utilizes one's expert level of knowledge and experience to apply the data to clinical situations. The goal of EBP is to improve patient care and outcomes by implementing the most current guidelines. It does not necessarily decrease nursing time spent caring for patients. It can facilitate communication between healthcare providers and may be used as a plan of care, but these are not the primary goals.

4. A) Feelings of helplessness

Families may experience all of these feelings (helplessness, guilt feelings, and denial), but the best answer, according to the presentation of the family in the scenario is feelings of helplessness. The suddenness of injury or illness may cause family members to have uncertainty about the situation. They may approach the ICU nurse with multiple questions and concerns. The family is thrown into a whirlwind of activity, and family members commonly experience feelings of helplessness. Asking questions and becoming agitated during the initial visit following a sudden illness or injury does not necessarily indicate poor coping skills. Family members are often unprepared for the whole impact of the injury or illness.

5. C) Explain to the family that they also need to get rest so that they can be more prepared when their loved one may require more of their care

Family members frequently react with a need for vigilance following a critical injury or illness of a loved one. Encourage the family to leave the hospital at times to take breaks and get some rest. Explaining to them that they need their rest in order to be prepared to assist with care when their loved one is ready sometimes helps the family understand the process. Reassuring the family that the patient will be okay is a false reassurance, and can lead to issues with trust. Telling the family there is nothing they can do fosters their feelings of helplessness. There is always something the ICU nurse can find for the family to do to assist with patient care, even if it is prayer in a religious family. Allowing a less restrictive visitation in the ICU has been found to benefit both the patient and family members, but encouraging a family member to remain 24 hours a day will lead to exhaustion of the family member.

6. A patient's family has asked the intensive care unit (ICU) nurse to accompany them in a prayer for their loved one. The nurse is uncomfortable with praying or providing spiritual support. Which of the following would be the most appropriate response by the ICU nurse?

   A. Perform the prayer anyway, as it is important to the family
   B. Tell the family she is too busy at this time and will do it later
   C. Ask the family if the chaplain could be called to assist them with their prayers
   D. Discuss with the family the need to focus on the medical issue instead of the spiritual issue

7. An intubated patient is attempting to communicate with the nurse. He is becoming frustrated. Which of the following would be the best response by the nurse?

   A. Reassure the patient that this is a short-term problem
   B. Administer sedation to calm the patient
   C. Use a communication board to facilitate communication
   D. Explain the difficulty of lip reading to the patient

8. Laughter has been found to have which positive effect?

   A. Improve a patient's spirituality
   B. Lower the risk of strokes
   C. Decrease pain
   D. Reorient the patient

9. While teaching the patient, the nurse uses a real or simulated example to demonstrate the importance of the lesson. This is using which of the following adult learning principles?

   A. Need to know
   B. Learner's self-concept
   C. Internal motivation to learn
   D. Life experiences

10. During visitation, the nurse observes that the patient's wife is just standing at the patient's bed. She is not talking to him or touching him. What would be the most appropriate response by the nurse?

    A. Recognize the wife's discomfort and do not force her to touch the patient
    B. Encourage the wife to touch the patient and talk to him
    C. Notify the physician of a potential conflict of interest with the wife
    D. Ask the physician for a psychological consultation to work with the wife

11. A group of night nurses has noticed that lab draws ordered for 2:00 a.m. interrupt sleep patterns. What is the best strategy for addressing this issue?

    A. Refuse to obtain routine labs at 2:00 a.m.
    B. Assemble a workgroup to research best practice and determine the best policy
    C. Perform a survey of nursing opinions regarding the current policy
    D. Request that the physicians form a committee to address the problem

12. The principle of double effect typically refers to which of the following situations?

    A. Disagreement between family members in regard to the removal of life support
    B. Stopping tube feeds but maintaining IV hydration
    C. Removal of life support even if the patient is awake
    D. Administration of opioids for pain even though they may cause respiratory depression

6. C) Ask the family if the chaplain could be called to assist them with their prayers
If the ICU nurse is uncomfortable with providing spiritual support for the patient or family, the most appropriate response would be to call the chaplain or the patient's spiritual advisor or representative. Spirituality is important to many people and is a part of the holistic care that should be provided to the patient and family.

7. C) Use a communication board to facilitate communication
Inability to communicate effectively while intubated and mechanically ventilated creates stress and anxiety in the patient. Using sign language, lip reading, or communication boards can facilitate communication with nonverbal patients. Merely reassuring the patient, or explaining the problem to the patient without attempting to improve the communication, just creates more anxiety. Administering a sedative is not indicated for a communication issue.

8. C) Decrease pain
Laughter has been found to reduce pain, even up to 15 mins after laughing. It has been reported to be the best self-prescribed pain management solution by oncology patients. Laughter increases the release of endorphins, the body's endogenous opioid. Laughter has not been found to lower the risk of strokes or affect patient orientation. Spirituality is a person's sense of belonging and belief in a higher being. Laughter has not been shown to affect spirituality.

9. A) Need to know
One of the most important principles of adult learning is the need to know what is being taught. By giving real or simulated examples pertinent to the patient, the nurse is explaining to the patient why he or she needs to know the knowledge being taught. Learner's self-concept is the self-motivation to learn and can be facilitated by providing more self-directed learning material. Internal motivation to learn is based upon a person's internal desire to learn or become motivated to improve quality of life. Adult education should also be focused upon the patient's life experiences. This would be facilitated by asking initial questions about the patient's current knowledge or skill level.

10. B) Encourage the wife to touch the patient and talk to him
Patients may be able to hear even if they are not responding or do not appear to be oriented. Families frequently do not know what to say to the patient or what to talk about at the bedside. Some families just stand at the bedside and are afraid to touch their loved ones due to all of the lines and tubes. intensive care unit (ICU) nurses can encourage them to talk to the patients directly and touch their loved ones. This behavior does not indicate a conflict of interest in the wife making decisions for the patient. This is a common response and does not require psychological work-up.

11. B) Assemble a workgroup to research best practice and determine the best policy
The first step in determining best practice is to become aware of the problem. In this situation, the problem identified was that lab draws caused sleep disruption in critical care patients. The next step is to assemble a workgroup to research current literature and studies regarding the formulated problem. Presenting a plan for changing current practice is received better if a best practice has been identified and is far more helpful than just refusing to do a particular practice. Obtaining other nurses' opinions is not basing the practice on research. This is not a situation or time in which physicians should be asked to form committees to institute change.

12. D) Administration of opioids for pain even though they may cause respiratory depression
The principle of double effect is commonly applied to the administration of opioids for pain management at the end of life. The principle applies when an action has two effects, one good and one bad. Providing analgesics to control pain is good, but opioids can cause respiratory depression, which is bad. It is ethically justifiable to provide opiates, even though the patient may develop respiratory depression, if the primary goal is to control pain. Disagreements between family members in decision-making and stopping tube feeds while maintaining hydration are not considered double effects. Life support may be removed even if a person is awake. Removal of life support can be considered to have both good and bad effects, but the hint in the question is the sentence regarding pain management.

13. When making a change in the intensive care unit (ICU), which of the following steps represents the acceptance and incorporation of change by the staff?

   A. Unfreezing
   B. Moving
   C. Mutual respect
   D. Refreezing

14. While teaching the patient to perform a dressing change, which of the following evaluations will determine the effectiveness of the learning?

   A. Do not ask for a demonstration if it embarrasses the patient
   B. Patient states the steps involved in performing a dressing change
   C. Patient states that the spouse can do the dressing change
   D. Patient demonstrates knowledge of the critical elements of the dressing change

15. A person has which of the following psychosocial concerns at the young adult stage of development?

   A. Integrity vs. despair
   B. Intimacy vs. self-isolation
   C. Generativity vs. self-absorption
   D. Body image vs. isolation

16. According to the synergy model, which of the following drives the nurse's characteristics or competencies?

   A. Educational level of nurse
   B. Experience as a critical care nurse
   C. Patient and family needs
   D. Collaboration with physicians

17. Your patient's liver enzymes have gone up, and the physician has ordered some diagnostic tests. The family is not there yet. Which of the following would be the best action of the nurse?

   A. Write down all of the diagnostics for the family so when they do come they can see what you have been doing
   B. Continue caring for the patient and obtain all of the diagnostics tests that were ordered. The family can be updated when they arrive
   C. Call the family and let them know the changes that have occurred while they were gone
   D. Tell the physician you would prefer to wait until the family arrives before taking the patient for diagnostics

18. Which of the following is the most common reason for an unhealthy work environment?

   A. Ineffective communication
   B. Lack of respect
   C. Knowledge deficits
   D. Stressful environment

13. D) Refreezing

Unfreezing is the initial step that restrains the forces that threaten the change. Moving is the step toward overcoming resistance and toward acceptance. Refreezing follows acceptance and establishes the change as a new habit. Mutual respect may be needed, but it is not a part of the change process.

14. D) Patient demonstrates knowledge of the critical elements of the dressing change

When teaching a psychomotor skill to a patient, the patient needs to perform the skill after having received verbal and written instructions regarding the steps involved in performing the skill. Critical elements of the skill must be identified, and those elements must be demonstrated by the patient when performing the skill. Just stating the steps of a skill does not demonstrate proficiency in actually performing the skill. Stating that the spouse can do the dressing change does not evaluate any learning, by either the patient or the spouse. Learning a new skill can be difficult and requires encouragement by the nurse. The demonstration of a skill by the patient should not be avoided for fear of embarrassing the patient. Learning has to be evaluated.

15. B) Intimacy vs. self-isolation

Young adults are challenged by the psychosocial concerns of intimacy versus self-isolation. This is the period of life when individuals establish both independence and intimate bonds with another. Generativity versus self-absorption is the challenge of middle-aged adults. This includes the balance between work and family roles. Older adults experience the challenge of integrity versus despair and need to adapt to changes such as the loss of spouse or end of life.

16. C) Patient and family needs

The needs of patients and families drive the competencies of the nurses. Synergy occurs when the nurse's competencies match the characteristics and needs of the patient. Optimal outcomes occur when the nurse and the patient are in synergy. The levels of competencies depend upon knowledge and experience, but synergy model is driven by patient's needs.

17. C) Call the family and let them know the changes that have occurred while they were gone

Establishing a trusting relationship immediately relieves some of the anxiety, then family members are more likely to feel comfortable enough to leave the hospital. When the family receives calls from the nurse with updates, they begin to develop a trust relationship. Writing down events in an ICU diary is good and recommended but in this case, letting the family know before they get to the hospital is the best intervention.

18. A) Ineffective communication

An unhealthy work environment can lead to increased medication errors and poor patient-care delivery. Poor communication is the most common reason for unhealthy work environments exist. Respect is important in healthy work environment but often comes with improved communication. Unhealthy work environments can lead to stressful workplace. Knowledge deficits are not reasons for unhealthy work environment but can be a result of poor communication.

19. Which of the following times of the day does most breakdowns in communication occur resulting in errors?

    A. Middle of the night
    B. Change of shift
    C. During family visiting hours
    D. During physician rounding

20. Holistic nursing care is centered on which relationship?

    A. Relationship with the family
    B. Relationship with the patient
    C. Relationship with the physician
    D. Relationship with leadership

19. B) Change of shift

Shift change is a common time for breakdown of communication to occur. This was quoted to be the "single largest source of medical error" due to a significant amount of information being passed along among nurses and change of patient care from one nurse to another. Middle of the night can cause some issues if the physicians are not readily available or the nurse is concerned about waking someone up, but it still is not as significant as change of shift. During family visitation and physician rounding, there can be increased distractions but still change of shift is considered the greatest time for communication errors to occur.

20. B) Relationship with the patient

Holistic nursing is patient-centered care directed toward healing, not diseases. It protects, promotes, and optimizes healing while attempting to alleviate suffering. It is comprehensive and recognizes the totality of the patient by interconnecting the body, mind, spirituality, energy, culture, relationships, and environment.

BIBLIOGRAPHY

AACN Certification Corporation, The AACN Synergy Model of Patient Care (www.certcorp.org)

American Association of Critical Care Nurses (AACN). (2005). Standards for establishing and sustaining healthy work environments. Retrieved from http://www.aacn.org

American Association of Critical Care Nurses Certification Corporation: General information regarding certification. Retrieved from www.certcorp.org

Becker, D., Kaplow, R., Muenzen, P. M., & Hartigan, C. (2006). Activities performed by acute and critical care advanced practice nurses: American Association of Critical-Care Nurses Study of Practice. *American Journal of Critical Care, 15*(2), 130–148.

Wilson-Stronks, A., & Glavez, E. (2007). *Hospitals, language and culture: A snapshot of the nation.* Washington, DC: The Joint Commission.

Practice Test

1. An arterial blood gas (ABG) is obtained on a patient with salicylate toxicity. Which of the following combinations would the intensive care unit (ICU) nurse expect to find in this patient?

   A. Metabolic acidosis-respiratory acidosis
   B. Metabolic alkalosis-respiratory acidosis
   C. Metabolic alkalosis-respiratory alkalosis
   D. Metabolic acidosis-respiratory alkalosis

2. Which of the following abnormal conductions can obscure the ECG signs of an acute myocardial infarction with elevated ST segments?

   A. Third-degree heart block (HB)
   B. Left bundle branch block (LBBB)
   C. Atrial flutter
   D. Prolonged QT interval

3. An increase in Creatine Kinase-MB (CK-MB) units without a significant increase in CK-MB percentage may be due to which of the following?

   A. Renal failure
   B. Skeletal injury only
   C. Both cardiac and skeletal injury
   D. Carbon monoxide poisoning

4. Which of the following findings would indicate the presence of dead space?

   A. Increase $EtCO_2$ with normal ventilation
   B. Abnormally low $PaCO_2$ for MV
   C. False high SaO_2 on pulse oximetry
   D. Elevated base excess

5. The intensive care unit (ICU) nurse on the previous shift reports that the patient is on noninvasive ventilation (BiPAP) and is restrained due to agitation. The patient had been trying to take the BiPAP mask off through the early evening. Which of the following would be the best response by the arriving nurse?

   A. I think that was a good idea. We need to make sure the patient is being ventilated
   B. Restraints would be better than an anxiolytic in this patient
   C. Restraining a patient on BiPAP is a safety issue. What other options do we have to assure compliance with BiPAP?
   D. I think we need to talk with the physician about intubation since the patient is not tolerating BiPAP

6. When assessing a pressure injury, it is noted that the eschar obscures the extent of injury or tissue loss. This is called

   A. Stage III
   B. Stage IV
   C. Deep tissue injury
   D. Unstageable Injury

7. Which of the following patients would be at the highest risk for developing stress-related mucosal disease and upper gastrointestinal (GI) bleeding complications?

   A. A patient who is immobilized for more than 24 hours
   B. A patient with a pelvic fracture
   C. A patient with meningitis
   D. A patient who has been on mechanical ventilation greater than 48 hours

8. A traumatic injury to your patient's lower extremities resulted in compartment syndrome and bilateral fasciotomies. When assessing the patient, the nurse notes their urine is "coke" colored. What would be the concern for this patient?

   A. Rhabdomyolysis
   B. Dehydrated
   C. Propofol syndrome
   D. Elevated Bilirubin

9. While caring for a patient with an acute episode of asthma with bronchospasm, which of the following findings should concern the intensive care unit (ICU) nurse the most, indicating that the patient's status is deteriorating?

   A. Hypercarbia
   B. Tachypnea
   C. Tachycardia
   D. FEV1 70% predicted

10. A non-intubated SCI patient is in the ICU to be monitored. His level of injury is C6. Which of the following is the most important parameter to monitor on this patient?

    A. Temperature
    B. Forced vital capacity (fVC)
    C. Blood glucose levels
    D. Serum osmolality

11. Which of the following statements is most accurate in describing cellulitis?

    A. It does not have purulent drainage
    B. Redness and warmth of an incision within 24 hours of surgery indicates cellulitis
    C. It is usually unilateral
    D. Cellulitis always presents with leaking fluid and drainage

12. Which of the following symptoms would be the most indicative of traumatic asphyxiation?

    A. Hypoxia and airway swelling
    B. Stridor and inspiratory wheezes
    C. Papilledema and conjunctival hemorrhage
    D. Facial cyanosis with chest petechiae

13. A patient is being admitted from the operating room (OR). The OR nurse reported that an annulo-plasty was performed. The intensive care unit (ICU) nurse should know that the valve abnormality prior to surgery was which of the following?

    A. Aortic stenosis
    B. Aortic regurgitation
    C. Mitral insufficiency
    D. Mitral stenosis

14. A patient is 2 days post cardiac surgery. He is extubated, weaned off all vasoactive infusions, and has adequate pain control. He is being assessed for transfer to the progressive care unit. It has been noted that no family has been in to see him since the surgery. He is awake and alert, and he has been following commands. At this time, which of the following characteristics should be the primary concern of the nurse caring for this patient?

    A. Vulnerability
    B. Complexity
    C. Participation in care
    D. Resource availability

15. During infusion of IV fluids, the vessel was damaged and fluid leaked into the tissue. Within 4 days, the site was swollen, red and blistering. Which of the following is the most correct terminology indicating the injury?

    A. Second-degree burns
    B. Infiltration
    C. Extravasation
    D. Leakage

16. Which of the following is an irreversible long-term complication of acute respiratory distress syndrome (ARDS) that follows acute recovery from ARDS?

    A. Pulmonary embolism
    B. Atelectasis
    C. Pulmonary edema
    D. Pulmonary fibrosis

17. A patient presents with HF. Upon admission to the ICU, the nurse notes the patient to have signs of reduced perfusion, but without hypotension or pulmonary congestion. Which of the following therapies is recommended based upon these findings?

    A. Inotropic therapy to improve contractility
    B. Ultrafiltration
    C. Diuresis with Lasix
    D. Reduce afterload with nitrates

18. Crepitus was noted when the ICU nurse was moving the trauma patient in the bed. What would be the nurse's best response?

    A. Call physician to obtain radiograph orders
    B. Medicate the patient prior to turning them
    C. Nothing, this is an incidental finding
    D. Pass this along in shift report so the following nurse will not be surprised

19. A patient is diagnosed with acute respiratory distress syndrome (ARDS). What chest X-ray (CXR) changes would the intensive care unit (ICU) nurse expect to find?

    A. Cardiomegaly
    B. Lobar consolidation
    C. Bilateral fluffy infiltrates
    D. Bilateral atelectasis in lower lobes

20. Following a bowel resection, a patient develops severe abdominal pain, rebound abdominal tenderness, and hypotension. Which of the following interventions would be considered the priority of care?

    A. Initiate vasopressors
    B. Aggressive volume resuscitation
    C. Place a nasogastric (NG) tube to low wall suction (LWS)
    D. Transport to abdominal computed tomography (CT) scan

21. Which of the following non-conventional modes of ventilation uses an esophageal balloon catheter to determine optimal PEEP levels?

    A. ECMO
    B. High-frequency oscillator ventilation (HFOV)
    C. Air pressure release ventilation
    D. Transpulmonary pressure-guided ventilation

22. An abdominal trauma patient, 24 hours post admission, is developing respiratory failure and acute renal failure. Which of the following is the MOST likely cause?

    A. Acute respiratory distress syndrome (ARDS)
    B. Abdominal compartment syndrome (ACS)
    C. Pulmonary embolism (PE)
    D. Congestive heart failure (CHF)

23. A patient presents with status asthmaticus. Which of the following acid-base abnormalities would be most expected?

    A. Respiratory acidosis
    B. Metabolic alkalosis
    C. Respiratory alkalosis
    D. Metabolic alkalosis

24. A patient in septic shock has received fluids and is now on Levophed (norepinephrine). Which of the following statements would be the most accurate?

    A. Dopamine is a better vasoconstrictor for managing blood pressures in patients with septic shock
    B. The goal for titrating norepinephrine is to maintain mean arterial pressure (MAP) greater than or equal to 65 mm Hg
    C. When managing septic shock patients, two vasopressors are recommended initially to utilize the synergistic effects of the drugs
    D. Norepinephrine may be started even if the patient is hypovolemic, since vasoconstriction is the priority of care

25. Your patient has been recently weaned off of the ventilator and is more awake. When you go in to bathe him, he becomes anxious and asks for you to do it at another time. What would be your best response?

    A. I'll let your family know and maybe they can help when they get here
    B. It is a really busy day and we need to do it now
    C. OK. I will document you refused your bath
    D. Of course. What time would you like your bath?

26. Lab results have come back on your patient indicating the cancer is back in their lungs after radiation treatment two years ago. Which of the following is the best approach by the healthcare providers?

    A. Wait to tell the patient and family the news until the patient is more stable
    B. If the family asks about the results, then tell them the cancer is back. Do not offer the information until the family is ready to hear it
    C. Let the physician tell the family when the physician has time
    D. Set up a conference with the family and the healthcare providers to review the results and make a plan together regarding the next step

27. Following a high-speed motor vehicle crash, a patient presented with hypoxia and respiratory distress. Bilateral chest tubes were inserted. Upon assessment, the nurse notes that the initial output was 2000 mL of blood. What would the nurse expect the appropriate treatment to be?

    A. Thoracotomy
    B. Continue to monitor
    C. Strip the chest tubes
    D. Replace the chest tubes

28. You overhear a nurse giving information to a family member, and you are aware that family member is not on the list of approved to obtain healthcare information by the patient. Which of the following is the best response?

    A. Allow the nurse to continue since this is a family member and would hear the information later anyway
    B. Wait until the nurse and family are done with the conversation, then take the nurse aside and tell her going forward not to discuss heath care issues with that family member
    C. Call risk management to come up and intervene in this situation
    D. Politely interrupt the conversation and explain to both the nurse and family members the issue

29. Orders have been received to get a bariatric patient out of bed and sitting in a chair. The patient weighs 450 pounds. The chair in the intensive care unit (ICU) has a weight limit of 400 pounds. Which of the following would be the most appropriate response by the nurse?

    A. Discuss purchasing chairs for bariatric patients with management
    B. Obtain an order to get a specialty bed company to bring a bariatric chair
    C. Refuse to get the patient out of bed due to the weight of the patient
    D. Use the chair available, as there is only a 50-pound difference

30. Which of the following interventions is the priority of care in early sepsis?

    A. Administer fluid bolus
    B. Initiate a vasopressor
    C. Administer a steroid
    D. Assist with arterial line placement

31. You are caring for a patient who is receiving continuous venovenous replacement hemodialysis (CVVHD). The low-pressure alarm is sounding. Which of the following would be your best response?

    A. Call the physician stat to replace the catheter
    B. Turn the patient to unkink the tubing
    C. Check for a disconnection
    D. Administer heparin

32. Which of the following management techniques is recommended for necrotizing fasciitis for source control of the infection?

    A. Daily wound dressing changes
    B. Oral broad-spectrum antibiotics
    C. Early ambulation
    D. Surgical debridement of necrosis

33. Which of the following is considered the most definitive diagnosis of Alzheimer's disease (AD)?

    A. Autopsy finding of Lewy bodies
    B. computed tomography (CT) scan demonstrating cerebral atrophy
    C. Magnetic resonance imaging (MRI) finding of ventricular enlargement
    D. Autopsy finding of neurofibrillary tangles and amyloid deposits

34. Upon assessment of your intensive care unit (ICU) patient, you note that the respiratory rate is 36, shallow and unlabored. Breath sounds are diminished in the bases with no adventitious sounds. The following arterial blood gas (ABG) results are obtained:

    pH 7.28
    $PaCO_2$ 25
    PaO_2 90
    SaO_2 96%
    Bicarb 18

    What is the most likely cause of the increased respiratory rate?

    A. Atelectasis
    B. Metabolic acidosis
    C. Metabolic alkalosis
    D. Pneumonia

35. Which of the following is recommended to decrease mortality in ARDS patients?

    A. Administration hypertonic saline
    B. Use of Pulmonary Artery Catheters (PAC) to monitor fluid status
    C. Negative fluid balance
    D. Maximize fluid balance

36. A patient presented in the emergency room with lower extremity fracture and developed compartment syndrome of the calf. A medical fasciotomy was performed. Upon assessment in the ICU, it is noted the patient is consistently complaining of pain despite pain medication. Which of the following is the best statement to explain this finding?

    A. Patient has a low tolerance for pain
    B. Patient probably is drug seeking
    C. Patient may require a second fasciotomy of the involved calf
    D. A missed injury may have occurred and requires radiographs

37. Which of the following is the most important discharge instruction regarding Vicodin?

    A. Only take Vicodin for 2–3 days to prevent addiction
    B. You may supplement Vicodin with other over-the-counter nonsteroidal anti-inflammatory drugs (NSAIDs) if you continue to have pain
    C. Always take Vicodin with food to prevent vomiting
    D. Do not combine Vicodin with other over-the-counter medications containing acetaminophen

38. Which of the following ethical principles promotes maximizing benefit and minimizing harm?

    A. Beneficence
    B. Nonmaleiience
    C. Justice
    D. Fidelity

39. Which of the following is a principle of adult learning?

    A. Adults require less time to perform a learned task
    B. Adults have greater flexibility in learning styles
    C. Adults are goal-oriented and can become impatient with isolated facts
    D. Adults must usually be coerced into learning

40. Which of the following patients may present with falsely low BNP levels while in HF?

    A. Obese patients
    B. End-stage renal disease
    C. Pulmonary embolism
    D. Elderly patients

41. Following treatment of acute asthma with an inhaled beta2 agonist, which of the following electrolyte abnormalities should the intensive care unit (ICU) nurse monitor?

    A. Hypercalcemia
    B. Hypokalemia
    C. Hypermagnesemia
    D. Hypoglycemia

42. Your patient was in a motor vehicle crash and sustained a traumatic amputation of his leg. The family is in the room, asking multiple questions and are getting angry. What would be the nurse's best response?

    A. I understand your grief, but if you continue to get angry we will have to have you escorted out
    B. I hear in your voice your anger. That is a normal reaction to an event like this. Let's take this one question at a time and I will help you through this
    C. I am trying to answer your questions, but I have to take care of your loved one as well. Can you save some of these questions for the physician?
    D. Remember your loved one can hear you. You need to be stronger for them and control your behavior

43. Haldol (haloperidol) is ordered for your patient in the intensive care unit (ICU) who is developing delirium. Which of the following should be recorded at the time of initiation and monitored throughout treatment?

    A. Magnesium level
    B. Lactate level
    C. QTc interval
    D. QRS width

44. Which of the following is not a cause of chloride wasting in a critically ill patient resulting in metabolic alkalosis?

    A. Chronic laxative abuse
    B. Aldosteronism
    C. Diuretic therapy
    D. Salicylate overdose

45. A patient is admitted with acute exacerbation of chronic obstructive pulmonary disease (COPD). The following blood gas results are obtained: pH 7.28, $PaCO_2$ 58, PaO_2 76, HCO_3 30. Which of the following statements by the nurse would indicate appropriate interpretation of the arterial blood gas (ABG) in this situation?

    A. This is a normal blood gas test result for a patient with COPD and does not require further intervention
    B. This blood gas test result indicates that the patient is severely hypoxic and needs oxygen to be administered
    C. This blood gas test result indicates a worsening in the patient's COPD and requires further intervention
    D. The patient's current alkalosis indicates a worsening of the ventilation

46. Which of the following signs may be found on CXR of a patient with a PE?

    A. Westermark sign
    B. Waterhammer sign
    C. Kernigs sign
    D. Kerley B signs

47. Anginal chest pain caused by coronary artery spasms is called:

    A. Variant embolic disease
    B. Prinzmetal's variant angina
    C. Esophageal spasms
    D. Microvascular angina

48. An intensive care unit (ICU) patient requires renal replacement therapy (RRT). He has the following vital signs and renal labs:

    BP 95/45
    HR 108
    RR 18
    Creatinine 6.2
    BUN 60

    Which of the following would be the most appropriate RRT at this time?

    A. Peritoneal dialysis
    B. Continuous venovenous hemodialysis
    C. Hemodialysis
    D. Ultrafiltration

49. Your patient has been in the intensive care unit (ICU) for 8 days following a motor vehicle crash. He has been receiving famotidine, heparin, morphine, and furosemide (Lasix). You note a sudden decrease in platelet count from 1,25,000 to 60,000. What is the most likely cause?

    A. Thrombocytopenia from excessive lab draws
    B. Dilutional thrombocytopenia
    C. Heparin-induced thrombocytopenia (HIT)
    D. Disseminated intravascular coagulation (DIC)

50. A nurse, being a moral agent, should emphasize which of the following principles?

    A. Natural law
    B. Justice
    C. Paternalism
    D. Autonomy

51. A patient presents to the hospital with an exacerbation of their coughing and shortness of breath. They have a significant history of smoking. Which of the following sputum assessments would most likely indicate the presence of a pulmonary infection?

    A. Tenacious, brown-tinged sputum
    B. Pink, frothy sputum
    C. Rust-colored sputum
    D. Yellow/green sputum

52. When your patient arrives in the intensive care unit (ICU) from surgery, his daughter is very demanding and wants to come in to see her father immediately. Which of the following statements by the ICU nurse is the most appropriate response?

    A. "I know it is very important for you to see your father to assure that he is OK. Give me 10 min to hook him up to the monitors and I will come get you"
    B. "You will just need to wait. There is a lot of work that needs to be done on patients coming from the OR"
    C. "We will call you when we are ready. It is our policy that visitors need to wait until we are ready"
    D. "We will have to ask you to leave if you do not follow our ICU policies"

53. Which of the following statements by the patient indicates that the patient understands the discharge instructions following a mechanical valve placement?

    A. I know I will have to take a blood thinner for the rest of my life
    B. I don't have any exercise restrictions at this time
    C. I will need to start taking a statin for my cholesterol
    D. I can drive my car within 2 weeks

54. A patient is diagnosed with Fournier gangrene. Where is the necrotizing fasciitis located?

    A. Submandibular and sublingual spaces
    B. Upper arm
    C. Perineum
    D. Oral cavity

55. A patient presents with history of hypoxia and is noted to have elevated pulmonary artery pressures (PAP) and elevated left atrial pressures (LAP). Which of the following best defines this patient's findings?

    A. Pulmonary arterial hypertension (PAH)
    B. Cor pulmonale
    C. Pulmonary venous hypertension (PVH)
    D. Primary pulmonary hypertension

56. Which of the following ventilator changes would best adhere to a lung protective ventilation strategy?

    A. Increase the respiratory rate
    B. Increase tidal volume
    C. Increase FiO_2
    D. Increase positive end-expiratory pressure (PEEP) levels

57. Which of the following symptoms will typically require urological imaging in a trauma patient?

    A. Flank pain
    B. Hematuria
    C. Kernig's sign
    D. Hypotension

58. Your patient is currently on 20 mg furosemide TID and has a positive fluid balance and decreasing urine output. Which of the following interventions would be most appropriate at this time?

    A. Initiate continuous venovenous hemodialysis (CVVHD)
    B. Change to or add a thiazide diuretic
    C. Increase the frequency to QID
    D. Administer low-dose dopamine

59. Which of the following acids will cause a non-anion gap metabolic acidosis?

    A. Lactate
    B. Chloride
    C. β-Hydroxybutyrate
    D. Glycolate

60. An intensive care unit (ICU) patient with sepsis and acute tubular necrosis (ATN) is on a bicarbonate continuous infusion. It is noted that he remains hyperkalemic (K^+ 5.8) and acidotic (7.26). Which of the following interventions would the intensive care unit (ICU) nurse expect to be ordered at this time?

    A. Renal replacement therapy (RRT)
    B. Glucose and insulin infusion
    C. Administer saline bolus
    D. Administer dopamine

61. A female patient from Saudi Arabia is admitted for acute coronary syndrome. Her husband has accompanied her to the intensive care unit (ICU) and is upset because a male nurse is attempting to perform an assessment. Which of the following is the most appropriate response to the situation?

    A. Explain to the husband that the male nurse is a professional and this is his assignment
    B. Call security to de-escalate the situation
    C. Ask the husband to leave the room while the assessment is being performed
    D. Change the assignment to a female nurse to accommodate the husband's wishes

62. Which of the following statements is the most appropriate regarding written patient education material for the patient or family?

    A. It should be used as a supplement to verbal explanation
    B. It is the best method for teaching patients and families
    C. It should be written at a college level to provide the most complete explanation
    D. It is used to provide immediate understanding but is not useful for later recall

63. Which of the following tools is used to assess for the severity of symptoms of alcohol withdrawal in the acute care setting?

    A. Clinical Institute Withdrawal Assessment for Alcohol scale (CIWA-Ar)
    B. ICU Confusion Assessment Method (ICU-CAM)
    C. Richmond Agitation Sedation Scale (RASS)
    D. Pasero Opioid-induced Sedation Scale (POSS)

64. Which of the following is the term in the synergy model used to describe the patient's capacity to return to a restorative level of functioning?

    A. Vulnerability
    B. Predictability
    C. Stability
    D. Resiliency

65. Which of the following is most recommended to improve oxygenation in acute respiratory distress syndrome (ARDS)?

    A. Increase the FiO_2
    B. Increase the positive end-expiratory pressure (PEEP)
    C. Decrease the ventilator rate
    D. Increase the flow rate

66. A patient with HF has an EF of 28% and prolonged QRS interval due to abnormal conduction. Which of the following would be the recommended therapy to manage this patient?

    A. Inotropic therapy
    B. Cardiac resynchronization therapy
    C. Diuretic management
    D. Vasopressor therapy

67. A patient receiving plasmapheresis should be monitored for which life-threatening electrolyte abnormality?

    A. Hypokalemia
    B. Hypoglycemia
    C. Hypocalcemia
    D. Hypernatremia

68. A patient is being treated for hyperglycemia and ketoacidosis. During the management, the following was found:

    serum pH 7.20
    anion gap 10
    osmolar gap 8

    Which of the following would be the most accurate statement regarding this patient's management?

    A. Continue treating the ketoacidosis with insulin
    B. Administer sodium bicarbonate
    C. Ketoacidosis has resolved and metabolic acidosis are not due to ketones
    D. Patient is normalized and requires no further treatment

69. Following extubation, your patient begins to have high-pitched wheezing audible without a stethoscope. Which of the following would be an appropriate initial intervention?

    A. Call anesthesia to reintubate the patient
    B. Place 40% FM and observe the patient
    C. Administer aerosolized racemic epinephrine
    D. Prepare the patient for a bronchoscopy

70. During your shift, another intensive care unit (ICU) nurse became angry and screamed at you regarding responsibilities in the unit. Which of the following would be the most appropriate response?

    A. Ignore the nurse; she will get over her anger in time
    B. Call the nurse manager and report the behavior immediately
    C. Ask other nurses if they think you were in the wrong
    D. Communicate with the angry nurse and discuss facts, not opinions

71. A patient has been on a sodium bicarbonate infusion to manage his metabolic acidosis following a toxic overdose. He has been diuresing 300–350 mL hour. Which electrolyte abnormality should be the greatest concern for the intensive care unit (ICU) nurse with this patient?

    A. Hypernatremia
    B. Hyperkalemia
    C. Hyperglycemia
    D. Hyperphosphatemia

72. Which of the following injuries most likely results in rapid peritonitis?

    A. Gastric rupture
    B. Duodenal rupture
    C. Liver laceration
    D. Splenic injury

73. Which of the following cardiovascular drugs is considered the gold standard for preventing sudden cardiac death from lethal ventricular arrhythmia?

    A. Lanoxin (digoxin)
    B. Lopressor (metoprolol)
    C. Cordarone (amiodarone)
    D. Covera-HS (verapamil)

74. A physician orders an alginate dressing for your patient's wound. Which of the following wound descriptions would you expect to find?

    A. Noninfected wound without drainage
    B. Wound with granulated tissue
    C. Large infected, draining wound
    D. Wound requiring autolytic debridement

75. A patient is admitted to the intensive care unit (ICU) in a myasthenic crisis. Which of the following would be the highest priority of the intensive care unit (ICU) nurse caring for this patient?

    A. Obtain electrolytes and replace as needed
    B. Hold the patient's anticholinergic drugs until the symptoms are alleviated
    C. Assess ventilation and provide ventilatory support as needed
    D. Intubate the patient immediately and initiate IV fluids

76. Your patient's cardiologist has a reputation for screaming and berating the nurses when being called for an issue. The patient was having arryhthmias, but the nurse was afraid to call the physician. The patient suffered a cardiac arrest. Which of the following would have changed this outcome?

    A. Zero tolerance for abusive behavior from the hospital's leadership
    B. Providing more disciplinary actions when nurses do not call physicians with updates
    C. Increase the inservicing and education to the nurses to recognize when a patient is deteriorating
    D. Develop a plan for charge nurses to round on the patients hourly to assure physicians are called in a timely manner

77. A patient has an ejection fraction (EF) of 30% following a myocardial infarction and has recently developed a third-degree heart block (HB). Which of the following interventions would most likely be recommended at this time?

    A. Biventricular pacemaker
    B. Intra-aortic balloon pump (IABP)
    C. Left ventricular assist device (LVAD)
    D. Ventricular pacemaker

78. A patient with a current history of substance abuse is in the intensive care unit (ICU) following a traumatic injury. The physician orders that normal saline be given as a "placebo," instead of an opioid, when the patient complains of pain. Which of the following ethical principles does this action most violate?

    A. Justice
    B. Fidelity
    C. Veracity
    D. Paternalism

79. Your patient's arterial blood gas (ABG) is the following: pH 7.50, $PaCO_2$ 25, bicarb 25. Which of the following would be the correct interpretation?

    A. Respiratory acidosis
    B. Respiratory alkalosis
    C. Metabolic acidosis
    D. Metabolic alkalosis

80. An automatic internal cardioverter defibrillator (AICD) may be indicated in which of the following cardiomyopathies to prevent sudden cardiac death?

    A. Dilated cardiomyopathy
    B. Constrictive cardiomyopathy
    C. Hypertrophic cardiomyopathy
    D. Restrictive cardiomyopathy

81. Which of the following terms best describes a research study using randomization to two groups to test the effect of an intervention?

    A. Quasi-experimental study
    B. Experimental study
    C. Descriptive study
    D. Qualitative study

82. An 82-year-old patient lives at home and is admitted with altered mental status. The brain computed tomography (CT) scan found multiple subdural hematomas of varying ages (acute, subacute, and chronic). The patient is awake in the intensive care unit (ICU) and has several of his family members with him at the bedside. The ICU nurse suspects elder abuse. Which of the following would be the most appropriate intervention by the nurse?

    A. Immediately call the police to question the family regarding elder abuse
    B. Tell the family about the abuse suspicions
    C. Have the physician talk with the patient and family together
    D. Ask the family to wait in the family room. Once the patient is alone, ask the patient directly about possible abuse

83. A patient is admitted to the intensive care unit (ICU) with a history of chronic renal failure and a new acute kidney injury (AKI) event. Her potassium level is 8.2 mEq/L, and she is extremely acidotic and unresponsive. Which of the following interventions would be most appropriate at this time?

    A. Peritoneal dialysis
    B. Continuous venovenous hemodialysis (CVVHD)
    C. Hemodialysis
    D. Ultrafiltration

84. Which of the following findings on a CXR may indicate presence of pericardial tamponade?

    A. Pleural effusion
    B. "Water-bottled" shape of cardiac silhouette
    C. Kerley B lines
    D. Widened-mediastinum

85. A patient is admitted to the intensive care unit (ICU) following an anterior myocardial infarction (MI). Within 24 hours, she develops sudden onset of new, loud, holosystolic murmur and demonstrates progressive shortness of breath, tachycardia, and pulmonary congestion. Which of the following is the most likely cause of these symptoms?

    A. Left ventricular (LV) wall rupture
    B. Ventricular septal wall rupture
    C. Aortic valve rupture and regurgitation
    D. Cardiogenic shock

86. A patient is being admitted to the ICU from the ED. He is hypothermic, bradycardic, hypotensive, and unresponsive. Which of the following would be the most likely diagnosis?

    A. Wilson's disease
    B. Myxedema coma
    C. Myelodysplastic syndrome
    D. Paraneoplastic syndrome

87. Which of the following statements is true regarding the management of acute respiratory distress syndrome (ARDS)?

    A. Tidal volumes are based upon actual body weight
    B. Recommended tidal volume is 6–8 mL/kg
    C. positive end-expiratory pressure (PEEP) can prevent the onset of ARDS
    D. The goal is peak inspiratory pressure less than 10 cm H_2O

88. Which of the following drug therapies is considered the treatment of choice for trigeminal neuralgia?

    A. Gabapentin
    B. Fentanyl
    C. Dilaudid
    D. Morphine

89. A patient in the intensive care unit (ICU) has a history of C6 complete spinal cord injury. He is admitted for cholecystitis and acute abdomen. While in the ICU, he develops a BP of 210/112. What should the nurse initially do for the patient?

    A. Elevate the head of the bed
    B. Administer an antihypertensive
    C. Turn the patient to the supine position
    D. Rehydrate the patient with a liter of fluid

90. A patient with an induced medical coma is in the intensive care unit (ICU). The family is at the patient's bedside, and they are talking over the patient's bed about the prognosis. Which of the following is the best response by the ICU nurse?

    A. Ask the family to step out in the waiting room to have their discussion
    B. Inform the family that patients in a coma are believed to still be able to hear
    C. Allow the family to discuss whatever they want at the patient's bedside, because it is their right
    D. Call the nurse manager to come and talk with the family regarding their behavior

91. Which of the following would more likely be an indication for a coronary artery bypass graft (CABG) procedure?

    A. Left anterior descending (LAD) occlusion
    B. Right ventricular (RV) infarction
    C. Left main occlusion
    D. Inferior wall infarction

92. In the adult patient, which of the following bones is more likely to be involved with osteomyelitis?

    A. Femur
    B. Vertebral bodies
    C. Knee joint
    D. Mandible

93. A patient with a tricyclic antidepressant overdose is admitted to the intensive care unit (ICU) for cardiac monitoring and treatment. Which of the following electrocardiogram (ECG) changes is monitored closely to recognize a potentially life-threatening complication of the overdose?

    A. Elevated ST segment
    B. Prolonged PR interval
    C. Wide QRS complexes
    D. Peaked T waves

94. A patient resuscitated from sudden cardiac arrest is improving. After extubation, the patient tells the nurse that he had a vivid dream and can recall being outside of his body watching the resuscitation. Which of the following is the best response by the nurse?

    A. Tell the patient that out-of-body experiences do not exist
    B. Ask the physician for a psychiatric referral for the patient
    C. Explain intensive care unit (ICU)–induced delirium to the patient and assure him that it was just a hallucination
    D. Listen to the patient and reassure him that many people have had this experience

95. A patient is in the ICU, intubated, foley, gastric tube to suction. An arterial bood gas (ABG) found: pH 7.52, $PaCO_2$ 50, Bicarb 30. Which of the following would be the correct interpretation?

    A. Respiratory acidosis
    B. Respiratory alkalosis
    C. Metabolic acidosis
    D. Metabolic alkalosis

96. A patient has been diagnosed with hypertrophied cardiomyopathy. He has an internal defibrillator. The wife is concerned about what to do if he collapses. What would be the best response by the nurse?

    A. Would you be interested in attending a CPR class?
    B. It will be OK. He has a defibrillator that will shock him if he collapses
    C. Would you like some assistance with case management to place him in an assisted living home?
    D. You will get used to it. There are many people that have this same issue

97. The following arterial blood gas values are obtained in a patient with acute respiratory distress syndrome (ARDS) who is being managed with lung protective strategies:

    pH 7.31
    $PaCO_2$ 58
    PaO_2 78
    SaO_2 90%

    Which would the nurse expect to be the most appropriate intervention?

    A. Increase FiO_2
    B. Decrease tidal volume
    C. Increase the respiratory rate
    D. No ventilator change recommended

98. Which of the following is the most likely cause of inadequate uptake of oxygen after blood transfusions?

    A. Metabolic acidosis
    B. High potassium
    C. Low levels 2,3 DPG
    D. Concentrated RBCs

99. What is the primary role of an intensive care unit (ICU) nurse who is caring for a patient enrolled in a medical research study being performed by the physician's group?

    A. Determine if the medical research study is feasible
    B. Obtain all the signed consent forms for the physicians
    C. Identify problems regarding the study format and inform the physician
    D. Protect the rights of the patients

100. A patient is admitted with the diagnosis of amyloidosis. Which of the following would best describe the cardiovascular effects of the disease process?

   A. Amyloidosis results in a diastolic dysfunction
   B. Amyloidosis is classified as a constrictive cardiomyopathy
   C. Postirradiation fibrosis is a direct cause of amyloidosis
   D. Amyloidosis is easily managed with an inotropic agent

101. Which of the following components of a fascia bundle is most susceptible to ischemic injury?

   A. Muscle
   B. Nerve
   C. Bone
   D. Vascular

102. Which of the following is a benefit of family presence during resuscitation?

   A. The family member will see that everything was done for the loved one
   B. The staff will try harder to resuscitate the patient
   C. The resuscitation time will be shorter if the family member is present
   D. The physician will interact better with the staff during the resuscitation

103. Which of the following best describes the ventilatory complication of volutrauma?

   A. Use of excessive airway pressures during ventilation
   B. Increased exudate and cytokines in alveoli
   C. Collapse of distal airways with small lung volumes
   D. Use of high tidal volumes during ventilation

104. A patient in the intensive care unit (ICU) has a history of congestive heart failure and is presently on the following medications:

   Captopril
   Digoxin
   Potassium replacement
   Furosemide (Lasix)

   Which of the following would be the most likely cause of angioedema?

   A. Captopril
   B. Digoxin
   C. Potassium
   D. Furosemide

105. Which of the following medications is most commonly used to prevent seizures in patients with eclampsia?

   A. Magnesium sulfate
   B. Phenytoin
   C. Keppra
   D. Calcium gluconate

106. Which of the following is an indication for thrombolytic therapy following an acute myocardial infarction when Cath lab is not immediately available?

    A. Non-ST segment elevation myocardial infarction (NSTEMI)
    B. Non-Q wave myocardial infarction (MI)
    C. ST segment elevation myocardial infarction (STEMI)
    D. Unstable angina

107. Which of the following diagnostics is the least effective in evaluating a patient with a potential blunt cardiac injury (BCI)?

    A. ECG
    B. Echocardiogram
    C. Chest CT scan
    D. Cardiac enzymes

108. Allowing a patient to make decisions will assist with giving control back to the patient and lowering anxiety. Which of the following would be an appropriate decision to assist with preventing loss of self-control?

    A. Whether the patient wants to be turned or remain supine
    B. Which family members can visit and for how long
    C. Whether the patient wants an IV or not
    D. Whether the patient wants to remain in the intensive care unit (ICU) or transfer to the progressive care unit

109. A thrombotic stroke patient in the intensive care unit (ICU) is within 24 hours of the stroke but did NOT receive tPA. The following are the current vital signs:

    Blood pressure (BP) 194/98
    Heart rate (HR) 88
    Respiratory rate (RR) 18
    Temperature 38.5 C (101.3 F)

    Which of the following would be the priority of care for this patient?

    A. Administer acetaminophen to reduce temperature
    B. Administer an antihypertensive to control blood pressure (BP)
    C. Prepare the patient for a follow-up computed tomography (CT) scan
    D. Notify respiratory therapy for assistance with patient's ventilation

110. Which of the following is a barrier to learning that the intensive care unit (ICU) nurse should recognize and make adjustments to before attempting to provide patient education?

    A. Small degree of anxiety
    B. Behaviors demonstrating that the patient is striving for recognition
    C. Need for confidence in a skill
    D. Poor language or reading skills

111. Which of the following parameters is used to measure the strength of respiratory muscles?

    A. FEV1
    B. Spontaneous tidal volume
    C. RR/Vt ratio
    D. Maximal inspiratory pressure

112. During the assessment of a casted arm, you note the patient complains of paresthesia. This could indicate which of the following?

    A. Muscle necrosis

    B. Nerve injury

    C. Irreversible tissue injury

    D. Compression of the vasculature

113. A patient is ready to transfer to your floor. She has a history of cardiovascular disease. The patient does not exercise and eats unhealthily. Which of the following would be the best focus for patient education at this time, using the holistic nursing approach?

    A. Harmful effects of alcohol

    B. Smoking cessation

    C. Family support groups

    D. Lifestyle changes

114. A patient presents with septic shock and a pulmonary artery catheter (PAC) is placed to monitor hemodynamics. Which of the following combinations of cardiac output (CO) and systemic vascular resistance (SVR) would the nurse expect to find?

    A. Increased CO and increased SVR

    B. Decreased CO and increased SVR

    C. Decreased CO and decreased SVR

    D. Increased CO and decreased SVR

115. Which of the following procedures is a less invasive surgical treatment of aortic stenosis?

    A. Aortic valve replacement

    B. Aortic valvuloplasty

    C. Percutaneous transaortic technique

    D. Transcatheter aortic valve replacement (TAVR)

116. What is the life-threatening complication of HELLP?

    A. Hemorrhage

    B. Acute liver failure

    C. Liver rupture

    D. Venous thromboembolism

117. While caring for a patient in septic shock, the physician places a central line to be used for $ScvO_2$ monitoring. The intensive care unit (ICU) nurse notes that the $ScvO_2$ is 60%. Which of the following interventions would be indicated at this time?

    A. Initiate broad-spectrum antibiotics

    B. Obtain lactate and procalcitonin levels

    C. Administer steroids

    D. Initiate dobutamine infusion

118. Which of the following is the most sensitive and specific diagnostic for aortic dissection?

    A. Chest x-ray (CXR)

    B. Magnetic resonance imaging (MRI)

    C. Transesophageal echocardiogram

    D. Ventilation perfusion (VQ) scan

119. The neurologist calls to schedule a lumbar puncture (LP) for a patient in the intensive care unit (ICU). The nurse caring for the patient notes that the patient is currently on a low molecular weight heparin (LMWH) to prevent venous thromboembolisms (VTEs). Which of the following is the most appropriate response by the nurse?

    A. Discuss the need to wait for 12 hours after the administration of LMWH with the physician
    B. Administer a dose of protamine sulfate prior to the LP
    C. Obtain a prothrombin time/partial thromboplastin time (PT/PTT) before the procedure
    D. Hold the next dose of LMWH for 24 hours

120. Which of the following types of cancer has the highest risk for the development of tumor lysis syndrome (TLS)?

    A. Glioblastoma multiform
    B. Multiple myeloma
    C. Acute leukemia
    D. Oat cell carcinoma

121. You are on a rapid response team that was called to a patient's room because of a decrease in the level of consciousness. Which is the initial lab you want to assist you with managing this patient?

    A. Sodium level
    B. Glucose level
    C. Complete blood count (CBC) with differential
    D. Ammonia level

122. Which of the following would be more diagnostic for the motor weakness found in PICS?

    A. MRI of brain
    B. Electromyography-Nerve Conduction Velocities (EMG-NCV)
    C. Peripheral nerve with Train of Four
    D. Vagal nerve stimulator (VNS)

123. A patient presents with a facial droop and arm weakness but resolves in the ED. The patient is admitted with TIA and during the diagnostic work-up, was found to have greater than 70% stenosis of carotid artery. Which of the following therapy is the more likely to be recommended?

    A. Endovascular thrombectomy
    B. Metformin
    C. Anticoagulation therapy
    D. Carotid endarcterectomy (CEA)

124. While caring for a patient being managed with therapeutic hypothermia, the patient's temperature is not reaching the goal of 34 °C. Which of the following is the most accurate statement regarding therapeutic hypothermia?

    A. If unable to obtain the goal temperature within 2 hours, therapeutic hypothermia should be discontinued
    B. Hypothermia below 36 °C is not recommended, and the nurse needs to notify the physician
    C. Surface cooling is a more rapid induction of hypothermia than intravascular cooling, and is the preferred route
    D. Shivering during induction can increase the body temperature and should be treated

125. A patient is admitted into your ICU with a recent history of being a kidney transplant recipient. Which of the following would be a sign of an infection in this patient?

    A. Purulent drainage from the incision

    B. Leukocytosis

    C. Fever

    D. Thrombocytopenia

126. Which of the following interventions has been found to decrease the incidence of post-intensive care syndrome (PICS)?

    A. Administer sedatives while in ICU

    B. ICU diary

    C. Limit visitation

    D. Maintain dark room 24 hours a day

127. A patient is one day post-myocardial infarction. He is being mechanically ventilated and has the following vital signs:

    BP 96/48

    HR 142

    RR 28 (IMV of 8)

His ABG results are:

    pH 7.38

    $PaCO_2$ 32

    PaO_2 68

    SaO_2 91% on 40% FiO_2

Which of the following statements best reflects the intensive care unit (ICU) nurse's correct understanding of the weaning process?

    A. The patient is not ready to be weaned from the ventilator due to his hemodynamic instability

    B. The patient should have spontaneous breathing trials started to decrease his number of ventilator days

    C. The patient needs more Ativan to improve his ventilation compliance and oxygenation

    D. The patient is ready to be extubated and monitored on a telemetry unit

128. Which of the following is an important step in providing family-oriented care in the intensive care unit (ICU)?

    A. Written information regarding expectations in the ICU

    B. An open visitation policy

    C. Encouraging patients to become involved in self-care

    D. Allowing autonomy of the patient

129. The intensive care unit (ICU) nurse notes serous-appearing drainage saturating the head dressing of a patient being monitored for intracranial pressure via intraventricular catheter. Which of the following would be the nurse's most appropriate response?

    A. Reinforce the dressing and continue to observe

    B. Notify the physician of the drainage

    C. Lower the drainage chamber to facilitate drainage through the catheter

    D. Discontinue the ICP monitor at this time

130. Which of the following is a symptom of central pontine myelinolysis that can occur with the administration of 3% saline?

    A. Quadriparesis
    B. Dysphagia
    C. Delirium
    D. Increased intracranial pressure (ICP)

131. Which of the following would be an indication to discontinue the intra-aortic balloon pump (IABP)?

    A. Tolerating a 1:1 inflation ratio
    B. Loss of sensorimotor function in the affected extremity
    C. Bleeding at the insertion site
    D. Development of fever

132. What is the hallmark of hypodynamic shock in sepsis?

    A. High cardiac outputs
    B. Elevated lactate levels
    C. Low cardiac outputs
    D. Elevated D-dimer

133. A Hispanic woman in the intensive care unit (ICU) requires immediate surgery, and the physician states that he will be there shortly to obtain consent from the patient. Which of the following would be the most appropriate intervention?

    A. Call the husband and tell him to come to the ICU to meet with the physician and his wife
    B. Encourage the patient to make her own decisions
    C. Suggest to the physician that he use a two-doctor signature for the consent form
    D. Delay the surgery until the conflict can be resolved

134. A patient presents with a diagnosis of lung cancer and has recently received chemotherapy. They are febrile on admission to the ICU. Lab work shows a significant neutropenia. Which of the following should the ICU nurse expect the physician to order?

    A. Exchange blood transfusions
    B. Corticosteroids
    C. Plasmapheresis
    D. Blood cultures

135. Following a traumatic brain injury, your patient develops the syndrome of inappropriate antidiuretic hormone secretion (SIADH). The patient has a serum sodium level of 124 and is asymptomatic. Which of the following would be the most appropriate treatment for this patient?

    A. Restrict fluid intake
    B. Administer a liter bolus of normal saline (NS)
    C. Administer 3% saline
    D. Diurese with mannitol

136. What is the best method for assessing a patient's sleep quality in an awake patient?

    A. Continuous video EEG
    B. Self-report
    C. BIS monitor
    D. Richmond agitation and sedation score (RASS)

137. Your hospital's policy is to allow family to remain in the patient's room during a code resuscitation. Which of the following has been found to be the most important intervention to improve this experience?

    A. Allow all family members to be at the bedside to support each other
    B. Keep the resuscitation time short to prevent extra trauma to the family
    C. Assure that one healthcare provider is present with the family throughout the resuscitation
    D. Allow the family to hold their loved one's hand during the resuscitation

138. A patient in the intensive care unit (ICU) has been noted to have problems with sleeping at night. Which of the following nursing interventions would be most beneficial to assist this patient with sleeping at night?

    A. Administer a sedative at 10:00 p.m
    B. Turn the television on for background noise
    C. No visitors after 8:00 p.m
    D. A 5-min back rub

139. Which of the following electrolyte abnormality is commonly associated with compartment syndrome?

    A. Hypocalcemia
    B. Hyperchloremia
    C. Hyperkalemia
    D. Hyponatremia

140. Following a coronary artery bypass grafting (CABG) procedure, the intensive care unit (ICU) is monitoring mediastinal CT output. During the immediate postoperative period, the CT output was noted to be 250 mL within 1 hour. Which of the following would the intensive care unit (ICU) nurse expect to happen?

    A. Immediate return to the OR
    B. Administer protamine
    C. Nothing, this is normal output
    D. Perform autotransfusions

141. Which of the following would be an appropriate intervention by the intensive care unit (ICU) nurse, working as a patient advocate, to lower the incidence of infection?

    A. Assure enteral feeding in the stomach
    B. Use peripheral intravenous (PIV) catheters only
    C. Remove the Foley catheter as soon as possible
    D. Use chlorhexidine mouthwash every 2 hours

142. Which of the following is the most accurate statement regarding sedation in a critically ill patient?

    A. Sedation should be avoided to improve number of ICU days
    B. Pain management is more important than sedation
    C. Goal is light sedation
    D. Heavier sedation improves outcomes

143. Following a hemorrhagic stroke, a patient is unresponsive and has a poor prognosis. A family conference is scheduled to talk about end-of-life care. Which of the following is the most appropriate response of the nurse to the family?

    A. Your loved one may improve, don't give up hope. You never know, he may respond
    B. Your loved one has no chance of survival and we need to stop providing him care at this time
    C. Everything will be fine with your loved one. We just need to talk about your feelings and wishes at this time
    D. Your loved one has a severe injury and has a very low chance of survival. At this time, we can provide him with comfort and pain management to help him at the end of life

144. A patient present with severe inspiratory wheezing, increased work of breathing, and hypocarbia. Which of the following drug and routes are most appropriate to initially manage this patient's condition?

    A. Albuterol, inhaled
    B. Ipratropium, inhaled
    C. Methylprednisolone, inhaled
    D. Aminophylline, IV

145. Which of the following patients with pancreatitis would most likely require surgical intervention?

    A. Edematous pancreatitis
    B. Hemorrhagic pancreatitis with sterile necrosis
    C. Pancreatic inflammation
    D. Hemorrhagic pancreatitis with infected necrosis

146. A patient is in the intensive care unit (ICU) following a motor vehicle crash (MVC). She had a traumatic brain injury (TBI) and a blunt chest injury. Her complication of acute respiratory distress syndrome (ARDS) is being managed with lung recruitment techniques. Which of the following interventions should be avoided to prevent further complications?

    A. High positive end-expiratory pressure (PEEP) levels
    B. Permissive hypercapnia
    C. Pressure control (PC) ventilation
    D. Diuretic therapy

147. Which of the following is a nursing intervention that would potentially prevent PTSD in critically ill patients?

    A. Restrict family visitation
    B. Tell the patient to try to forget the ICU experience
    C. Reassure the patient frequently they will survive
    D. Maintain an ICU diary for the patient

148. A patient presents with an altered level of consciousness and blood glucose level of 650 mg/dL. The following lab values were obtained on admission:

    K^+ 3.1
    Na^+ 126
    Mg^+ 3.0
    $PO4^+$ 4.0

Based on these findings, which of the following interventions should be the initial treatment?

A. Administer bolus dose of insulin

B. Initiate a continuous low-dose infusion of insulin

C. Bolus 1-liter IV fluids over 30 min

D. Administer potassium IV

149. A patient is being evaluated for treatment options following the diagnosis of normal pressure hydrocephalus (NPH). A lumbar drain is placed and orders are to drain 10 mL/hour of CSF. Which of the following would be the greatest concern for the intensive care unit (ICU) nurse?

A. Loss of cerebral autoregulation

B. Subdural hematoma

C. Seizure

D. Anoxic brain injury

150. Which of the following diagnostic studies is considered the most informative tool for risk stratification for anginal chest pain?

A. 12-lead electrocardiogram (ECG)

B. Echocardiogram

C. Cardiac catheterization

D. Computed tomography angiogram (CTA)

Practice Test: Answers

1. **D) Metabolic acidosis-respiratory alkalosis**
   Salicylate (aspirin) is converted to salicylic acid, but it is a weak acid and does not typically cause the acidosis seen with the toxicity. The metabolic acidosis is more likely caused by uncoupling oxidative phosphorylation and the resultant increased anaerobic metabolism. The typical ABG of salicylate toxicity is metabolic acidosis with compensatory respiratory alkalosis. Increased respiratory rates are also caused by direct stimulation of the brainstem by salicylic acid.

2. **B) Left bundle branch block (LBBB)**
   Patients presenting with signs of angina with the presence of LBBB makes the diagnosis of STEMI more difficult because of the ECG changes of the LBBB. The ST-T wave changes in LBBB can obscure the findings of ischemia and infarction on a 12-lead ECG. Third-degree HB, atrial flutter, and prolonged QT interval may be present in AMI but do not obscure or make the diagnosis more difficult.

3. **C) Both cardiac and skeletal injury**
   CK-MB should be reported in both units and as the ratio of CK-MB to total CK. Following an injury to both cardiac and skeletal muscle (e.g., perioperative MI), the ratio of CK-MB to total CK may not be elevated, but the CK-MB units will be elevated. Skeletal injury only will result in a significant increase in CK, but will have less effect on the ratio of CK-MB to total CK. Renal failure and carbon monoxide poisoning may falsely elevate the ratio of CK-MB to total CK.

4. **A) Increase EtCO$_2$ with normal ventilation**
   An increase in end-tidal CO$_2$ (capnography) during normal ventilation may indicate the presence of dead space. Dead space is normal alveolar ventilation without perfusion. Abnormally high PaCO$_2$ for MV, not low, occurs in dead space. False high SaO$_2$ on pulse oximetry is a sign of carbon monoxide poisoning. Elevated base excess is a sign of hypovolemia and hypoperfusion.

5. **C) Restraining a patient on BiPAP is a safety issue**
   What other options do we have to assure compliance with BiPAP? Restraining a patient who is on BiPAP is a safety issue. If the patient vomited, she would not be able to remove her own mask due to the restraints and could aspirate. Looking at the fit of the mask, orientation of the patient, and education are other options that may enhance compliance. It may not be necessary to intubate until all other options are reviewed.

6. **D) Unstageable injury**
   If slough or eschar obscures the extent of tissue loss, it is called unstageable pressure injury. If eschar is removed, a stage III or IV would be revealed. Stage III has eschar but visibility of adipose. Stage IV is exposed fascia, muscle, tendon, ligament, cartilage, and bone. Deep tissue injury is intact skin with localized area of non-bleachable deep red or purple discoloration.

7. **D) A patient who has been on mechanical ventilation greater than 48 hours**
   Mechanical ventilation greater than 48 hr and coagulopathies are the two highest risk factors for stress ulceration and upper GI bleed. Pelvic fracture and immobilization are higher risks for venous thromboembolism (VTE). Meningitis presents a lower risk for GI complications.

8. **A) Rhabdomyolysis**

   Crush syndrome is a condition in which prolonged muscle compression leads to muscle necrosis and the releasing of myoglobin. Rhabdomyolysis is a form of acute kidney injury in which there is a large amount of injured muscle releasing myoglobin in the blood (myoglonemia) and is filtered through the kidneys (myoglobinurea). The urine would be dark amber if the patient was dehydrated.

9. **A) Hypercarbia**

   Hypercarbia is an ominous sign in asthma patients. It indicates a greater severity of airway obstruction and the need for close observation to determine the need for intubation. Tachypnea and tachycardia are commonly associated with asthma. An FEV1 of 70% of predicted is considered mild airway obstruction and would not be as concerning as hypercarbia.

10. **B) Forced vital capacity (fVC)**

    The fVC and negative inspiratory force (NIF) are two important assessments of a SCI ability to maintain own ventilation. They monitor ability of the respiratory muscles to generate a breath. C6 level of injury may require intubation and ventilation initially due to swelling of the cord. C4 level innervates the diaphragm. Temperature is important to assess for Poikliothermia, but airway and breathing are most important. Blood glucose levels are important to prevent further injury to the cord, but airway and breathing are priority. Serum osmolalities is not commonly monitored in an SCI patient.

11. **C) It is usually unilateral**

    Cellulitis is almost always unilateral. If bilateral skin findings are present, it is more likely a result of venous stasis. Cellulitis can be non-purulent or purulent (evidence of fluid collections or abscesses). Postoperative wounds, typically within the first 24 hr, may appear warm, red, and tender. This is inflammation and is a normal postoperative finding

12. **D) Facial cyanosis with chest petechiae**

    Severe crush injury to the chest can result in traumatic asphyxiation. The patient presents with craniofacial congestion, purple discolorations, petechial hemorrhages, and edema of the upper thorax and face. Papilledema indicates cerebral swelling and may not be present initially in traumatic asphyxiation. Stridor and inspiratory wheezes may be heard in partial airway obstructions but are not necessarily caused by traumatic asphyxiation. Hypoxia can occur but is not associated with airway swelling.

13. **C) Mitral insufficiency**

    Mitral insufficiency may be treated with annuloplasty if annular dilation is the cause of the regurgitation. Aortic valve abnormalities requiring surgical intervention involve valve replacement surgeries. Mitral stenosis may be surgically managed with commissurotomy or valve replacement.

14. **D) Resource availability**

    The patient has been weaned from the ventilator, extubated, and is off of all vasoactive infusions. This indicates that he is less vulnerable and complex now than he was immediately following the cardiac surgery. He is awake, alert, and follows commands, so he is likely to be able to participate in his own care. He has had no family members visit him since his surgery. This indicates that the area of concern is resource availability. He has minimal to no personal/psychological supportive resources or social system resources.

15. **C) Extravasation**

    Extravasation is the term used when the IV fluid that has leaked into the tissue damages tissues, causing cellular death and necrosis. Signs of extravasation include swelling, redness, and blistering. Infiltration is fluid leaking into the tissue, but the fluid is non-damaging. It can cause swelling and redness but does not usually result in blistering of the skin. Second-degree burns are described as redness and blistering, but IV infiltration/extravasation are not classified as burns. Leakage is not a formal term used to describe this event.

16. **D) Pulmonary fibrosis**
ARDS has a fibrin proliferative phase that eventually results in irreversible pulmonary fibrosis. This can lead to frequent respiratory infections and exercise intolerance in some patients. Atelectasis and pulmonary edema are short-term complications. Pulmonary embolism may be a complication, but is not considered an irreversible long-term complication.

17. **D) Reduce afterload with nitrates**
A patient with signs of being "cold and dry" is managed with afterload reduction. This includes medications such as nitrates or hydralazine. Since the patient does not have signs of hypotension, an inotropic therapy is not recommended. Ultrafiltration and diuresis are recommended with "wet" HF patients with signs of congestion.

18. **A) Call physician to obtain radiograph orders**
Crepitus noted during palpation of an extremity indicates the possibility of an underlying fracture, and a radiograph should be obtained. This scenario does not indicate the patient was in pain. Crepitus should not be ignored or considered an incidental finding.

19. **C) Bilateral fluffy infiltrates**
One of the criteria for the diagnosis of ARDS is the presence of bilateral fluffy infiltrates on the CXR. A consolidated lobe indicates lobar pneumonia. Cardiomegaly is found in heart failure, typically with pulmonary edema. Atelectasis occurs frequently with hypoventilation.

20. **B) Aggressive volume resuscitation**
The patient is hypotensive with abdominal pain following a bowel resection. A likely cause is generalized peritonitis, and aggressive fluid resuscitation is required to replace vascular losses due to third-spacing of fluid. Avoid vasopressors if possible, due to splanchnic vasoconstriction and worsening the ischemic condition of the bowel. An abdominal CT scan may be indicated, but the hypotension should be managed prior to transport. Placing a NG tube to low wall suction may not be indicated in this patient.

21. **D) Transpulmonary pressure-guided ventilation**
Transpulmonary pressure-guided ventilation is a non-conventional technique that uses an esophageal balloon catheter to measure pleural pressures and is used to determine the optimal PEEP and pressures for the individual. ECMO is used in severe ARDS or refractory hypoxemia. It brings the blood out through an external "artificial lung" to facilitate adequate gas exchange. HFOV delivers very rapid (high frequency), small tidal volumes with the goal to maintain mean airway pressure.

22. **B) Abdominal compartment syndrome (ACS)**
Early-onset respiratory failure and renal involvement following abdominal trauma are most likely due to abdominal compartment syndrome (ACS). The increased pressure in the abdomen contributes to respiratory and renal failure. ARDS can cause respiratory failure, but typically not in the first 24 hr. PE is a complication that can occur within 24 hr, but is less likely to be the result of the renal involvement. CHF is not a common complication of abdominal trauma.

23. **A) Respiratory acidosis**
Status asthmaticus can result in acute respiratory acidosis and can indicate a worsening of the patient's airway.

24. **B) The goal for titrating norepinephrine is to maintain mean arterial pressure (MAP) greater than equal to 65 mm Hg**
The goal with vasoconstrictors in septic shock patients is to maintain the MAP at or above 65 mm Hg. Fluid administration should be initiated before the vasopressor to fill the vessels. Norepinephrine is the vasoconstrictor of choice in managing septic shock patients. Dopamine is not strongly recommended in the current guidelines. One vasoconstrictor is recommended first; if this is ineffective, a second vasoconstrictor may be started.

25. **D) Of course**

What time would you like your bath?. Patients in the ICU commonly experience a loss of control that creates anxiety. Providing order and predictability can create an illusion of some control by the patient. This is called anticipatory guidance that keeps the patient from being surprised at a routine. Once the patient is able to make simple decisions, allow the patient to make small choices. Give some control back to the patient in areas in which he or she can make decisions.

26. **D) Set up a conference with the family and the health care providers to review the results and make a plan together regarding the next step.**

The number one identified need of the family members is the need for information. Families experience increased frustration when they get different information from different health care providers. Most families do not want "sugar-coated" answers; they want to be told the truth. Honesty and full disclosure of prognosis are recommended. Setting up a meeting with all of the health care providers is proactive and helps that the family hear one message.

27. **A) Thoracotomy**

Blood output greater than 1500 mL upon initial insertion of chest tubes indicates a massive bleed and is usually an indication for a surgical thoracotomy. Continued monitoring without treatment may result in severe blood loss and death. Stripping or replacing the chest tube is not indicated.

28. **D) Politely interrupt the conversation and explain to both the nurse and family members the issue**

When discussing a patient's health care information with a family member, make sure that the family members involved has the patient's approval to obtain health care information regarding the patient. Allowing the conversation to continue is a HIPPA violation.

29. **B) Obtain an order to get a specialty bed company to bring a bariatric chair**

Obtaining a bariatric chair that has an appropriate weight limit would be the best response. Refusing to get the patient out of bed would not benefit the patient. The nurse needs to be an advocate for the patient. Discussing the need to purchase chairs for bariatric patients is a good response but will not benefit this patient at this particular time. Using a chair that is not approved for the weight is an inappropriate answer. The nurse would be legally liable for injury incurred if the chair broke and the patient was injured.

30. **A) Administer fluid bolus**

Volume resuscitation is a priority in early sepsis because venodilation and fluid third-spacing cause a decrease in cardiac filling pressures. If fluid does not improve the patient's hemodynamics, vasopressors are recommended next. Steroids are not recommended until late in septic shock. Arterial and central lines are recommended but would not be a priority over administering fluids.

31. **C) Check for a disconnection**

A low-pressure alarm frequently indicates a disconnect. A kink or an obstruction would result in a high-pressure alarm. The catheter would not necessarily have to be replaced. There is no indication that heparin is required at this time.

32. **D) Surgical debridement of necrosis**

Surgical debridement is used to remove the infectious source and is the primary treatment of necrotizing fasciitis. Antibiotics may not be completely effective without the removal of necrotic tissue. Daily dressing changes of the wound may be ordered but is not the intervention used to control the source of the infection. Early ambulation is a recommendation for intensive care patients but is not a management technique specific to necrotizing fasciitis.

33. **D) Autopsy finding of neurofibrillary tangles and amyloid deposits**
AD is definitively diagnosed on autopsy with the findings of neurofibrillary tangles and amyloid deposits. AD does cause cerebral atrophy and enlarged ventricles, but this is not the definitive diagnosis. Lewy bodies are found in patients with dementia from Parkinson's disease.

34. **B) Metabolic acidosis**
The ABG interpretation reveals a partially compensated metabolic acidosis. The respiratory system compensates for metabolic acidosis by increasing the respiratory rate to blow off CO_2 (an acid), thus lowering the pH. Even though there are diminished breath sounds, the patient is unlabored with normal oxygenation, so atelectasis and pneumonia are the less likely causes of this patient's respiratory changes. This patient does not have metabolic alkalosis.

35. **C) Negative fluid balance**
Conservative fluid management in patients is recommended in patients with stable hemodynamics and adequate urine output. Current studies have shown a higher mortality in patients with a positive fluid balance. Use of PAC has been found to increase complications and mortality in some studies. Hypertonic saline is not indicated in ARDS patients.

36. **C) Patient may require a second fasciotomy of the involved calf**
Opening of the fascia will release the pressure in the muscle fascia and can prevent injury to muscle, nerves, and vessels within the compartment. Each extremity has two or more compartments and varies in numbers based upon the compartment. The calf has four compartments. Opening only one compartment may not have relieved the compression and a second fasciotomy may be recommended. Always look for a physiological cause before stating the patient has a low tolerance of pain or is drug seeking. Patient has a known fracture so radiographs would not be indicated.

37. **D) Do not combine Vicodin with other over-the-counter medications containing acetaminophen**
Acetaminophen is the most common cause of acute liver injury and acute liver injury is commonly caused by taking more than one drug containing acetaminophen. Taking Vicodin with food can limit some of the nausea and vomiting, but may not prevent it. Restricting to 2–3 days is probably inadequate for pain relief, and there is a low risk for addiction when taking opioids for acute pain management. Supplementing with NSAIDs is not recommended when the patient is taking a combined opioid and acetaminophen such as Vicodin.

38. **A) Beneficence**
Beneficence is the obligation to promote the welfare of others by maximizing benefits and minimizing harm. Beneficence is frequently used in ethical dilemmas in the hospital and refers to the health care practitioner's responsibility to benefit the patient, usually through acts of kindness, compassion, and mercy. Nonmaleficence requires that actions do not inflict harm. Justice is that every person is to be treated similarly, avoiding discrimination on the basis of age, sex, perceived social worth, financial ability, or cultural/ethnic background. Fidelity is the duty to be faithful to others by keeping promises and fulfilling contracts and commitments

39. **C) Adults are goal-oriented and can become impatient with isolated facts**
Adults are goal-oriented and may become impatient when presented with isolated facts instead of the whole picture. This is a part of the "need to learn" of an adult learner's motivation. Adult learners are usually less flexible and require more time to learn new tasks. Learning is usually on a voluntary basis, and the learner wishes for mutual construction of the learning plan.

40. **A) Obese patients**
Obese patients may present with falsely low BNP levels in HF. Advancing age, renal failure, and pulmonary embolism may cause a falsely high level of BNP.

41. **B) Hypokalemia**

    A beta2 agonist can cause hypokalemia by driving the potassium into the cells. Other electrolyte abnormalities that may occur following the administration of inhaled beta2 agonists include hyperglycemia, hypomagnesemia, and hypophosphatemia.

42. **B) I hear in your voice your anger**

    That is a normal reaction to an event like this. Let's take this one question at a time, and I will help you through this. The suddenness of injury or illness may cause family members to have uncertainty about the situation. They may approach the ICU nurse with multiple questions and concerns. The family is thrown into a whirlwind of activity and commonly experience feelings of helplessness. They are often unprepared for the whole impact of the injury or illness. Family members may ask "unanswerable" questions and usually do not expect an answer. It shows their deep and inner fears. Using a reflection helps to clarify the emotions and then offering to address all of their issues tells the family you are there for them. Using the words "I understand" can actually make families even more upset because you are not experiencing what they are at this time.

43. **C) QTc interval**

    Haldol's life-threatening complication is a prolonged QTc interval that can lead to ventricular tachycardia (torsades de pointes). It is recommended to note a baseline QTc and to monitor the QTc on a regular basis throughout treatment. Other drugs and electrolyte abnormalities can contribute to the prolonged QTc.

44. **C) Diuretic therapy**

    Diuretics can cause chloride wasting through the renal system. Aldosteronism or Cushing diseases result in loss of chloride through renal system. Chronic abuse of laxatives results in loss of chloride through the GI system. Salicylate overdose causes metabolic acidosis, not alkalosis.

45. **C) This blood gas test result indicates a worsening in the patient's COPD and requires further intervention**

    The ABG results indicate a worsening of the patient's COPD. Even though COPD can cause CO_2 retention and hypercarbia, the low pH (respiratory acidosis) indicates that the $PaCO_2$ is higher than usual and the CO_2 retention and hypercarbia are no longer compensated. A PaO_2 of 76 is low but is not considered severely hypoxic in a COPD patient. This is an acidosis. not an alkalosis.

46. **A) Westermark sign**

    Westermark sign, which is the dilation of the pulmonary vessels with a sharp cut-off, is a sign found on CXR suggestive of a PE. A Waterhammer sign is a bounding pulse followed by collapsing carotid pulse and is found in patients with aortic regurgitation. Kernigs sign is found in patients with meningitis and is a sign of meningeal irritation. Kerley B lines are found on CXR but are more indicative of pulmonary edema.

47. **B) Prinzmetal's variant angina**

    Prinzmetal's variant angina or vasospastic angina is presentation with typical anginal chest pain but caused by spasms of coronary arteries. This typically occurs at rest and bedtime hours. Esophageal spasms present like anginal chest pain but are actually caused by spasm of the esophagus. Microvascular angina is spasm caused by spasms within walls of small arterial blood vessels not the significant coronary arteries. Variant embolic disease is not coronary artery spasms.

48. **B) Continuous venovenous hemodialysis**

    Due to the patient's signs of hemodynamic instability (hypotension and tachycardia), continuous venovenous hemodialysis would be the most appropriate RRT at this time. Neither the K^+ or pH is considered life threatening at this time. Hemodialysis is intermittent and removes fluid more rapidly. This can lead to further hypotension and hemodynamic instability. Peritoneal dialysis is not indicated in acute renal failure. Ultrafiltration primarily moves water (removes excessive volume), but this patient also needs toxins removed (elevated creatinine and BUN).

49. C) Heparin-induced thrombocytopenia (HIT)

HIT is the most common cause of a drug-induced thrombocytopenia. The highest incidence of thrombocytopenia due to HIT occurs between day 5 and day 10 of heparin administration. This patient is 8 days post admission and has been receiving heparin. DIC can also decrease a platelet count, but there is nothing in the scenario to indicate DIC. This patient is on Lasix, not aggressive fluid resuscitation or blood administration, so dilutional thrombocytopenia is not the cause. Excessive lab draws have been associated with anemia, not with a sudden decrease in platelets.

50. D) Autonomy

Autonomy is a very important principle when a nurse is working as a moral agent for the patient or family. The nurse should respect, and not interfere with, choices and decisions made by the autonomous individual (patient and/or family member). Paternalism is when physicians overrule the family's or patient's wishes for the patient's own welfare. This principle is appropriately applied in certain situations, but it is not the primary principle used by moral agents for patients. Justice is the principle of fairness to everyone and is frequently applied in the distribution of scarce resources. Natural law is when actions are morally right because they are in accordance with the end purpose of human nature and goals. Natural law takes precedence over man-made law, but this principle is not commonly used to resolve ethical dilemmas in health care.

51. D) Yellow/green sputum

Evaluation of the color and consistency of sputum can be used to assist with identifying the underlying physiology of a patient with pulmonary complications. Yellow/green colored sputum indicates the presence of a pulmonary infection and can predict a positive culture. Tenacious brown tinged sputum is found in patients with asthmatic episodes. Pink, frothy sputum is a sign of pulmonary edema, typically associated with left heart failure. Rust colored sputum can be associated with Tuberculosis (TB).

52. A) "I know it is very important for you to see your father to assure that he is OK. Give me 10 min to hook him up to the monitors and I will come get you."

Avoid being defensive, and be positive when confronted by demanding patients and/or their families. Empathize with the daughter's experience and acknowledge her needs, then explain the situation. Just explaining or telling the family member that it is a "policy" can escalate the situation.

53. A) I know I will have to take a blood thinner for the rest of my life

A patient who has had mechanical valve replacement surgery will be on an anticoagulant for the rest of their life. There are typically exercise restrictions in the early postoperative phase, and such patients typically will not be allowed to drive for 4–6 weeks. Statins may be prescribed, but are not necessarily indicated following valve surgery.

54. C) Perineum

Necrotizing fasciitis can be classified based upon the anatomical site of infection. Fournier gangrene is necrotizing fasciitis that affects the perineum. Anaerobic bacteria are the typical cause of this infection. Ludwig's angina involves the submandibular and sublingual spaces.

55. C) Pulmonary venous hypertension (PVH)

Elevation of both the PAP and LAP indicates the pulmonary hypertension is probably secondary to left ventricular failure. This is called PVH. PAH has elevation of PAP but normal LAP. This is a primary pulmonary hypertension and can result in Cor pulmonale (right ventricular failure).

56. D) Increase positive end-expiratory pressure (PEEP) levels

The goal in lung protective ventilation is to ventilate the patient with a lower tidal volume (6 mL/kg) and to use PEEP to open collapsed airways. Increasing the respiratory rate can increase atelectrauma, increasing tidal volume can result in volutrauma injury, and increasing the FiO_2 can contribute to oxygen toxicity.

57. **B) Hematuria**
Hematuria is a common sign of GU trauma and would be a trigger for obtaining renal series of imaging. Flank pain would be more of a suspicious sign than abdominal pain with palpation. Kernig's sign is present in meningitis, not renal trauma. Hypotension in a trauma patient can be from multiple different injuries and does not necessarily indicate renal involvement.

58. **B) Change to or add a thiazide diuretic**
When furosemide no longer has the desired effect, the next step is to change to a thiazide diuretic. The dose or frequency should not be increased. Continued use of furosemide can cause a resistance to diuresis. Changing to a thiazide diuretic may improve diuresis. Furosemide is a loop diuretic, whereas thiazide diuretics block sodium reabsorption in distal renal tubules. Dopamine is an inotropic agent, not a diuretic. CVVHD is not required at this time.

59. **B) Chloride**
Hyperchloridemia is a cause of non-anion gap metabolic acidosis. Two common acids resulting in an anion gap are lactate (lactic acidosis) and β-hydroxybutyrate (ketoacidosis). Glycolate elevates anion gap and is caused by ethylene glycol poisoning.

60. **A) Renal replacement therapy (RRT)**
Renal replacement therapy (RRT) is indicated in acute renal failure patients who have refractory hyperkalemia and/or metabolic acidosis. Glucose and insulin are used to treat hyperkalemia, but the bicarbonate currently being used does the same and is not correcting the potassium overload. Fluid is administered in early sepsis, but this patient is already in intrarenal failure and may be at a higher risk for volume overload. Volume is not typically a treatment for intrarenal injury. Dopamine is not recommended in acute renal failure.

61. **D) Change the assignment to a female nurse to accommodate the husband's wishes**
Changing the assignment to allow a female nurse to care for this patient demonstrates cultural sensitivity and competency. Arab culture values female purity and maintains gender segregation. Their belief system involves extreme modesty for women and would require the woman to be kept completely covered if a male enters the room. Explaining to the husband that the male nurse is a professional does not address the issue of a male exposing the woman to perform an assessment. Requiring the husband to leave the room or calling security would escalate the situation and might interfere with patient care and well-being.

62. **A) It should be used as a supplement to verbal explanation**
Written material is a supplement to verbal instruction, and should not be used alone in most situations. It is useful for later review or as a reference. It should be written at a fourth-grade level.

63. **A) Clinical Institute Withdrawal Assessment for Alcohol scale (CIWA-Ar)**
CIWA-Ar (revised version) is currently the best tool to assess for the severity of alcohol withdrawal and can be used to titrate benzodiazepines. ICU/CAM assesses delirium. RASS and POSS assess for sedation.

64. **D) Resiliency**
Resiliency is the patient's capacity to return to a restorative level of functioning. Vulnerability is the level of susceptibility. Predictability allows one to expect a certain course of events or illness.

65. **B) Increase the positive end-expiratory pressure (PEEP)**
Increasing the PEEP will assist with improving the intrapulmonary shunt. The oxygenation of a patient with a significant shunt (e.g., ARDS) will not be significantly improved by increasing the FiO_2, so this is not considered the best intervention to improve oxygenation. Changing the ventilator rate and flow rate affects the $PaCO_2$ greater than the oxygenation.

66. **B) Cardiac resynchronization therapy**
   HF patients with EF below 35% and prolonged QRS interval requiring a pacemaker will benefit from cardiac resynchronization therapy to improve EF. Inotropic therapy has not been found to significantly improve outcomes in HF. Diuretic therapy is indicated in HF patients with signs of congestion but is not the recommended therapy for improving EF. Vasopressor therapy is not recommended and will worsen EF by increasing afterload.

67. **C) Hypocalcemia**
   During the external removal of blood, the risk of clotting increases. Citrate is commonly added to the blood to bind calcium and lower the clotting risk. This can lead to life-threatening hypocalcemia, so calcium levels should be monitored closely.

68. **C) Ketoacidosis has resolved and metabolic acidosis are not due to ketones**
   The patient continues to have metabolic acidosis despite a normal anion gap (12–15) and osmolar gap (<10). This indicates the ketoacidosis has resolved, but the patient has a metabolic acidosis caused by another underlying mechanism. It may be due to the treatment or lactic acidosis if patient was hypoperfused. Insulin may still be required if the patient is hyperglycemia, but it is not required to manage the acidosis at this time. Sodium bicarbonate is not indicated at this time because the pH is not less than 7.00. Patient still requires some treatment because they remain in metabolic acidosis.

69. **C) Administer aerosolized racemic epinephrine**
   The presence of audible wheezing (stridor) is a sign of laryngeal obstruction and may be due to laryngospasm after extubation. Aerosolized racemic epinephrine is the drug of choice for post-extubation stridor. The patient may also be placed on 100% FiO_2 to assist with managing the laryngospasm. Other interventions are tried before the patient is reintubated. A bronchoscopy is not indicated in this situation.

70. **D) Communicate with the angry nurse and discuss facts, not opinions**
   Conflict resolution begins by discussing the issue with the person directly in a nonthreatening manner. Use facts, not opinions, and discuss without anger. Ignoring the person or asking other people's opinions are not a part of conflict resolution. Attempt to resolve the conflict directly first, before involving a higher organizational level.

71. **A) Hypernatremia**
   The administration of sodium bicarbonate can cause a gain of sodium, and the resulting diuresis contributes to the hypernatremia by hemoconcentration. Hypernatremia would be the greatest concern with this patient. Hyperglycemia can also cause diuresis, but in this case hypernatremia is the greater concern. Hypokalemia would be a greater concern than hyperglycemia due to the diuresis. Hyperphosphatemia would be a concern in acute kidney injury (AKI).

72. **A) Gastric rupture**
   The fluid in the stomach is acidic and when spilled into the peritoneal cavity causes a rapid, severe peritonitis. Duodenal tears, however, may have minimal signs of peritonitis with mild irritation or tenderness of the abdomen initially. This is because the fluid in the duodenum and small bowel is alkaline, which causes less irritation. Liver laceration and splenic injury cause acute blood loss in the abdomen but not peritonitis.

73. **C) Cordarone (amiodarone)**
   Amiodarone is the only agent to date known to reduce the incidence of arrhythmogenic sudden cardiac death. Metoprolol, digoxin, and verapamil can affect conduction rates, but are not as effective in prevention of lethal arrhythmias.

74. **C) Large infected, draining wound**
Alginate dressings are used in large, draining, infected wounds. Hydrocolloids are used for non-infected wounds without drainage. Wounds with granulated tissue may require hydrogels. Transparent dressings are used for autolytic debridement.

75. **C) Assess ventilation and provide ventilatory support as needed**
In a myasthenic crisis, progressive weakness of the chest wall and diaphragm leads to ventilatory failure. The ICU nurse should assess ventilation closely, in case intubation and mechanical ventilation are needed. Not all myasthenia gravis crisis patients require intubation, so evaluation is the better answer. In an anticholinergic crisis, the patient's medications are held until symptoms resolve, at which time they are restarted at a lower dose. Breathing is a priority over electrolytes.

76. **A) Zero tolerance for abusive behavior from the hospital's leadership**
One aspect of skilled communication in a healthy work environment is zero tolerance for abusive or disruptive behavior. Outbursts and disruptive behavior may prevent a nurse from calling a physician to report patient changes or question an order. This may lead to medication or patient-care errors. Discipline and education are not the issues in this scenario; it is the fear of being abused by the nurse when calling a particular physician. Developing a plan for charge nurses to round may have changed the outcome but does not address the underlying issue of the physician's behavior.

77. **A) Biventricular pacemaker**
The use of a ventricular or AV pacemaker is indicated in patients with a third-degree HB, whereas in patients with a low EF, a biventricular pacemaker is indicated. This pacemaker paces in both the left and right ventricles, thus resynchronizing the ventricles and improving EF, stroke volume (SV), and cardiac output (CO).

78. **C) Veracity**
Veracity is the best answer because this principle refers to an individual's (nurse's) obligation to tell the truth and not to intentionally mislead the patient. By administering a placebo instead of an opioid, the nurse is not being truthful and is misleading the patient. Justice is the patient's right to be treated equally with other patients. Failing to inform the patient that he or she is receiving a placebo could also violate the justice principle. However, veracity is the main ethical principle being violated in this situation. The ethical principles of fidelity and paternalism would not be used to determine if placebos are ethical in this situation.

79. **B) Respiratory alkalosis**
A pH of 7.50 is alkalosis. A low $PaCO_2$ indicates respiratory alkalosis, and the bicarbonate is normal. This indicates the blood gas is respiratory alkalosis.

80. **C) Hypertrophic cardiomyopathy**
Hereditary hypertrophic cardiomyopathy has a high incidence of sudden cardiac death due to ventricular arrhythmias and may be an indication for placement of an AICD. The other cardiomyopathies listed do not present as high a risk for ventricular arrhythmias.

81. **B) Experimental study**
Experimental studies utilize both a control group and an experimental group to test the effects of an intervention Quasi-experimental studies involve the manipulation of variables but lack the control group. A descriptive study is non-experimental and describes situations or experiences. Qualitative studies include case studies and participant observations.

82. **D) Ask the family to wait in the family room**
Once the patient is alone, ask the patient directly about possible abuse. Establishing a good rapport and trusting relationship with elderly patients will allow them to feel safer about disclosing

mistreatment and abuse. Most of the time, they will not talk about the abuse while the family is present. Once the family leaves, opening the conversation about abuse may help the patient to discuss the situation. Then report the suspected abuse directly to adult protective services or to the ICU manager or social worker. Nurses should know their hospital's policy, and whether there is a protocol in place for reporting suspected or confirmed cases of elder abuse. Legally and ethically, nurses have a responsibility to protect the patient from further harm or injury.

83. **C) Hemodialysis**
This patient requires the rapid removal of life-threatening solutes and toxins. Her potassium level, "extreme" acidosis, and unresponsiveness are hints indicating the need for a more rapid clearance of solutes. CVVHD and peritoneal dialysis are slower methods for removing solutes and are not indicated in life-threatening situations. Ultrafiltration primarily removes excessive fluids.

84. **B) "Water-bottled" shape of cardiac silhouette**
The cardiac silhouette in pericardial tamponade appears as a "water-bottle" shape on CXR. Lack of the change on CXR does not rule out pericardial tamponade. Pleural effusions and Kerley B lines may accompany HF but are not typically used for identifying pericardial tamponade. A widened mediastinum is found with aortic transections, while an enlarged cardiac silhouette is found with pericardial tamponade and other cardiomyopathies.

85. **A)Left ventricular (LV) wall rupture**
A severe but uncommon complication of an anterior MI is rupture of the LV wall. Symptoms present as acute-onset cardiogenic shock and a holosystolic murmur. Ventricular septal wall rupture presents with systolic murmur but is not commonly associated with pulmonary congestion. It will demonstrate changes in oxygen saturation on the right side of the heart. Aortic valve rupture and regurgitation will cause a diastolic murmur with pulmonary congestion. Cardiogenic shock would not typically occur as a sudden onset with a systolic murmur.

86. **B) Myxedema coma**
Myxedema coma is severe prolonged hypothyroidism in which the patient can present with altered mentation, hypothermia, bradycardia, and hypotension. Myelodysplastic syndrome involves abnormal or low cells in the blood. Paraneoplastic syndrome can present with altered mentation but without hypothermia and bradycardia. It is a syndrome found in cancer patients and affects the central nervous system (CNS). Wilson's disease is an inherited disorder, which causes copper to accumulate in organs. It may affect the neurological system but does not present like this patient.

87. **B) Recommended tidal volume is 6–8 mL/kg**
The recommended tidal volume ventilator setting in ARDS patients is 6–8 mL/kg of ideal body weight. PEEP is used to improve oxygenation, but does not prevent ARDS. The goal is to maintain a peak inspiratory pressure of less than 40 cm H_2O pressure.

88. **A) Gabapentin**
Neuropathic pain is best managed with antiepileptic drugs or antidepressants. Opioids, such as fentanyl, dilaudid, and morphine, are not effective with neuropathic pain.

89. **A) Elevate the head of the bed**
The patient has significant hypertension. Elevating the head of the bed assists with lowering the patient's blood pressure while the cause of the hypertension is determined. The cause of the hypertension is most likely autonomic hyperreflexia (AH). In patients with spinal cord injury, this is frequently caused by an obnoxious stimulus below the level of injury (e.g., overfull bladder). Administering an antihypertensive before the source of the stimulation is found can cause hypotension once the stimulus is removed. Turning the patient supine and rehydrating with IV fluids do not manage the AH.

90. **B) Inform the family that patients in a coma are believed to still be able to hear**
Families may not be aware that patients in a coma, or medically induced coma, may still be able to hear. It is important to encourage the family to speak directly to the patient and not to discuss inappropriate issues over the patient's bed. Explaining the situation to the family is a better initial option than asking them to step out of the patient's room or involving the nurse manager.

91. **C) Left main occlusion**
The left main coronary artery is a small arterial segment but provides blood to both the left anterior descending (LAD) and left circumflex (LCX) arteries. It is more difficult to stent and occlusion can result in a loss of blood flow to the majority of the left ventricle.

92. **B) Vertebral bodies**
Vertebral bodies of the spine are more likely to be involved with infection in adult patients. Pediatric patients are at higher risk for long bone osteomyelitis. Knee joint is not commonly involved unless following knee replacement. Mandible is not a common location for osteomyelitis.

93. **C) Wide QRS complexes**
A cyclic antidepressant overdose can cause wide QRS complexes (>0.10 sec) and can result in ventricular tachycardia (torsades de pointes). The intraventricular delays are caused by the cyclic antidepressant slowing the influx of sodium into myocardial cells.

94. **D) Listen to the patient and reassure him that many people have had this experience**
There are many reports of patients having near-death experiences following periods of clinical death. The best response is to listen to the patients, be nonjudgmental, and reassure them. A report of such an experience does not mean the patient needs a psychiatric evaluation. There are support groups, though, if the patient desires them. Do not deny or disregard the experience.

95. **D) Metabolic alkalosis**
A pH of 7.52 is an alkalosis. High bicarb level (30) can cause an alkalosis. High $PaCO_2$ (50) causes an acidosis, not an alkalosis. This ABG is interpreted as a metabolic alkalosis partially compensated with elevation in $PaCO_2$.

96. **A) Would you be interested in attending a CPR class?**
Acknowledging the wife's fear and providing her with an option that will assist her to feel less helpless in this situation. Just reassuring a person or telling them how many other people have the same issue is not helping the wife to gain some confidence in caring for her husband. Assisted living might be an option but based upon the question the wife just needed some knowledge on what to do if he collapsed.

97. **D) No ventilator change recommended**
Lung protective ventilation allows hypercarbia without making a change in the respiratory rate or tidal volume. In ARDS patients, maintaining a saturation greater than 90% is an adequate goal and would not require increasing FiO_2 levels. A decrease in tidal volume can cause a further increase in $PaCO_2$.

98. **C) Low levels 2,3 DPG**
Administration of blood causes a decrease in 2,3 DPG levels and a shift in the oxyhemoglobin curve resulting in an increased affinity of hemoglobin for oxygen. This causes the inadequate uptake of oxygen at the tissue level. Metabolic acidosis actually can increase oxygen release at the tissue level. High potassium and concentrated RBCs do not affect the tissue oxygenation.

99. **D) Protect the rights of the patients**
The nurse's primary role in research studies is to protect the rights of the patients involved in the study. Working with the physician on feasibility, obtaining informed consents, and identifying issues at the bedside may be a part of the role, but the nurse's primary role is to remain a patient advocate.

100. **A) Amyloidosis results in a diastolic dysfunction**
Amyloidosis is a restrictive (not constrictive) cardiomyopathy that results in a diastolic dysfunction. The myocardial muscle is infiltrated by amyloid material, limiting elasticity and filling capabilities of the ventricles. Postirradiation fibrosis is also a type of restrictive cardiomyopathy but does not cause amyloidosis. An inotropic agent is not recommended to treat a diastolic dysfunction.

101. **A) Muscle**
An osteofascial compartment is a sheath of fascia, which binds the muscle and the neurovascular bundles. Compartment syndrome is an elevated pressure within the osteofascial compartments, which results in ischemic injury to muscle, nerve, and vascular structure. Of the components, muscle is most susceptible to ischemia.

102. **A) The family member will see that everything was done for the loved one**
Having a family member present during a resuscitation has been shown to be a benefit for the family. One of the commonly expressed benefits is that the family member is able to see that everything that could have been done for the loved one was done. This is better than being on the other side of the door and not knowing what is happening. Family presence should not make the staff try harder, improve physician interactions with staff, or decrease the resuscitation (which may not be a benefit in many cases).

103. **D) Use of high tidal volumes during ventilation**
Volutrauma occurs when large tidal volumes cause overdistention of the alveoli. Pressure-related injury is called barotrauma. Atelectrauma involves the collapse of the alveoli at the end of expiration. Increased levels of proinflammatories in the alveoli is called biotrauma.

104. **A) Captopril**
Angiotensin-converting enzyme (ACE) inhibitors, such as Captopril, may have an adverse effect of angioedema. Digoxin, potassium, and furosemide are not high-risk drugs for angioedema.

105. **A) Magnesium sulfate**
Magnesium sulfate infusions prior to cesarean delivery may be used for seizure prophylaxis and prevention of additional seizures. It has been found to be a better preventive in severe eclampsia than antiepileptic medications (phenytoin and Keppra) Calcium gluconate is not used for seizure prevention in eclampsia

106. **C) ST segment elevation myocardial infarction (STEMI)**
Indications for thrombolytic therapy include ST elevation, new-onset left bundle branch block (LBBB), and posterior wall MI. Thrombolytics are not indicated in NSTEMI or unstable angina. A non-Q wave MI may be either a STEMI or NSTEMI. The elevation of the ST segment determines whether a thrombolytic may be administered.

107. **C) Chest CT scan**
CT or MRI typically do not play a role in the initial evaluation of the blunt chest trauma patients for BCI. An ECG to evaluate for arrhythmias is recommended initially as well as cardiac enzymes (troponin levels). If ECG or cardiac enzymes are abnormal or the patient is hemodynamically unstable, an echocardiogram is recommended to assess the function of the heart.

108. **B) Which family members can visit and for how long**
Patients in the ICU commonly experience a loss of control that creates anxiety. Once the patient is able to make simple decisions, allow small choices to be made by the patient. Give some control back to the patients in areas in which they can make decisions. Patients should have the right to make decisions about visitors, such as who can visit and for how long. Patients need to be turned to prevent pressure sores. Giving them the choice of which side to be turned to is appropriate, but not whether they want to be turned or not. An IV is also a safety issue. Patients may assist by stating which arm they prefer but not whether they want an IV. When patients are ready to be

transferred to the PACU, they may require reassurance but are not given the choice to remain in the ICU.

109. **A) Administer acetaminophen to reduce temperature**
In this patient, the fever is the most important finding that requires immediate intervention. Fever (increased body temperature) has been found to worsen neurological outcomes. The BP is high but the patient did not receive a thrombolytic and is within 24 hr of the stroke. The BP is allowed to be elevated in such patients unless systolic is greater than 220 mmHg and diastolic is greater than 120 mm Hg. The patient may receive a follow-up CT scan in 24 hr, but this is not the priority of care. A respiratory rate of 18 by itself is not an indication that the patient needs assisted ventilation.

110. **D) Poor language or reading skills**
Poor language or reading skills are barriers to learning and should be recognized by the ICU nurse before attempting patient education. Materials should be presented in format and language the patient can understand. A small degree of anxiety is needed to learn, and an adult's tending to strive for recognition is not considered a barrier. Most people require confidence in a new skill, and a skill can be arranged from simple to complex, but these are not considered barriers to learning.

111. **D) Maximal inspiratory pressure**
Maximal inspiratory pressure (also called negative inspiratory pressure) is the standard clinical measurement of respiratory muscle strength. It is the negative pressure generated by maximum inspiratory pressure against a closed airway. FEV1 is the forced expiratory volume in 1 sec and is used to measure airway obstruction. Spontaneous Vt and the RR/Vt ratio are weaning parameters that are used to predict weaning success, but do not specifically measure respiratory muscle strength.

112. **B) Nerve injury**
When assessing using the 5 Ps, paresthesia is a finding of nerve injury as well as paralysis and pain. Muscle necrosis and irreversible tissue injury can occur with compartment syndrome but not a result of nerve compression. Compression of the vasculature would result in loss of pulse and pallor.

113. **D) Lifestyle changes**
Holistic nursing focuses on lifestyle changes, prevention, and overall well-being. The scenario gave the information that the patient does not exercise and eats unhealthy. This indicates a need for lifestyle changes to improve her health and to prevent further complications of cardiovascular and cerebrovascular disease. Education on smoking and alcohol can also benefit patients, but there was no indication in this scenario that the patient was a smoker or used alcohol. Family support groups are important, but the focus of this scenario was on the patient.

114. **D) Increased CO and decreased SVR**
Septic shock is classified as a type of distributive shock. In septic shock, the patient has significant vasodilation, which decreases the SVR. The decrease in afterload (resistance) causes the high CO that occurs in septic shock.

115. **D) Transcatheter aortic valve replacement (TAVR)**
TAVR is a less invasive route for replacing the aortic valve. An aortic valvuloplasty is more invasive and is not typically recommended because of the restenosis rate of the aortic valve. Percutaneous transaortic technique is not a procedure used for aortic valve replacement.

116. **C) Liver rupture**
Liver rupture is a severe complication of HELLP that requires immediate surgery. Emergency surgery is not delayed for diagnostic imaging studies. Low platelet counts occur but rarely low enough to cause hemorrhage. VTE are a risk of pregnancy but not of the HELLP.

117. **D) Initiate dobutamine infusion**
Dobutamine is one of the recommended interventions to be initiated in patients with sepsis/septic shock with low venous oxygenation. Dobutamine increases myocardial contractility and ejection fractions. Antibiotics should have already been initiated at the onset of sepsis, and are not used to increase venous saturations. Steroids are considered in septic shock to improve blood pressure. Obtaining lactate and procalcitonin levels is not an intervention and will not improve tissue oxygenation.

118. **B) Magnetic resonance imaging (MRI)**
An MRI is the most sensitive and specific diagnostic test for an aortic dissection (98% for both). A transesophageal echocardiogram has only a 77% specificity. CXR is more of a screening device, and VQ scan is used to diagnose a PE, not an aortic dissection.

119. **A) Discuss the need to wait 12 hr after the administration of LMWH with the physician**
LMWH should be held 12 hr prior to a LP or placement/removal of an epidural catheter, to prevent epidural hematoma. Administering protamine sulfate prior to the procedure may not be effective in reversing the LMWH. LMWH does not affect the PT or PTT levels. The next dose of LMWH may be administered within 12 hr of the procedure.

120. **C) Acute leukemia**
Acute leukemia associated with a high WBC count is one the highest risk cancers for the development of TLS. Chemotherapy triggers the rapid lysis of the neoplastic cells. The lowest risk is multiple myeloma and solid tumors. Glioblastoma and oat cell carcinoma are not considered a risk for TLS.

121. **B) Glucose level**
A glucose test is a point-of-care test that can be readily obtained at the bedside. Hypoglycemia is a common cause of a decreased level of consciousness and is manageable with glucose. Sodium, white blood cell (sepsis), and ammonia are also differentials, but not as immediate as glucose level.

122. **B) Electromyography-Nerve Conduction Velocities (EMG-NCV) studies**
Electromyography-Nerve Conduction Velocities (EMG-NCV) studies are used to evaluate muscle and nerve function. Patients with PICS and neuromuscular involvement will have EMG-NCV studies that demonstrate decreased amplitudes of sensory and motor nerve action potentials. MRI brain does not evaluate muscle function. Train of four is used with evaluating affect of the neuromuscular blocking agent not PICS. VNS is a treatment for seizures, not a diagnostic study.

123. **D) Carotid endarterectomy (CEA)**
CEA is typically recommended in symptomatic carotid stenosis. In this patient, they presented with neurological deficits and were found to have high-grade stenosis greater than 70% obstruction of the carotid artery so CEA or carotid artery stent (CAS) would be recommended. Endovascular thrombectomy is not recommended because the neurological symptoms are resolved. Metformin is not appropriate in the above scenario. Antiplatelets are the medical management of carotid stenosis, not necessarily anticoagulation therapy.

124. **D) Shivering during induction can increase the body temperature and should be treated**
During the induction phase, the body temperature is lowered to the goal range. The typical range ordered is 34–36 °C. Shivering is a common complication during the induction and maintenance phases. It increases body metabolism and generates heat. This is counterproductive and thus should be treated. Intravascular cooling has been found to be a more rapid route for induction than surface cooling. Combination routes can be used as well. Cooling for more than 2 hr to reach the temperature goal is not a reason to discontinue therapeutic hypothermia.

125. **C) Fever**
A recipient of a kidney transplant will be taking immunosuppressive agents. An immunosuppressed patient cannot increase WBCs so will not present with leukocytosis or purulent drainage even with an infection. Fever is the primary presenting symptom of an infection in an immunosuppressed patient. Thrombocytopenia is not a sign of infection.

126. **B) ICU diary**
ICU diary is initiated upon admission and may be written by both staff and family. It has been found to decrease PICS, post-traumatic stress disorder, and depression. Limiting visitation, dark rooms, and sedation may actually increase PICS.

127. **A) The patient is not ready to be weaned from the ventilator due to his hemodynamic instability**
The patient has a heart rate of 142 and a low BP of 92/48, one day post-Mi. Thus, he does not meet hemodynamic criteria to begin the weaning process from mechanical ventilation. He is also hypoxic with a rapid respiratory rate. Spontaneous breathing trials should be started when the patient is stable. Sedation with a benzodiazepine is not going to improve his oxygenation. He is definitely not stable enough for extubation at this time.

128. **B) An open visitation policy**
ICUs have been changing to become more family oriented. An important step is to allow family members more time at the patient's bedside. For facilitation of family-oriented care, visitation should be encouraged, not strictly limited, as has been previous practice in ICUs. Written information regarding the ICU is appropriate, but this is not the main focus of providing family-oriented care. Encouraging the patient to be more involved in self-care and allowing autonomy are also encouraged in the ICU, but these actions are not focused on the family.

129. **B) Notify the physician of the drainage**
The serous-appearing drainage is probably cerebrospinal fluid (CSF) and indicates an uncontrolled CSF leak. Notifying the physician is the most appropriate response. A saturated dressing may indicate the need to discontinue or change the catheter, but that decision should be made by the neurosurgeon. The nurse should not discontinue the catheter without a physician's order. Lowering the drainage chamber may actually increase the loss of CSF and worsen the patient's clinical status. Reinforcing the dressing will not address the problem of the CSF leak and can cause significant complications.

130. **A) Quadriparesis**
Correcting a serum sodium too rapidly can result in severe complications. Central pontine myelinolysis (CPM) is a potential complication of correcting serum sodium levels too quickly with the administration of 3% saline. Signs of CPM include quadriparesis, dysarthria, and loss of consciousness.

131. **B) Loss of sensorimotor function in the affected extremity**
The principal concern with an IABP procedure is vascular injury. Pulses and sensorimotor assessments should be performed frequently to recognize a loss of perfusion distal to insertion site. Loss of sensorimotor function in the affected extremity should always result in immediate discontinuation of the IABP catheter. Fever does not necessarily indicate infection of the catheter, and bleeding at the insertion site will not always require discontinuation of the IABP catheter.

132. **C) Low cardiac outputs**
Hypodynamic shock (formerly called cold shock) in sepsis indicates a low cardiac output with an increased systemic vascular resistance (SVR). Early septic shock is typically hyperdynamic, with increased cardiac outputs and low SVRs. Sepsis and septic shock elevate lactate levels, but that does not differentiate between hypo- and hyperdynamic shock. D-dimer is not used in the diagnosis of sepsis.

133. **A) Call the husband and tell him to come to the ICU to meet with the physician and his wife**
Being aware of cultural differences, the nurse knows that Hispanic women typically view their husbands as decision-makers. The nurse is demonstrating patient advocacy by taking the initiative to call the husband and arrange for him to meet with the physician and his wife to discuss the surgery and obtain a consent form. This honors the cultural belief system of the patient and family and facilitates care. Encouraging the patient to make her own decisions may delay the required surgery. A two-doctor signature is not required in this situation. The patient has the legal and ethical right to receive information about the proposed surgery and the ability to make her own decisions. To delay the surgery while attempting to resolve the conflict may cause complications and poor outcomes if the patient requires immediate surgery.

134. **D) Blood cultures**
Febrile neutropenia in cancer patients who have recently received chemotherapy are at high risk for bacterial or fungal infections. Blood cultures should be obtained and patient should be started on antibiotics. Corticosteroids may actually depress the immune system more with higher risks of infections. Plasmapheresis and exchange blood transfusions are not indicated in febrile neutropenia.

135. **A) Restrict fluid intake**
In SIADH, the patient's fluid status is usually euvolemic to hypervolemic, and the low sodium is primarily due to hemodilution. Fluid restrictions and diuresis with furosemide (Lasix) is the treatment of choice, if the patient is asymptomatic. Administering a hypertonic 3% saline may be indicated if the patient has a symptomatic hyponatremia. Giving a large bolus of fluid may dilute the patient's sodium further. Mannitol is not typically the diuretic of choice.

136. **B) Self-report**
Self-report of sleep quality is the best assessment if the patient is able to communicate. Using the patient's own appraisal of their sleep is beneficial because they are able to compare usual sleep quantity and quality to usual sleep. If patient is unable to communicate, continuous EEG or BIS monitors can be utilized. RASS score can also be used in intubated, nonverbal patients.

137. **C) Assure that one health care provider is present with the family throughout the resuscitation**
In "family presence during resuscitation" programs, one family member is usually allowed to remain in the room during resuscitation. The success of the program depends upon the ability to keep a support person with the family member to explain what is happening, provide emotional support, and evaluate the person's response. In some situations, allowing the family member to hold the patient's hands may benefit the family, but this is not possible in all resuscitations and is not essential for a good experience. Shortening the resuscitation time may not be in the patient's best interest.

138. **D) A 5-min back rub**
Studies have found that a 5-min back rub may increase sleep by 1 hr. Administering sedatives or hypnotics may actually decrease the REM sleep that has the most benefit for the patient. Having a familiar person with the patient at night may actually improve the patient's sleep. Noise is one of the factors contributing to inability to sleep, so turning the television on will just increase the noise level, unless the patient states that his or her normal routine is to fall asleep with the television on at night.

139. **C) Hyperkalemia**
Compartment syndrome can result in a crush injury. Potassium elevates following crush injuries due to the release of intracellular components following cellular injury. Potassium is primarily intracellular and is released with traumatic crush injuries. Hyperkalemia is most commonly found early and will typically peak within 12–36 hr after a crush injury.

140. **B) Administer protamine**
Mediastinal CT output greater than 200 mL/hr may require administration of protamine following a CABG. Output greater than 500 mL/hr indicates surgical bleeding and requires surgical re-exploration. An expected normal range in the immediate postoperative period is 100–200 mL/hr. Auto-transfusion is not routinely recommended for mediastinal CT.

141. **C) Remove the Foley catheter as soon as possible**
Removing the Foley catheter has been found to lower the incidence of urinary tract infections (UTIs). Enteral feeding is recommended to lower the incidence of gram-negative septicemia, but feeding in the stomach may increase the risk of aspiration pneumonia. PIV catheters have a lower incidence of infection, but patients in ICU frequently require central lines for certain drug administration. Chlorhexidine is used in oral care but should not be used more often than every 12 hours.

142. **C) Goal is light sedation**
Sedation is an important aspect of critical care and should be administered as needed. The goal is to maintain light sedation, if tolerated, to improve length of ICU stay, ventilator days, and outcome. Sedation and pain management are commonly used and may not always be used exclusively. Heavier sedation can lengthen number of ventilator days and negatively affect outcomes.

143. **D) Your loved one has a severe injury and has a very low chance of survival**
At this time, we can provide him with comfort and pain management to help him at the end of his life. It is important to be honest with the family and not provide false reassurance regarding recovery. Offering to provide comfort and pain management assures the family that you will still be caring for their loved one.

144. **A) Albuterol, inhaled**
The patient is experiencing a bronchospasm. A short-acting beta2 agonist delivered via the inhaled route is recommended for the first-line management of acute asthma (the oral route is less effective). Ipratropium is an anticholinergic and can be added later to the beta2 agonist, but is not considered as first-line management in asthma. Methylprednisolone may be added to the regimen in acute asthma but is administered IV. Aminophylline is not recommended to manage acute asthma.

145. **D) Hemorrhagic pancreatitis with infected necrosis**
Hemorrhagic pancreatitis with infected necrosis typically requires multiple surgeries for debriding the pancreas. If the necrosis is sterile (non-infected), surgery is not typically recommended even in hemorrhagic pancreatitis patients. Edematous pancreatitis or inflammatory do not require surgical intervention. Typically self-limiting.

146. **B) Permissive hypercapnia**
Permissive hypercapnia is frequently used in combination with lung recruitment to manage ARDS. Permissive hypercapnia allows higher CO_2 levels without manipulating ventilator settings to lower the CO_2 to protect the lungs from further injury. However, this patient also has a TBI. Hypercapnia can increase intracranial pressure (ICP) and should be avoided in TBI patients. Permissive hypercapnia is contraindicated in neurological patients. High PEEP levels are used in lung recruitment techniques. Pressure control therapy and even diuretic therapy are used at times to manage ARDS and would not be contraindicated in TBI patients.

147. **D) Maintain an ICU diary for the patient**
ICU diaries maintained with accurate events that occurred during the ICU stay can help the patient identify the real from delusional events. Opening family visitation can help improvement with development of PTSD. Encourage the patient to talk about the ICU stay and their memories. False reassurance does not protect the patient from fear of death.

148. **D) Administer potassium IV**

Initiation of insulin should be delayed until potassium is administered, if potassium levels are less than 3.5 mEq/L initially. Once potassium is above 3.5 mEq/L, IV fluids and insulin infusions may be initiated. Administration of insulin, either bolus or continuous infusion, will drive the potassium back into the cells, causing an even greater decrease of potassium that may initiate arrhythmias.

149. **B) Subdural hematoma**

Too rapid or too large of a CSF loss can cause a shift that results in the tearing of the dura. This can cause a subdural or epidural hematoma. Seizure, anoxic injuries, and loss of autoregulation are not complications of overly rapid removal of CSF.

150. **A) 12-lead electrocardiogram (ECG)**

The 12-lead ECG is the primary diagnostic tool for the risk stratification of anginal chest pain. The presence of T-wave inversion, ST elevation. or a Q wave differentiates injury, ischemia, and infarction. An echocardiogram may be used to evaluate heart failure. Cardiac catheterization and CTA are diagnostic tools, but are not the primary risk stratification tools for anginal chest pain.

Index